T0264624

SEXUAL ABUSE OF MALES

SEXUAL ABUSE OF MALES
THE SAM MODEL OF THEORY AND PRACTICE

Josef Spiegel

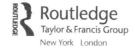
Routledge
Taylor & Francis Group
New York   London

First published in 2003 by
Brunner-Routledge
29 West 35th Street
New York, NY 10001
www.brunner-routledge.com

Published in Great Britain by
Brunner-Routledge
27 Church Road
Hove, East Sussex
BN3 2FA
www.brunner-routledge.co.uk

This edition published 2012 by Routledge

Routledge	Routledge
Taylor & Francis Group	Taylor & Francis Group
711 Third Avenue	27 Church Road
New York, NY 10017	Hove East Sussex BN3 2FA

Library of Congress Cataloging-in-Publication Data
  Spiegel, Josef.
    Sexual abuse of males : the SAM model of theory and practice / Josef Spiegel.
      p. cm.
    Includes bibliographical references and index.
    ISBN 1-56032-403-1 (Hardcover)
      1. Male sexual abuse victims—Mental health. 2. Adult child sexual abuse
victims—Mental health 3. Sexually abused children—Mental health. 4. Psychotherapy.
    I. Title.

RC569.5.A28 S65 2003
619.9'285836'0081—dc21
                                                              2002014088

CONTENTS

FOREWORD vii

SAM ACKNOWLEDGMENTS xi

PART I

Chapter 1   INTRODUCTION   3

Chapter 2   THE DEVELOPMENT OF THE SAM MODEL   19

Chapter 3   ASSUMPTIONS OF THE SAM MODEL   109

Chapter 4   THE SAM MODEL OF DYNAMICS AND EFFECTS   137

Chapter 5   APPLICATION OF THE SAM MODEL   245

PART II

Chapter 6   THE SAM MODEL OF PHILOSOPHY OF PRACTICE   317

Chapter 7   PREPARATORY EMPATHY   333

Chapter 8   THE SAM MODEL OF TREATMENT AND OBJECTIVES   363

Chapter 9   THE SAM PRACTICE MODEL: AN ANALOGY   405

Chapter 10   INTERVENTIONS FOR SAM   411

Chapter 11   FROM SAM   453

REFERENCES   461
ADDITIONAL RESOURCES   503
INDEX   521

FOREWORD

IN CONTEMPORARY SOCIETY, the sexual abuse of males is massively denied, misunderstood, and trivialized. This has much to do with the stereotypes and myths that abound about being male and about the possibility of being sexually abused by either a male or female—each carries its own negative connotations and burden of incredulity. Unfortunately, the neglect of this topic has also been at the professional level, professionals themselves not immune from social stereotypes, and their viewpoints further reinforced by the findings of research studies that the sexual abuse of boys occurs less often than that of girls and may be less damaging. This widespread neglect, at both societal and professional levels, is enormously unfortunate and is of great consequence to the sexually abused male (or SAM as he is referred to in this book, a term I will adopt here). I offer two examples of how SAM incorporates this neglect as well as the societal myths on which it is built. These occurred, quite ironically, during the time that I was reading this manuscript and so are contemporary examples. One of my male patients, abused by a male camp counselor, lamented to me that *if only he had been abused by a female*, he would be able to talk (and maybe even boast!) about it because he wouldn't really consider it abuse and he wouldn't have any of those "homosexual connotations" to worry about. In the second case, a man furtively contacted me by email because he couldn't tolerate making contact by phone. In his correspondence, he described ever-increasing daily distress that made him feel like he was having a breakdown, for which he was seeking information and assistance. He had been surfing the net for resources and had come to the conclusion that, *if only he were female*, services would be readily available and he wouldn't be so isolated and feel like such a freak.

That male victims of sexual abuse still struggle today in silence, secrecy, and shame is itself shameful, for much is now known about the devastating consequences such abuse can have. And much has been learned over the course of this past year (albeit often with reluctance and repugnance) as the scope of the scandal of abuse by Catholic priests and the cover-up at the diocesan level has unfolded, abuse mostly perpetrated against young boys. *Sexual Abuse of Males: The SAM Model of Theory and Practice* was written with the explicit goal of setting the record straight about the abuse of males and presenting a comprehensive conceptual framework from which to understand effects and to organize treatment. Dr. Josef Spiegel describes the problem and what is needed in compelling terms:

> Gender has come to have jurisdiction over childhood sexual abuse because social imperatives have made it so. Most treatment programs, research endeavors, and social policies continue to promote the feminization of victimization and the masculinization of perpetration. To do so is to present, identify, treat, and study CSA as a function of gender, thereby negating the substantial numbers of males with abuse histories and females who perpetrate against both boys and girls. To do so is to be dictated to by cultural and social myths, and consequently to contradict the life histories of both the abusers and the abused.
>   The traditional male perpetrator/female victim paradigm, with its mutually exclusive, dichotomous categories, must give way to a model that allows for the recognition of male traumatization and female perpetration. The stark reality of childhood sexual abuse is that neither gender is exempt from either role. Therefore, the term *childhood sexual abuse* is a misnomer unless the plight of sexually abused boys is acknowledged. (p. 15)

Strong words, but words that are sorely needed as a major correction of faulty perceptions and beliefs. Dr. Spiegel further notes that "sexual abuse professionals are in a unique position to tell the truth" and with this book, it is clear that he is taking a leadership role in dong so. *Sexual Abuse of Males: The SAM Model of Theory and Practice* is a major addition to the literature on the abuse of males and a breakthrough in understanding the complexity of its aftermath. It not only sifts through and presents huge volumes of up-to-date research from disparate sources and fields of study but it integrates the information with clinical observations and treatment models. Dr. Spiegel further integrates this information with first-person accounts of a diverse group of seven male victims who were interviewed in depth about their experiences of abuse and their efforts to recover from its effects. Throughout the manuscript, he uses their words to effectively and poignantly illustrate the dynamics of their abuse and their response to treatment. Dr. Spiegel is not content to superimpose his research and observations about males over the extant models developed primarily for females; rather, he has extensively researched the unique experiences of male victims in order to develop "The SAM Model" of dynamics and effects and of treatment objectives and anticipated outcome. The SAM Model is comprehensive in its scope and detail and quite unique in its approach, although it is clearly grounded in the accumulated clinical and research knowledge base developed over the past quarter century.

The book begins with a broad review of the many and unique ways that abuse effects can be manifested in order to develop an understanding of the unfolding of dynamics over the life span. These effects are continuously presented from the perspective of SAM and are, at times, compared and contrasted with the effects on females. The numerous permutations, gradations, and interactions of effects at the various systems levels, from the individual, to family, to community, to society are detailed to illustrate how SAM is affected subjectively, influenced by his family's teachings, perspectives, and responses and by the messages that are sent by his community and culture and by the larger society. A major strength of the presentation is the state-of-the-art biopsychosocial perspective that pervades this material. In particular, Dr. Spiegel describes the psychobiology of the stress response and how the traumatized body and mind are impacted directly by abuse that, in turn, impacts and skews SAM's total psychosexual development, including the ability to relate to and be intimate with others. Also presented in detail are the following dynamics of the cycle of abuse: *subjection* to boundary and role confusion; intrapsychic, interpersonal, and social *concealment; invalidation* of the experience; *reconciliation* of the abuse by taking responsibility, *compensatory measures* to separate from the abuse, *continuing this cycle* throughout the life span, often with great pain and anguish. Each of these dynamics is amply illustrated with the words of all seven boys and men. Each is then analyzed and explained with accompanying clinical notes, an effective vehicle that simultaneously sensitizes readers to the plight of SAM and desensitizes them to some of the common and horrific abuse details that they can expect to hear in the clinical setting. The SAM treatment model is also presented extensively beginning with an emphasis on the philosophy of practice. The treatment process is multimodal and is conceptualized comprehensively so as to respond to the biopsychosocial dynamics and effects of abuse, that is, with interventions that are oriented toward all three dimensions (physiological, psychological, and relational).

As I hope is evident from this brief introduction and overview, this book has much to offer and I highly recommend it to therapists and male survivors alike. It fills a void in the literature and fills it impressively. It offers SAM a model by which to understand his unique responses as a male to events that heretofore have been mostly explained from the perspective of the female. It amply documents the struggle of SAM to make sense of events that are contradictory to gender expectations and stereotypes and that serve to compound traumatic reactions that are bad enough without these additional gender complications. However, these must be understood by SAM and by professionals who seek to assist him because they make up his uniquely male response and perspective. To understand these differences and the male perspective is to offer treatment that is comprehensive and specialized in its response to the shamed and often silent and isolated sexually abused male. It also offers that most important component of treatment, hope, a lifeline to those whose everyday burdens include feelings of despair and hopelessness.

Christine A. Courtois, Ph.D.
Psychologist, Independent Practice and
Co-Founder and Clinical and Training Director
The CENTER: Posttraumatic Disorders Program
The Psychiatric Institute of Washington
Washington, DC
Author: *Recollections of sexual abuse: Treatment principles and guidelines* (1999)
 Adult survivors of child sexual abuse: A treatment model (1993)
 Healing the incest wound: Adult survivors in therapy (1988)

SAM ACKNOWLEDGMENTS

I DIDN'T SET OUT TO WORK in the field of childhood sexual abuse nor did I seek to write a book about the sexual abuse of males. I simply wanted to find a way to be of service. From the first day of my first internship, I inquired into the lives of those assigned to me—intravenous drug users, the homeless, sex workers, Native Americans, Asian Americans, Hispanic Americans, illegal aliens, grandmothers, sons, wives, partners, the elderly and toddlers, professors, prostitutes and priests, the mentally ill, prisoners on death row—all member of my human family. I learned of horrific histories of childhood sexual abuse at almost every turn, solely by asking and listening. Throughout my career, I continue to discover that in this world, there are no spare parts; we each have a guiding purpose and a rightful place. My purpose at this moment in time is to tell their stories. That is why I am writing this book.

There are many others who could have written "SAM." While drafting the manuscript, I focused on the "message" rather than the "messenger." As I acknowledge those who have directly and indirectly contributed to this process, I cannot separate the two so easily.

First and foremost, I thank God for blessing me with life. I am grateful to be a part of this world. I'm proud to be the son of Lawrence and Dolores Lagona Spiegel. Thank you, Mom and Dad, for teaching me by example about working hard serving others, and honoring God. I appreciate more than ever the lessons I've learned from you. And thank you for believing in me.

I am indebted to the countless number of boys, adolescent males, and adult males with histories of childhood sexual abuse who participated in the national study or who engaged in individual, couples, group, and family therapy. While I am unable to acknowledge you by name, I thank you from the bottom of my heart for sharing your stories with me. Your contributions represent the foundation of this book.

I am beholden to the leaders of the field, many of whom I've yet to meet. I thank Dr. David Finkelhor for believing in my work and for encouraging me to continue. Our meetings and conversations are highlights of my career and the actualization of a longheld dream. I would also like to acknowledge the impeccability of Dr. Christine Courtois, the eloquence of Dr. Judith Lewis

Herman, the sensitivity of Mike Lew, the wisdom of Dr. David Spiegel, the pioneering efforts of Dr. J. Douglas Bremner, and the holistic philosophy of Dr. Daniel Spiegel, among so many others. I am fortunate to be one of the many recipients of your vast knowledge and skill. And, an extra note of gratitude to Dr. Christine Courtois: Thank you for writing the foreword to this book. Wishes do come true!

I owe a resounding note of gratitude to the hundreds of students who entered my classroom. Your desire for excellence as well as your aspiration to help ameliorate biopsychosocial inequities continue to inspire me. I thank you for entrusting me with your educational goals and objectives. At the same time, I pay tribute to my professors—Dr. Richard Tate (multivariate statistics, structural equation modeling), Dr. Dianne Harrison Montgomery (dissertation chair), Dr. J. Neil Abell (clinical theory), Dr. Robert Schilling (research methods), Dr. William Stanton (human sexuality), and to many others at Columbia Univeristy, the University of Pennsylvania, and Florida State University—for actualizing your passions, sharing you wisdom, and helping me to discover my path.

I would also like to recognize those who attended local, state, national, and international conferences. Your interest in the "SAM Model" remains a constant source of incentive for me. A special thank you to the New York State Department of Corrections, the New York State Department of Substance Abuse Services, the Medical College of Pennsylvania, Hahnemann University School of Medicine, Boston University, the State of Florida, the State of West Virginia, the Philadelphia Department of Social Services, Orange County, California, and the Florida State University School of Law among other private and public agencies and institutions for seeking knowledge that will ultimately help professionals to understand and better serve males with histories of childhood sexual abuse.

I treasure the support and encouragement so consistently and freely extended by my colleagues. I am buoyed by Dr. Cathy Foister's empathy, Dr. Margaret Weschner's support, Dr. Noreen LeGare's mettle, and Blace Nalavany's unwavering belief in this project. While I cannot mention all by name, I thank you for believing in SAM. On a more personal note, I cherish the friendships that blossomed along my life path. In particular, I thank Annie Hughes, Janet Dubin, Joy Dolan, Ellen Olk Hamilton, and Dennis Haynes. Thank you for unknowingly creating precious moments in my life. Many others offered their encouragement and support—my sister, Andrea Spiegel Rask, and nephew Jeffery Rask, my cousins, Stacy Newman and Lisa Newman, relatives, Bill and Audrey Spiegel Linton and Sophia Vukovich Cisco, friends, David and Denise Yelton, Andrew Gentry, Robert Clark and Andrew Gall, and my neighbors, Mr. Charles and Mrs. Anna Garabedian. I would also like to acknowledge a very special family whose generous and anonymous gift to the SAM Project made this book possible.

So many have directly impacted the outcome of "SAM." Special thanks to Brunner-Routledge for taking an interest in the sexual abuse of males. My editor, George Zimmar, is a writer's advocate. Enough cannot be said of his assistant, Shannon Vargo. George, thank you for believing in the utility of this book. Shannon, your interest, encouragement, and steadfast manner refresh my spirit. I wish every writer experiences the support and encouragement of such a team. To those who helped with reading and editing—Annie Hughes, John Yelton, Dr. Ann Hughes, and Dr. Rick Pyeritz—your generosity, thoughfulness and red ink contributed significantly to this publication. Thank you again, John Yelton, for the figures, tables and charts.

Additionally, a number of others associated with the SAM Project, particularly Nicholas Dudding, Jean Sandler, Elizabeth Molina Romo, Charlotte Bassett and Alison Goldstein—worked on the foundational elements. Thank you for the brainstorming sessions and for all the laughter. A special note of appreciation to Erica Rosen Jourdan for the late nights, early mornings, long weekends and for helping me to find my voice. Your contributions will not be forgotten.

I would not be who and where I am today without the generosity and giftedness of my mentor, Susan Stoller, MS, PsyT. Thank you, Susan, for leading me, walking beside me and helping me to forge a path of my own. The depth of your wisdom, the breadth of your facility and the bounteousness of your integrity inspire me, professionally and personally. You are one of the greatest and most serendipitous gifts of my life. I hope I can give to others of kernel of what you've so abundantly given me.

On a more personal note, I prize the blessing that is my life partner, John Richard Yelton. Thank you, John, for welcoming "SAM" into your life. Thank you for gracing my life with your love, patience, kindness, and understanding. You, my friend, are an unsung ally of this project. Your imprint lies in this book and in my heart. Thank you for giving me the greatest gift of all.

Finally, I would like to acknowledge my maternal grandparents, Albert and Martha Vukovich DeMarino. Nanny, thank you for the many special conversations about life and love; for encouraging me to seek the truth and for accepting me and all I am. PapPap, thank you for teaching me that boys can play football and play the violin, for showing me that blood is not thicker than water and for encouraging me to live my life with passion, humility, and gratitude. Even though you left this earth long ago, your kindred spirits echo in all I do.

Josef Spiegel, Ph.D.
February 22, 2003
Asheville, NC
Aboutwellsprings@aol.com

PART ONE

CHAPTER ONE

INTRODUCTION

EMPIRICAL RESEARCH, clinical reports, the media, and social movements soundly maintain that childhood sexual abuse (CSA) is one of the most serious forms of interpersonal violence among both boys and girls (see, e.g., Boney-McCoy & Finkelhor, 1995b; De Bellis, 2001; Gartner, 1999; National Committee to Prevent Child Abuse, web page [www.childabuse.org]; National Organization on Male Sexual Victimization, web page [www.malesurvivor.org]; SNAP: Survivors Network of those Abused by Priests, web page [www.survivorsnetwork.org/~snapper/SNAP]). Data and messages from these same sources, historically and currently, minimize and, in some cases, promote the incidence of CSA by way of muting its occurrence and abridging to the smallest degree its effects (see, e.g., Masson, 1984; the North American Man/Boy Love Association, web page [www.nambla.org]; Riegel, 2000; Rind, Tromovitch & Bauserman, 1998). These two contributaries of information merge to produce a confusing history. Following is a brief (and noninclusive) synopsis.

1849 The Texas Supreme Court rules in favor of a father who allegedly incested his daughter. The court can not conceive that incest occurs in this day and age in the United States of America (Ashby, 1997).

1889 Pierre Janet authors *L'automatisme psychologique*, one of the first books to introduce and expound upon dissociation as a reaction to, and as a means of coping with, psychological trauma. He asserts that "merely uncovering memories [is] not enough; they need to be modified and transformed, i.e., placed in their proper context and reconstructed into neutral or meaningful narratives" (Janet, 1889, cited in van der Kolk & van der Hart, 1989).

1891 By the mere exclusion of the word "feloniously," the Mississippi Supreme Court reverses an incest conviction (Ashby, 1997).

1896 In two separate but related publications, "The Aetiology of Hysteria" and "Studies on Hysteria," Sigmund Freud offers what comes to be known as the seduction theory to account for the dynamics and effects experienced by female patients with histories of childhood sexual abuse. Based on actual cases from his practice, he takes great risk and goes to great lengths to demonstrate how CSA is a causal factor in the manifestation of traumatic effects, such as adult hysteria, fear, obsessiveness, and compulsive sexual behavior (Freud, 1896/1962; Gay, 1988; Masson, 1984). However, his presentation of a paper on hysteria at a professional conference is less than appreciated by members of the Vienna Circle, his network of colleagues and followers.

1897 Freud shifts paradigms, moving, within a period of a year, from the seduction theory to the development of the oedipal theory. Unable to reconcile the pervasiveness of CSA, he attributes the source of the vast numbers of sexual abuse disclosures to the fantasy lives of the women under his care. What were once viewed as repressed traumatic memories from childhood are now perceived as the emergence of unconscious childhood wishes for sex. Further, while the seduction theory was deduced from his clinical practice, the oedipal theory is based on self-analysis (Freud, 1896/1962; Gay, 1988).

1900 The Georgia Supreme Court rules in favor of a stepfather accused of sexually abusing his stepdaughter. The stepdaughter alleges that she has repeatedly tried to stop him from having intercourse with her but to no avail. The Court concludes that the stepdaughter consented to sexual relations with her stepfather; however, she must have done so with a sense of reluctance given her need to simultaneously maintain a viable relationship with the woman who was both her mother and her stepfather's wife (Ashby, 1997).

1930 The White House sponsors a conference on child health and protection. The organizing committee contends that physical cruelty is much less prevalent today than it was at the turn of the century. In response, Theodore Lothrop, General Secretary of the Massachusetts Society for the Prevention of Cruelty to Children, argues that the sexual abuse of young males is far more common than purported and that it amounts to a serious national problem. His comments cannot be found in the committee's final report (Costin, Karger, & Stoesz, 1996).

1932 Sandor Ferenczi presents his paper, "Confusion of Tongues Between Adults and the Child" (1932/1949) at the International Psychoanalytic Congress in Wiesbaden, Germany. He emphatically asserts that CSA must not be underestimated as it has been in the past. "The real rape of girls . . . similar acts of mature women with boys, and also enforced homosexual acts, are far more frequent occurrences than has hitherto been assumed" (p. 201). He calls attention to CSA's debilitating effects, highlighting personality fragmentation, dissociation, and identification with the aggressor, in addition to the core consequences of guilt and shame. Shortly thereafter, and in response to taking such a stand, Ferenczi is ostracized from his professional network and rejected by his mentor, Sigmund Freud.

1937 Drs. Lauretta Bender and Abram Blau, after investigating females with histories of childhood sexual abuse, assert that girls play a very active role in initiating sexual relationships with adult males, characterizing them as "bold, flaunting and even brazen" (Bender & Blau, 1937, p. 510). They conclude that adult males are victims of the girls' seductive and precocious behaviors and that girls experience little if any negative consequences as a result of sexual interactions with adults.

1941 The sexual abuse of boys and girls living in orphanages during World War II is corroborated. The children are often blamed by intervening professionals (Ashby, 1997).

1942 Sloane and Karpinski (1942) maintain that girls subjected to CSA evidence few, if any, negative effects since children "often unconsciously desire the sexual activity and become more or less a willing partner in it" (p. 666).

1950 Raskovsky and Raskovsky (1950) report that sexual relations between an adult and a child advance the child's psychosocial adaptation capacities.

1953 The Kinsey Institute releases an account of their landmark study, *Sexual Behavior in the Human Female* (Kinsey, Pomeroy, Martin, & Gebhard, 1953). In spite of the study's rendered childhood sexual abuse prevalence rate of 25% among females, the Kinsey team states: "It is difficult to understand why a child, except for cultural conditioning, should be disturbed at having its genitalia touched, or disturbed at seeing the genitalia of other persons, or disturbed even at more specific sexual acts" (p. 121). In fact, childhood sexual abuse is "not likely to do the child any appreciable harm " (p. 122).

1955 Weinberg delineates a childhood sexual abuse incidence rate of nine cases per million population (1955).

1962 The slogan "Sex before year eight or it's too late," coined by the René Guyon Society, is employed to advocate for social policy sanctioning sex between an adult and a child as well as sex between children. This society is founded by seven lay persons after attending a seminar in Los Angeles on human sexuality. The group is named in honor of the French jurist and Freudian psychologist who advocated for adult–child sex. The René Guyon Society encourages sexual relations between parents and their own children (de Young, 1989).

1962 Dr. Henry Kempe and colleagues publish the seminal article, "The Battered Child Syndrome" (Kempe, Silverman, Steele, Droegmueller, & Silver, 1962). In it, they not only bring public attention to the devastating effects of physical abuse, but also reprimand physicians for not detecting and treating it and parents and caretakers for not preventing and reporting it.

1970 The National Commission on Obscenity and Pornography, in a published report, deduces the following: (a) Children are not victimized by pornography; (b) pornography does not promote criminal activity; therefore (c) pornography should not be a matter of social concern (Report of the Commission on Obscenity and Pornography, 1970).

1971 Henry Giaretto develops "Parents United," a self-help model for the treatment of incest. Conceived on family systems theory and humanistic psychology, this model views incest as symptomatic of dysfunctional family dynamics and conflictual marriage interactions wherein parents and daughters unconsciously actualize the abhorrent behavior.

1971 The Childhood Sensuality Circle is established in San Diego, California. This new group argues in favor of sexual self-determination for adults and children alike. Members champion the early initiation of children into sexual relationships, sexual relations between parents and their children, and the repeal of age of consent laws (de Young, 1989).

1974 The Child Abuse Prevention and Treatment Act (42 USC 5101-5106), sponsored by Senator Walter Mondale of Minnesota, is signed into law. It requires states to initiate mandatory reporting procedures as a prerequisite to obtaining federal funding for combating child abuse (Moore, 1992).

1975 *The Comprehensive Textbook of Psychiatry*, edited by Freedman, Kaplan, and Sadock (1975) supports the current incidence estimate of sexual abuse cases: 1 per million.

1976 The New York Gay Activist Alliance is the first gay group to sponsor a public forum on man/boy love (Thorstad, 1991).

1977 Dr. Henry Kempe and associates establish the International Society for Prevention and Treatment of Child Abuse and Neglect.

1978 Louise Armstrong authors the book, *Kiss Daddy Goodnight: A Speak-Out on Incest*, and produces the first feminist documentary on the sexual abuse of girls within their families.

1978 A conference entitled "Man–Boy Love: Age and Consent" is held in Boson at a community church. One hundred fifty people attend. Afterwards, 30 man–boy lovers and youth form the North American Man Boy Love Association (NAMBLA). As a sociopolitical organization, NAMBLA seeks to: (a) advocate sex with boys; (b) lobby for the legalization of adult–child sexual activities; and (c) provide legal assistance to its members. It espouses sexual freedom for all, not just for gays and lesbians (de Young, 1989).

1980 Maria Nasjleti authors the journal report, "Suffering in Silence: The Male Incest Victim." It is the first major article to address the sexual abuse of males as it interfaces with gender role socialization and social mythology.

1982 The social concealment and the clinical misperceptions around CSA up to the recent past comprise a period known as the "Age of Denial." Based on the publication of a number of works recognizing and authenticating the sexual abuse of females — *Father–Daughter Incest* (Herman, 1981), *Incest: A Psychological Study of Cause and Effects with Treatment*

Recommendations (Meiselman, 1979), and *The Best Kept Secret: Sexual Abuse of Children* (Rush, 1980)—a new period emerges: the "Age of Validation" (Armstrong, 1982).

1983 "The Child Sexual Abuse Accommodation Syndrome," written by Orlando Summit, is perhaps the most referenced work in the CSA literature. Based on the responses of children, particularly females, to CSA, this article highlights the child's perspective vis-à-vis adult assumptions and sensibilities. In the years ahead, it will become a subject of controversy within the judicial system.

1985 The Reverend Giblet Gauthe, a Catholic priest in Lafayette, Louisiana, is sentenced to 20 years for sexually abusing numerous children. He was accused of molesting children since 1972. When church authorities were informed of his perpetration, he was moved from one parish to the next (Jenkins, 1996).

1987 A confidential report, authored by two priests, Thomas Doyle and Michael Peterson, as well as the Reverend Gauthe's attorney, F. Ray Moulton, is submitted to the Catholic hierarchy. Entitled "The Problem of Sexual Molestation by Roman Catholic Clergy: Meeting the Problem in a Comprehensive and Responsible Manner," this report warns against delayed reactions to abuse allegations, the destruction of evidence, and meetings held in secret (Jenkins, 2001).

1986 David Finkelhor and colleagues Sharon Araji, Larry Baron, Angela Browne, Stefanie D. Peters, and Gail E. Wyatt produce *A Sourcebook on Child Sexual Abuse*. It contains one of the most cited references in the CSA field, "Traumagenic Dynamics," a conceptual framework based on the sexual abuse of females knowledge base.

1986 Based on data generated from a random probability sample, Diana E. H. Russell authors *The Secret Trauma: Incest in the Lives of Girls and Women.* This study will come to be a model in terms of its research methodology, particularly in the areas of defining sexual abuse, sampling procedures, and enhancing internal and external validity.

1986 Rieker and Carmen, in their seminal paper, "The Victim-to-Patient Process: The Disconfirmation and Transformation of the Abuse Process," underscore the importance of "recontextualizing" the abuse experience of females. Their model "emphasizes the fragmented identity that derives from victims' attempts to accommodate or adjust to the judgments that others make about the abuse" (1986, p. 360). Thus, the victims' reality, embedded beneath denial and fragmented by dissociation, must emerge to the fore.

1988 *Healing the Incest Wound: Adult Survivors in Therapy*, authored by psychotherapist Christine Courtois, is published to great acclaim. It is the most comprehensive text on the dynamics and effects associated with, and the treatment of, the incestual experiences of females.

1988 *The Courage to Heal: A Guide for Women Survivors of Child Sexual Abuse,* written by Ellen Bass and Laura Davis, is released. In 4 years it will spawn controversy, particularly in terms of the false memory disputation; however, it will remain a popular resource guide for adult females with histories of CSA.

1988 Mike Lew authors the landmark book, *Victims No Longer: Men Recovering from Incest and Other Sexual Child Abuse*. His intention is to "provide as much information as possible to as many people as possible about a subject that seems to be ignored as much as possible" (1988, p. 3). This is the first published book written directly for males with histories of childhood sexual abuse.

1990 In the first national childhood sexual abuse study to employ state-of-the-art research methodology, including a random probability sample and a definition of sexual abuse restricted to respondents' perceptions, Finkelhor, Hotaling, Lewis, and Smith (1990) report that 16% of American males have histories of CSA.

1990 *The Sexually Abused Male: Volume 1, Prevalence, Impact and Treatment* and *Volume 2, Application of Treatment Strategies* is published. Edited by Mic Hunter (1990a, 1990b), it encompasses a review of the literature, individual and group interventions, and practice guidelines.

1990 Sandfort, Bronfersma, and van Naerssen, three members of the editorial board of *Paidika: The Journal of Paedophilia*, are selected to be guest editors for a special issue of the *Journal of Homosexuality*. The theme of this special issue is "Male Intergenerational Intimacy." In it, the editors suggest that rather than use the term "pedophilia," they prefer "man/boy love" and "intergenerational intimacy" because the latter phrases "give man–boy contacts a less dangerous outlook" (1990, p. 8).

1992 "Primetime Live," the ABC network news magazine, conducts a thorough investigation of Father James Porter, a Catholic priest accused of abusing between 200 and 300 children in the Massachusetts diocese of Fall River prior to retiring from the priesthood in 1974. His attorney argues: "You've got a church that knew as early as 1963 that there had been 30 to 40 reports of what this man had done, and they kept him supervising altar boys for four more years in this state" (Jenkins, 2001, p. 47).

1993 President William Jefferson Clinton signs the "National Child Protection Act of 1993" on December 20. The stated purpose of this act is to mandate "States to report information of arrests and convictions for child abuse crimes to the national criminal history record system maintained by the Federal Bureau of Investigation " (House Report No. 103-393).

1994 Psychologist Elizabeth Loftus and researcher Katherine Ketcham compose the controversial text, *The Myth of Repressed Memory: False Memories and Allegations of Sexual Abuse*. The authors assert that rather than being victims of CSA, female patients are victimized by their therapists' zeal in linking isolated symptoms to repressed memories of childhood trauma. Therapists are accused of diagnosing a history of CSA without reason and of implanting false recollections of CSA that lack corroboration.

1995 The National Organization of Male Sexual Victimization (NOSMV) is officially established and incorporated by a Founding Congress composed of therapists and laypersons with histories of CSA. Its mission is to advance understanding, treatment, research, and social policy with respect to the sexual abuse of males.

1996 The people of the State of New York, as represented by their State Senate and Assembly, render null and void Zymurgy, Inc., a not-for-profit organization, because it "has acted fraudulently . . . on behalf of . . . the North American Man/Boy Love Association (NAMBLA), whose members engage in and actively promote illegal sexual activity between adults and children, without revealing its affiliation with that organization. Such misrepresentation is known to have enabled NAMBLA to gain access to facilities from which it would otherwise have been excluded, and to have otherwise misled the public about the true nature of Zymurgy, Inc." (bill number S7879).

1997 "The Boylove Manifesto" is released on the Internet. Its demands include freedom of speech in the media, promotion of a boy's rights to pursue a sexual relationship with an adult male, reconsideration of the term "pedophile," as it is polemic, and the freedom of sexual expression between and among boys and boylovers (Mahoney & Faulker, 1997).

1997 Sheldon Kennedy, a National Hockey League player, discloses a history of childhood sexual abuse. His perpetrator was his mentor and coach. Numerous others, in response, disclose their histories of abuse by the same perpetrator-coach (Kornheiser, 1998).

1998 Rind, Tromovitch, and Bauserman (1998) author a review of 59 studies on the effects of childhood sexual abuse. In "A Meta-Analytic Examination of Assumed Properties of Child Sexual Abuse Using College Samples," the authors contend that researchers of late have greatly overstated the harmful potential of CSA and that the sexual abuse of males does not correlate with negative effects or maladjustment. Further, the authors encourage researchers to study a young male's appraisal of his sexual encounter with an adult. In doing so, investigators would likely discover that such an encounter would not constitute childhood sexual abuse but rather be viewed "simply [as] adult–child sex" (p. 46). Their article will come to be employed by a number of defense lawyers in their quest to minimize the effects of CSA and by numerous pedophile groups in their fight to lower or rescind age-of-consent laws (Dallam, 2001).

1999 The U.S. Congress and the House of Representatives, for the first time in history, denounce a study by unanimously passing a resolution that condemns the conclusions of Rind, Tromovitch, and Bauserman (House Cong. Res. 107).

1999 The federal publication "Child Maltreatment 1999," based on data from the 50 states and the National Child Abuse and Neglect Reporting System, calculates the sexual abuse rate for male children: 0.4 per 1,000.

2001 Researchers Richard Estes and Neil Alan Weiner of the School of Social Work at the University of Pennsylvania assert that cases of child pornography and prostitution are on the rise. In their report, "The Commercial Sexual Exploitation of Children in the U.S., Canada and Mexico," the authors reveal that of the estimated 766,686 missing juveniles in the United States last year, including abductees, runaways, and abandoned "throwaways," approximately 16% were victims of sexual exploitation (Estes & Weiner, 2001).

2001 Congress members Robert Simmons and Nancy Johnson introduce the "Cybermolesters Enforcement Act." This bill establishes 5-year mandatory prison sentences for adults who use the Internet to entice and entrap children for sexual activity. In a statement, Simmons explains: "convicted child pornographers receive 10-year mandatory sentences, but those who use the Internet to meet children and commit criminal sexual acts can receive no jail time at all." The "Cybermolesters Enforcement Act" confronts opposition from Congress member Bob Barr (MacMillan, 2001).

2002 Bishop Wilton Gregory, president of the U.S. Conference of Catholic Bishops, releases a statement on the sexual abuse of children and young people by priests. In it he remarks: "In recent weeks our attention has again been turned to the issue of sexual abuse of minors by priests. Though the renewed focus on this issue is due largely to cases of priest abusers that were not dealt with appropriately in the past, it gives me the occasion as a pastor and a teacher of faith and morals to express, on behalf of all of the bishops, our profound sorrow that some of our priests were responsible for this abuse under our watch."

2002 The Federal Bureau of Investigation launches "Operation Candyman," a nationwide crackdown on the trafficking of child pornography on the Internet. Charges are filed against 89 people in 20 states, including a foster care worker, Little League coaches, a teacher's aide, a guidance counselor, a law enforcement officer, and a school-bus driver (Thompson, 2002).

2002 J. Douglas Bremner authors the book *Does Stress Damage the Brain?* Based on a number of recent studies and imaging techniques, he evidences the ways in which subjection to childhood sexual abuse impacts various regions of the brain, including the amygdala, a substructure vital to implicit memory, and the hippocampus, a limbic system component central to explicit memory.

From this brief digest, a number of points are readily apparent. First, two streams of thought and action work against each other, one striving to bring to light or authenticate the prevalence, dynamics, and effects of CSA, and the other attempting to conceal or mythologize them, thereby exacerbating the uncertainty surrounding an already bewildering biopsychosocial problem. For example, segments of the women's movement tend to conceptualize CSA as a function of the patriarchal social structure of American society (Brownmiller, 1975; Herman, 1981; Russell, 1986), demarcating the roles of the abuser and the abused by gender. A minority division of the gay movement seeks to normalize sexual relations between men and boys (Mahoney & Faulkner, 1997; White, 1989), characterizing man–boy sex as a normative stage of the coming-out process. A burgeoning age-of-consent movement strives to eliminate age restrictions altogether (Americans for a Society Free from Age Restrictions, web page [www.asfar.org]; Brongersma, 1988), acting as if children hold immunity from the power, status, authority, and detrimental intentions of some adults. If an adult's sexual relations with a boy is considered abusive from one vantage point, benign from another, and barely recognized by another still, concealment, confusion, and controversy become mainstays. How does this serve the children?

Second, while a number of studies, publications, and social movements have attempted to uncover and document the realities of CSA in general, and the sexual abuse of males in particular, the preponderance of data elicited and consequently analyzed and disseminated stem from investigations into the dynamics and effects of CSA as they relate to female children perpetrated by adult men (Roane, 1992). A comparable focus on the sexual abuse of males lags behind (Spencer & Tan, 1999). One might ask: In light of the estimated prevalence rates, typically ranging between 15% and 25%, and given the reported incidence ratios, often falling between 1/5 and 1/7 (Allard-Dansereau, Haley, Hamane, & Bernard-Bonnin, 1997; DiIorio, Hartwell, & Hansen, 2002; Faller & Henry, 2000; Finkelhor et al., 1990; Leverich et al., 2002; Paul, Catania, Pollack, & Stall, 2001; Ratner et al., in press) (and in many reports, approaching rates, if not comparable to, within the proximity of female incidence and prevalence indices), what then deters the sexual abuse of males knowledge base from keeping pace with its counterpart? Certainly, a convincing argument cannot employ for support the sporadic incidence of CSA among males (Gold, Elhai, Lucenko, Swingle, & Hughes, 1997).

Within the knowledge base, childhood sexual abuse and the sexual abuse of females are typically viewed synonymously. Essentially, they are not only associated with each other, but suggestive of each other as well. Further, the dynamics and effects around the sexual abuse of males are often minimized, denied, or otherwise downgraded, as evidenced by social perceptions (Korbin, Coulton, Lindstrom-Ufuti & Spilsbury, 2000; McCauley & Parker, 2001; Pintello & Zuravin, 2001; Spencer & Tan, 1999) and the perceptions of professionals in the field (Holmes, Offen, & Waller, 1997; Lab, Feigenbaum, & De Silva, 2000; Gore-Felton, Arnow, Koopman, Thoreson, & Spiegel, 1999; Richey-Suttles & Remer, 1997). And across studies, males tend to be outnumbered by a ratio of

5 to 1 in mixed-gender samples; moreover, mixed-gender studies are not the norm. For example, the latest comprehensive review of the sexual abuse of males knowledge base, about the fourth of its kind, held as a criterion studies that employed at least 20 male subjects (Holmes & Slap, 1998). The rendered pool, of course, included samples that were disproportionately represented by females and incommensurate with prevailing prevalence rates by gender. This is not a reflection of the reviewers' strategies; rather, it is a reflection of the very social environment in which the sexual abuse of males is addressed, prevented, detected, investigated, treated, invalidated, and concealed. The point is not to criticize investigators, research endeavors, or funding sources, but only to highlight the state of the knowledge base. On the contrary, it is vital that we support researchers striving to conduct conceptually, methodologically, and ethically sound studies in spite of funding, sampling, and sociopolitical challenges.

Perhaps the lack of focus on the sexual abuse of males and difficulties in identifying this population may be due to any combination of the following: (a) the extensive use of the male perpetrator/female victim paradigm to conceptualize research, treatment, and prevention protocols; (b) a social aversion to even considering, let alone acknowledging, that male children are susceptible to CSA; (c) the socially constructed allocation of aggression to the male gender (and passivity to the female gender) and the resultant unwillingness of males to acknowledge such an experience, even to themselves; (d) inhibitions stemming from the gender-based proscription of male self-reliance even as a boy confronts age, power, role, stature, size, and developmental discrepancies between himself and the perpetrator; (e) the prohibiting authority of social stigma associated with homosexuality; and (f) the socially constructed notion that a young male's sexual "encounter" with an older female is positive and the consequent assumption that female perpetration is rare and unusual, among others (see, e.g., Allen, 1990; Dziuba-Leatherman & Finkelhor, 1994; Lisak, 1995; Mendel, 1995; Nasjleti, 1980; Paul, Catania, Pollack, & Stall, 2001; R Roane, 1992; Struve, 1990; Weinstein, Levine, Kogan, Harkavy-Friedman, & Miller, 2000).

To be sure, social constructions and personal assumptions reach far beyond Main Street. The dynamics and effects of childhood sexual abuse remain concealed even from professionals in the helping fields (Lab, Feigenbaum, & De Silva, 2000). The vast majority of graduate programs in social work, psychology, psychiatry, medicine, nursing, marriage and family therapy, and mental health counseling fail to impart to students the knowledge and skill necessary to understand and work with traumatized individuals, families, and groups (Sgroi, 1992). Within the arenas of CSA prevention, assessment, and treatment, scholarship remains inadequate (Hibbard & Zollinger, 1990), moreover, the available knowledge remains undisseminated (Conte, Fogarty, & Collins, 1991) and ultimately, unassimilated (Holmes & Offen, 1996; Spiegel, 1998b).

A majority of allied-service professionals report no prior training in the evaluation and treatment of CSA, notwithstanding an average of 7 years of practice experience in their respective disciplines (Hibbard & Zollinger, 1992). Nearly twice as many professionals have received training around the sexual abuse of females than training highlighting the sexual abuse of males (Campbell & Carlson, 1995). When asked to rate their self-assurance level in treating sexual abuse cases, a majority of child psychiatrists, clinical psychologists, and social workers fell between the categories of "somewhat" and "not very" confident (Zellman, 1990). Perhaps this is why mental health professionals routinely fail to ask about a male's history of CSA (Mills, 1993). For example, one study reported that among psychotherapists and allied professionals, only a limited minority (6%) routinely seek information about possible histories of CSA (Lab, Feigenbaum, & De Silva, 2000). Fewer than half of individuals working in the field have received training specific to the sexual abuse of males, yet of these, 80% recognize a need for more training. Prior training is more common among social workers and law enforcement officials than among physicians, nurses, lawyers, and psychologists (Hibbard & Zollinger, 1990).

Without question, these data endorse a need for basic education across all helping professions and continued education for all professionals associated with the field of CSA (Hibbard & Zollinger, 1990). Decades from now, as psychohistorians analyze the state of sexual abuse prevention, treatment, and research conducted today, they may find themselves baffled by the following questions (Sgroi, 1992): Why was it that the sexual abuse of males received relatively little attention in both investigatory and therapeutic domains? Why did so many practitioners lack the preparatory knowledge and skill necessary to impede, ameliorate, and investigate sexual trauma? How could it have been that physicians, psychiatrists, psychologists, and social workers, among others, working in the field of childhood sexual abuse, found themselves isolated and away from traditional therapeutic ideology and practice?

Perhaps historians will ultimately discover that the allied professions considered and actualized the calls of Suzanne Sgroi, David Finkelhor, and Mike Lew: a call for accurate and adequate education and training in assessing, treating, and preventing CSA (Sgroi, 1992); a call for model development that encompasses the dynamics and effects of CSA and that employs more general psychological and sociological theories to elucidate sexual trauma (Finkelhor, 1988); and a call to help males with histories of CSA discover the freedom to makes choices in their lives—choices regulated by their birthright, not by the abuse (Lew, 1990). These calls, first heard decades ago, still echo today.

THE SEXUAL ABUSE OF MALES

Coercion. Forced anal intercourse. Foreboding around disclosure. Fear of being viewed as deviant, feminine, and gay. The dynamics around, and the effects of, the sexual abuse of males reach notably beyond physical violation. What's more, sexual abuse is far from an uncommon phenomenon in the

United States today. It is estimated that 16% of males—or roughly 1 of every 6—are sexually abused prior to the age of 18 (Ryan, Kilmer, Cauce, Watanabe, & Hoyt, 2000; Simpson & Miller, 2002; Tyler, Hoyt, Whitbeck, & Cauce, 2001). Contrary to social mythology, the vast majority of these boys, nearly 100%, are abused by perpetrators known to them (Feiring, Taska, & Lewis, 1999; Fondacaro, Holt, & Powell, 1999; Fontanella, Harrington, & Zuravin, 2000; Huston, Prihoda, Parra, & Foulds, 1997; McLeer et al., 1998). Additionally, a majority of males abused by one perpetrator will subsequently be abused by others (Gold, Elhai, Lucenko, Swingle, & Hughes, 1997; Harrison, Fulkerson, & Beebe, 1997; Hunter, 1991).

The realities of childhood sexual abuse of girls, once shrouded from public awareness, were revealed during the 1970s as a result of the Women's Movement. Through pioneering efforts, and with little or no support from their male counterparts, female activists, clinicians, researchers, and others brought family violence, rape, and sexual abuse into social consciousness. Since that time, the vast majority of philosophical inquiry into, and the scientific investigation and clinical presentation of, sexual traumatization and its repercussions has emerged from the male perpetrator/female victim paradigm.

Now the same must be done for males with histories of CSA, particularly boys. The prevailing model for identifying, preventing, treating, studying, and adjudicating this social problem serves only to disserve. To begin, the male perpetrator/female victim paradigm renders the disclosures of boys null and void; it holds no place for their reality, their truth. Second, it promotes dichotomous thinking in both clinical and empirical domains. Far too often, externalizing behaviors, such as aggression, sexual reactivity, sexual compulsivity, risk taking, and drug use, are ascribed to males, while internalizing behaviors, including withdrawal, depression, suicidality, eating disorders, and repression, are apportioned to females. If this paradigm, or social lens, is the vantage point of psychotherapeutic and investigatory observations, the realities of CSA, as well as prevention, detection, treatment, and research efforts directed toward children, will continue to be contravened by socially constructed notions of masculinity and femininity.

Unquestionably, from a sociocultural standpoint, masculinity, as the ultimate outcome of gender role socialization, demands the recoiling from femininity—that is, a repudiation of any thoughts, feelings, and behaviors that are socially allocated to women. Given the contradictory and oppositional social blueprints around gender, it is currently unlikely that males will disclose histories of CSA when the only role available to them is that of perpetrator, and the only other role is that of victim. To be a victim is to be female, powerless, vulnerable, and abused by a male (Duncan & Williams, 1998; Gill & Tutty, 1999). To be a perpetrator is to be male, aggressive, compulsive and manipulative, and a victimizer of female children (Hislop, 2001). The result of this social prescription is that males cannot be victims, and victims are not males (Lew, 1990).

Gender has come to have jurisdiction over childhood sexual abuse because social imperatives have made it so. Most treatment programs, research endeavors, and social policies continue to promote the feminization of victimization and the masculinization of perpetration. To do so is to prevent, identify, treat, and study CSA as a function of gender, thereby negating the substantial numbers of males with abuse histories and females who perpetrate against both boys and girls. To do so is to be dictated to by cultural and social myths, and consequently to contradict the life histories of both the abusers and the abused.

The traditional male perpetrator/female victim paradigm, with its mutually exclusive, dichotomous categories, must give way to a model that allows for the recognition of male traumatization and female perpetration. The stark reality of childhood sexual abuse is that neither gender is exempt from either role. Therefore, the term *childhood sexual abuse* is a misnomer unless the plight of sexually abused boys is acknowledged.

Sexual abuse professionals are in a unique position to tell the truth. This necessitates a reframing of, and a sensitivity to, the ways in which gender role socialization impinges upon childhood sexual abuse as a social problem and a life event. Such reframing can enhance the gender sensitivity, cultural competency, and developmental appropriateness of prevention, detection, intervention, and investigatory strategies. We are equipped with evolving knowledge and skill; now, it's time for a new view.

THIS BOOK

Sexual Abuse of Males: The SAM Model of Theory and Practice is both original and unique. There is little or no question that sexual abuse brings authentic change to a child's life (Browne & Finkelhor, 1986; Garnefski & Diekstra, 1997). These changes may occur within a two-year period following the abuse (Gully, Hansen, Britton, Langley, & McBride, 2000; Leverich et al., 2002), or persist for years, even into adulthood (Black, Dubowitz, & Harrington, 1994; Cohen, Brown, & Smaile, 2001). Based on a comprehensive review of the literature and supported by data generated from the grounded theory model of research presented by Strauss (1987), the content analytic procedures suggested by Lofland and Lofland (1984), and multivariate strategies outlined by Stevens (1992), this book describes a conceptual link between clinical observations and an integration of the biological, psychological, and social sequelae experienced by males who have been sexually abused as children. While both anecdotal and empirical data, such as measures of attributional tendencies regarding responsibility (Dimock, 1988; Lisak, 1994a), neurophysiological dysfunction (Bremner et al., 1997; van der Kolk & Fisler, 1995), aggression (Chandy, Blum, & Resnick, 1997; Friedrich, Beilke, & Urquiza, 1988), conflict regarding sexual orientation (Johnson & Shrier, 1985; Spiegel, 1997), and self-mutilating behavior (McClellan, Adams, Douglas, McCurry, & Storck, 1995; Woods & Dean, 1985), have been cited in the literature, these phenomena have not yet been classified and ordered into a conceptual framework that addresses the relationship between sexual trauma and its impact on males. The impact issues or initial effects discussed herein include gender identity confusion, traumatic rage, blame, shame and responsibility, and physical findings; dynamics include abusive acts, use of force, coabuse, and suspicion of abuse without confirmation. This framework, guided by practice and informed by research, can be utilized toward the development of assessment and intervention protocols.

Although many publishing houses have disseminated books on the topic of the sexual abuse of girls, a mere handful have published books on their male counterparts. Indisputably, it is important to acknowledge, read, and appreciate all publications in this burgeoning field. At the same time, it is critical to produce a work that does not superimpose constructs founded upon female victimology, such as the male perpetrator/female victim paradigm or the father/daughter incest model, onto the population of sexually abused males. To do so is to misrepresent, misunderstand, misinform, and thereby disserve. Hence, "SAM" is based on the life histories of more than 1,000 boys, adolescent males, and adult males with histories of CSA.

The purposes of this book are to:

1. Present the Sexual Abuse of Males (SAM) model of dynamics and effects.
2. Apply the SAM model to seven cases representing a diverse group of males with histories of childhood sexual abuse.
3. Translate the SAM model into a practice philosophy and a stepwise treatment framework.
4. Operationalize the SAM model treatment objectives into a number of systematic interventions, each with a definition of the strategy, a systematic description of its execution, and its anticipated outcomes.

Part I of this book is conceptual in nature. The next chapter presents a comprehensive inventory of the dynamics and effects associated with the sexual abuse of males. It also describes the developmental process of the SAM model. Chapter 3 addresses the working assumptions and concepts undergirding this conceptual framework. The SAM model of dynamics and effects is introduced in Chapter 4. Chapter 5 applies the SAM model to seven diverse cases.

Part II of this book focuses on treatment. Chapter 6 highlights philosophical assumptions and principles that support, guide, and sustain practice. Chapter 7 addresses preparatory empathy, or ways in which a therapist can anticipate and contemplate issues prior to treatment, such as psychic trauma, memory, the therapeutic alliance, client expectations, and potential transference and countertransference interactions. Chapter 8 proposes seven treatment objectives that comprise an initial phase of therapy. Chapter 9 characterizes a client-centered treatment analogy based on the anthropological concept of excavation. Chapter 10 proffers a number of intervention strategies and rationales that operationalize the treatment objectives. Chapter 11 highlights the experience of males with histories of CSA in therapy.

Thus, as a book, "SAM" strives to provide:

1. A conceptual framework integrating the numerous and seemingly unrelated dynamics and effects deduced by a number of studies and now lying disparate in the knowledge base.
2. A vantage point from which to view in detail and reflect on the sexual abuse of males within a biopsychosocial context.
3. A frame of reference that facilitates the preparation for and the sustainment of a therapeutic relationship with boys, adolescent males, and adult males with histories of CSA.
4. A systematic way of approaching treatment and actualizing treatment objectives.
5. A number of interventions that are theory driven, modifiable to client age, and amenable to evaluation.
6. A foundation from which to develop, pilot, and empirically validate gender-sensitive assessment and treatment protocols.
7. A theoretical framework for future research endeavors.
8. Perhaps most importantly, SAM strives to provide a voice of understanding, empathy, and hope.

Finally, the SAM model of dynamics and effects and its corresponding philosophy of treatment, practice framework, and selected interventions represent attempts to answer three common questions among social workers, psychologists, psychiatrists, pastoral counselors, mental health counselors, and those interested in understanding the sexual abuse of males as a biopsychosocial problem, and those striving to help males with histories of CSA: What can I do? How do I do it? Why am I doing it? This book dedicates itself to attempting a few answers. I hope it is helpful to you.

Josef Spiegel, Ph.D.

CHAPTER TWO

THE DEVELOPMENT
OF THE SAM MODEL

I've been through the system—foster care, child protection workers, social workers, guardians, family court—and as an adult, I've tried to go to mental health clinics, therapists. I wanted the abuse to stop. I want to get help for the problems from the abuse. But whenever I talk to people who are supposed to help me, they seem to forget that I was the one who was abused. They treat me like I was the abuser or like I'm going to turn into one. Can't they see that the two are very different? Can't they keep their information straight? (Palo, a young Native American male with a history of childhood sexual abuse)

THIS CHAPTER FOCUSES on the evolution of the SAM (Sexual Abuse of Males) model of dynamics and effects. Beginning with a brief explanation of a conceptual model, it presents three frameworks that continue to be instrumental in delineating the experience of sexual assault, particularly as it pertains to females. Next, this chapter transitions to a lengthy summary of the sexual abuse of males knowledge base, concluding with a description of the strategies employed to develop the SAM model of dynamics and effects.

WHY A MODEL?

In this context, a model is a conceptual framework composed of a discerning set of various facts, concepts, propositions, and hypotheses together with beliefs, values, and assumptions. As for data, a model contains both assumptive or theoretical knowledge and confirmed or empirical knowledge, with emphasis on the latter. The ultimate goal of a model is to select, organize, and present data within a parsimonious yet comprehensive framework in order to consider in a meaningful way data that might otherwise remain disparate and of limited utility. Moreover, a model reflecting human behavior in the social environment must validate and authenticate the realities as experienced by individuals, families, and groups. In other words, a model must tell their stories, tell their truths.

19

CURRENT THEORETICAL MODELS

The vast majority of philosophical inquiry into and the scientific investigation and clinical presentation of childhood sexual abuse (CSA) and its repercussions have arisen from the foundation of the male perpetrator/female victim paradigm. This section addresses three models based on that perspective: (a) the *rape trauma syndrome* (Burgess & Holmstrom, 1974, 1979), (b) the *child sexual abuse accommodation syndrome model* (Summit, 1983), and (c) the *traumagenic dynamics model of child sexual abuse* (Browne & Finkelhor, 1986; Finkelhor & Browne, 1985; Finkelhor, 1988). Although the first model focuses on rape and the second and third on the sexual abuse of girls, all three were generated and/or supported by empirical research, all are dimensional or phasic in nature, and all three have palpably and extensively contributed to the advancement of the field.

The Rape Trauma Syndrome

The *rape trauma syndrome* is included here because it was one of the first models in the sexual abuse field to parsimoniously explain the effects of sexual violence. Burgess and Holmstrom (1974, 1979) based this conceptual framework on the issues and consequences typical of women following a single, violent sexual assault. This research team studied the effects of rape among 92 female victims.

According to their model, there are two phases of rape trauma (Burgess & Holmstrom, 1974, 1979). The first, identified as the acute phase, begins immediately after the rape and may continue for days, weeks, or months. The victim's immediate reaction is one of shock, anger, fear, and disbelief. The effects experienced during the acute phase are diverse, spanning the psychological, emotional, behavioral, and physiological. Such effects may include a sense of powerlessness, cognitive or emotional suppression, humiliation, feelings of guilt and shame, sleeplessness, headaches, nausea, gastrointestinal irritability, genito-urinary disturbances, and genital bruising. Many of these initial effects overlap into the next stage, characterized as the long-term reorganization phase.

The reorganization phase may last from several months to several years (Burgess & Holmstrom, 1974, 1979), during which time women who experienced rape potentially endure a number of personal and relational conflicts. Fears once associated with the rape have now generalized to other situations. Fear of being alone, fear of strangers, fear of crowds, and fear of retaliation by the rapist may instigate frequent changes in residency and phone numbers throughout this extended period. Within the domain of intimacy and sexuality, anxiety-based effects may encompass inhibited sexual desire and arousal. Activities of daily living, such as parenting, school work, housework, and employment, may also be negatively impacted.

Talking about the rape experience and its after-effects in an empathic and supportive atmosphere is fundamental to recovery. Doing so often helps women who survived rape to gain an understanding of and sense of control over the initial and long-term effects. Consequently, knowledge and a viable sense of empowerment are two primary treatment outcomes.

The Child Sexual Abuse Accommodation Syndrome

To help explain the female child's life context following sexual abuse, Summit (1983) conceptualized the child *sexual abuse accommodation syndrome*. The child's reaction is typically characterized by secrecy and helplessness (two prerequisites of sexual abuse), entrapment and accommodation (the sexual abuse itself), and delayed disclosure and retraction (two common consequences of sexual abuse).

Secrecy, the first stage, is fundamental. Sexual abuse occurs when the girl is alone with the perpetrator; secrecy must be maintained. For the child, secrecy around the sexually abusive relationship is both a source of fear and a haven of safety. In terms of the former, a sexually abused girl often fears the actualization of the perpetrator's threats if and when the abuse is disclosed, and she remains fearful of the potential responses of others who may react negatively upon disclosure. As for the latter, a sexually abused girl often receives assurances that all will be well as long as the sexually abusive relationship remains hidden from others. Secrecy stigmatizes a child with a sense of shame even when there is little or no pain from the sexual experience itself (Summit, 1983).

Helplessness is the second stage or category. Even though a child is three times more likely to be abused by a known and seemingly trustworthy adult than by a stranger (Summit, 1983), this same child, when confronted with childhood sexual abuse, faces a dilemma, for she also is taught to be biddable and affectionate with any adult entrusted with her care. Children are, and often remain, relatively vulnerable and defenseless with adults and within authoritarian relationships. That the perpetrator is often in an apparently trustful and caregiving position only serves to exacerbate the power imbalance within the sexually abusive relationship and the sense of helplessness within the child.

The next category is *entrapment and accommodation*. When childhood sexual abuse is not prevented, or when the child does not receive protection and care immediately following its initial occurrence, her only viable option, then, is to strive to accept the abuse and to cope with it to the best of her ability (Summit, 1983). Entrapped by secrecy and bound by helplessness, a child often accommodates to the abuse by assuming responsibility for its occurrence and preservation, viewing herself as the provocateur, the one to be punished. She thereby safeguards an illusion of goodness, if not virtue, around the perpetrator, both for herself and for others. In order to accomplish this— that is, in order to survive—the child often relies on a number of ego defense mechanisms that allow her to cope with the abuse while simultaneously projecting a mirage of normalcy.

Delayed disclosure follows as the fourth category. According to Summit (1983), CSA is rarely disclosed, but if it is, chances are knowledge of it will silently abide within the immediate family circle. If and when disclosure occurs, it is often delayed, perhaps resulting from a chance discovery by a third party, the child's exposure to a prevention education campaign in the community, or as an attempt to stop a seemingly irrepressible family conflict.

Retraction is the fifth and final category. No matter what the scenario, a child of any age often confronts disbelief, blame, and punishment as a counterblast to her acknowledgment of the abuse. In response, she often retracts what was initially revealed, repeatedly bearing the responsibility not only for the abuse but for its aftermath as well, and discovering that she holds the key to either family preservation or family destruction. She learns once and again not to complain, and adults learn, over and again, not to listen. Retraction consequently actualizes the cycle of accommodation, leaving the sexually abused girl as bearer of the burden of childhood sexual abuse (Summit, 1983).

The Traumagenic Dynamics Model of Child Sexual Abuse

Based on their review of the empirical literature associated with the sexual abuse of female children, Browne and Finkelhor (1986) developed the traumagenic dynamics model. According to these authors, the sexually abusive experience alters the sexually abused girl's cognitive, affective, and behavioral orientation to the world. The four factors generating trauma are based on the subjective reactions of the female child, rather than on external criteria. They are traumatic sexualization, betrayal, powerlessness, and stigmatization.

Traumatic sexualization is described as the facilitative and formative conditions that impact a child's sexual thoughts, feelings, and behaviors in a developmentally inappropriate and relationally dysfunctional manner. In essence, the perpetrator sexualizes the child beyond her developmental capacities. Traumatic sexualization, as a dynamic, is unique to child sexual abuse. Generated effects may include a distorted sexual self-concept, confusion and misconceptions around sexual norms and knowledge, preoccupation with sex, aversion to sex, sexual dysfunction, phobic reactions to sexual intimacy, and sexual compulsivity (Browne & Finkelhor, 1986; Finkelhor, 1988).

Betrayal occurs when children recognize that they are being harmed by trusted individuals on whom they are also dependent. Betrayal occurs again when, upon disclosure, nonoffending caretakers disbelieve, blame, and/or denigrate the child. Thus, the child's faith and trust in the expectation of care are shattered irrespective of what role the perpetrator holds in her life; in fact, betrayal extends beyond the sexually abusive relationship, encircling nonoffending family members and collateral as well. With the occurrence and aftermath of this dynamic, a girl may experience corresponding effects such as depression, anger, lack of trust, clinging behavior, and antisocial behavior, as well as vulnerability to subsequent abuse and conflictual relationships (Browne & Finkelhor, 1986; Finkelhor, 1988).

Powerlessness is conceptualized as the outcome of a process whereby a child's sense of efficacy and self-determination are steadfastly overruled as her body, person, and place are repeatedly trespassed against her will. Additionally, the sexually abused girl, in the midst of perpetration and disclosure, finds herself confronting threats of injury or annihilation as this form of child abuse exposes her to coercion, bodily invasion, and violence (Browne & Finkelhor, 1986; Finkelhor, 1988). Fear and anxiety, a victim identity, identification with the aggressor, and academic and workplace problems are examples of engendered effects of this traumagenic dynamic.

Stigmatization involves the means by which negative reactions, messages and implications associated with the child's sexually abusive experiences are subsequently incorporated into her self-concept. For example, subtle or blatant messages from the perpetrator and nonoffending caretakers may convey that the sexually abused girl is evil, worthless, shameful, and guilty. Maintaining secrecy, and the burdens that come with it, contribute to this dynamic as well. Guilt, shame, drug and alcohol misuse, self-injurious behavior, and suicidal ideation are examples of the impact of stigmatization (Browne & Finkelhor, 1986).

Burgess and Holmstrom's (1974, 1979) conceptualization of the *rape trauma syndrome* was derived from a research study intended to assess the effects on women generated by a single episode of rape. Summit's (1983) child sexual *abuse accommodation syndrome* was founded upon the aggregate experiences of a number of sexual abuse treatment centers. Browne and Finkelhor's (1986) *traumagenic dynamics* model was based on a comprehensive review of the literature around the effects of childhood sexual abuse associated with girls. All three of these models have contributed significantly to the field of childhood sexual abuse, undergirding research conceptualizations and questions, guiding practice-based articles, chapters, and books, impacting social policy, informing professors in the classroom and students in the field, and validating individuals who know rape and sexual abuse firsthand.

LITERATURE ON THE SEXUAL ABUSE OF MALES

In 1986, when Browne and Finkelhor published their seminal review of the literature on the initial and long-term effects of sexual victimization and proposed the traumagenic dynamics model, they, like others before them, limited their efforts to studies that focused on females because "few clinical and even fewer empirical studies have been done on boys, and it seems premature to draw conclusions at this point" (p. 144). Since that time, there has been an increase in published literature addressing the sexual abuse of males.

Given next is a report of the literature on the sexual abuse of males. It is not a review of the literature, such as those presented by Holmes and Slap (1998), Mendel (1995), Urquiza and Capra (1990), and Watkins and Bentovin (1992). Rather, it is a consolidation of more than 75 studies focusing, in whole or in part, on the sexual abuse of males. It is not a critique of the literature but rather a summarized presentation of the data to date, spanning the years 1981–2002.

Summary of Sexual Abuse Dynamics

Since the majority of studies conducted thus far can be characterized as lacking various degrees of methodological rigor, drawing any firm conclusions regarding the dynamics and effects of the sexual abuse of males is premature. At this time, however, the following tentative propositions can be presented. Whenever possible, three or more citations are employed to substantiate a finding. In some cases, only two are utilized, and in fewer instances, only one. The latter findings are typically generated from studies focusing on peripheral or new areas of research such as professional perceptions of CSA, repression and memory, and CSA fatalities, among several others.

In this context, dynamics refer to the physical, temporal, psychological, interpersonal, familial, and social forces that produce and impact, or initiate and maintain, the sexually abusive relationship and/or the context in which it occurs. Effects are defined as the biological, psychological, and sociological consequences rendered by individual or collective dynamics. A system is utilized to represent the rendered statistics across studies. Throughout the upcoming section, a "limited minority" represents values between 1% and 19%, "minority," 20% to 34%, "considerable minority," 35% to 45%, "near majority," 46% to 50%, "narrow majority," 51% to 59%, "majority," 60% to 69%," "substantial majority," 70% to 84%, "vast majority," 85% to 99%, and "virtual majority," 100%. For example, under the category of "social perceptions," the reader will find the following: The substantial majority (75%) of potential jurors of both genders endorse the idea that people can and do repress memories of traumatic events such as childhood sexual abuse. Following are a broad spectrum of dynamics and effects that delineate the sexual abuse of males.

THE FAMILY

Boys who experience childhood sexual abuse are more likely than nonabused boys to reside in a single-parent household or a reconstructed household with parents who are separated or divorced (Conte & Schuerman, 1987; Feiring, Taska, & Lewis, 1999; Gellert, Durfee, Berkowitz, Higgins, & Tubiolo, 1993; Hall, Mathews, & Pearce, 1998; Hibbard, Ingersoll, & Orr, 1990; Janus, Burgess, & McCormack, 1987; Mian, Wehrspann, Klajner-Diamond, LeBaron, & Winder, 1986; Ray & English, 1995; Spencer & Dunklee, 1986; Tjaden & Thoennes, 1992; Wells, McCann, Adams, Voris, & Dahl, 1997). Within such households, there are more absent biological mothers, more absent biological fathers, larger families of origin, more frequent relocations, and more children in foster care (Fontenella, Harrington & Zuravin, 2000; Gale, Thompson, Moran, & Sack, 1988).

The majority (approximately 60%) of sexually abused boys have multiple or shifting caregivers, are separated from a primary caregiver for more than 6 months, and experience the absence of a father for 3 or more years (Bagley, Wood, & Young, 1994; Fontanella et al., 2000; Pierce & Pierce, 1985). These boys are more likely to experience the death of a father than nonabused boys (Janus, Burgess, & McCormack, 1987). They are more likely than nonabused males to experience insecure attachments dynamics and effects with both parents, but particularly with their mothers (Hall, Matthews, & Pearce, 2002; Styron & Janoff-Bulman, 1997). Males reporting an unhappy family life are more than twice as likely to have a history of CSA than counterparts without such family dynamics and perceptions (Finkelhor, Hotaling, Lewis, & Smith, 1990).

Boys subjected to CSA often experience the following in terms of family dynamics, and significantly more so than nonabused children:

1. More biological parents (or caretakers) with criminal histories and more family arrests and court appearances (De Bellis, Broussard, Herring, Wexler, Moritz, & Benitez, 2001; Gale, Thompson, Moran, & Sack, 1988; Hall, Matthews, & Pearce, 2002; Janus et al., 1987; Ryan, Kilmer, Cauce, Watanabe, & Hoyt, 2000; Urquiza & Crowley, 1986; Widom, 1999).
2. Illicit drug use in the home with one or more alcoholic parents and/or family members (Bartholow et al., 1994; Brown & Anderson, 1991; De Bellis et al., 2001; Estes & Tidwell, 2002; Gellert et al., 1993; Friedrich & Luecke, 1988; Hernandez, 1995; Little & Hamby, 2001; McClellan, Adams, Douglas, McCurry, & Storck, 1995; Nelson et al., 2002; Roane, 1992; Robin, Chester, Rasmussen, Jaranson, & Goldman, 1997; Ryan, Kilmer, Cauce, Watanabe, & Hoyt, 2000; Widom, 1999).
3. Antisocial behavior among the parents (Janus, Burgess, & McCormack, 1987; McClellan et al., 1995).
4. A greater frequency of parental psychiatric history characterized by comorbidity, for example, mood disorders, anxiety disorders, and posttraumatic stress disorder due to domestic violence (Brown & Anderson, 1991; De Bellis, Broussard, et al., 2001; Friedrich & Luecke, 1988).
5. A greater likelihood of a CSA history among the parents (Elwell & Ephross, 1987; Estes & Tidwell, 2002; Kelley, 1990; Newberger, Gremy, Waternauz, & Newberger, 1993; Sansonnet-Hayden, Haley, Marriage, & Fine, 1987).
6. An unstable home life, including serious arguments within the family, an inability to manage and express anger productively, marital discord, domestic violence, and the witnessing of violence between the parents (Brown & Anderson, 1991; De Bellis, Broussard, et al., 2001; Estes & Tidwell, 2002; Friedrich & Luecke, 1988; Gold et al., 1997; Hall et al., 2002; Janus et al., 1987; Krug, 1989; Lisak, 1994a; Ray & English, 1995).

Additional family dynamics are likely to include the following:

1. Deficient family income, parental unemployment, annual family income less than $25,000, and receipt of social welfare entitlements (Cappelleri, Eckenrode, & Powers, 1993; Feiring et al., 1999; Hall et al., 1998; Janus et al., 1987; Tjaden & Thoennes, 1992; Violato & Genuis, 1993; Widom, 1999).
2. Confused parental roles, inappropriate attitudes toward sex, and inappropriate limits around privacy (Hall et al., 2002; Ray & English, 1995).
3. Lack of positive parental involvement (Ryan et al., 2000; Salmon & Calderbank, 1996), including disinterest and/or inconsistent interest conveyed regarding the personal concerns of children, erratic monitoring of the boy's involvement in school and community activities, and unavailability of the parents in educating and discussing concerns around human sexuality (Woods & Dean, 1985).
4. Inappropriate sexual attitudes and sexualized interactions within the home (Hall et al., 2002).
5. Isolating, scapegoating, and blaming the boy for the abuse (Friedrich & Luecke, 1988).
6. At times, a history of child neglect and abandonment (De Bellis, Broussard, et al., 2001; Ray & English, 1995).

THE PERPETRATOR

Childhood sexual abuse perpetrators of boys tend to be well-educated, employed, and socially-economically diverse (Abel et al., 1987). Across many life domains, they tend to evidence a well-versed adeptness in presenting themselves as psychologically and relationally "normal" (Bagley et al., 1994); however, for at least a segment of the perpetrator population (undetermined at this time), the reverse is more accurate (Cullen, Smith, Funk, & Haaf, 2000).

A history of CSA appears to be a common element among perpetrators. Childhood sexual abuse perpetrators are approximately two times more likely than nonsexual offenders and three times more likely than nonoffending males to have reported histories of CSA (Romano & De Luca, 1996). In a major study, a majority of perpetrators (68%) experienced at least one negative sexual encounter as a child, with the same number reporting a history of CSA (Elliott, Browne, & Kilcoyne, 1995). The mean age at which their abuse experience began was 9.75, within the age range of, but definitely older than, the boys they target for abuse. However, other studies show a smaller proportion, in the range of 20% (Dhawan & Marshall, 1996). A considerable minority (approximately 40%) of adolescent male perpetrators report histories of CSA (Ryan, Miyoshi, Metzner, Krugman, & Fryer, 1996; Worling, 1995). Although samples of female perpetrators tend to be small, a near majority (50%) to virtual majority (100%) report histories of CSA (see, e.g., Fehrenbach & Monastersky, 1988; Mathews, 1989; Wolfe, 1985). The percentage of those with sexual abuse histories decreases (22%) among incarcerated women and men convicted of sexual offenses against children (U.S. Department of Justice, 1996).

Developmental risk factors for the perpetration of CSA include histories of childhood sexual abuse, childhood physical abuse, childhood emotional abuse, and behavioral problems, all within the context of family dysfunction (Baker, Tabacoff, Tornusciolo, & Eisenstadt, 2001; Becker & Hunter, 1997; Briggs & Hawkins, 1996; Knight & Prentsky, 1993; Lee, Jackson, Pattison, & Ward, 2002; Ryan, 1996). Even though male perpetrators are significantly more likely to have a history of CSA than nonabused adult males, with odds ranging from 5 to 13 (Haywood, Dravitz, Wasyliw, Goldberg, & Cavanaugh, 1996), a history of CSA, separate and apart from other personal and ecological factors, cannot fully explain the path from abused to abuser (Bagley et al., 1994; Garland & Dougler, 1990; McGee, Wolfe, & Wilson, 1997). Rather, a number of coalescing factors contribute to this cycle.

Among perpetrators, insecure childhood attachments, and, more specifically, maternal anxious attachment and paternal avoidant or insecure attachment, in addition to caregiver inconstancy, are correlates and predictors of the perpetration of sexually coercive and abusive activities (Smallbone & Dadds, 2000). With histories of anxious, avoidant, and insecure parent–child attachment configruations (Marshall, 1993; Saradjian, 1996; Ward, Hudson, & Marshall, 1996), and with greater security in their attachments to mothers as opposed to fathers, perpetrators tend to evidence problematic dynamics and ineffectual coping within interpersonal relationships as adults (Marshall, Serran, & Cortoni, 2000). As a group, they tend to exhibit inadequate social and relational skills, low self-esteem, anxiety, impulsivity, inability to trust others, and problems with anger management (see, e.g., Marshall & Mazzucco, 1995a; Prentsky & Knight, 1993; Prentsky, Knight, & Lee, 1996). However, these qualities and characteristics may be undetectable as perpetrators strive to build rapport with children and their parents alike.

A substantial majority (74%) of perpetrators have chemical dependency problems (Cavaiola & Schiff, 1988), while a limited minority (12%) of perpetrators are known to have a prior sexual perpetration history (Spencer & Dunklee, 1986). With regard to psychiatric comorbidity, the vast majority (93%) of perpetrators in sex offender treatment programs meet criteria for a *DSM–IV* Axis I disorder (in addition to pedophilia) as well as an Axis II disorder. Mood disorders, anxiety disorders, psychoactive substance use disorders, other paraphilia diagnoses, and sexual function disorders represent the most common mental disorders whereas the most prevalent personality disorders are obsessive-compulsive, narcissistic, antisocial, avoidant, and paranoid (Cavaiola & Schiff, 1988; Prentsky, Knight, & Lee, 1997; Raymond, Coleman, Ohlerking, Christenson, & Miner, 1999). In one study, perpetrators indicated or had the appearance of signs and symptoms of HIV in a narrow majority (58%) of cases (Gellert et al., 1993). More often than not, perpetrators tend to be of the same racial origin as the boy (DeJong, Hervada, & Emmett, 1983).

A majority (66%) of perpetrators report that stress often precipitates their offenses, including stress associated with work, sexual problems, conflicts within the home, and/or psychological problems (Elliott, Browne, & Kilcoyne, 1995). In preparing for an abusive episode, they often use drugs and alcohol, view pornography, and fantasize about previous encounters with children, all of which serve to disinhibit the perpetrator (Finkelhor, 1984; U.S. Department of Justice, 1996; Lambie, Seymour, Lee, & Adams, 2002; Wurtele & Miller-Perrin, 1992).

CSA perpetrators hold a keen instinct for not only discovering, but also exploiting, a child's vulnerabilities, such as the need to feel loved, validated, and valued by primary caretakers (Berliner & Conte, 1990; Saradjian, 1996). They tend to experience sex with children as less threatening than sex with a peer (Elliott, Browne, & Kilcoyne, 1995). Relative to rapists of adults, perpetrators of children are twice as likely to sexually abuse multiple numbers of individuals (U.S. Department of Justice, 1997b). In 1995, the substantial majority (70%) of sexual offenses involving physical force and the vast majority (95%) of sexual offenses without reported physical force were committed against individuals between the ages of 0 and 17 (Crimes Against Children Research Center, 1998).

A substantial majority of male perpetrators (70%) commit abusive acts against 1–9 children, a minority (23%) commit offenses against 10–40 children, and a limited minority (7%) commit offenses against 41–450 children (Elliott, Browne, & Kilcoyne, 1995). On average, however, a perpetrator if intrafamilial is likely to abuse 1.7 children whereas if extrafamilial is likely to subject an average of 150 boys and approximately 20 girls to CSA. Perpetrators abuse boys with an incidence that is five times greater than the molestation of young girls. More specifically, in one study of 561 sexual abuse offenders, 224 nonincestuous perpetrators documented 5,197 sexual acts against 4,435 girls whereas 153 non-incestuous perpetrators disclosed 43,100 acts against 22,981 boys. The frequency of perpetrator-reported CSA offenses is vastly greater than the number of crimes for which perpetrators are arrested. The ratio of arrest to commission of CSA is approximately 1:30 (Abel et al., 1987).

Among convicted sexual abuse perpetrators, those who abuse children are significantly more likely than those who rape adults to have a history of childhood physical and/or sexual abuse (Greenberg, Bradford, & Curry, 1993; U.S. Department of Justice, 1996). Further, the vast majority (86%) of state prison inmates convicted of sexual assaults perpetrated against a child under the age of 18 while a considerable minority (39%) of state prison inmates convicted of rape targeted a child within that same age range (U.S. Department of Justice, 1996). Men who initially offended against an extended family member, an acquaintance, or a stranger are significantly more likely to reoffend and be charged with a new sexual crime than convicted perpetrators who initially abused their biological children (Firestone, Bradford, McCoy, Greenberg, & Curry, 1999; Greenberg, Bradford, Firestone, & Curry, 2000). Recent studies suggest that a limited minority (6% to 22%) of convicted adolescent and adult male perpetrators, monitored for periods spanning from 5 to 36 years, evidence sexual reoffense rates within the range of 13% to 20% (Firestone et al., 2000; Hanson & Bussière, 1998; Prentsky, Lee, Knight, & Cerce, 1997; Proulx, Pellerin, Paradis, McKibben, Aubut, & Quimet, 1997; Rasmussen, 1999; Sipe, Jensen, & Everett, 1998). A meta-analytic study revealed the following predictors of sexual offense recidivism: (a) a negative relationship with mother during childhood; (b) juvenile delinquency; (c) disruptions and dysfunction in the family of origin; (d) the relational status of "single," (e) a history of prior offenses and incarcerations; (f) a sustained sexual preference for children; (g) a sexual preference for children outside the family; and (h) a sexual preference for male children (Hanson & Bussière, 1996). However, recidivism rates, as well as many other variables associated with CSA research, are difficult to measure because most sexually abusive acts, episodes, and relationships remain undetected and undisclosed.

PEDOPHILES

Central to pedophilia is a sexual orientation toward prepubescent children. Pedophiles with a sexual interest in boys are significantly more likely to have mothers of a higher maternal age and to possess intellectual deficits in contrast to pedophiles with a sole sexual interest in female children (Blanchard et al., 1999). As for personal characteristics, when compared to nonsexual offenders, pedophiles who perpetrate against boys and pedophiles who perpetrate against girls exhibit more fragile body images and manifest significantly more indicators of social introversion (Tardi & Gijseghem, 2001). They are more likely than normal controls to evidence impulsivity, inhibition, passive-aggression, and harm avoidance (Cohen et al., 2002). In one study, the vast majority (93%) of perpetrators met the *DSM* diagnostic criteria for an Axis I disorder in addition to pedophilia and a majority (60%) fulfilled the diagnostic requisites for Axis II disorders (Raymond, Coleman, Ohlerking, Christenson, & Miner, 1999). Within this sample, a number of diagnostic categories reached majority proportions: mood disorder (67%), anxiety disorder (64%), psychoactive substance abuse disorder (60%), paraphilia comorbidity (53%), and alcohol abuse (51%). The most common personality disorders included obsessive compulsive, narcissistic, avoidant, and antisocial.

Relative to male pedophiles who abuse young girls, adult male perpetrators of boys display significantly weaker ego structures. Regarding emotional congruence, pedophiles with a preference for male children are significantly more likely to align with the boy at his developmental level, thereby psychologically and relationally fixating themselves on, and ultimately personifying, the role of a child, whereas incest perpetrators are significantly more likely to elevate the child into the role of an adult. When compared to these two perpetrating groups, male pedophiles who hold a preference for female children tend to be motivated by sexual gratification as opposed to emotional or relational interests (Wilson, 1999).

Neurologically, male pedophiles, when compared to normal controls, exhibit significant alterations in serotonergic, catecholaminergic, and hormonal activity. For example, pedophiles manifest significantly greater cortisol responsivity and significantly lower degrees of serum cortisol, prolactin, and body temperature. Additionally, pedophiles, as well as other paraphiliacs, render significantly higher levels of plasma norepinephrine than normal controls (Kogan et al., 1995, cited in Maes, De Vos, Van Hunsel, Van West, Westenberg, Cosyns, & Neels, 2001). And, relative to normal male controls, adult male pedophiles show significantly higher levels of plasma epinephrine and norepinephrine. These results, in aggregate, suggest that serotonergic and catecholaminergic alterations may contribute to a pedophile's pathophysiology and may underlie his heightened sense of impulsivity, aggression, and violence (Maes, van West, De Vos, Westernberg, Van Hunsel, Hendriks, Cosyns, & Sharpé, 2001).

ADOLESCENT SEX OFFENDERS

Juvenile CSA offenders, as a group, commit their first sexual offense before age 15 (Araji, 1997) and, in a considerable minority (46%) of cases, before the age of 12 (Burton, 2000). Adolescent male and adolescent female offenders are similar with regard to the types of CSA acts they perpetrate and in their tendencies to select and abuse children of the other gender (Mathews, Hunter, & Vuz, 1997). Babysitting appears to be the context in which adolescent sex offending is most likely to occur. With regard to characteristics related to the self, adolescent offenders are significantly more likely than controls to evidence academic difficulties in addition to neurological, cognitive, and/or intellectual impairment (Miner, Siekert, & Ackland, 1997; Fehrenbach, Smith, Monastersky & Deischer, 1986; Knight, & Prentsky, 1993; Ferrara & McDonald, 1996). Further, they are significantly more likely to exhibit substance abuse problems, behavioral problems, inappropriate sexual boundaries, deviant sexual fantasies, uncontrollable sexual urges, impulse control problems, depression, and anxiety, as well as avoidant, antisocial, and dependent personality disorders (Carpenter, Peed, & Eastmen, 1995; Becker & Hunter, 1997; Kahn & Chambers, 1991).

In terms of family dynamics, common characteristics include a mother with a history of CSA, the presence of domestic violence, the witnessing of domestic violence, a home environment with insufficient sexual and personal boundaries, exposure to pornography, the child's emotional detachment or physical separation between the child and parents, and subjection of the child to sexual abuse, physical abuse, emotional abuse, and neglect (Baker et al. 2001; Becker & Hunter, 1997; Kahn & Chambers, 1991; Fehrenbach, Smith, Monastersky, & Deischer, 1986; Kobayashi, 1995; Ryan, 1996). As for social dynamics, juvenile perpetrators, when compared to controls, are significantly more likely to demonstrate impaired social skills, conflictual peer relations, and a fragmented, dysfunctional, or nonexistent system of social support (Knight & Prentsky, 1993; Miner & Crimmins, 1995; Prentsky & Knight, 1993).

Adolescent sex offenders tend to have histories of engaging in criminal and antisocial behaviors of a nonsexual nature and significantly more so than nonabused peers (Ryan, Miyoshi, Metzner, Krugman, & Fryer, 1996; Weinrott, 1996). Adolescent males with histories of sexually abusing children are significantly more likely to commit adult sexual offenses as well as more adult violent nonsexual offenses than a comparison group of violent males without histories of sexual offending (Rubinstein, Yeager, Goodstein, & Lewis, 1993). A comprehensive review of the literature highlighted the fact that the vast majority (up to 90%) of adolescent sex offenders have sexual abuse histories, with "very few having no abuse history if physical, sexual and emotional abuse are considered collectively" (Ryan, 1995, p. 6).

THE SIBLING OFFENDER

Relative to nonsibling sexual offenders, adolescent offenders of siblings are significantly more likely to be the oldest child or an only child (Pierce & Pierce, 1990). In comparison with adolescents who sexually offend against children other than siblings, adolescent perpetrators of siblings report significantly more distressing family dynamics, such as more physical punishment, more negative communication patterns within the family, greater marital discord, and less satisfaction with family relations. Further, adolescent sibling-incest perpetrators tend to have greater rates of sexual and physical abuse histories than nonsibling adolescent perpetrators and greater numbers of younger siblings within the home (see, e.g., O'Brien, 1991; Pierce & Pierce, 1990; Worling, 1995).

CHILD SEX OFFENDERS

If sexual abuse is conceptualized as sexual actions perpetrated against another without his or her consent, without a sense of equality, and/or with some form of coercion (National Task Force on Juvenile Sexual Offending, 1993), then children under the age of 12 can sexually abuse other children (Araji, 1997; Johnson, 1999). Although sexual aggression has been documented in children as young as 3, the mean age of onset appears to be between the ages of 6 and 9 (Araji, 1997). Whether a child's sexual aggression is identified as CSA perpetration or abuse reactivity remains unclear at this point in time.

When comparing adult and adolescent perpetrators in relation to the child, the greatest dyadic differences appear to be that of age and gender. The mean age difference between a juvenile sex offender and child is significantly less than the age difference between an adult perpetrator and child (Shaw, Lewis, Loeb, Rosado, & Rodriguez, 2000). More specifically, the average age difference between a juvenile perpetrator and child is three years and the average age difference between an adult perpetrator and child is 30 years. As for gender, among young juvenile perpetrators, prepubescent females outnumber males whereas among adult perpetrators, males outnumber females (Araji, 1997; Shaw et al., 2000). Child offenders and adolescent offenders are similar in terms of their personality characteristics, personal histories, family environment, family background, and histories of abuse and neglect (Araji, 1997; Pithers & Gray, 1998; Ray & English, 1995). With regard to sexual abuse dynamics, child, adolescent, and adult sex offenders are equally likely to use force and bribery to ensure compliance of the target child, to perpetrate similar types of sexual acts, and to use weapons to convey threats of injury or death (Shaw et al., 2000).

FEMALE PERPETRATORS

Females comprise a minority (an estimated 24%) of CSA perpetrators who offend against boys (Finkelhor & Russell, 1984). Female perpetrators are significantly more likely to offend against younger children than their male counterparts (Anderson, 1996; Finkelhor & Ormrod, 2001; Rudin, Zalewski, & Bodmer-Turner, 1995), and female perpetrators tend to be younger than male perpetrators, at least in terms of their age at state intervention (Allen, 1991; Faller, 1995; Finkelhor & Ormrod, 2001). Further, female perpetrators, relative to male perpetrators, do not evidence significant differences in terms of the number of children they abuse nor in terms of the proportions of incestual mother and father offenders they encompass (Faller, 1987). Female perpetrators tend to abuse equivalent numbers of boys and girls or to show a preference toward female children (Faller, 1987, 1995; Fehrenbach & Monastersky, 1988; Mayer, 1992; Rudin et al., 1995; Travin, Cullen, & Protter, 1990), whereas, on the contrary, male perpetrators are significantly more likely to abuse girls over boys, at a rate of two to one or more Finkelhor, Williams, & Burns, 1988; Finkelhor & Ormrod, 2000; Rudin ey al., 1995). These studies show that, of sexual abuse episodes perpetrated by females, a narrow majority (51%) to majority (67%) involve girls and a considerable minority (33%) to near majority (49%) involve boys. With regard to abuse dynamics, female perpetrators and male perpetrators alike subject children to comparable numbers of abusive sexual acts that include similar degrees of coercion, intrusion, and severity (Kelley, Brant, & Waterman, 1993; Snow & Sorenson, 1990).

Few studies, let alone comparative investigations, have been conducted on female perpetrators of CSA. Thus, only attributes, traits, and characteristics found among female perpetrators will be highlighted here. For example, female perpetrators of CSA show a trend toward evidencing (a) a history of CSA; (b) a history of abusing children within and outside the family; (c) a history of committing severe sexual abuse (e.g., episodes involving penetration, exploitation); (d) displays of aggression during the abusive episodes; (e) a pattern of perpetrating ritualistic sexual activities; (f) low self-esteem; (g) interrupted education; (h) a history of mental illness; (i) mental retardation; (j) a history of substance abuse; (k) early marriage and pregnancy; (l) conflictual relations with adult males; (m) a sexual history characterized by numerous sexual partners and sexual compulsivity; (n) intimate relationships exemplifying isolation and separation; and (o) a history of using children as "substitute" partners and confidants (see, e.g., Allen, 1991; Faller, 1995; Johnson, 1989; Matthews, Matthews, & Speltz, 1991; McCarty, 1986; Rowan, Rowan, & Langelier, 1990; Travin, Cullen, & Protter, 1990; Wolfe, 1985).

ALONE OR IN TANDEM

Although the vast majority of perpetrators act alone (Brown & Anderson, 1991), dyadic perpetration is not unusual (Woods & Dean, 1985), as evidenced by the knowledge base frequency range of 7% to 26% (Elliott, Browne, & Kilcoyne, 1995; Gale, Thompson, Moran, & Sack, 1988; Gellert et al., 1993; Gully, Hansen, Britton, Langley, & McBride, 2000; Huston, Parra, Prihoda, & Foulds, 1995; Kelly, Wood, Gonzalez, MacDonald, & Waterman, 2002). Gang perpetration is reported at levels varying from 4% to 22% (Gold et al., 1997; Kellogg & Hoffman, 1995, 1997; Richardson, Meredith, & Abbot, 1993). In contrast to male perpetrators, female perpetrators are significantly more likely to have a co-offender (Allen, 1991; Faller, 1995; Fehrenbach & Monastersky, 1988; Finkelhor et al., 1988; Saradjian, 1996).

PERPETRATOR/BOY RELATIONSHIP

The vast majority of perpetrators (up to 100% in many studies) are known to the child (Cupoli & Sewell, 1988; Doll et al., 1992; Hutchings & Dutton, 1993; Kisiel & Lyons, 2001; Mian et al., 1986; Nutall & Jackson, 1994) but are outside of the immediate nuclear family or unrelated (Dimock, 1988; Levesque, 1994; Lodico, Gruber, & DiClemente, 1996; McLeer et al., 1998; Ratner et al., in press; Robin et al., 1997; Sigmon, Greene, Rohan, & Nichols, 1996; Spencer & Dunklee, 1986; Wolfe, Sas, & Wekerle, 1994; Wells et al., 1997; Woods & Dean, 1985). Among adults imprisoned by their state for rape or sexual assault, a considerable minority (33%) perpetrated against their own children (U.S. Department of Justice, 1997b).

In general, a greater proportion of male children are abused by perpetrators outside the family whereas a greater proportion of female children are abused by perpetrators within the nuclear family (Finkelhor et al., 1990; Gold, Elhai, Lucenko, Swingle, & Hughes, 1998; Gordon, 1990; Thomlinson, Stephens, Cunes, & Grinnell, 1991), although a majority (63%) of boys are abused by family members as well (Faller, 1989). Among younger boys, parents tend to represent the most common perpetrator group (Bradley & Wood, 1991; Feiring et al., 1999; Gellert et al., 1993; Kelly et al., 2002; Spencer & Dunklee, 1986) followed by other immediate family members. In some studies, this order is reversed but by only a few percentage points. Collectively, the largest category of perpetrators of boys older than 12 comprise known nonrelatives. Following nonrelatives, as a perpetrator category, typically are parents, including both mother and father figures, other relatives, siblings, and strangers (Feiring et al., 1999; Huston et al., 1995; Levesque, 1994; Mendel, 1995; Olson, 1990; Richardson et al., 1993; Sigmon et al., 1996; Wolfe et al., 1994). In studies of female perpetrators, mothers, baby-sitters, other relatives, and teachers, all in caretaking positions, commonly constitute the most prevalent relational roles vis-à-vis the boy (Faller, 1987, 1995; Mathews, Mathews, & Speltz, 1991; Saradjian, 1996).

It is not uncommon for unrelated perpetrators to hold formal and, at times, professional roles with respect to the boys (Burgess, Hartman, McCausland, & Powers, 1984; Faller, 1989; Gold et al., 1997; Roane, 1992), for example, group or organizational leaders such as Scout masters, youth ministers, and Little League coaches, and school employees, such as teachers, principals, coaches, and bus drivers. Informal roles include friends of the family, neighbors, sexual partners of caretakers, and others who attempt to befriend the family.

STRANGERS

Few perpetrators of CSA are true strangers to the sexually abused boy. Although several studies have documented the prevalence of stranger perpetration at 0% (e.g., Gale, Thompson, Moran, & Sack, 1988; Mian et al., 1986; Robin et al., 1997; Sigmon, Greene, Rohan, & Nichols, 1996; Wells et al., 1997), the preponderance of investigators and research teams report a stranger cohort of approximately 10% or less (Doll et al., 1992; Feiring et al., 1999; Fondacaro, Holt, & Powell, 1999; Huston, Parra, Prihoda, & Foulds, 1995; Huston, Prihoda, Parra, & Foulds, 1997; Levesque, 1994; Lisak & Luster, 1994; McLeer et al., 1998; Wolfe et al., 1994) with others noting rates of less than 5% (Conte & Schuerman, 1987; Deblinger, McLeer, Atkins, Ralphe, & Foa, 1989; Holmes, 1997; Kisiel & Lyons, 2001; Reinhart, 1987; Woods & Dean, 1985). Still, a few investigators document higher frequencies of stranger perpetration, ranging from 40% to 50% (DeJong, Hervada, & Emmett, 1983; Finkelhor et al., 1990; Little & Hamby, 2001).

SELECTION CRITERIA

Perpetrators characteristically hold a preference for the gender of their target child; a narrow majority (58%) target girls, a limited minority (14%) target boys, and a minority (28%) target both boys and girls. In terms of perpetrators' preferences for age or developmental stage, the mean age of boys at the onset of abuse is 8.5 years whereas the mean age of boys at abuse cessation is 13. Although the vast majority (85%) of perpetrators offend against one child at a time, a limited minority (15%) abuse several children at the same time (Elliott, Browne, & Kilcoyne, 1995), individually and in small groups.

Perpetrators target children who appear to possess the following qualities or characteristics: sensitivity, insecurity, low-self esteem, quietness, passivity, curiosity, and blind trust. They also tend to seek boys who appear to be vulnerable, who appear to be experiencing problems within the family, who appear to lack secondary sex characteristics, or who they perceive to have qualities typically allotted to females (see, e.g., Budin & Johnson, 1989; Conte, Wolfe, & Smith, 1989; Elliott et al., 1995; Harry, 1989, in Doll et al., 1992).

PERPETRATOR SELECTION STRATEGIES

Perpetrators gain access to children through the neighborhood, the family, or work (Burgess et al., 1987). Common selection strategies include playing games with boys, teaching them the skills required to play various sports, and teaching them how to play a musical instrument. Some perpetrators use affection, understanding, and love as subjection strategies while others focus on establishing rapport with a boy's family members and, ultimately, securing greater access to and control of the boy (Budin & Johnson, 1989; Conte et al., 1989). They may also invite children for outings or offer them rides to and from home. A near majority (48%) of perpetrators locate and isolate children by gaining supervision of them through roles such as babysitter, coach, minister, and teacher (Elliott et al., 1995).

To establish first sexual contact, the abusers employ coercion and persuasion, discussion of sexual matters, "accidental" touching or rubbing, and the use of bribery and gifts (Elliott et al., 1995). Other predispositional strategies involve introducing the boy to pornography, drugs, and alcohol (Burgess et al., 1987). At times, perpetrators coerce or threaten current and older abused boys to recruit other children (Burgess et al., 1987; Elliott et al., 1995). For example, perpetrators instruct older siblings to use threats and acts of violence against younger boys (Burgess et al., 1987). To further entice the new "recruits," bribes and gifts are frequently utilized (Elliott et al., 1995).

The vast majority (85%) of perpetrators state that once a particular strategy appears to achieve the intended goal, they are apt to use the same methods every time (Elliott et al., 1995). A narrow majority (56%) also report that they are unaware as to what initially prompts their use of specific strategies, although a limited minority (14%) suggest that pornographic materials, television programs, films, and various media hold influential roles.

RITUAL ABUSE

This is, perhaps, one of the most controversial areas of CSA research. As a form of sexual abuse, it is most often associated with groups, organizations, or institutions, such as underground perpetrator networks, child sex rings, day care centers, and churches. Ritual abuse may be broadly defined as "abuse that occurs in the context linked to some symbols or group activities that have a religious, magical or supernatural connotation, and where the invocation of these symbols or activities are repeated over time and used to frighten and intimidate the children" (Finkelhor, Williams, Burns, & Kalinowski, 1988, p. 59). It is important to note that "ritual," under these circumstances, does not necessarily imply satanism, although satanic worship and indoctrination may be dynamics of this form of CSA.

Ritual abuse may encompass group sex, circle sex (wherein the child in the middle of the circle is perpetrated by the adults in the inner circle while those in the outer circle watch and encourage), sadomasochistic transactions, and the generation and dissemination of pornography. In some factions, activities may include ritualized killings of animals and other children, the mandatory intake of blood, urine, feces, drugs, and alcohol, forced sex between children and animals, torture chambers, confinement, and coerced child-on-child sexual encounters. Ritualistic abuse often involves brainwashing strategies as well (see, e.g., Saradjian, 1996; Snow & Sorenson, 1990; Waterman, Kelly, Oliveri, & McCord, 1993; Weir & Wheatcroft, 1995).

One study reported that a limited minority (15%) of female perpetrators were involved in ritual abuse at various day care centers and that a limited minority (6%) participated in this form of CSA in church settings (Faller, 1995). Another study noted ritual abuse across a limited minority (13%) of CSA cases in day care settings, all with female perpetrators (Finkelhor, Williams, & Burns, 1988).

THE ROLE OF THE INTERNET

Perpetrators who use the Internet as a subjection modality are in an unparalleled position to devise and reveal self-representations that might otherwise remain dormant or inoperative (Quayle & Taylor, 2001). Further, the relative anonymity proffered by the Internet supports perpetrators in their expression of illegal, immoral, and disinhibited sexual behavior. According to a recent national survey conducted by Finkelhor, Mitchell, and Wolak (2001) and the U.S. Department of Justice, children and adolescents are routinely subjected to sexual harassment, sexual solicitation, and pornography on the Internet. Within a 1-year period, 1 in 5 youth received a solicitation for sex, including requests from adults to reveal personal sexual information, to engage in sexual talk, and to participate in sexual activities. A minority (25%) of children or adolescents were exposed to digital photographs of naked people and/or people performing sexual acts. One in 33 youths was subjected to an aggressive solicitation. A minority (25%) of aggressive episodes were incited by females. Perpetrator strategies included asking a child or adolescent to meet, calling him or her on the telephone, and sending him or her letters, money, or gifts by way of the U.S. Postal Service. One in 17 children or adolescents were sexually threatened or harassed during the past year. Sexual harassment was indicated by an offender's threats of physical harm and his or her posting of defamatory remarks about or embarrassing information related to, the child. Internet users, including other perpetrators, can easily access, view, and transmit these defamatory postings.

LOCATION OF ABUSE

The child's home and/or the perpetrator's home are the most likely places in which the sexual abuse of children occurs. Together, they account for the vast majority (85%) of common locales, whereas public places and commercial sites represent narrow minorities (8% and 3%, respectively) (U.S. Department of Justice, 1997). In general, the abuse occurs in the perpetrator's home (61%) or in the child's home (49%) (Elliott et al., 1995) or in both homes (76.7%) (Dubé & Hebert, 1988). The preponderance of extrafamilial abusive episodes take place during the day and the plurality of intrafamilial abusive episodes ensue after dark. Both types of CSA occur in locations customarily perceived as safe for and by the boy (DeJong, Hervada, & Emmett, 1983). Abuse by relatives occurs disproportionately in the boy's home or in the perpetrator's home whereas abuse by known nonrelatives and strangers takes place more frequently outside the home (Dubé & Hebert, 1988; Gordon, 1990).

More specifically, the vast majority (89%) of infant, toddler, and preschooler abuse occurs in a family setting (Gellert et al., 1993). School-aged boys are more likely to be abused in the perpetrator's home or in a community setting (Gold et al., 1997; Gordon, 1990; Levesque, 1994). A substantial amount of abuse, particularly among boys, occurs in public places where boys would be expected to go, such as shopping malls, video arcades, playgrounds, amusement parks, swimming pools, carnivals, public parks, camp sites, beaches, and restrooms (Elliott et al., 1995).

PERPETRATOR GENDER

Although the percentage of male perpetrators typically exceeds that of female perpetrators, and in many cases by a wide margin (Bartholow et al., 1994; Doll et al., 1992; Hunter, 1991; Reinhart, 1987; Roesler & McKenzie, 1994; Sansonnet-Hayden et al., 1987), across a number of studies females account for substantial percentages of the perpetrator population under investigation—20% (American Humane Association, 1993; Kelly et al., 2002), 25% (Dimock, 1988; Finkelhor & Russell, 1984), 27% (Gray, Pithers, Busconi, & Houchens, 1999; Romano & De Luca, 1996), 29% (Violato & Genuis, 1993), 35% (Spiegel, 1995; Urquiza & Crowley, 1986), 37% (Ramsey-Klawsnik, 1990), 42% (Lisak, 1994a), 44% (Johnson & Shrier, 1987), 51% (Duncan & Williams, 1998), 58% (Lisak & Luster, 1994), 60% (Mendel, 1995), 61.5% (Olson, 1990), 72% (Fromuth & Burkhart, 1987), and 75% (Woods & Dean, 1985)—making it more heterogeneous than previously assumed. A limited minority (19%) of boys experience abuse by lone male and lone female perpetrators (Duncan & Williams, 1998). Researchers commonly assert that female perpetration remains substantially underrecognized, underreported, and consequently underestimated (Elliott,1994; Jennings, 1993; Mendel, 1995; Rudin, Zalewski, & Bodmer-Turner, 1995; Saradjian, 1996). Compounding the issue is the fact that definitions of perpetration and sexual abuse vary across studies just as information technologies and reporting procedures vary across the 50 states.

PERPETRATOR SEXUAL ORIENTATION

The vast majority (approximately 98% across studies) of perpetrators of boys appear to be heterosexual (Groth & Birnbaum, 1978; Groth & Gary, 1982; Jenny, Roesler, & Payer, 1994; Spencer, Dunklee, & Stevenson, 2000). In one study, only 4% of male perpetrators were known homosexuals (Spencer & Dunklee, 1986). In another study, a substantial majority (74%) of boys were abused by a male who was, or had been, involved in a heterosexual relationship with a boy's mother, foster mother, grandmother, or other female relative. A boy's risk of being sexually abused by a relative's heterosexual partner is over 100 times greater than someone who could be identified as having a homosexual, lesbian, or bisexual orientation (Jenny, Roesler, & Poyer, 1994).

PREVALENCE

Incidence, in this context, refers to the number of sexual abuse cases reported during a circumscribed time period; prevalence corresponds to the number or percentage of individuals within a circumscribed population who have been subjected to sexual abuse. While prevalence rate, as well as any other variable, is subject to and materially impacted by a study's conceptual, definitional, and methodological processes, the greater portion of empirical investigations, including those employing national and regional random samples, university samples, clinical samples, race-specific samples, hospital samples, and abuse registry samples render rates within an approximate range of 15% to 25% (Allard-Dansereau et al., 1997; Bagley et al., 1994; Briere, Smiljanich, & Henschel, 1994; Debruyn, Lujan, & May, 1992; DiIorio, Hartwell, & Hansen, 2002; Dubé & Hebert, 1988; Ellason, Ross, Sainton, & Mayran, 1996; Faller & Henry, 2000; Feldman-Summers & Pope, 1994; Finkelhor, 1994; Finkelhor et al., 1990; Glover, Janikowski, & Benshoff, 1995; Gordon, 1990; Huston, et al., 1995; Huston et al., 1997; Jenny et al., 1994; Holmes, 1997; Hutchings & Dutton, 1993; Kellogg & Hoffman, 1995, 1997; Leverich et al., 2002; Melchert & Parker, 1997; Neisen & Sandall, 1990; Paul et al., 2001; Ratner et al., in press; Rew, Esparza, & Sands, 1991; Robin et al., 1997; Rosetti, 1995; Rohsenow, Corbett, & Devine, 1988; Ryan et al. & Hoyt, 2000; Simpson & Miller, 2002; Tyler et al., 2001; U.S. Department of Justice, 1997b; Violato et al., 1993; Zierler et al., 1991). A few studies report rates as low as 6% to 12% (Cupoli & Sewell, 1988; Deykin, Buka, & Zeena, 1992; Dunn, Ryan, Paolo, & Van Fleet, 1995; Grice, Brady, Dustan, Malcom, & Kilpatrick, 1995; Gutierres, Russo, & Urbanski, 1994; Harrison, Hoffman, & Edwall, 1989; Priest, 1992; Simpson, Westerberg, Little, & Trujillo, 1994; Wallen & Berman, 1992; Windle, Windle, Scheidt, & Miller, 1995) and as high as 37% (Bagley, 1988; Bartholow et al., 1994; Blood & Cornwall, 1996; Clark, Lesnick, & Hegedus, 1997; Convoy, Weiss, & Zverina, 1995; Doll et al., 1992). However, a stable summary statistic for the sexual abuse of males has yet to emerge, due in large part to the variability in definitions, sample pools, sampling procedures, and items of inquiry across studies. To date, the most commonly cited prevalence rate is 16% (see, e.g., Finkelhor et al., 1990; Simpson & Miller, 2002). Based on a review of nine studies, Finkelhor (1994) concluded that 10% represents a conservative estimate of males subjected to CSA. Calculations among these and other studies suggest that males comprise 25% to 35% of individuals with histories of CSA (Holmes et al., 1997).

In general, statistics reflect reported cases of CSA. Nationally, it is estimated that reported cases account for approximately 20% of the projected incidence of sexual abuse in the United States today (Okamura, Heras, & Wong-Kernberg, 1995; Tzeng & Schwarzin, 1990). For example, the 1993 National Incidence Study revealed that 300,200 children in the United States met the criteria for CSA, rendering a rate of 45 cases per 10,000 children (Sedlak & Broadhurst, 1996). Although the 1993 rate is approximately 100% greater than the 1986 rate, it is much lower than the rates reported by way of the national, local, random, and convenience samples just highlighted.

AGE AT ONSET OF ABUSE

Among boys, the mean age at the onset of abuse is usually between 8 and 11 years (Briere, Evans, Runtz, & Wall, 1988; DeJong, Emmett, & Hervada, 1982; Doll et al., 1992; Finkelhor et al., 1990; Fondacaro et al., 1999; Holmes, 1997; Hunter, 1991; Lisak, 1994a; Mraovich & Wilson, 1999; Nutall & Jackson, 1994; Pierce & Pierce, 1985; Risin & Koss, 1987; Robin et al., 1997; Ryan et al., 2000; Sarwer, Crawford, & Durlak, 1997; Spiegel, 1995; Stein et al., 1988; Young, Bergandi, & Titus, 1994), prior to the physical manifestation of puberty and the development of secondary sex characteristics (Johnson & Shrier, 1987; Sansonnet-Hayden, et al., 1987). While this is the mean age range, a minority (a mean of 28% across studies) of boys are abused between the ages of 0 and 7 (Cupoli & Sewell, 1988; Fontanella et al., 2000; Gold, Elhai, Lucenko, & Swingle, 1998; Gray et al., 1999; Kelly et al., 2002; Mendel, 1995; Richardson et al., 1993; Roesler & McKenzie, 1994; Sigmon et al., 1996), and often when they are preverbal (Huston et al., 1995).

Boys abused by intrafamilial perpetrators tend to be substantially younger than boys abused by nonfamily perpetrators. On average, 7 is the age of onset for boys abused within the family whereas 10 is the age of onset for boys abused outside the family (DeJong et al., 1983; Fischer & McDonald, 1998; Mian et al., 1986). Although it remains unclear whether boys tend to be younger than girls when first abused, a greater proportion of males are represented in younger age categories across a number of studies (Cupoli & Sewell, 1988; Fischer & McDonald, 1998; Pierce & Pierce, 1985; Thomlinson et al., 1991). In general, sexual abuse increases, just as neglect decreases, as a function of the child's chronological age (Mraovich & Wilson, 1999; National Center on Child Abuse and Neglect, 1998).

AGE AT EVALUATION

If a boy is evaluated, it will most likely occur between the ages of 6 and 8 (Jenny et al., 1994; Roane, 1992). However, as with age of onset, frequency, duration, and a number of other variables, there is considerable variability as evidenced by relatively large standard deviations.

AGE ABUSE TERMINATES

On average, a boy's abuse experience ends between the ages of 12 and 13 (Briere, Evans, Runtz, & Wall, 1988; Gold et al., 1997; Kendall-Tackett & Simon, 1992; Ryan et al., 2000; Sigmon et al., 1996). However, among boys abused by perpetrators with a sexual orientation toward postpubescent males, the abuse may not commence until the male's secondary sex characteristics have emerged.

PERPETRATOR AGE

The majority of perpetrators are adults (Doll et al., 1992; Gale et al., 1988; Ray, 1996; Spencer & Dunklee, 1986), often ranging between the ages of 20 and 60 (Fondacaro et al., 1999; Fontanella et al., 2000; Gray et al., 1999), with a mean age interval of 26 to 31 (Hibbard & Hartman, 1992; Johnson & Shrier, 1987; Tjaden & Thoennes, 1992). Even so, a limited to considerable minority (10%–40%) of perpetrators are adolescents under the age of 20 (DeJong et al., 1983; Gray, Busconi, Houchens, & Pithers, 1997; Gray & Pithers, 1993; Mathews, 1994; McLeer et al., 1998), and boys are more likely than girls to have an older adolescent perpetrator (Finkelhor et al., 1990; Hunter, 1991). For example, of sexual assaults reported to state agencies, a considerable minority (43%) of offenses against children 6 and under, a minority of offenses against children ages 7 through 11, and a minority of offenses against adolescents between the ages of 12 and 17 are perpetrated by juvenile sex offenders (U.S. Department of Justice, 2000). Still, children under the age of 13 comprise a limited minority (18%–20%) of sexual abuse offenders (Gray & Pithers, 1993; Gray et al., 1999). Among youth under the age of 15, the rates of arrest for forcible rape increased 190% between the years 1980 and 1995.

AGE DIFFERENCE

By and large, male and female perpetrators are significantly older than the boys they abuse (Finkelhor et al., 1990), with some studies indicating a mean age difference of at least 11 to 20 years (Fondacaro et al., 1999; Gordon, 1990; Gray et al., 1999; Lisak & Luster, 1994; Paul et al., 2001). The age difference is significantly higher for boys under the age of 6 and over the age of 15 (Doll et al., 1992). Incest tends to be intergenerational, in that when boys are abused by a relative, the relative tends to be closer to them in age (Gordon, 1990).

COABUSE

Boys are likely to be one of several children being abused by one sexual offender (Farber, Showers, Johnson, Joseph, & Oshins, 1984; Levesque, 1994). They are 15 times more likely than nonabused males to have a family member who was abused as well (Holmes & Slap, 1998). A considerable minority (40%) of perpetrators abusing male children are also abusing at least one other child in the family (Pierce & Pierce, 1985). If a boy is abused within the home, another abused child resides in the same home a majority (60%) of the time (Finkelhor, 1994). A documented history of a female sibling's abuse often leads to the discovery of her brother's abuse by the same perpetrator (Spencer & Dunklee, 1986). One study found that, in regard to fathers, a substantial majority (approximately 80%) of biological fathers and a majority (approximately 66%) of noncustodial fathers sexually abused more than one child within the same family. In fact, a narrow majority (approximately 53%) of biological fathers as well as stepfathers abused all children in their household (Faller, 1990).

FREQUENCY

Few studies report on abuse frequency, but rather on abuse duration and/or multiple episodes of abuse. Of the relatively few investigative teams that have disseminated reports highlighting abuse frequency, it appears that the substantial majority (approximately 70% across studies) of abusive acts are not isolated incidents (Briere et al., 1983; Feiring et al., 1999; Hutchings & Dutton, 1993; Johnson & Shrier, 1987; Lisak & Luster, 1994). A near majority to narrow majority (49%–61%) of sexually abused males experience abuse on a weekly basis, while approximately one-sixth to one-fourth confront daily abuse (Gold, et al., 1997; Kisiel & Lyons, 2001; Woods & Dean, 1985).

DURATION

The sexually abusive relationship often lasts from 1 to 3 or more years (Nutall & Jackson, 1994). The mean duration of these relationships generally extends from 2.5 to 4 years (Briere et al., 1994; Gold et al., 1998; Kelly et al., 2002;

Kendall-Tackett & Simon, 1992), with a typical range extending from one episode to 7 or more years (Briere et al., 1994; Gellert et al., 1993; Gold et al., 1997; Spencer & Dunklee, 1986). On average, abuse occurring within the family tends to last longer than abuse perpetrated by a nonfamily member, given the sustaining conditions of access, relational proximity between the perpetrator and child, and family injunctions against disclosure even after the abuse has been witnessed (DeJong et al., 1983; Fischer & McDonald, 1998; Gomes-Schwartz, Horowitz, & Cardarelli, 1990; Mian et al., 1986).

MULTIPLE EPISODES

Multiple episodes of abuse by the same perpetrator are the norm. A narrow majority to vast majority (54%–94%) of boys are subjected to 5 to 20 episodes of CSA (Allard-Dansereau et al., 1997; Doll et al., 1992; Gale et al., 1988; Feiring et al., 1999; Gellert et al., 1993; Gully et al., 2000; Hibbard & Hartman, 1992; Hutchings & Dutton, 1993; Kellogg & Hoffman, 1995; Levesque, 1994; Little & Hamby, 1997; Lisak, 1994a; Lisak & Luster, 1994; Spencer & Dunklee, 1986; Wolfe et al., 1994; Woods & Dean, 1985), and a minority (15% to 25%) experience more than 20 episodes of CSA (Kellogg & Hoffman, 1995; Wolfe et al., 1994). In a recent study, the mean number of abuse incidents among males was 53.75 (Kelly et al., 2002).

OTHER FORMS OF CONCURRENT OR HISTORIC CHILD ABUSE

Physical abuse and neglect are strong correlates of chronic childhood sexual abuse (McClellan et al., 1995). More specifically, those subjected to childhood sexual abuse are much more likely to experience physical abuse (Nutall & Jackson, 1994) as well as emotional abuse (Melchert & Parker, 1997), psychological abuse (Sigmon et al., 1996), and neglect (Ray & English, 1995). One-fifth of males with histories of CSA experience three forms of abuse, for example, sexual, physical, and emotional (Melchert & Parker, 1997). In a study of intergenerational abuse, a narrow majority (53%) of children were subjected to a minimum of three forms of maltreatment during their lives (De Bellis et al., 2001).

The proportion of males with histories of CSA who also experience physical abuse, historically or concurrently, ranges from 21% to 72% (Gale et al., 1988; Garnefski & Diekstra, 1997; Kelly et al., 2002; Kolko, Moser, & Weldy, 1988; Leverich et al., 2002; Lisak, 1994; MacMillan et al., 2001; Mendel, 1995; Sigmon, Greene, Rohan, & Nichols, 1996). In fact, children and youth confronting CSA are 11 times more likely to experience physical abuse than nonabused peers (Hibbard et al., 1990). Further, males are more likely to be physically abused by their sexual abuse perpetrator than females (Gold et al., 1997; Sansonnet-Hayden et al., 1987) and more likely to be physically abused by someone other than their sexual abuse perpetrator than females (Gold et al., 1998). Among mothers and fathers who sexually abuse and physically abuse their male children, the most common physically abusive behaviors reported include slapping, pulling hair, hitting with objects, throwing objects at the boy, hitting with the back of the hand across the face, kicking, punching, and hitting with a belt or whip (Mendel, 1995).

EXPOSURE TO PORNOGRAPHY

Adult pornography is employed to teach children about, and induce them into, sexual activity (Burgess et al., 1984; Roane, 1992). Boys are more likely than girls to be exposed to pornography (Levesque, 1994). Exposure to heterosexual and homosexual forms of pornography are equally common (Roane, 1992). At times, boys are used as pornographic objects (Gold et al., 1997; Woods & Dean, 1985). For example, in a study of underground pederasty sex rings, male children were coerced into becoming objects of pornography, and offending adults used the generated materials for personal stimulation and trade; sometimes these materials were sold commercially, with the child receiving, from the adult, some of the derived income (Burgess et al., 1984).

BRIBES

In many instances, children are rewarded for the abuse and its concealment (Conte & Schuerman, 1987). A common abuse dynamic involves seduction and coercion in the form of money or gifts offered by the perpetrator. Other forms of bribery include withdrawal of allurements, such as special privileges, attention, affection, and care, as well as the withdrawal of tangible items, particularly those employed to entice the boy, including toys, pets and outings to special events (see, e.g., Dubé & Hebert, 1988; Gold et al., 1997; Pipe & Goodman, 1991; Saradjian, 1996) . A narrow majority (58%) of runaway adolescent males with histories of CSA are offered money to have sex with an adult (Janus et al., 1987).

COERCION

Given the needs of perpetrators to secure cooperation and ensure concealment, it follows that virtually all sexually abused boys experience some form of coercion (Berliner & Conte, 1990). The vast majority (96%) of perpetrators coerce in a stepwise manner, carefully and subtly testing a boy's reaction to increasing levels of sexualized talk, sexual materials, and sexual touching (Elliott et al., 1995).

Emotional coercion is another predominant strategy. Emotional coercion frequently and ordinarily involves subjecting the child to labels such as "fag," "queer boy," "whore," and "sissy." The perpetrator manipulates the boy into believing that he will be judged harshly if anyone were to find out, employing injunctions such as "If you tell, people will think you're a slut" and "If anyone finds out, you'll be scum for life." Emotional coercion may also take the form of the perpetrator convincing the boy to conceal the abuse in order to emotionally protect the parent(s) from learning of their son's activities (Berliner & Conte, 1990; Kaufman, Hilliker, & Daleiden, 1996; Kelley et al., 1993; Spiegel, 1997).

Types of coercion apart from strategies requiring a perpetrator's physical force include plea bargaining, bribery, trickery and game playing in addition to the use of a perpetrator's status or authority to engender the child's compliance (Pipe & Goodman, 1991; Wolfe et al., 1994). Female perpetrators tend to use persuasion tactics over threats or force (Johnson & Shrier, 1987; Wolfe, 1985). Thus, coercion can be expressed verbally and physically (Dubé & Hebert, 1988), each with emotional undertones and implications. The anticipated and, quite often, rendered outcome of a perpetrator's coercive strategies is the illusion that the boy is, in essence, consenting, thereby rendering the perpetrator less responsible for his or her own actions (Berliner & Conte, 1990).

THREATS

Threats and intimidation are the means by which perpetrators initiate and maintain the sexually abusive relationship and the concealment surrounding it (Berliner & Conte, 1990). Quite commonly, something or someone important to the child is threatened (Gully et al., 2000; Kelley et al., 1993; Pipe et al., 1991). For example, threats often involve actual physical harm to the boy, threats against the lives of his parents and grandparents (i.e., if the sexual abuse is disclosed), threats of abandonment or rejection (e.g., mother will leave, family will separate, father will be angry), and consequences to the perpetrator (e.g., he or she will get into trouble with the law, will commit suicide) (Berliner & Conte, 1990; Furniss, 1991; Kaufman et al., 1996; Kiser et al., 1988; Pipe & Goodman, 1991; Robin et al., 1997; Roesler & McKenzie, 1994). Homicidal threats appear to escalate with the age of the boy (Roane, 1992). In essence, threats and persuasion often bypass the need to say anything about the abuse itself (Berliner & Conte, 1990), only the consequences of its disclosure.

FORCE

Threats and acts of violence are common perpetrator strategies (Friedrich et al., 1988) used to commence and conceal the sexually abusive relationship. Actual force is more routinely brought to bear against males than females (Pierce & Pierce, 1985) and is executed in 15% to 50% of the cases (Briere et al., 1994; Doll et al., 1992; Feiring, Taska, & Lewis, 1999; Finkelhor et al., 1990; Levesque, 1994; Paul et al., 2001; Sarwer et al., 1997) with the rate reaching majority proportions (e.g., 51% to 65%) in a number of studies (DeJong et al.,

1982; Finkelhor, 1981; Gully et al., 2000; Gold et al., 1997; Ratner et al., in press; Roesler & McKenzie, 1994; Wolfe et al., 1994). Physical coercion tends to be a more routine strategy of unrelated perpetrators than those within the boy's family and, consequently, force engenders more physical injury for boys abused by nonfamily members (Dubé & Hebert, 1988; Fischer & McDonald, 1998).

If and when a boy resists or expresses fear, a considerable minority (39%) of perpetrators are prepared to use violent force or weapons to silence the child and control his anxiety (Elliott et al., 1995; Paul et al., 2001). Knives and handguns are the two most common weapons employed by adults who rape and sexually assault children (U.S. Department of Justice, 1997). Frequent physical beatings are employed to intimidate the boy, render him vulnerable, and ensure his concealment of the sexually abusive relationship (Robin et al., 1997). In one study, 8% of the perpetrators murdered or attempted to murder a male child during or after an abusive episode (Elliott et al., 1995). Between the years 1976 and 1994, sexual assault murders accounted for 1.5% or 4,807 of all murders across the United States within that time period. With the exception of adults aged 60 or older, children 12 and younger and adolescents between the ages of 13 and 17 account for the highest percentages of individuals murdered during sexual assault, with males comprising a limited minority (18%) of the total (U.S. Department of Justice, 1997).

PERPETRATOR RATIONALES

Perpetrators customarily rationalize the abuse with the intention of minimizing their responsibility and maximizing the boy's consent and benefit. Consequently, CSA is often reframed as sex education, developmental preparation for sex, a common yet private family activity, and/or as an expression of love (Berliner & Conte, 1990; Elliott et al., 1995). A perpetrator's general distortions regarding sex between adults and children, for example, "A child who doesn't physically resist an adult's sexual advances really wants to have sex with that adult," correlates with his or her inability to recognize, let alone empathize with, a child's distress upon subjection to CSA and the harm generated by the sexually abusive relationship (Marshall, Hamilton, & Fernandez, 2001).

PERPETRATOR DRUG AND ALCOHOL ABUSE USE AND ABUSE

A minority (22%) of perpetrators drink alcohol and/or use drugs subsequent to and during sexually abusive episodes (Elliott et al., 1995). There is a high incidence (37%) of perpetrator alcohol and/or drug abuse throughout the sexually abusive relationship (Mendel, 1995). In general, a substantial majority (74%) of perpetrators have chemical dependency histories and a narrow majority (56%) experience moderate to severe levels of alcohol abuse (Abracen, Looman, & Anderson, 2000; Cavaiola & Schiff, 1988).

SEXUALLY ABUSIVE ACTS

Childhood sexual abuse typically follows a gradual progression from noncontact behaviors to contact behaviors (Sgroi, Blick, & Porter, 1982; Berliner & Conte, 1990). Once the behaviors or activities advance to the sexual abuse stage, boys, in great measure, experience three or more types of sexual acts (Conte & Schuerman, 1987; Pierce & Pierce, 1985), the three most common being anal penetration of the boy, fellatio of the boy, and fellatio of the perpetrator (Richardson et al., 1993; Roane, 1992; Sarwer et al., 1997; Sigmon et al., 1996). These sexual behaviors are often conceptualized by investigators as the most serious forms of abuse (see, e.g., Dubé & Hebert, 1988; Lisak & Luster, 1994; Mendel, 1995).

Among boys, penetrating sexual acts are more common than nonpenetrating acts irrespective of perpetrator gender (Allard-Dansereau et al., 1997; Etherington, 1997; Feiring et al., 1999; Kellogg et al., 1995; McLeer et al., 1998; Paul et al., 2001). Boys tend to confront more serious sexual abuse than girls and are up to 2.5 times more likely to be subjected to actual or attempted intercourse (Dubé & Hebert, 1988; Huston et al., 1997; Levesque, 1994), whereas girls are more likely to experience fondling and exhibitionism (Dubé & Hebert, 1988; Gordon, 1990). Boys also experience more anal penetration with objects than females (Gold et al., 1997) and more anal penetration with a penis than females (Kendall-Tackett, 1992; Robin, 1997). In fact, the mean act and/or modal act experienced by boys is coercive receptive rectal intercourse (Briere, 1994; Cupoli & Sewell, 1988; DeJong, 1983; Doll et al., 1992; Elliott, 1995; Gellert et al., 1993; Gold et al., 1998; Gully et al., 2000; Holmes, 1997; Hunter, 1991; Huston et al., 1995; Hutchings et al., 1993; Kellogg & Hoffman, 1995; Kelly et al., 2002; Kisiel & Lyons, 2001; Roane, 1992; Robin et al., 1997; Roesler & McKenzie, 1994; Sigmon et al., 1996; Spencer & Dunklee, 1986; Spiegel, 1997a, 1997b; Wells et al., 1997; Woods & Dean, 1985). A limited minority (15%) report rectal bleeding at the time of the abuse (Wells et al., 1997).

The likelihood of genital (or genital versus digital) penetration increases with age (Allard-Dansereau et al., 1997; Gomes-Schwartz, Horowitz & Sauzier, 1985; Huston et al., 1997; U.S. Department of Justice, 1996). For boys 8 and above, anal intercourse is the most prevalent form of sexual abuse. For boys younger than 8, anal contact and anal penetration with an object occur more often than penile penetration (Reinhart, 1987). A near to substantial majority (48%–80%) of boys, regardless of age, experience oral intercourse (Friedrich & Leucke, 1988; Gold et al., 1998; Hunter, 1991; Kendall-Tackett & Simon, 1992; Paul et al., 2001; Sigmon et al., 1996; Woods & Dean, 1985). Children abused by strangers experience much higher rates of penetration (Huston et al., 1995; Huston et al., 1997).

A substantial majority (78%) of boys are coerced into performing sexual acts on the perpetrator (Gold et al., 1997; Moisan, Sanders-Philips, & Moisan, 1997), including vaginal penetration (Kelly et al., 2002; Lisak & Luster, 1994; Mendel, 1995; Paul et al., 2001; Richardson et al., 1993; Sigmon et al., 1996). In fact, vaginal intercourse is the modal abusive act involving boys and their female perpetrators (Duncan & Williams, 1998; Lisak & Luster, 1994; Mendel, 1995). Coerced fellatio upon the perpetrator is higher for boys than girls (Huston et al., 1997).

In terms of sexually abusive acts, a preponderance of boys have to perform oral sex on their perpetrator, fondle him or her, masturbate him or her, digitally penetrate him or her, or perform either penile/anal or penile/vaginal penetration on him or her (Gold et al., 1997; Kelly et al., 2002; Lisak & Luster, 1994; Spiegel, 1997a, 1997b). A limited minority (10%) of boys are subjected to sadomasochistic bondage (Richardson et al., 1993; Woods & Dean, 1985). Last, but not least, genital violence and mutilation, a particular and relatively undisclosed form of child abuse, may be even more common than CSA among boys (Boney-McCoy & Finkelhor, 1995b).

SUBSEQUENT ABUSE

A prior experience of CSA serves as a risk factor for subjection to CSA by a perpetrator other than the first (Boney-McCoy & Finkelhor, 1995a; Swanston et al., 2002). Reports of subsequent abuse among boys range from 25% to 65% (Deblinger et al., 1989; Gold et al., 1997; Hunter, 1991; Hutchings & Dutton, 1993; Kellogg & Hoffman, 1995; Lisak & Luster, 1994; Richardson, et al., 1993; Robin et al., 1997; Spiegel, 1995; Violato & Genuis, 1993; Woods & Dean, 1985). In a number of studies, the preponderance of boys were abused by two or more perpetrators (Kelly et al., 2002; Mendel, 1995; Roesler & McKenzie, 1994; Sansonnet-Hayden et al., 1987) prior to the age of 18. Approximately two-thirds of males reporting sexual abuse by a family member also experience sexual abuse by a nonrelative outside of the nuclear family home (Harrison et al., 1997). Finally, homeless adolescent males with histories of CSA are significantly more likely to be subjected to rape than nonabused homeless youth (Ryan et al., 2000).

PERPETRATOR CONCEALMENT

The majority (61%) of perpetrators are fearful of the child disclosing, and such fear intensifies when the boy says "no," or expresses fear, distress, sadness, or pain (Elliott et al., 1995). Perpetrator generated and enforced concealment strategies customarily include: specifically informing the child not to disclose, framing the abuse as education or as a game, using threats of dire consequences, threatening the boy with physical aggression and force, expressions of anger, blaming the child, and/or threatening the loss of a loved one.

When perpetrators are not caught after a particular episode, some feel anxious, some feel apathetic, and some, although fewer, justify their actions to themselves (Elliott et al., 1995). Younger children are more easily pressured into secrecy due to the perpetrator's illusion of care (DeJong et al., 1983).

DISCLOSURE

The sexual abuse of females is significantly more likely to be disclosed and reported while, on the contrary, the sexual abuse of males is significantly more likely to remain concealed and, consequently, underreported (Boney-McCoy & Finkelhor, 1995a; Dhaliwal, Gauzas, Antonowicz, & Ross, 1996; Feiring et al., 1999; Finkelhor et al., 1990; Gordon, 1990; Holmes et al., 1997; Rew et al., 1991; Risin & Koss, 1987; Roesler & McKenzie, 1994; Salter, 1992). Younger children tend to disclose accidentally (Campis, Hebden-Curtis, & Demaso, 1993; Fontanella et al., 2000; Mian et al., 1986; Sorenson & Snow, 1991), for example, by means of evocative, developmentally advanced, and/or inappropriate expressions of sexual knowledge and behavior. Observation by an unanticipated third party, the manifestation of a medical injury or sexually transmitted disease and recognition of abuse-reactive sexual behavior may also indirectly or accidentally lead to disclosure. In general, younger children, when compared to older children, are less likely to deliberately initiate the disclosure process (Nagel, Putnam, Noll, & Trickett, 1997). Adolescent boys, on the other hand, when compared to girls and when compared to younger boys, are significantly less likely to disclose under any conditions (Hecht & Hansen, 1999; Lamb & Edgar-Smith, 1994).

In contrast to the indirect disclosure of younger boys, older children, if and when they reveal the abuse, tend to do so by way of purposeful self-disclosure and they are more likely to disclose directly to a parent or caretaker (Campis et al., 1993; Sorenson & Snow, 1991). Purposeful disclosure may be prompted by the child's anger toward the perpetrator, attempts to stop the abuse, exposure to a prevention module or television program highlighting CSA, anticipation of an upcoming meeting with the perpetrator and support and motivation from friends (Lamb & Edgar-Smith, 1994; Paine & Hansen, 2002; Roesler & Wind, 1994; Sorenson & Snow, 1991). Among children with supportive parents and caretakers—that is, adults who express a willingness to consider the possibility that their child was abused and who refrain from coercing the child to deny the abuse or to recant its occurrence and from punishing the child in any way—disclosures occurred at a rate 3.7 times greater than among children with caretakers identified as unsupportive (Lawson & Chaffin, 1992), Still and all, the substantial majority (74%) of disclosures across ages 3 to 17 tends to be accidental or indirect, with someone reporting the abuse after a child utters a suggestive statement or exhibits sexualized behavior (Sorenson & Snow, 1991) or after someone witnesses the abuse or overhears a discussion about the abuse and makes an anonymous report to police or Department of Social Service officials (Levesque, 1994). The sexual abuse of males is most often disclosed by a third party witness to the abuse (Reinhart, 1987).

Boys who do not disclose their abuse experience directly evidence significantly lower levels of anxiety and hostility when compared with those who purposefully reveal their abuse immediately or subsequently (Gomes-Schwartz,

Horowitz, Cardarelli, & Sauzier, 1990). For example, boys who purposefully disclose yield higher levels of symptomology as per the "Trauma Symptom Checklist for Children," particularly in the areas of anxiety, dissociation, and sexual concerns. Ironically, from the perspective of caretakers, family members, and child protection professionals, the purposeful disclosure of boys signifies a greater level of psychological functioning and, consequently, a lesser need for therapy when compared to boys who disclose indirectly or accidentally (Nagel et al., 1997).

Reports involving males are significantly and substantially more likely to come from an anonymous source than revelations involving females (Dersch & Munsch, 1999). When the reporter is anonymous, a case worker cannot, by definition, contact or interview the reporter about any information associated with the case (Dersch & Munsch, 1999). However, sexual abuse is only witnessed and reported by another person in a minority (25%) of cases (Gellert et al., 1993).

By and large, the sexual abuse of boys is more likely to come to the attention of officials by means of indirect disclosure (Johnson & Shrier, 1985; Reinhart, 1987) and to come to the attention of police as opposed to child protection teams or hospitals (Finkelhor, 1984; Levesque, 1994). Other-initiated disclosure far outweighs self-disclosure, including another abused child disclosing, a nonstranger overhearing, a hospital or school detecting, or anonymous individual reporting (Levesque, 1994). The unintentional disclosure and confirmation of abuse for males is likely to be associated with the preceding disclosure of a female victim. Essentially, the suspicion of CSA along with the subsequent reporting of alleged sexual abuse is more common among females than males (Reinhart, 1987). Even when abuse is disclosed and a case is referred to the police or other state agencies, boys and girls are significantly inclined to deny, minimize, and depreciate their experiences, even after the identification of positive physical findings (Bradley & Wood, 1996; Lawson & Chaffin, 1992; Sjöberg & Lindblad, 2002; Sorensen & Snow, 1991). In one study, a narrow majority (57%) of children with physical symptoms subsequently diagnosed as a sexually transmitted disease (STD) denied any history of CSA (Lawson & Chaffin, 1992). Denial and reluctance reach majority proportions in the substantial range (72% and 78%, respectively), certainly before, but sometimes after, abuse confirmation (Bradley & Wood, 1996).

Males with histories of CSA tend to keep the abuse concealed for decades, with 27 as the mean number of years since the abuse began to when it was disclosed to anyone (Sigmon et al., 1996; Woods & Dean, 1985). In studies of adults that investigate the disclosure rates and delays between and among both genders, the mean age at disclosure tends to be younger and the mean delay in years tends to be less for females (Lamb & Edgar-Smith, 1994).

In the *Los Angeles Times* national prevalence study, only 3% of the sexual abuse incidents were reported to police departments or social service agencies (Timnick, 1985). When abuse involves threats of harm to the boy and/or his family, disclosure, if it occurs at all, is long delayed. In many instances, the duration between the last abusive episode and disclosure is twice as long for boys who were subjected to aggression than for children who were not exposed to physical violence (Paine & Hansen, 2001).

In studies employing adult males abused as boys, investigators report, as a matter of course, that few, if any, cases were brought to the attention of social or legal authorities at the time of the abuse and only in rare instances were males referred to counseling or therapy of any kind (Collings, 1995; Spiegel, 1995; Woods & Dean, 1985). In another study, one involving children with abuse histories and STDs, a narrow majority (57%) denied any history of CSA (Lawson & Chaffin, 1992).

Abuse disclosure may, in part, be a function of abuse severity and the age of the child. To illustrate, children subjected to intercourse are less likely to disclose than children subjected to other forms of abuse (Gomes-Schwartz et al., 1990). Regardless of abuse dynamics, it is not uncommon for researchers to note that a considerable minority to vast majority (39% to 89%) of sexual abuse cases involving males remain unreported until boys, adolescent males, and adult males with histories of CSA participate in a study or find themselves in a treatment facility that is conducting an empirical investigation (Brannon, Larson, & Doggett, 1991; Cavaiola & Schiff, 1988; Finkelhor et al., 1990; Gomes-Schwartz et al., 1990; Mendel, 1995; Woods & Dean, 1985). As a side note, within the context of treatment centers, reports of CSA are 4.5 times more frequent when clients are directly asked by therapists whether or not they have experienced abuse (Lanktree, Briere, & Zaidi, 1991). Within the context of schools, even though such institutions identify the greatest number of children exposed to child abuse, only a limited minority (16%) are investigated by state social service agencies (U.S. Department of Health and Human Services, 1996b). If and when the abuse is disclosed outside of such circumstances, the recipient of the disclosure is most often the mother or other caretaker (Berliner & Conte, 1995; Lamb & Edgar-Smith, 1994; Levesque, 1994; Roesler & Wind, 1994; Woods & Dean, 1985).

Approximately one-sixth of boys with histories of CSA disclose to an adult (Kendall-Tackett & Simon, 1992). Upon disclosure, these adults tend to disbelieve the boy and often attempt to silence him (Carballo-Dieguez & Dolezal, 1995). In fact, a majority (68%) of disclosing males state that nothing was actually done about the abuse or the perpetrator (Gordon, 1990). Parents may, after their son's disclosure, choose not to make a report in order to avoid the stigmatization the child or family may experience; this can be very harmful to the boy in terms of his self-concept and his opportunities for resolving the trauma generated by CSA and its effects (Carballo-Dieguez & Dolezal, 1995). In responding to a child's or an adult's disclosure of CSA, family members, peers, school officials, treatment professionals, forensic professionals, and legal professionals can significantly contribute to the positive or negative effects experienced by the child or adult, in that the reactions of others can either help ameliorate the traumatic effects or exacerbate them depending on the degree to which a CSA disclosure is validated or invalidated (Hartman & Burgess, 1993).

Still, even if the abuse is disclosed, a limited to considerable minority (8% to 33%) of children recant their accidental or purposeful disclosures (Faller, 1988; Gonzalez, Waterman, Kelly, McCord, & Oliveri, 1993; Jones & McGraw, 1987; Sorenson & Snow, 1991). A near majority (50%) of recanting children in one study did so in response to pressure from adults (Bradley & Wood, 1996). In cases under state investigation, a substantial majority (72%) initially denied the abuse. Of those who initially disclosed, a minority (25%) recanted. However, the vast majority (92%) of children who initially disclosed and subsequently recanted ultimately reclaimed their initial allegations (Sorenson & Snow, 1991). The variability in disclosure and recantation rates may be, in part, a function of context in which assessment and evaluation, be it clinical, medical or forensic, interviewer style, question construction and format and the number and relationship of attending collaterals. Still, a substantial to vast majority (71% to 93%) of children who make an initial disclosure are significantly more likely to disclose again during subsequent formal interviews relative to children who have not officially disclosed (Bradley & Wood, 1996; DeVoe & Faller, 1999; Gries, Goh, & Cavanaugh, 1996; Keary & Fitzpatrick, 1994). Finally, it must be noted that current incidents of CSA are most likely reported when the child's parents also have histories of CSA (Finkelhor, Moore, Hamby, & Straus, 1997).

NONDISCLOSURE

Males are significantly more likely than females to conceal the abuse from everyone (Finkelhor et al., 1990; Gordon, 1990; Gries et al., 1996; Keary & Fitzpatrick, 1994; Lamb & Edgar-Smith, 1994; Lynch, Stern, Oates, & O'Toole, 1993; Ray, 1996) at the time of its occurrence and long thereafter as well. For example, at an adolescent medical facility, a virtual majority (100%) of abused males did not disclose their abuse and no reports were filed with authorities on their behalf until commencement of the study (Johnson & Shrier, 1985). Nondisclosure and denial predominated despite the fact that males with histories of CSA were significantly more likely to evidence psychological trauma, physical symptomology, and sexual dysfunctions relative to nonabused male patients.

Reasons for nondisclosure, in the form of factor analytic items with significant and functional loadings, include, under the category of "shame," "I was scared," "I didn't want to get in trouble," "No one would believe me," "I was embarrassed," and "I didn't want to get anyone else in trouble." Items associated with "ambivalence" include "I still like/love the other person," and "It was my fault as much as the other person's." Males with abuse histories who feel responsible and/or possess some positive feelings or concerns about the perpetrator are even more reluctant to disclose the abuse experience to anyone (Kellogg & Hoffman, 1997).

To be sure, boys, adolescents, and adult males with histories of CSA experience an overwhelming fear of disclosing the abuse to others (Kiser et al., 1988; Robin et al., 1997). The vast majority (up to 99% in some studies) of males, independent of age, do not disclose out of fear of negative consequences (Bagley et al., 1994; Carballo-Dieguez & Dolezal, 1995; Gordon, 1990; Sebold, 1987; Sorenson & Snow, 1991; Spiegel, 1997b; Woods & Dean, 1985), including, but not limited to, fear of being perceived as gay, fear of being perceived as "feminine," fear of being perceived as a potential perpetrator, fear of disbelief, fear of being blamed, fear of being viewed as abnormal or deviant, fear of bearing the responsibility for accusing the perpetrator and for any repercussions experienced by the family such as turmoil, shame, separation, and divorce, fear of negative repercussions experienced by the perpetrator, because he or she may be loved and respected by many, fear of perpetrator harm, fear of scandal, fear of being placed in foster care, with or without siblings, feelings of shame and guilt, guilt for experiencing pleasure, shame for failing to prevent the abuse from occurring, guilt and shame for receiving money gifts or special privileges in exchange for sex, fear of the attitudes of others, fear of familial and peer rejection, and fear that the perpetrator's threats will become a reality.

FALSE ALLEGATIONS

Among boys reporting abuse to local, county, or state officials, only 1.3% of alleged sexual abuse cases are assessed to be false (Everson & Boat, 1989). A 12-state investigation of approximately 9,000 divorce cases revealed that false allegations of CSA occurred in a very limited minority (<2%) of contested divorces involving the parental custody of children (Association of Family Conciliation Courts, 1990). Finally, in a study of CSA at a major children's hospital, investigators noted that a child's disclosure is more reliable than medical examinations (Cincinnati Children's Hospital Medical Center, 2000).

FAMILY RESPONSES TO DISCLOSURE

Disclosures of CSA frequently render negative outcomes for the child (Lamb & Edgar-Smith, 1994). If and when a boy discloses, families tend to deny the abuse (Ray, 1996). In mixed-gender studies, approximately 1 in 10 boys and girls confront disbelief on their disclosure of CSA (Berliner & Conte, 1995; Gomes-Schwartz et al., 1990). It follows that recantation is significantly more likely to occur among abused boys with nonsupportive parents when compared to children with supportive families (Elliott & Briere, 1994). Males with histories of CSA, in comparison to abused females, report less family protectiveness after disclosure and less support from parents and siblings (Stroud,

1999). Nonoffending mothers are significantly more likely to believe and support a child's disclosure if they deferred the birth of their first child until reaching adulthood, if they were not sexually active with the perpetrator at the time of disclosure, they remained unaware of the child's sexual abuse prior to disclosure, if the child reported less than five episodes of abuse, if the abuse lasted less than 1 year, if the disclosure occurred within a year of the last episode, and if the child does not exhibit sexualized behavior (see, e.g., Gomes-Schwartz et al., 1990; Elliott & Briere, 1994; Pintello & Zuravin, 2001). A nonoffending mother is significantly less likely to believe and support her son if she or another caretaker neglected or physically abused the boy, if she has a history of domestic violence, and if she or another caretaker has substance abuse problems (Elliott & Briere, 1994).

The seriousness of the sexual abuse of males is often minimized by adults, with many believing that boys in general and adolescents in particular are not psychologically harmed (Burgess et al., 1984). Many parents are unable to effectively respond to and cope with their child's disclosure and/or acknowledgment of CSA (Ray & English, 1995). Parents of sexually abused boys appear to be less concerned about the effects of CSA on their sons than parents of female children with similar experiences or histories (Gill & Tutty, 1997). In one study, a virtual majority (100%) of parents of abused boys became preoccupied with their concerns about homosexuality and, more specifically, in viewing CSA as a determinant of their sons' sexual orientations (Davies, 1995). For these and many other reasons, parents of sexually abused boys are often opposed to seeking help of any kind for their sons (Schwartz, 1994). Yet problems persist, as the parents, upon disclosure of their son's abuse, tend to experience intrusive thoughts, depression, anxiety, relational difficulties, sexual problems, conflicts with their abused son, and the loss of a significant relationship as a consequence of disclosure (Davies, 1995).

While a majority to substantial majority (65% to 79%) of parents believe their sons, claiming that once a boy discloses, they tend to eventually accept the likelihood of his statements (Faller & Henry, 2000; Gully et al., 2000), a limited minority of nonoffenders, approximately 1 in 6, refuse to believe the boy. Impediments to considering a boy's disclosures include fear of the perpetrator's violent reaction, fear of lost income, and fear of losing emotional support if the abuse is disclosed or reported. In more than a few instances, a limited minority (12%) of nonoffending parents encourage the abuse (Pierce & Pierce, 1985).

Parents, perhaps unknowingly, employ the defense of projective identification, wherein the boy is perceived as deviant or as a "bad seed," like the perpetrator (Friedrich & Luecke, 1988). After disclosure, mothers of abused children perceive a number of personality problems in their sons. Typical responses of families upon abuse disclosure include: (a) denial of the abuse; (b) reframing the abuse as normal child behavior; (c) acknowledging the abuse but blaming or punishing the child; and (d) acknowledging the abuse but neglecting to protect the child from further abuse (Weihe, 1990). Perhaps most importantly, from the boy's perspective, and in terms of family reactions to the abuse, males often feel pressured, threatened, or rejected for disclosing the abuse, feel blamed for causing the abuse, and feel punished by their parents for the abuse (Burgess et al., 1987). That notwithstanding, children receiving support, even after a substantial period of no support, fare better psychically; their experience is validated, their sense of personal autonomy is enhanced, and they are more able to place blame and responsibility on the perpetrator (Adams-Tucker, 1985).

SOCIAL RESPONSES

Despite growing attention, public perceptions of children's allegations of CSA are increasingly more likely to be viewed with doubt and suspicion for a number of reasons, including the highly publicized and sensationalized nature of childhood sexual abuse trials, the overuse of the "abuse excuse," the dramatic and often fatalistic depictions of sexually abused children, the media's presentation of abuse mythology as fact, the divisive conflicts between abuse-related memory proponents, and the irreconcilable ideologies of social workers, psychologists, and sociologists as to the positive and negative effects of CSA (Myers, 1995). Peers and classmates, when informed of the abusive experiences of a boy, tend to ridicule, label, and stigmatize him (Burgess et al., 1984). Adults may fail to take immediate and preventive action as well. For example, in a study involving substantiated cases of CSA, a minority (24%) of adults to whom children disclosed histories of CSA neglected to contact the appropriate authorities (Paine & Hansen, 2002). Women, married partners, and individuals with children are significantly more likely to believe and make efforts on behalf of the child to prevent further abuse than are men, nonmarried individuals, and individuals without children (Calvert & Munsie-Benson, 1999).

SOCIAL INTERVENTION

Social and medical intervention directed toward children with histories of CSA is inadequate (Cupoli & Sewell, 1988). Both the general public and helping professionals interfacing with sexually abused children tend to minimize the prevalence, severity, and effects of this biopsychosocial problem. For example, professionals on the front lines of abuse identification and prevention, namely, social workers and police, are significantly more likely to contact the jurisdiction's abuse registry when the perpetrator is male and significantly less likely to do so when the perpetrator is female (Hetherton & Beardsall, 1998). Further, the public school system is both the single greatest source of CSA reports nationwide and the single greatest source of failures to report, as the vast majority (85%) of cases in public schools are not directly conveyed to state agencies (Sedlak & Broadhurst, 1996; U.S. Department of Health and Human Services, 1999). Although teachers tend to report suspected abuse, they do so indirectly to other school officials, such as nurses, guidance counselors, and principals, rather than directly to child protection agencies (Abrahams, Casey, & Daro, 1992). Teachers working in Catholic schools are significantly more likely to recognize and report suspected CSA and other forms of child abuse than teachers at other types of academic institutions (O'Toole, Webster, O'Toole, & Lucal, 1999). All in all, approximately 28% of suspected child abuse is formally reported to state abuse registries by school officials (Abrahams et al., 1992; Reinger, Robinson, & McHugh, 1995).

Cases involving boys are substantiated at a significantly lower rate than cases involving girls (Dersch & Munsch, 1999; Eckenrode, Munsch, Powers, & Doris, 1988; Haskett, Wayland, Hutcheson, & Tavana, 1995). An average of four protective service reports per child are registered prior to a boy receiving an emergency treatment referral (Cupoli & Sewell, 1988). In advance of a medical examination, virtually all children are interviewed by law enforcement officers or child protection team workers (Gully et al., 2000) and a determination of probable cause must be submitted by a representative of the state (Cupoli & Sewell, 1988). The mean length of time from the last episode of CSA to evaluation is 113 days for boys, a substantially longer duration than that for girls (Huston et al., 1995).

Among professionals mandated to report and/or participate in the evaluation of suspected cases of CSA, social service involvement is significantly more likely to be initiated and the suspected abuse cases are significantly more likely to be presented to the abuse registry if the alleged perpetrator is male (Hetherton & Beardsall, 1998). Moreover, one study revealed that even when reports of female perpetration were filed with the designated abuse registry, neither child protection services nor the police selected to investigate a limited minority (14%) of the cases (Faller, 1995).

When compared to girls, boys who experience sexual abuse are more likely to come to the attention of police departments (Dersch & Munsch, 1999) than child protective agencies, hospitals, or schools (Gordon, 1990). Female law enforcement officers are more likely than their male counterparts to believe the child's disclosures (Froum & Kendall-Tackett, 1998; Kendall-Tackett & Watson, 1991). Reports made directly to law enforcement officials are more common when CSA occurs outside the home and by a unrelated perpetrator (Dubé & Hebert, 1988). When such reports are made, boys are less likely to receive counseling or to be placed in protective custody (Gordon, 1990). Disproportionately fewer males than females are removed from the home as a preventive strategy against further abuse (Pierce & Pierce, 1985). In one study, only a minority (28%) of children between the ages of 2 and 5 were removed from the home (Fontanella et al., 2000). The likelihood of such a preventive and ameliorative intervention by the state decreases with age.

Before a case can be considered for criminal prosecution, the alleged sexually abused boy must make an explicit disclosure to child protective workers or to law enforcement officials. Among cases involving adult perpetrators, a child protection services (CPS) agency, upon registration of the allegation, did not conduct an investigation or did not substantiate the case (Gray et al., 1999). However, even after disclosures and even after cases are presented to the district attorney's office, a considerable minority (up to 40%) are declined (Chapman & Smith, 1987; Cross, Whitcomb, & De Vos, 1995; Gray, 1993). When a case is declined, it becomes ipso facto. At that point, it is officially expelled from the criminal justice system; however, charges may be pursued by way of civil proceedings. Of the accepted CSA cases, the vast majority (88% to 99%) do not go to trial (Cross et al., 1995; Faller & Henry, 2000; Gray, 1993; Gray et al., 1999). Thus, the preponderance of perpetrators are neither charged with nor tried for a sexual offense. Rather, the charges are frequently dropped or a plea bargain to a lesser, nonsexual charge is filed. Only a limited minority (8% to 9%) result in criminal court conviction (Bradley & Wood, 1996; Gray et al., 1999). When perpetrators are prosecuted, less than two-fifths of their cases result in conviction (Cross et al., 1995; Faller & Henry, 2000).

If a guilty verdict is rendered, the most common sentence involves jail, with or without probation, for 2 to 11 years (Faller & Henry, 2000). Even when a jail term of 2 to 11 years is rendered, most are suspended at some point in time (Cheit & Goldschmidt, 1997; Cullen et al., 2000; Gray et al., 1999; Stroud, Martens, & Barker, 2000). Among CSA cases adjudicated in court, the disparity between warrants of guilt and actual incarceration ranges from 25% to 42% (Chapman et al., 1987; Cheit & Goldschmidt, 1997; Goodman et al., 1992; Gray, 1993; Smith & Elstein, 1993). For example, although the vast majority (86%) of perpetrators in one study pled guilty, once the case was accepted and carried forward by the district attorney's office, only a narrow majority (53%) were incarcerated (Goodman et al., 1992). A recent archival study found that in the state of Rhode Island, judges and juries are 64 times more likely to convict and incarcerate an individual charged with murder than an individual charged with first-degree CSA (Cheit & Goldschmidt, 1997).

In terms of actual prison sentence, adults who sexually abuse children are significantly more likely to receive shorter periods of incarceration than adults who rape adults. Further, sexual perpetrators of teens are significantly more likely to serve less time than perpetrators against children and adults (Finkelhor & Ormrod, 2001). For example, in state prisons across America, the median sentence for the rape or sexual assault of a child is approximately 5 years less than the equivalent offense against an adult. Additionally, sexual perpetrators on adults are approximately three times more likely to receive a life sentence than sexual perpetrators on children (U.S. Department of Justice, 1996). Moreover, sentences rendered for CSA tend to be more clement than the suggested sentences mandated by law (Cheit & Goldschmidt, 1997; Gray, 1993).

Cases alleging the sexual abuse of a female child are significantly more likely to involve court action than reports involving a male child, even though the number of investigative interviews and reports for males and females tend to be equivalent (Dersch & Munsch, 1999; Stroud et al., 2000). Further, male perpetrators, once arrested and charged, are significantly more likely to have their cases referred to the district attorney than accused female perpetrators (Stroud et al., 2000). When considering CSA cases in aggregate, only a limited minority (1% to 13%) reach the prosecution stage (Cross et al., 1995; Stroud et al., 2000; Tjaden & Thoennes, 1992). Even then, if the boy is 12 or older, the chance of a case resulting in a conviction is significantly less likely than if he were 11 or younger (Isquith, Levine, & Scheiner, 1993). Even when cases are substantiated by Child Protective Services, a substantial majority (83%) are not criminally adjudicated (Tjaden & Thoennes, 1992).

Prosecutors report a number of reasons for deciding against the filing of a case. These include: (a) lack of viable corroborating evidence; (b) a family's unwillingness to prosecute; (c) the young age of a child; and (d) inconsistencies in the child's story (Gray, 1993). Even when perpetrators are arrested, two-thirds are released on bail or on their own recognizance. Imprisonment tends to be viewed by social service workers and police officers as more appropriate for male perpetrators than for female perpetrators (Hetherton & Beardsall, 1988). Perpetrators identified as racial/ethnic minorities are significantly more likely to be prosecuted than their Caucasian counterparts. Even in cases involving children who acquired HIV disease as a result of CSA, the perpetrator was found "not guilty" a substantial majority (70%) of the time (Gellert et al., 1993).

As for sexual abuse reenactments, boys are significantly more likely to be charged with a sexual offense than girls. Girls who sexually abuse are significantly more likely to receive victim-specific CSA assessment, crisis intervention, and counseling (Ray & English, 1995). Regarding adult female perpetrators with substantiated sexual offenses, one study noted that, of the 72 reported to state authorities, only a limited minority (4%) had criminal charges filed against them. Although all attempts to prosecute female perpetrators failed, some of their male co-offenders were criminally adjudicated (Faller, 1995). Another study, this one reporting on the perceptions of professionals who are mandated reporters, found that incarceration for charges or convictions associated with CSA was viewed as significantly more appropriate for male, as opposed to female, perpetrators (Hetherton & Beardsall, 1998). To illustrate this further, of the adolescent female perpetrators mandated to attend a sexual abuse treatment program, the majority (61%) were not adjudicated for their sexual offense even though a narrow majority (54%) of sexual acts involved vaginal and anal penetration. The modal age of the boys they abused was 5 (Fehrenbach & Monastersky, 1988).

In the courtroom, female jurors are significantly more likely to support the plaintiff while male jurors are significantly more likely to favor the defendant. Further, a substantial majority (75%) of potential jurors of both genders endorse the idea that people can and do repress memories of traumatic events such as childhood sexual abuse. However, this point of view is not upheld when rendering a verdict. In cases involving the repression of memories, support for the defendant redoubles (Tsai, Morsback, & Loftus, 1999, cited in

Schwarz, 1999). Even in cases unrelated to memory repression, jurors tend to attribute at least partial responsibility to the child for encouraging and provoking the sexual abuse or, at the very least, for failing to prevent the abuse from occurring in the first place (Isquith et al., 1993).

Across the United States, judges compel only a limited minority (<13%) of child abuse perpetrators to engage in a sexual offender treatment program or to enter into psychiatric or psychological counseling programs (Cullen et al., 2000; U.S. Department of Justice, 1996). Even when allegations are corroborated and confirmed as "legitimate" sexual abuse cases, the majority (65%) are assessed to be without a need for services (Tjaden & Thoennes, 1992), and especially so if the perpetrator is female (Hetherton & Beardsall, 1988). Such services might include counseling for the boy and his family, parenting classes for the nonoffending caretaker, and drug and alcohol testing and treatment for the perpetrator. Caseworkers tend to give greater priority to services for the parents or family as opposed to services especially designed for the child (Holder & Corey, 1993; Kolko, Seleyo, & Brown, 1999).

In terms of female perpetrators, one of the few peer-reviewed quantitative studies in this area found that after confirmation and/or adjudication by the state, a considerable minority (39%) of case outcomes failed to include provisions that could protect children from further abuse. Children were characterized as "unprotected" when the female perpetrator had unsupervised access to the children she had already abused and unimpeded access to other children as well. Incestual perpetrators were significantly more likely to have continued access to the children they abused than extrafamilial offenders, whereas the extrafamilial perpetrators were significantly more likely to have access to children outside the family than incestual offenders (Faller, 1995).

The legal mandate to report suspected cases of childhood sexual abuse engenders reluctance and resistance and, consequently, inconsistency among professionals and institutions. One study reported that a narrow majority (58%) of psychiatrists, a narrow majority (51%) of social workers, and a considerable minority (44%) of psychologists failed to report a case of child abuse at least one time during their professional careers (Zellman, 1990a). A U.S. Department of Health and Human Services study (1988) revealed that a majority (69%) of all cases of child abuse and neglect detected by mandated professionals was not reported to state or local child protection agencies. Another study documented failure-to-report rates of suspected child abuse across a number of mandated institutions: day-care facilities (88%), public and private schools (76%), local, county, and state social service agencies (70%), community mental health organizations (42%), and hospitals (31%) (National Center on Child Abuse and Neglect, 1988).

With respect to child abuse professionals, the most common reasons for reporting abuse are as follows: (a) compliance with the legal requirement to report; (b) fear of lawsuit or liability if a report is not made; (c) adherence to the reporting policy of the agency or workplace; (d) a desire to obtain intervention for the child or for the family; (e) an interest in helping the family understand the seriousness of CSA; (f) ensuring continuation of treatment for the child or family; (g) a desire to stop the abuse; (h) an interest in bringing the expertise of child protection services to the case; and (i) protecting the child through law enforcement (Zellman, 1990a). Generally speaking, helping and service professionals, such as physicians, nurses, psychiatrists, and psychologists, evidence greater knowledge with regard to indicators of child abuse when compared to their knowledge of social policy and reporting mandates and procedures (Reiniger et al., 1995; Zellman, 1990b).

Conditions that facilitate reporting of subsequent cases include the following. The social worker at the abuse registry (a) acted professionally; (b) was receptive to the report; and (c) did not ask too many questions, while the mandated reporter (a) was treated in a professional manner; (b) sensed that a viable action would be taken; (c) received feedback on the case after investigation; (d) found the written report to be satisfactory; and (e) believed the child would be safer as a result of the report (Vulliamy & Sullivan, 2000).

The most common reasons for declining to report include, but are not limited to, the following: (a) personal concerns, such as unfamiliarity with reporting or fear of a legal counterstrike; (b) a reluctance to get involved; (c) unwillingness to breach confidentiality or the seal of confession; (d) loyalty to the child's parents; (e) perceptions that the abuse is not serious enough to merit a report; (f) the belief that evidence of abuse, rather than suspicion, is essential to registering a report; (g) the student, patient, or client denies the abuse or recants; (h) a fear of making a false or inexact report; (i) considerations around the effects such an intervention might have on the child, for example, risk for additional abuse or disruption of the family unit; (j) a fear of damaging the clinical, professional, or pastoral relationship with the family; (k) a fear of parental or familial retaliation; (l) the client is of legal age; (m) the prior reporting of the case by another party; and (n) system concerns, such as the potential poor quality of child protection services, the insensitivity of law enforcement officers, and the unlikelihood that authorities would do anything constructive (see, e.g., Abrahams et al., 1992; Crenshaw, Crenshaw, & Lichtenberg, 1995; Fortune, 1988; Grossoehme, 1998; Kenny, 2001; Vulliamy & Sullivan, 2000; Zellman, 1990a).

That being said, the most common response pattern is one of reporting some incidents of suspected CSA while choosing not to report others. The majority of mandated reporters are cognizant of and accept their responsibility to report suspected cases of child abuse and neglect (Zellman, 1990a, 1990b). However, the fact remains that mandated female professionals are more likely to suspect and report abuse, regardless of its severity, than their male counterparts (Crenshaw et al., 1995; Finlayson & Koocher, 1991). And even though all 50 states mandate the reporting of CSA, mandated reporting has not increased the identification of children subjected to CSA (Berlin, Malin, & Dean, 1991).

SOCIAL PERCEPTIONS

In terms of social perceptions, physical abuse, lack of food, lack of cleanliness, inadequate supervision, emotional abuse, and verbal maltreatment are viewed more definitively as "child abuse and neglect" than sexual abuse, across a number of demographics, including gender, race, socioeconomic status, and neighborhood profile (Korbin et al., 2000). Within a statewide representative sample of households, a narrow majority (53%) of adults were unable to define the term "childhood sexual abuse" and a substantial majority (73%) were unable to identify characteristics of an adult who sexually abuses children (Centers for Disease Control, 1997). In another statewide study ascertaining public perceptions of and attitudes concerning child abuse, a substantial majority (75%) of citizens were cognizant of their duty to report suspected child abuse to state authorities; however, a only a minority (32%) of individuals who suspected child abuse actually made formal reports to designated agencies (Dhooper, Royce, & Wolfe, 1991).

With regard to social perceptions of CSA, women, individuals who are married, and individuals with children are significantly more likely than their respective counterparts to be more knowledgeable about the dynamics and effects of CSA and to perceive children as truthful when disclosing a history of CSA (Calvert & Munsie-Benson, 1999). However, if the child is male, the perpetrator is viewed as less responsible for the abuse (Broussard & Wagner, 1988). It is not uncommon for some to view a boy's subjection to CSA as educational, a developmental milestone, or even harmless (Broussard, Wagner, & Kazelskis, 1991; Spencer & Tan, 1999).

In general, adult males, relative to adult females, are apt to perceive the abused child more negatively and the perpetrator less negatively. Specifically, males tend to attribute more responsibility for the abuse on the boy's characteristics and behavior and, accordingly, less responsibility on the perpetrator (Spencer & Tan, 1999). In addition, males generally find allegations of CSA less credible than females (Bottoms & Goodman, 1994; Crowley, O'Callaghan, & Ball, 1994; Golding, Sanchez, & Sego, 1997; McCauley & Parker, 2001; O'Donohue & O'Hare, 1997). On the whole, adults discern the male child/female perpetrator pairing as less harmful than other child/perpetrator dyads. Further, the male child/female perpetrator pairing and the male child/male perpetrator pairing are viewed as less representative of childhood sexual abuse than other possible combinations involving a female child (Broussard et al., 1991).

Adult males and females alike are inclined to perceive older children as more responsible for their abuse than younger children (Back & Lips, 1998; Waterman & Foss-Goodman, 1984) and are more likely to perceive older boys as less masculine than younger boys vis-à-vis the sexually abusive experience (Spencer & Tan, 1999). However, as the child progresses in age, the balance of responsibility shifts from the nonoffending parents to the child. Both males and females are apt to regard a female perpetrator of young children as relatively immune from responsibility. In general, the degree to which an observer perceives himself or herself as personally dissimilar to the child is the degree to which he or she will place responsibility on the child (Back & Lips, 1998).

Children who respond to CSA in a passive way are held significantly more culpable than children who resist. Additionally, when children react to CSA in what may be perceived as an encouraging manner—in other words, if they do not clearly convey passivity or resistance—they are viewed as significantly more accountable for their abuse whereas adult perpetrators are perceived as less responsible (Broussard & Wagner, 1988). Further, according to the social perceptions of adults, it is more reasonable for a boy to respond in an encouraging manner to a female perpetrator than it is for the same reaction to occur among male children of male perpetrators, female children of male perpetrators, or female children of female perpetrators (Broussard et al., 1991).

Overall, adult females, in comparison to adult males, tend to hold and express stronger pro-child or validational attitudes, beliefs, and emotional responses to CSA as a psychosocial problem and to the plight of abused children (Back & Lips, 1998; Jackson & Nutall, 1993; Wellman, 1993; Zellman & Bell, 1989). American males, on the other hand, tend to evidence greater levels of homophobia and hostility toward homosexuals, especially toward gay men, than do females (Kite, 1985, cited in Cochran & Peplau, 1991).

PERCEPTIONS OF CHILD ABUSE PROFESSIONALS

The dissemination and implementation of CSA knowledge is incomplete (Conte et al., 1991). This may be evidenced in the following. Akin to the perceptions of the general public yet contrary to the CSA knowledge base, allied professionals, including social workers, physicians, nurses, psychologists, and psychiatrists, tend to view (a) father/daughter incest as more serious than father/son or mother/son incest (Eisenberg, Owens, & Dewey, 1987), (b) male perpetrators as more harmful than female perpetrators (Eisenberg et al., 1987; Hetherton & Beardsall, 1988), and (c) older children as more responsible for the occurrence of CSA than younger children (Kalichman, 1992; Wagner, Aucoin, & Johnson, 1993). In considering indicators of CSA, for example, fear of the perpetrator, provocative behavior, sexualized language, and aggression against anatomical dolls, law enforcement officials are significantly more inclined to find indicators like these more convincing than mental health professionals. Similarly, female professionals tend to find such indicators more persuasive than their male counterparts (Kendall-Tackett & Watson, 1991).

In terms of education, a narrow majority (51%) of professionals in the CSA field report no prior formal training in the evaluation of alleged child abuse cases, even after an average of more than 10 years of practice in various disciplines, including law enforcement, social work, psychology, nursing, and law (Hibbard & Zollinger, 1992). A considerable minority (38%) of more than 1,000 mandated reporters—psychiatrists, psychologists, social workers, medical professionals, principals, and child care workers—received no formal training in CSA (Zellman, 1990b). Among psychologists, nurses, and psychiatrists, only a minority (31%) received training in the assessment and treatment of CSA (Lab et al., 2000). Of those who participate in some form of training, continuing education courses after entry into their profession dominate. The average length of total training is 28.5 hours (Hibbard & Zollinger, 1992).

The preponderance of mental health professionals, including psychiatrists, psychologists, and nurses, fail to routinely inquire into the possible histories of CSA in male clients and patients (Holmes et al., 1997). For example, one study reported that among mental health professionals, only a limited minority (6%) routinely ask about histories of CSA. A considerable minority (46%) inquire only when the client presents the topic, and a minority (34%) pursue this line of questioning when the topic of CSA comes to mind (Lab et al., 2000). Further, mental health professionals are less likely to conceptualize a male's presenting problems as potential effects of CSA, relative to the presenting problem of a female patient (Holmes & Offen, 1996).

Male professionals are significantly more likely than female professionals to believe that false allegations of childhood sexual abuse are relatively common (Marshall & Locke, 1997). They are more inclined to perceive perpetrators as individuals who, by virtue of their offenses, are well differentiated from and quite visible within the general population (Trute, Adkins, & MacDonald, 1992). Further, male professionals are significantly more likely than their female colleagues to attribute greater responsibility to the child and his nonoffending caretakers (Back & Lips, 1998; Waterman & Foss-Goodman, 1984). Among therapists and child abuse professionals, male and female, there is a trend toward placing greater responsibility on perpetrating fathers who admit abusing their child and a greater responsibility toward nonoffending mothers if the father denies the abuse. When the father disputes the child's abuse disclosure, the mother is identified as a collaborator and, as such, is held more responsible for the abuse of her son (Kalichman, Craig, & Follingstad, 1990).

Female professionals working in the CSA field are more likely to view childhood sexual abuse as a critical psychosocial problem and to conceptualize its effects as more detrimental than their male counterparts (Eisenberg et al., 1987). Males also tend to view CSA as less prevalent (Gore-Felton et al., 1999; Trute et al., 1992). More specifically, professional males are more apt than females to underestimate the prevalence of father/daughter incest and to overestimate the numbers of children who make false allegations of CSA (Eisenberg et al., 1987). Additionally, male professionals are significantly more likely than female professionals to believe that the sexual abuse of children is on the decline and that sexual abuse during childhood is rare, whereas female professionals are significantly more likely than their male counterparts to believe that a client's suspicions of an abuse history suggest a history of abuse and that many psychological problems can be attributed to a history of CSA (Gore-Felton et al., 1999).

In general, therapists are more likely to perceive sexual abuse as the most prominent issue to address in therapy when working with females with histories of CSA; this is not the case with males who have similar histories. Regarding females with histories of CSA, clinicians new to the field and therapists working from a psychodynamic knowledge base, as opposed to a cognitive-behavioral orientation, are more likely to identify sexual abuse within a case (Hibbard & Zollinger, 1992). Among the various theoretical orientations of therapists, only those working within a behavioral framework are significantly less likely to have strong beliefs in the prevalence of CSA (Gore-Felton et al., 1999).

Professionals with histories of CSA are more likely to believe sexual abuse allegations than colleagues without such histories (Gore-Felton et al., 1999; Nutall & Jackson, 1994). However, akin to public perceptions, a minority (33%) of child abuse professionals believe that a girl is more impacted and affected by CSA than a boy (Eisenberg et al., 1987). Perceiving the sexual abuse of males as critical and as generating negative effects may call into question the perceiver's masculinity (Hunter, 1991; Smith, Fromuth, & Morris, 1997).

Mental health professionals acceding to and complying with traditionally prescribed attitudes associated with gender role socialization tend to blame males more than females for their abuse and tend to perceive sexual contact between a boy and an adult, relative to a girl and an adult, less definitively as sexual abuse. When a boy responds to the abuse with passivity or with resistance, they tend to be more definitive as to their perceptions of the event as abuse. Further, they are more apt to assign less blame to the perpetrator if the boy reacts to the abuse in a passive way (Richey-Suttles & Remer, 1997). The age of the child is also an influential factor in perceptions around indicators of CSA (Kendall-Tackett & Watson, 1991), with older boys perceived as more responsible than younger boys. Professionals working within the field of CSA are not immune from bias (Hibbard & Hartman, 1993; Levesque, 1994).

All in all, male and female professionals across a number of disciplines fail to inquire about sexual abuse when working with male patients or clients. Professionals are more likely to ask a female about a history of CSA, more likely to believe a female's disclosure, less likely to conceptualize a link between a male's biopsychosocial problems and a history of CSA, and more likely to align with the male patient by responding to his disclosure in a manner that invalidates his history of abuse (Holmes, Offen, & Waller, 1997; Lab, Feigenbaum, & Silva, 2000). The knowledge base evidence indicates that the social perceptions of the general public and the perceptions of professionals within or on the periphery of the field of CSA are essentially one and the same.

EFFECTS

Current Reactions to Abuse

Boys abused by females respond in the same way as boys abused by males (Woods & Dean, 1985) and, irrespective of whether the perpetrator is a child, adolescent or adult, abused boys evidence comparably high levels of physiological, psychological, emotional, sexual, and behavioral problems (Shaw et al., 2000) although physical effects may be more apparent among boys abused by older perpetrators (Allard-Dansereau et al., 1997). Moreover, regardless of perpetrator gender and age, boys experience childhood sexual abuse as having an intense impact on their lives, both at the time of its occurrence and at the time of reporting it to research teams. The plurality of males with histories of CSA characterize the immediate impact as strong, devastating, and negative. Years later, the same characterizations still hold (Doll et al., 1992; Hutchings & Dutton, 1993; Johnson & Shrier, 1987; Ray, 1996).

Initial reactions center around fear (Carballo-Dieguez & Dolezal, 1995; Dubowitz, Black, Harrington, & Verschoore, 1993; Garnefski & Diekstra, 1997)— of the perpetrator, that the abuse will be discovered, and that the boy will be blamed—as well as shock and surprise, which later turn to anger, worry, and confusion (Mendel, 1995; Woods & Dean, 1985). Relatively few respond to CSA with curiosity, interest, and pleasure; however, even when they do, such reactions tend to be coupled with and compounded by guilt, shame, disgust, and confusion (Gilgun & Reiser, 1990; Gill & Tutty, 1999; Johnson & Shrier, 1987; Lisak, 1994a; Risin & Koss, 1987; Woods & Dean, 1985).

Adult males, in retrospect, find the abuse to be harmful (Hutchings & Dutton, 1993). The immediate effects continue to be viewed as negative at a rate of 100%, and the long-term and overall effects are perceived as negative by a vast majority (96%) (Ray, 1996). In contrast, even though adult males report having only somewhat recovered from the experience of CSA (Hutchings & Dutton, 1993), they perceive only a modest association between the abuse and their present problems such as anxiety, depression, generalized stress response, substance abuse, sexual addiction, and relational difficulties.

Perceptions of Abuse

Even though many childhood experiences are congruent with, and even surpass, the formal criteria for CSA, it is not uncommon for boys, adolescent males, and adult males with histories of CSA to gravitate toward describing the sexually abusive relationship as consensual or otherwise nonabusive (Duncan & Williams, 1998; Fondacaro et al., 1999; Kelly et al., 2002). For example, among adults with histories of court-substantiated CSA, males are significantly less likely than females with similar histories to label and characterize their subjection to sexual abuse as "sexual abuse." In fact, less than 16% of males with documented histories of CSA, compared to 64% of females, identify their abusive histories in accordance with state statutes (Widom & Morris, 1997). Upon retrospect, however, a vast majority (86%) of adult males with histories of CSA now perceive their sexual interactions as abusive (Mendel, 1995).

In a few studies employing university samples, a majority (60%) of respondents view the sexually abusive experience, at the time of its occurrence, as positive, whereas a considerable minority (40%) view the sexually abusive relationship as having a positive life impact (Fromuth & Burkhart, 1987). In general, however, both males and females tend to retrospectively assess the abuse as negative, although a minority (21%) of males, as young adults, view it as positive or mostly positive; as boys, a considerable minority (40%) perceive the abuse to be positive or mostly positive. Thus, there appears to be a trend toward perceiving one's subjection to CSA more negatively as an adult (Urquiza & Crowley, 1986).

Among males who meet criteria for childhood sexual abuse, those who do not consider themselves to have been sexually abused are significantly more likely to experience current or lifetime alcohol abuse or dependence, while males who identify their abuse histories as CSA are significantly more likely to manifest current and/or lifetime posttraumatic stress disorder (PTSD) and obsessive-compulsive disorder (Fondacaro et al., 1999; Kelly et al., 2002; Kilpatrick & Saunders, 1997). Further, adult males with abuse histories who initially report positive perceptions of CSA are significantly more likely than abused males with negative perceptions of their abuse histories to have committed and be incarcerated for a sexual offense (Briggs & Hawkins, 1996) and to evidence indicators of dissociation aggression, self-destruction, interpersonal problems, sexual dysfunctions, and a sense of stigmatization (Kelly et al., 2002).

Effects Across Time

The knowledge base contains studies that assess CSA effects within 30 days of abuse cessation and studies that identify abuse-generated effects across the life span (see, e.g., Conte & Schuerman, 1987; McLeer et al., 1998; Schaaf & McCanne, 1998; Silverman, Reinhert, & Giaconia, 1996; Stein, Walker, Anderson et al., 1996). Childhood sexual abuse substantially disrupts the anticipated course of human development (Pynoos & Eth, 1985) and correlates with both initial and long-term effects experienced across the life span (Briere, 1992; Cohen et al., 2001). Among children, adolescents, and adults with histories of CSA, self-perceptions, that is, the meanings emanating from the abuse dynamics and effects, vary by developmental stage and change across time (Black et al., 1994). A meta-analytic investigation of community, university, and clinical studies assessing the relationship between exposure to CSA and adult symptomology supports the long-standing clinical notion that childhood sexual abuse is significantly related to adult psychological adjustment (Jumper, 1995). That a history of CSA predicts risk for the subsequent development of psychiatric symptomology at some point across the life span, that it contributes to the vulnerability of succeeding life stressors, and that it predisposes one to the materialization of other life stressors (including subsequent abuse) are strongly supported by a number of studies (Boney-McCoy & Finkelhor, 1996; Cohen, Brown, & Smaile, 2001; Fergusson, Lynskey, & Horwood, 1996a, 1996b; Leverich et al., 2002).

Boys, adolescent males, and adult males with histories of CSA evidence more negative symptomology with the progression of time, thereby suggesting an additive outcome of CSA effects (Boney-McCoy & Finkelhor, 1995a, 1996; Gomes-Schwartz, Horowitz, & Cardarelli, 1990). For example, in a longitudinal study, children who were asymptomatic at the initial evaluation manifested a number of abuse effects by the 18-month follow-up and significantly more so than children who were highly symptomatic from the start (Gomes-Schwartz, Horowitz, & Cardarelli, 1990). In another study assessing sexual abuse effects 4 weeks, 9 months, and 2 years after state detection, substantial increases in anxiety, depression, somatic complaints, academic and school difficulties, eating problems, running away, substance abuse and suicide attempts, for example, exacerbated with the passage of time (Calam, Horne, Glasgow, & Cox, 1998).

It has been asserted that one's perception and experience of CSA intensifies with time, rendering a self-concept imbued with the negativity of the abusive relationship and its aftermath (Lisak, 1994a, 1994b). That adolescents with abuse histories are significantly more likely to manifest pervasive biopsychosocial distress and, consequently, more symptomology than sexually abused children is a function of the developmental trajectory, not abuse characteristics. The socially imposed stressors of CSA subjection, coping, concealment, and disclosure, cross-cutting with the normative stressors of adolescent development, heighten the vulnerability and risk associated with each one independently as well as conjointly (Feiring et al., 1999), thereby engendering a number of sexual abuse-related developmental effects (Finkelhor, 1995). Localized effects are abuse generated and circumscribed by the abuse experience: fear of disclosure, hyperarousal, guilt, and shame, for example. Developmental effects, on the other hand, generalize across microenvironments; more pervasive, they trespass upon developmental tasks such as identity consolidation, educational attainment, relational interaction, and career development. While some localized or initial effects may abate with time, developmental and long-term effects, in conjunction with the abuse-related coping strategies employed for progressive adaptation, tend to generalize and amplify with time (Briere & Elliott, 1994).

Severity of Effects

Males with histories of CSA manifest more emotional and behavioral problems than males without abuse histories and report such problems with greater frequency than females with histories of CSA (Garnefski & Diekstra, 1997). For example, a considerable minority (43%) of males with histories of CSA often exhibit problems in the clinical range (Dubowitz et al., 1993) as indicated by significantly higher scores than nonabused boys for both the internalizing and externalizing scales of the Child Behavior Checklist (e.g., Hibbard & Hartman, 1992), the Personality Inventory for Children (e.g., Kiser et al., 1988), the Piers-Harris Self-Concept Scale (e.g., Janus et al., 1987), the Tennessee Self-Concept Scales (e.g., Cavaiola & Schiff, 1989), the Adolescent Sexual Concerns Questionnaire (e.g., Hussey, Strom, & Singer, 1992), the World Assumptions Scale (e.g., Mendel, 1995), the Trauma Symptom Checklist (e.g., Briere et al., 1988), the Minnesota Multiphasic Personality Inventory (e.g., Olson, 1990), and the Sexual Self-Esteem Scale (e.g., Finkelhor, 1981), as well as clinical screening measures (e.g., Bartholow et al., 1994; Gellert et al., 1993) and other scales employed in sexual abuse research.

As for sexually abused boys, the vast majority (95%) exhibit at least one symptom related to CSA and a majority (61%) experience at least three correlated symptoms (Gale et al., 1988). In general, boys initially present more clinically significant symptoms than girls (Kiser et al., 1988). Adolescents males with histories of CSA exhibit a greater tendency toward self-destruction than nonabused youth (Cavaiola & Schiff, 1988). Adult males abused as boys also evidence significantly higher rates of substance abuse/dependence and a myriad of Axis I and Axis II diagnoses such as affective disorder, major depressive disorder, anxiety disorder, phobia, panic disorder, and antisocial personality disorder when compared to their nonabused counterparts (Stein et al., 1988; Windle et al., 1995). In essence, boys, adolescent males, and adult males with histories of CSA experience more psychological, emotional, behavioral, adaptational, and social problems than nonabused males (Olson, 1990). Finally, across the life span, a history of CSA statistically holds significant links with a number of indicators of current mental health and general well-being. The strongest correlations are with anxiety, depression, suicidal ideation and action, psychoneurosis, posttraumatic stress, and dissociative experiences (Bagley et al., 1994).

History of Treatment

Individuals with abuse histories comprise a substantial proportion of the patient population. It is estimated that more than a narrow majority (>50%) of outpatients and a substantial majority (50% to 70%) of inpatients have histories of CSA (Carmen, Riker, & Mills, 1984). Males with histories of CSA are more likely than nonabused males to be, or to have been, involved in psychotherapy (Lisak, 1994a; Urquiza & Crowley, 1986) with unsuccessful outcomes (Brown & Anderson, 1991) and to have reported a mental health hospitalization at some time. Of those with an inpatient psychiatric admission, the vast majority (94%) were hospitalized after the first sexual abuse episode (Bartholow et al., 1994).

The mean number of years between the cessation of abuse and entry into treatment is 17 (Kendall-Tackett & Simon, 1992). The lifetime duration of psychotherapy for adult males abused as boys is approximately 5 years (Mendel, 1995). Even so, across treatment settings, males are much less likely than females to participate in therapy, and if they do, are much less likely to disclose a history of CSA to their therapist (Brown & Anderson, 1991; Jacobson & Richardson, 1987). As a sidenote, prevalence estimates suggest that one of every three adults with histories of CSA is male; treatment programs show otherwise, evidencing a 1:5 ratio (Gold et al., 1997, 1998).

Physical Findings

Girls are more likely to evidence definitive findings indicative of CSA than boys (Huston et al., 1995). Older children tend to evidence more definitive physical findings than younger children (Gully et al., 2000). Age progression is significantly correlated with more episodes of CSA, more perpetrators, the use of force and, consequently, the presence of injury. That notwithstanding, the majority (67%) of boys who experience multiple episodes of abuse exhibit physical findings consistent with a history of childhood sexual abuse. In one study, even after a single episode, physical findings were identified in the vast majority (86%) of cases (Spencer & Dunklee, 1986); however, such outcomes are not the norm.

Across studies, the frequencies of reported and definitive anogenital findings among boys tend to range from 15% to 80% (Bays & Chadwick, 1993; Bowen & Aldous, 1999; DeJong et al., 1983; Dubé & Hebert, 1988; Gully et al., 2000; Kellogg, Parra, & Menard, 1998; Levesque, 1994; Mian et al., 1986; Reinhart, 1987, Spencer & Dunklee, 1986). Such physical findings commonly include: anogenital bleeding, anogenital bruising, bite marks, penile erythema, rash, urethal discharge, perianal erythema, perianal hyperpigmentation, anal lacerations, anal fissures, anal laxity, rectal scarring, fecal impaction, and skin tags. In one study, abnormal physical findings led to diagnosis in 57% cases of children with HIV disease (Gellert et al., 1993).

Among boys, anal abnormalities are more common than genital abnormalities. Anal abnormalities are most evident in boys between the ages of 0 and 2. Chronic, or old findings, significantly outnumber acute findings (Reinhart, 1987). For example, superficial lacerations tend to heal within 1 to 11 days. Deep lacerations may persist for several weeks, leaving narrow bands of scar tissue. Anal sphincter dilation may persist for several months. Distended veins tend to remain longer than most other abnormalities (Hobbs & Wynne, 1989; McCann & Voris, 1993; McCann, Reay, Siebert, Stephens, & Wirtz, 1996). If a boy is not evaluated immediately, only vague and unascertainable signs of historic injury may persist. The presence of contusions, abrasions, and lacerations suggest the use of force and restraint (DeJong et al., 1983). However, it must be noted that the preponderance of medical evaluations render normative or inconclusive findings despite the presence of abnormalities (see, e.g., Bays & Chadwick, 1993; Claytor, Barth, & Shubin, 1989; Cupoli & Sewell, 1988; Elliott & Peterson, 1993; Gully et al., 2000; Slusser, 1995). Abused children with genital findings secondary to CSA are most often abused by postpubescent perpetrators (Allard-Dansereau et al., 1997).

Other Physical Effects

Additional physical effects, reported by boys, adolescents, and adult males with histories of CSA and/or observed by parents of sexually abused children, include: (a) generalized body pain; (b) chronic pain; (c) headaches and migraines; (d) gastrointestinal problems, loss of appetite, and abdominal pain; (e) nausea; (f) rectal pain and irritation; (g) hemorrhoids; (h) penile soreness; (i) urinary tract infections; (j) overactive gag reflex; (k) weight problems; and (l) lethargy (see, e.g., Allard-Dansereau et al., 1997; Burgess et al., 1984; Janus et al., 1987; Linton, 1997; Mian et al., 1986; Ray, 1996; Wells et al., 1997; Wurtele, Kaplan, & Keairnes, 1994). Generally speaking, males with histories of CSA tend to experience these effects significantly more and to a greater degree than their nonabused counterparts.

Gastrointestinal Effects

Males with histories of CSA are significantly more likely than nonabused peers of both genders to experience functional gastrointestinal disturbances without structural, metabolic, or infectious properties (Berkowitz, 1998; Leserman, Drossman, Li, Toomey, Hachman, & Glogau, 1996; Locke, 1996; Wells, McCann, Adams, Voris, & Ensign, 1995). These include irritable bowel syndrome, nonulcer dyspepsia, and chronic abdominal pain. A near majority to narrow majority (50% to 55%) of males with irritable bowel syndrome also report histories of CSA (Talley, Fett, Zinmeister, & Melton, 1994; Walker, Gelfand, Gelfand, & Katon, 1995; Walker, Katon, Roy-Byrne, Jemelka, & Russo, 1993). In both clinical and population-based studies, a history of CSA is associated with an odds ratio of 2.3 for irritable bowel syndrome and 2.0 for dyspepsia (Longstreth & Wolde-Tsadik, 1993; Talley et al., 1994).

Neurological Effects

Subjection to childhood sexual abuse may give rise to adverse and enduring effects for the boy, including impairment of his biological stress systems as well as his brain (De Bellis, Baum, et al., 1999; De Bellis, Keshavan, et al., 1999; McEwen, 2000b; Saplonksy, 1993) In response to internal and external stressors, the brain discharges epinephrine, norepinephrine, dopamine, serotonin, cortisols, and opioids, among other stress-responsive chemicals, into the bloodstream. These neurotransmitters may circulate for hours, perhaps days, after an episode of CSA and, in some cases, long after the cessation of the sexually abusive relationship. Over time, the regulating systems that modulate hormone levels begin to malfunction (Yehuda, 2000). Protracted subjection to CSA and, consequently, protracted discharge of stress-responsive chemicals incite hyperresponsivity within the hypothalamic–pituitary–adrenal (HPA) axis as well as the upregulation of the corticotropin releasing factor (CRF) system (Nemeroff et al., 1999), thereby increasing a sexually abused boy's risk for a number of psychiatric disorders, such as depression, PTSD, and anxiety (Roy, 2002; Yehuda, 2000).

With respect to circadian rhythm, the daily 24-hour periodicity of body temperature, hormone levels, urine production, cognitive activity, motor performance, and wake/sleep cycle, abused boys with PTSD and abused boys without PTSD manifest different patterns. Boys with histories of CSA and the diagnosis of PTSD evidence a robust and normal circadian rhythm with activity profiles similar to those of children with attention-deficit hyperactivity disorder (ADHD), whereas abused boys without a PTSD diagnosis yield a protracted circadian amplitude with activity profiles more comparable to those of depressed children (Glod & Teicher, 1996).

After the initial stress, wherein the brain and particularly the limbic system are flooded with cortisol, the levels drop significantly (Hart, Gunnar, & Cicchetti, 1995, 1996). Thus, it follows that severely abused boys with trauma symptomology secondary to CSA yield significantly greater baseline urinary free cortisol concentrations than nonabused boys (De Bellis, Baum, et al., 1999; De Bellis, Hall, Boring, Frustaci, & Moritz, 2001), whereas adult males with histories of CSA tend to emit lower values of 24-hour urinary output of urinary-free cortisol (UFC) than males without histories of abuse (Bremner, 1999; Roy, 2002). Excessive and protracted discharge of cortisol in response to stress produces HPA dysregulation, hypocortisolemia, disinhibition of CRF secretion, and damage to the hippocampus (Bremner, 1999). Additionally, subjection to CSA may render functional deficits in the cerebellar vermis, a brain substructure with a key role in the regulation of limbic system functioning and various states of attention and emotionality, thereby impacting blood volume and flow to this region of the brain (Anderson, Teicher, Polcari, & Renshaw, 2002). Children with abuse histories, when compared to nonabused peers, evidence increased blood flow in the cerebellar vermis and, as a result, a disruption in emotional equilibrium (Teicher, 2000).

Subjection to CSA alters the development of the brain (Perry, 1999; Schore, 2001), and especially so within the limbic system (Bremner et al., 1997; van der Kolk & Fisler, 1995). A history of CSA is associated with a 49% increase in somatic, sensory, behavioral, and memory symptoms akin to temporal-lobe epilepsy; when coupled with a history of physical abuse, the manifestation of limbic-system symptomology increases to 113% (Teicher, Glod, Surrey, & Swett, 1993). The neurotoxicity of hypercortisolemic states generates damage to the hippocampus, the chief neural destination of glucorticoids (De Bellis, Baum, et al., 1999; De Bellis et al., 1994). This limbic system substructure is central to the establishment of short-term memory and the spatial and contextual encoding and retrieval of episodic and declarative long-term memory (Phillips & LeDoux, 1992; van der Kolk & Fisler, 1995). Adults with histories of CSA evidence a 12% reduction in the size of the left hemispheric hippocampi; decreases in volume appear to be a function of abuse duration, with longer duration rendering greater reduction (Bremner et al., 1997). Hippocampal atrophy correlates with a number of psychiatric disorders, including depression, anxiety, and PTSD; and in many cases is accompanied by deficits in declarative, contextual, and spatial memory recall (McEwen, 2000b). Yet, when compared with nonabused controls, boys with histories of CSA and trauma symptomology do not evidence reductions or alterations in hippocampal, amygdaloid, or temporal lobe volume (De Bellis, Keshavan, et al., 1999b; De Bellis, Hall, et al., 2001). Thus, within the context of CSA, hippocampal atrophy may be classified as a long-term or developmental effect. At this stage of research, the question of whether decreases in hippocampal volume precede sexual abuse or manifest as an effect of sexual abuse has yet to be fully elucidated (Bremner, Southwick, & Charney, 1999).

Adolescents and adults with histories of CSA, when compared to nonabused peers, exhibit significant electrophysiological abnormalities, particularly in the left hemisphere of the frontal, temporal, and anterior regions of the brain (Ito et al., 1993; Teicher et al., 1997). Abused children, in contrast to controls, demonstrate higher levels of left-hemispheric coherence in addition to a reversed asymmetry. In one study, a substantial majority (72%) of adolescents with histories of severe CSA rendered abnormal electroencephalograph (EEG) readings of the frontotemporal or anterior regions of the brain, compared to a minority (27%) of nonabused controls. Left-hemispheric coherence significantly surmounts right-hemispheric coherence, suggesting abnormalities in left cortical differentiation (Ito, Teicher, Glod, & Ackerman, 1998). Within the realm of left-hemispheric abnormalities, limbic-system dysregulation may correlate with panic disorder and PTSD, diminished growth with depression, and hippocampal atrophy with dissociative disorders and memory impairments (Teicher, 2000). For example, when adults with histories of CSA recall a neutral memory, they employ the left hemisphere, whereas when they recall an evocative memory from childhood, they significantly activate the right hemisphere, indicating a problem with hemispheric integration (Teicher et al., 1997).

Finally, children with histories of CSA, when compared to nonabused controls, evidence significantly smaller brain structures, particularly in terms of cerebral and prefrontal cortex volumes including both gray matter and white matter, right and left amygdala and their corresponding gray matter, right and left temporal lobes, and the corpus callosum (De Bellis, Keshavan, et al., 1999). The corpus callosum is the substructure connecting the two hemispheres of the brain and responsible for communication between them (De Bellis, 2001; Teicher, 1997, 2000; Teicher, Anderson, Polcari, Anderson, & Navalta, 2002).

Impairment in the corpus callosum is linked to symptoms of ADHD, as well as to dramatic shifts in personality characteristics and mood. This last finding holds special significance. In general, nonabused boys and adolescent males, when compared to nonabused females, exhibit greater age-related decreases in cerebral gray matter and greater age-related increases in white matter volume in the corpus callosal area (De Bellis, Keshavan, et al., 2001). With regard to the corpus callosum and the cerebral cortex, the opposite is true for abused boys and when compared to abused girls (De Bellis, Keshavan, et al., 1999; Teicher, 2000).

Anxiety Among Boys

Compared to nonabused boys and norming samples, sexually abused boys exhibit significantly more anxiety, state and trait (De Bellis, Broussard, et al., 2001; Fontenella et al., 2000; Friedrich, Urquiza, & Beilke, 1986; Gale et al., 1988; Kiser et al., 1988; Kolko et al., 1988; McLeer et al., 1998). Separation anxiety disorder and overanxious disorder of childhood are common diagnoses among these boys (Livingston, Lawson, & Jones, 1993). Additionally, sexually abused boys experience heightened levels of fear, worry, and rumination; they are anxious to please and try very hard to do so (Conte & Schuerman, 1987; Hibbard & Hartman, 1992; Kiser et al., 1988; Sebold, 1987). They exhibit fearful states and anxious behaviors, including fear of disclosure, fear of disparaging responses to disclosure, suspiciousness of others, fear of being alone with others, and discomfort in the bathroom (see, e.g., Gomes-Schwartz et al., 1985; Kolko et al., 1988; Mian et al., 1986; Spiegel, 1995). Finally, relative to nonabused peers, boys with histories of CSA evidence significantly more psychological, biological, and physiological manifestations of anxiety (McLeer et al., 1998).

Anxiety Among Adolescent Males

Higher levels of anxiety and greater frequencies of worries and phobic symptoms are more common among adolescent males with histories of CSA than among abused females and nonabused males (De Bellis, Broussard, et al., 2001; Gomes-Schwartz et al., 1985; McClellan et al., 1995; Rew et al., 1991). Not only are abused adolescent males anxious about the sexual abuse that has already happened, they are also more concerned than nonabused counterparts about future rape and sexual abuse (Hussey et al., 1992).

Anxiety Among Adult Males

Among adult males, anxiety is one of the most common symptoms associated with a history of childhood sexual abuse (McKelvey & Webb, 1995; Stein et al., 1988; Urquiza & Crowley, 1986). Adult males abused as boys are significantly more likely than nonabused peers to have higher lifetime rates of generalized anxiety disorder and panic disorder (Fondacaro et al., 1999; Friedman et al., 2002). They are also more likely to experience heightened levels of fear, worry and rumination, particularly in terms of identity issues and conflicts (Hunter, 1991). For boys, adolescent males and adult males with abuse histories, fear is pervasive and enduring, from the onset of the abuse and long thereafter (Bagley et al., 1994; Briere et al., 1988; Collings, 1995). Fear emanating from the exposure and disclosure of the sexually abusive relationship and fear of the effects of abuse alienates them, confines them, and undermines their self-confidence, self-worth, and self-esteem (Lisak, 1994a, 1994b).

Depression Among Boys

When compared to nonabused groups and normative samples of children, abused boys evidence more depressive symptoms, greater rates of major depression as a diagnosis, more feelings of isolation, more mood swings, and more crying spells (Burgess et al., 1984; De Bellis, Keshavan, et al., 1999; De Bellis, Broussard, et al., 2001; Friedrich et al., 1986; Gale et al., 1988; Hibbard & Hartman, 1992; Kiser et al., 1988; Livingston, Lawson, & Jones, 1993; McLeer et al., 1998; Sansonnet-Hayden, Haley, Marriage, & Fine, 1987; Young et al., 1994). In one study of effects over time, boys with histories of CSA were 4.5 times more likely than nonabused peers to experience depression during a 2-year follow-up (Boney-McCoy & Finkelhor, 1996).

Depression Among Adolescent Males

Adolescent males with histories of CSA are significantly more likely than nonabused peers and norming samples to exhibit higher levels of depression (Grilo et al., 1999; Janus et al., 1987; Meyerson, Long, Miranda, & Marx, 2002; Ryan et al., 2000) and to receive the diagnosis of major or bipolar depression (Cavaiola & Schiff, 1988; De Bellis, Broussard, et al., 2001; Forbey, Ben-Porath, & Davis, 2000; Grilo et al., 1999). Common manifestations include sadness, despondency, self-criticism, mood lability, and the belief that the future is hopeless and that life, in general, will not improve (Boney-McCoy & Finkelhor, 1995b; Grilo et al., 1999; Hibbard et al., 1990; Hussey et al., 1992; McClellan et al., 1995). In light of the additive nature of CSA effects, adolescents, when compared to younger children with abuse histories, are more often depressed and suicidal (Adams-Tucker, 1985).

Depression Among Adults

Depression is among the most prevailing symptoms exhibited by adult males with histories of CSA (Roesler & McKenzie, 1994; Stein et al., 1988). A history of CSA is significantly associated with the diagnosis of major depression

(Fondacaro et al., 1999; Nelson et al., 2002; Windle et al., 1995) with reversed neurovegetative features, including hypersomnia, increased appetite, and weight gain (Levitan et al., 1998). Adult males abused as boys are significantly more likely to feel depressed than nonabused peers (Bagley et al., 1994; Briere et al., 1988; Collings, 1995; McKelvey & Webb, 1995; Styron & Janoff-Bulman, 1997; Urquiza & Crowley) and abused females (Janoff-Bulman, 1989; Robin et al., 1997). Finally, the experience of and hospitalization for depression is more common among adult males abused as boys than nonabused adult males (Bartholow et al., 1994).

Suicidality

Suicidality is reported nearly 5 times more often among males with histories of CSA than among sexually abused females and nearly 11 times more often among nonabused males (Garnefski & Diekstra, 1997; Molnar, Berkman, & Buka, 2001). When compared to nonabused adults with histories of suicidality, adult males with histories of CSA evidence an earlier age of onset of suicidal ideation and behavior, with the highest probability of initial suicide attempt occurring at ages 12 and 15 (Brodsky et al., 2001; Leverich et al., 2002; Molnar et al., 2001). Suicidal ideation and suicidal behavior tend to be the most prevailing symptoms reported upon admission to an inpatient psychiatric facility. Further, they are more commonly associated with abused males than with nonabused psychiatric inpatients, a subpopulation with established rates of higher suicidality than the general population (Brown & Anderson, 1991).

The rate of suicidal behavior among males with histories of CSA generally ranges from 10% to 55% (Bagley et al., 1994; Briere et al., 1988; Chandy, Blum, & Resnick, 1997; Friedman et al., 2002; Hibbard et al., 1990; Lisak, 1994a; Livingston et al., 1993; Mendel, 1995; Molnar et al., 2001; Ratner, et al., in press; Roane, 1992). The lower figures correspond to samples composed of boys and the higher percentages coincide with adult populations. Among boys and adolescents subjected to multiple forms of abuse, a majority (68%) experience clinically significant suicidal ideation and a considerable minority (34%) report a history of suicide attempts (De Bellis et al., 2001).

With respect to abused boys experiencing depression and suicidality, their parents observe a constellation of indicative behaviors, among them withdrawal from family members, estrangement from peers, crying spells, malaise, and mood swings (Burgess et al., 1984). Abused adolescent males are significantly more likely than their nonabused peers to experience suicidal ideation and attempts at least once during their lifetime (Cavaiola & Schiff, 1988; Grilo et al., 1999; Janus et al., 1987; Ryan et al., 2000), more likely to report at least one suicide attempt within the past year (Sansonnet-Hayden et al., 1987), and, compared to younger children with histories of CSA, are more often depressed and suicidal (Adams-Tucker, 1985). Attempted suicide rates among this group often reach majority proportions. Similarly, adult males with histories of CSA are significantly more likely to consider suicide than nonabused males (Urquiza & Crowley, 1986), more likely to attempt suicide than nonabused males and abused females (Nelson et al., 2002; Robin et al., 1997), and more likely than nonabused males to have experienced hospitalization for suicidal ideations and actions (Bartholow et al., 1994). Finally, when compared to abused females, males with histories of CSA are significantly more likely to hold weaker survival and coping beliefs and less likely to fear suicide (Peters & Range, 1995; Spencer & Dunklee, 1986).

Psychiatric Diagnosis

The manifestation of psychiatric symptomology is not uncommon among boys, adolescent males, or adult males with histories of CSA. Comorbidity of psychiatric disorders is significantly more prevalent among abused males than their nonabused counterparts (Friedman et al., 2002; Swett, Surrey, & Cohen, 1990). As for boys, many do not warrant a *DSM* Axis I mental disorder, but rather a "Phase of Life or Other Life Circumstance Problem." The modal clinical syndrome tends to be adjustment disorder with depressed mood, followed by adjustment disorders with mixed disturbance of emotions and conduct, atypical features, mixed emotional features, disturbance of conduct, or anxious mood (Sirles, Smith, & Kusama, 1989). Of those with a mental disorder or clinical syndrome, cognitive, behavioral, and adjustment disorders greatly outnumber other diagnostic categories. Typically included are ADHD, oppositional defiant disorder, and conduct disorder (Ackerman, Newton, McPherson, Jones, & Dykman, 1998). Still, when compared to nonabused groups, abused boys evidence more schizoid/psychotic symptoms (Sansonnet-Hayden et al., 1987) and ideas of reference (Livingston et al., 1993).

With respect to adolescent males, they are more likely to be diagnosed with a clinical syndrome than younger children with similar abuse histories (Sirles et al., 1989) and more likely to experience obsessive tendencies to a greater extent than younger counterparts (Gomes-Schwartz et al., 1985). Relative to nonabused peers, male adolescents with histories of CSA evidence an earlier onset of Axis I and Axis II disorders as well as more rapid cycling frequencies (Leverich et al., 2002).

In keeping with the additive effects of CSA, adult males with abuse histories, on average, are more likely to evidence more comorbidity, that is, more lifetime Axis I and Axis II disorders (Leverich et al., 2002), more likely to be diagnosed with three or more psychiatric disorders, excluding alcohol dependence or abuse, than nonabused males (Robin et al., 1997), and more likely to experience somatization, obsessive-compulsive disorder, and paranoia well into the clinical range (Collings, 1995). Higher lifetime rates of PTSD and obsessive-compulsive disorder correlate with males who consider themselves to have been sexually abused, while higher lifetime rates of substance abuse correspond to males (with histories of abuse) who do not consider themselves to have been abused (Fondacaro et al., 1999). Additionally, a considerable minority (45%) of adult males are prescribed psychotropic medication with antidepressants, tranquilizers, and/or antianxiety drugs as the most frequently identified categories. Finally, a minority (21%) of adult males with histories of CSA have been hospitalized for psychiatric purposes (Mendel, 1995).

Personality Disorders

The diagnoses of personality disorders are significantly more prevalent among adult males with histories of CSA than nonabused contemporaries. Within this population, the most common *DSM* Axis II diagnoses are borderline personality disorder, antisocial personality disorder, and avoidant personality disorder, as well as other personality disorders with self-defeating features (Ackerman et al., 1998; Brown & Anderson, 1991; Fondacaro et al., 1999; Leverich et al., 2002; Robin et al., 1997; Stein et al., 1988).

Posttraumatic Stress Disorder

Boys, adolescent males, and adult males with histories of CSA are significantly more apt to develop and manifest symptoms associated with posttraumatic stress disorder (PTSD) (and not necessarily the disorder itself) than nonabused males (Ackerman et al., 1998; Bagley et al., 1994; Boney-McCoy & Finkelhor, 1995a, 1996; Briere et al., 1988; Brown, Lourie, Zlotnick, & Cohn, 2000; De Bellis, Keshavan, et al., 1999; Fondacaro et al., 1999; McClellan et al., 1995; McLeer et al., 1998; Robin et al., 1997; Widom, 1999). Upon traumatization, children and adolescents are approximately 1.5 times more likely to manifest PTSD symptomology than adults (Fletcher, 1996). However, CSA, in and of itself, is neither necessary nor sufficient for the development of PTSD (Widom, 1999). Although it is not uncommon for sample rates of PTSD to approximate or exceed majority proportions, this diagnosis is substantially more common among females with abuse histories than among their male counterparts (Ackerman et al., 1998; Kessler, Sonnega, Bromet, Hughes, & Nelson, 1995; Kiser, et al., 1988; Livingston et al., 1993; Wolfe et al., 1994; Zlotnick, Zimmerman, Wolfsdorf, & Mattia, 2001). Still, PTSD remains the most frequently applied diagnosis for males with histories of CSA, with most studies rendering rates between 25% and 35% (Ackerman et al., 1998; Brown et al., 2000; Forbey et al., 2000; Kilpatrick & Saunders, 1997; McLeer et al., 1998; Mulder, Beautrais, Joyce, & Fergusson, 1998; Ruggiero, McLeer, & Dixon, 2000; Widom, 1999). Even when a male with an abuse history does not meet the requirements for frank PTSD, he is still likely to manifest a constellation of its reexperiencing, avoidance/numbing, and/or hyperarousal symptomology.

Traumatic stress incites the following threats among children: threats against the child's life, fears about physical harm, concerns over the safety of attachment figures, threats to the self-image, and a sense of isolation surrounding these threats and fears (Kiser, et al., 1988). A history of CSA, the experience of physical assault by a family member, and a prior kidnap attempt are all associated with greater levels of PTSD-related symptomology. In terms of CSA dynamics and effects, the following are correlated with higher levels of PTSD-related symptomology: fear of serious injury or death during a CSA episode, penetration, the severity of injuries sustained, the perpetrator's use of drugs or alcohol at the time of the abuse, and the occurrence of perpetrator threats (Boney-McCoy & Finkelhor, 1995a).

Common PTSD symptomology experienced by boys (Roane, 1992; Wolfe et al., 1994), adolescent males (Boney-McCoy & Finkelhor, 1995a, 1995b; Burgess et al., 1987), and adult males with histories of CSA (Briere et al., 1988; Roesler & McKenzie, 1994) includes intrusive thinking, trouble falling asleep due to intrusive imagery, dreams or nightmares with abuse content, wanting to cry when thinking about the abuse, avoidance of thinking, avoidance of associations to the abuse, anticipation of deteriorating life circumstances, lack of trust, and social withdrawal from family and friends. Both individuals with PTSD in full operation and individuals with partial symptomology evidence significantly greater interference with workplace functioning, educational pursuits, family relations, and social functioning than individuals with fewer manifestations of PTSD symptomology (Stein, Walker, Hazen, & Forde, 1997). In general, females are at least twice as likely to meet the full criteria for PTSD than males whereas males are significantly more likely to experience comorbidity, particularly with mood, affective, and attention-deficit hyperactivity disorders, than females (Ackerman et al., 1998; Kessler et al., 1995; Zlotnick et al., 2001). Finally, PTSD is more likely to be diagnosed among older sexually abused children who experienced a greater frequency of sexual abuse, longer duration of sexual abuse, perpetration by a nonparent, subjection to other forms of child abuse, disclosure to someone other than their mother, and abuse-related guilt and self-blame (see, e.g., Ruggiero et al., 2000; Wolfe et al., 1994).

Trauma Symptoms

Trauma symptoms commonly detected among males with histories of CSA, although not necessarily sufficient in scope or number to render a diagnosis of PTSD, include the following: (a) reexperiencing the abuse through intrusive thoughts and flashbacks; (b) vivid memories and dreams of the abuse with content revolving around the return and/or retaliation of the perpetrator and actualization of the threats made during the abuse; (c) excessive autonomic arousal and hyperalertness; (d) thinking, feeling, and/or acting as if the abuse is recurring in response to benign stimuli; (e) avoidance of activities that trigger recollections about the abuse; (f) intensification of symptoms upon exposure to events that symbolize or resemble the abuse; (g) distress reactions to demonstrations of affection from parents or loved ones; (h) abuse-specific and generalized fears; (i) diminished responsiveness to others; (j) blanking out; (k) internalized and externalized stress reactivity; and (l) acute or generalized panic responses. Males with histories of CSA are significantly more likely to experience these trauma symptoms than nonabused males and corresponding normative samples (see, e.g., Burgess et al., 1984; Burgess et al., 1987; Deblinger et al., 1989; Gomes-Schwartz et al., 1985; Janus et al., 1987; Kiser et al., 1988; McLeer et al., 1998; Roesler & McKenzie, 1994). Finally, in a study assessing trauma symptomology (by category) among sexually abused children within 1 to 2 months following disclosure and termination of CSA, a majority (65%) reported a minimum of one reexperiencing symptom, 58% disclosed at least two symptoms of autonomic hyperarousal, and a considerable minority (44%) experienced three or more avoidant symptoms. Further, sexually abused children were significantly more likely to manifest symptomology across all three categories than two nonabused control groups, one comprised of psychiatric patients and the other nonclinical in nature (McLeer et al., 1998). Trauma symptoms emerge quickly and may amplify, recede, and surge up again over time (van der Kolk & Fisler, 1995).

Dissociative Experiences

In both clinical and nonclinical samples, boys, adolescent males, and adult males with histories of CSA experience and exhibit more dissociative symptoms and states than nonabused males, with many studies reporting results well into the clinical range, especially when the abuse involved attempted or actual intercourse and/or when coupled with a history of physical abuse (see, e.g., Bagley et al., 1994; Briere et al., 1988; Chu & Dill, 1990; De Bellis et al., 1999b; Deblinger et al., 1989; Draijer & Langeland, 1999; Fontenella et al., 2000; Gill & Tutty, 1999; Kirby, Chu, & Dill, 1993; Kisiel & Lyons, 2001; Macfie, Cicchetti, & Toth, 2001; Mulder et al., 1998; Roesler & McKenzie, 1994; Sanders & Giolas, 1991; Zlotnick et al., 1994). In fact, childhood trauma, including CSA, predicts dissociative experiences at all developmental levels (Ogawa, Stroufe, Weinfield, Carlson, & Egeland, 1997). Further, dissociation is associated with abuse-generated internalizing and externalizing symptomology among both girls and boys (Macfie et al., 2001; Wherry, Jolly, Feldman, Balkozar, & Manjanatha, 1994). Such symptomology appears to increase with age (Hornstein & Putnam, 1992). Nevertheless, subjection to CSA is a necessary but not fully sufficient condition for the development of a dissociative diagnosis (Ogawa et al., 1997).

Peridissociation is a common coping strategy unconsciously employed during the abuse and shortly thereafter (Adams-Tucker, 1985). As a matter of course, it manifests in memory lapses, conversion symptoms, trancelike episodes, derealization, and depersonalization (McClellan et al., 1995). Symptoms like these significantly correlate with the ways in which a boy interprets and consequently responds to CSA (Morgan et al., 2001). Dissociation, between sexually abusive episodes and long after the last, correlates with sensory, kinesthetic, and affective reexperiencing of the abuse history and is often associated with gaps in narrative autobiographical memory and self-soothing behaviors that promote coping in the short term but self-destruction in the long term. Finally, the depth and degree of peridissociation at the time of the abuse is a risk factor for the subsequent manifestation of PTSD (Bremner et al., 1999; van der Hart & Nijenhuis, 1999); further, dissociation appears to be a mediating factor between subjection to CSA and numerous mental health outcomes, particularly in terms of risky, injurious, and destructive behaviors (Chu, Frey, Ganzel, & Matthews, 1999; Kirby et al., 1993; Kisiel & Lyons, 2001). In essence, the boy's response to CSA will significantly condition the composition of his psychobiological reactions to subsequent stressors (Morgan et al., 2001). Among dissociative symptomology, derealization, depersonalization, identity alteration, and identity confusion tend to significantly outnumber severe amnesia symptoms (Carrion & Steiner, 2000).

Recovered Memories

Amnesia and delayed recall transpires across a number of traumatic events but significantly more so for experiences involving interpersonal maltreatment such as childhood sexual abuse (Brown, Scheflin, & Hammond, 1998; Elliott, 1997). An evolving body of more than 40 studies, including case, clinical, and nonclinical samples, as well as those with prospective and random-selection designs (with the later investigations addressing the methodological weaknesses and criticisms of the earlier ones), every study reported the occurrence of at least one case of full or partial amnesia for childhood sexual abuse. What's more, substantial to vast proportions of participating males, usually in the range of 75% to 100%, are able to authenticate their abuse histories with historic and/or contemporaneous corroboration (Brown et al., 1998; Burgess, Hartman, & Baker, 1995; Feldman-Summers & Pope, 1994; Scheflin & Brown, 1996; van der Kolk & Fisler, 1995; Widom & Morris, 1997). Accuracy rates of CSA memories also tend to be the same whether continuously remembered or delayed (Dalenberg, 1996; Scheflin & Brown, 1996; van der Kolk & Fisler, 1995). Delayed memories are most commonly triggered by intrapersonal, relational, or environmental cues reminiscent of the historic abuse experience (Elliott, 1997; Feldman-Summers & Pope, 1994).

Independent of childhood trauma, it is normative to recall once-forgotten memories from childhood (Melchert, 1996; Melchert & Parker, 1997; Melchert, 1998). Adults with abuse histories, in general, do not evidence an inferior capacity to recall childhood memories when compared to adults without such histories. Approximately one-fifth of individuals with histories of CSA give an account of recovering at least one memory related to the abuse (Elliott & Briere, 1995). However, there is a greater tendency among females, as opposed to males, to experience full or partial amnesia and to report recovering sexual abuse memories (Grassian & Holtzen, 1996; Melchert & Parker, 1997).

At this time, there is no evidence to support the social perception that a history of childhood sexual abuse is correlated with inferior or faulty memories of such trauma (Brown et al., 1998; Melchert, 1996; Melchert & Parker, 1997). In one recent study, only 7.4% of adults with histories of CSA reported memory impairment; the vast majority (93%) did not report problems with memories of their histories of CSA (Freyd, DePrince, & Zurbriggen, 2001). Although the bulk of studies on memories of CSA exclusively employ female paticipants, a growing number are incorporating males as well.

Across nonclinical and/or randomly selected and/or prospective samples incorporating a moderate cohort of males, the base rate of those with continuous memory ranges from 58% to 70% with a aggregate mean of 66%. Of studies reporting partial amnesia for some period prior to disclosure, rates range from 14% to 28% with a mean of 17%. Finally, the rates of amnesia, or significant periods of time without memories of CSA, range from 5% to 37% with an aggregate mean of 17% (see, e.g., Belicki, Correy, Boucock, Cuddy, & Dudlop, 1994; Bernet, 1993; Burgess et al., 1995; Dale & Allen, 1998; Elliott & Briere, 1995; Elliott & Fox, 1994; Fish & Scott, 1999; Gold, Hughes, & Hohnecker, 1994; Grassian & Holtzen, 1996, cited in Brown, Scheflin, & Hammond, 1998; Feldman-Summers & Pope, 1994; Melchert, 1996; Polusny & Follette, 1996; Widom & Morris, 1997). Thus, the most commonly reported type of abuse-related memory process is that of knowing about it but keeping it "out of mind" (Dale & Allen, 1998, p. 808). On average, the most frequently noted cues for the emergence of abuse memories include a sexual experience and observing a child of an age similar to the reporter's age at the onset of abuse, whereas the least frequently noted cues include psychotherapy. In fact, adults with delayed recall of their histories of CSA are no more or less likely than adults with continuous recall of their abuse histories to be in psychotherapy (Elliott & Briere, 1995). And individuals in therapy are just as likely and able to find corroborating evidence for their stories as are individuals whose memories return in other contexts and by other means (Feldman-Summers & Pope, 1994).

In terms of brain hemispheric activity, adults with histories of CSA, when compared to nonabused counterparts, evidence significant left-dominant asymmetry while recalling a neutral memory, with an abrupt shift to right dominance while recalling a traumatic memory. Nonabused adults do not exhibit significant asymmetry while recalling neutral or unpleasant memories, nor do they manifest significant shifts between neutral and unpleasant memories (Schiffer, Teicher, & Papanicolaou, 1995). CSA is associated with long-term deficits in verbal but not visual short-term memory (Bremner et al., 1995).

Upon recall, however, studies consistently reveal children and adults are able to specify the particulars of autobiographical memories and often with corroboration (Burgess et al., 1995; van der Kolk & Fisler, 1995; Widom & Morris, 1997). In many instances, the initial memories emerge implicitly, that is, in the form of sensory perceptions, somatic sensations, mental images, and affective states (Terr, 1996). Accordingly, the early narratives of the explicit-autobiographical memories tend to be fragmented (Grassian & Holtzen, 1996). Further, explicit-autobiographical memories, or memories of the facts of CSA as well as memories of the fear emanating from them, tend to be relatively accurate and remain constant over time (Christianson & Safer, 1996). The implicit memory of other emotions as well as dissociative intensity show a trend toward fluctuating with time (Zoellner, Sacks, & Foa, 2001).

Upon the emergence and acknowledgment of once dissociated abuse-related memories of childhood sexual abuse, adolescents and adults are likely to report an increase in symptomology, including cognitive and emotional intrusion, hyperarousal, depersonalization, derealization, panic, fear, and shame. (Burgess et al., 1995; Elliott & Fox, 1994; Grassian & Holtzen, 1996; van der Kolk & Fisler, 1995). However, when abuse-related memories emerge, the process is more akin to a reconnection with the past rather than the remembrance of once forgotten facts and meanings (Dale & Allen, 1998).

Perceptions of Others and the World

Adult males with histories of CSA are significantly more likely than nonabused males and abused females to perceive the world as a random, malevolent and hurtful place in which to live (Janoff-Bulman, 1989; Mendel, 1995). Males sexually abused as children are more likely than nonabused males to conclude that others don't care if they hurt you (Lisak, 1994a), are more likely to hold a general mistrust of others (Hunter, 1991; Kiser et al., 1988; Kolko et al., 1988), are more likely to feel as if they don't need anyone (Burgess et al., 1984), and are more likely to experience greater difficulty in identifying and interacting with supportive adults, male and female (Bartholow et al., 1994).

Self-Injurious Behavior

Self-injurious ideations and behaviors are more common among boys, adolescent males and adult males with histories of CSA than among their nonabused male counterparts (Hibbard et al., 1990; McClellan et al., 1995). These behaviors include mutilation, disfigurement, cutting, burning, excessive tattooing, scratching, biting, pounding, hairpulling, daredevil behavior, reckless behavior, repeated accidents, and self-destructive ideation (Pescosolido, 1989).

Substance Abuse and Smoking

Among males with histories of CSA who experience substance abuse as an effect, the vast majority (89%) begin to abuse drugs and alcohol after the first episode of sexual abuse (Holmes, 1997). Abused boys in elementary school and adolescent males with abuse histories, in comparison to nonabused peers, are significantly more likely to evidence substance abuse problems (Clark et al., 1997; Deykin et al., 1992; Grilo et al., 1999; Harrison et al., 1989; Rohsenow et al., 1988). Adult males with histories of CSA are significantly more likely to experience lifetime alcohol abuse/dependence than nonabused males (MacMillan et al., 2001; Nelson et al., 2002; Ratner et al., in press; Windle et al., 1995) as well as problematic substance abuse (DiIorio, Hartwell & Hansen, 2002). In fact, males abused as boys evidence an increased risk of substance abuse for all routes of administration. For example, they are up to 12 times more likely to inject drugs intravenously than their nonabused counterparts (Zierler et al., 1991). Finally, adolescent and adult males with abuse histories are significantly more likely than nonabused males to smoke cigarettes and begin to do so at an earlier age (Disorbio & Bruns, 1998; Nelson et al., 2002).

Eating Disorders

Adolescent and adult males with histories of CSA are more likely than nonabused males to encounter difficulties around compulsive eating behaviors and patterns (Chandy et al., 1997; Hernandez, 1995; Nagy, Adcock, & Nagy, 1994; Neumark-Sztainer & Hannon, 2000; Olson, 1990; Smolak & Murnen, 2002). More specifically, adult males with histories of CSA are significantly more likely to be diagnosed with full or partial-syndrome bulimia nervosa than nonabused adult females and significantly more likely to express a vulnerability for mood and anxiety disorders (Garfinkel et al., 1995). Compared to adolescent and adult females abused as children, adolescent and adult males with histories of CSA evidence a later age of onset, higher rates of premorbid obesity and greater frequencies of homosexual or asexual orientations (Carlat & Camargo, 1991; Carlat, Camargo, & Herzog, 1997). Common manifestations of eating disorders include compulsive eating rituals, worries about weight, bingeing, purging, erratic dieting, overeating, fasting, vomiting, and using laxatives, diuretics, and diet pills (Hernandez, 1995; Hibbard et al., 1990). Males with histories of CSA tend to be more underweight or overweight than nonabused peers (Hernandez, 1995) and are more apt to have excessive concerns about body image and masculinity presentation (Dimock, 1988; Pescosolido, 1989; Sansone, Gaither, & Songer, 2001; Wells et al., 1997).

Enuresis and Encopresis

Enuresis, or the involuntary discharge of urine, and encopresis, the involuntary impaction or discharge of fecal matter, are commonly reported in empirical literature focusing on the sexual abuse of boys (see, e.g., Allard-Dansereau et al., 1997; Burgess, et al., 1984; Dubowitz et al., 1993; Elliott & Peterson, 1993; Fontenella et al., 2000; Roane, 1992); however, rates and frequencies are rarely presented. In one study, a limited minority (16%) of encopretic patients had a history of CSA (Boon, 1991). More recently, a considerable minority

(36%) of boys with abuse histories in residential treatment experienced encopresis, 27 times the reported prevalence rate found within the general population of boys between the ages of 10 and 12 (Morrow, Yeager, & Lewis, 1997). Boys who experience encopresis also evidence physical findings of anal hyperpigmentation, loose anal sphincter, and poor anal tone (Spencer & Dunklee, 1986).

Self-Image and Self-Concepts Among Boys

Changes in a boy's self-concept during and following CSA are overwhelmingly negative (Adams-Tucker, 1985), as indicated by a loss in self-esteem, lack of self-confidence, and feelings of guilt and shame (Conte & Schuerman, 1987). As psychosexual development progresses, fears around body image and gender-related tasks and expectations increase and intensify (Sebold, 1987; Wells et al., 1997). There is also a tendency among abused boys to imitate and assume effeminate mannerisms (Spencer & Dunklee, 1986) long after a sense of masculine gender identity has been established.

Self-Image and Self-Concepts Among Adolescent Males

Adolescent males with histories of CSA experience more negative self-concepts, more negative self-worth, and more concerns about their appearance than nonabused males in the same age cohort (Hussey et al., 1992; Janus et al., 1987). Many male teens are ashamed of and frightened by the developmental processes and normative functioning that occur after the abuse (Pescosolido, 1989). Fear and shame in response to the growth and maturation of secondary sex characteristics and confusion between sexual orientation and gender identity are commonplace. Such negativity, fear, and confusion underlie one adolescent male's projection of an aggressive masculine identity and another's strident efforts toward presenting a neutral or desexualized self (Gill & Tutty, 1999; Pescosolido, 1989). A lack of self-confidence (Gomes-Schwartz, et al., 1985) coupled with a sense of gender inferiority (Spiegel, 1995) exist beneath the superficial aspects of obsession with physique, compulsive attention to a masculine, feminine, or desexualized presentation to the world, cross-dressing, overpowering peers, heightened homophobia, and preoccupation with teasing effeminate boys (Pescosolido, 1989).

Self-Image and Self-Concepts Among Adult Males

Negative self-concepts are the norm among adult males with histories of CSA (Mendel, 1995; Ray, 1996; Woods & Dean, 1985). Common images include "misfit," "outsider," "queer," "whore," "vulnerable," and "damaged" (Dimock, 1988; Gill & Tutty, 1999; Janoff-Bulman, 1989; Spiegel, 1997). A boy abused by a male perpetrator may not only feel stigmatized but come to label himself a "homosexual" as well (Finkelhor, 1981). A boy abused by a female perpetrator frequently marks himself as a gender outcast because he did not fulfill his socialized role expectations of initiation and desire (Etherington, 1997; Kasl, 1990). Such socially constructed labels adulterate a male's self-concept and promote a prolonged and enduring sense of alienation from self, others, and life tasks, goals, and aspirations (Lisak, 1994a).

Men abused as boys evidence a significantly lower sense of sexual self-esteem than abused females and nonabused males (Finkelhor, 1981). Further, they experience increased sexual self-concept confusion in terms of masculine, feminine, and androgynous/undifferentiated selves (Richardson et al., 1993). Low self-esteem and a diminished sense of self-efficacy are found well into the clinical range (Rew et al., 1991; Roesler & McKenzie, 1994).

Identity conflicts persist. Adult males abused as boys report and evidence more opposite gender trait identification than nonabused men (Hunter, 1991). An internalized sense of "badness" is expressed in core beliefs including "I am unacceptable," "My life is meaningless," and "I am unlovable," and through core feelings such as inferiority, shame, and dishonorment (Lisak, 1994a).

Academic Effects

Boys, adolescent males, and adult males with histories of CSA are significantly more likely to experience academic problems and difficulties than nonabused counterparts of both genders (Boney-McCoy & Finkelhor, 1995b; Burgess et al., 1984; Hibbard & Hartman, 1992; Wells et al., 1997; Wells et al., 1995). Additionally, abused boys evidence a significantly greater risk of performing poorly on IQ and other standardized tests and repeating a grade than abused girls and nonabused boys (Eckenrode, Laird, & Doris, 1993; Rogeness, Amrung, Macedo, & Harris, 1986; Rowe & Eckenrode, 1999; Sadeh, Hayden, McGuire, Sachs, & Civita, 1994). Further, when compared to abused girls, sexually abused boys are significantly more likely to meet the criteria for, and/or receive the diagnosis of, attention-deficit hyperactivity disorder (ADHD) (Ackerman et al., 1998; Famularo, Fenton, Kinscherff, & Augustyn, 1996).

For boys and teens, school-related problems and difficulties include attention deficits, cognitive deficits, difficulty concentrating, a significant and abrupt decline in grades, behavioral problems, problems with teachers and school officials, fear of showers and restrooms, withdrawal from school and extracurricular activities, delinquency, and truancy. Further, they are more likely to experience consequences such as placement into remedial or special education classes even with average or above-average intelligence scores, corporal punishment for misbehavior, the repetition of a grade or course, rejection by peers, and suspension or expulsion from school (see, e.g., Adams-Tucker, 1985; Dubowitz et al., 1993; Eckenrode, Laird, & Doris, 1993; Friedrich & Luecke, 1988; Friedrich, Urquiza, & Beilke, 1986; Hibbard et al., 1990; Janus et al., 1987; Lisak & Luster, 1994; Olson, 1990; Perez & Widom, 1994; Robin et al.,

1997; Ryan et al., 2000; Straus & Smith, 1990; Wells et al., 1997). Despite lower achievement scores than controls, boys with histories of CSA are significantly more likely than abused girls and nonabused peers of both genders to overestimate their competence in a number of academic areas in order to compensate for perceptions of low self-worth (Kinard, 2001).

Academic problems in childhood persist through adulthood as a history of abuse correlates with a record of undermined educational goals and substandard academic outcomes, both incongruent with potential (MacMillan, 2000). Problems in college encompass the following: withdrawing from classes, taking too many pass/fail classes, changing majors frequently, and dropping out (Lisak & Luster, 1994). Finally, adult males with histories of CSA, when compared to nonabused adults, evidence lower IQ scores, lower reading ability, lower intellectual ability, and lower educational accomplishment (Perez & Widom, 1994).

Attention-Deficit Hyperactivity Disorder

Recent studies suggest that attention-deficit hyperactivity disorder (ADHD) and PTSD are two of the most common disorders diagnosed among children with histories of CSA (Famularo et al., 1996; McLeer, Deblinger, Henry, & Orvaschel, 1992; McLeer, Callaghan, Henry, & Wallen, 1994; McLeer et al., 1998; Merry & Andrews, 1994; Rowan & Foy, 1993), with rates significantly higher than those found among nonabused children. More often than not, PTSD is reported as secondary to CSA, with ADHD as secondary to PTSD. The high rates of PTSD and ADHD comorbidity may be a function of extensive symptom overlap as well as the absence of differential diagnoses guidelines in the *Diagnostic and Statistical Manual-IV* (Weinstein, Staffelbach, & Baggio, 2000).

Workplace Effects

A sexually abused male's undermined academic performance holds implications for advanced educational and occupational achievement. Across a number of occupations and workplaces, males with histories of CSA earn approximately 14% less per hour than nonabused counterparts (MacMillan, 2000). In addition to academic challenges, fear and avoidant behaviors, two common effects of CSA, tend to generalize into the workplace as well (Gill & Tutty, 1999), making employment and careers difficult to initiate and maintain. In comparison to nonabused males, adolescent and adult males with histories of CSA are more likely to anticipate failure in the workplace, work compulsively, underachieve, hold a lower level position, experience conflicts with colleagues, supervisors, and administrators, generate an insufficient income, be terminated, and/or be unemployed (see, e.g., Bagley et al., 1994; Gill & Tutty, 1999; Janus et al., 1987; Lisak & Luster, 1994; Olson, 1990).

Relational Effects Among Boys

Interpersonal sensitivity, that is, a hypersensitivity to the attitudes and rejections of others, is more common among boys, adolescent males and adult males with histories of CSA than nonabused peers (see, e.g., Collings, 1995; Gomes-Schwartz et al., 1985; McLeer et al., 1998; Young et al., 1994). In contrast to nonabused children, and in terms of personal–social development, sexually abused boys exhibit significantly more problems with social interaction, negative and conflictual peer relations, and more social withdrawal (Adams-Tucker, 1985; Burgess et al., 1984; Conte & Schuerman, 1987; Dubowitz et al., 1993; Friedrich et al., 1986; Gale et al., 1988; Kolko et al., 1988; Young et al., 1994). Sexually abused boys also tend to be fearful of other males, play alone, and avoid group activities (Kiser et al., 1988; Wells et al., 1997).

Relational Effects Among Adolescent Males

Adolescent males with histories of CSA are significantly more likely than nonabused peers to experience difficulties, such as social discomfort and social alienation, with same-gender and other-gender relationships (Ben-Porath & Davis, 2000; Hibbard et al., 1990; Young et al., 1994), including a generalized fear of adult men (Briere & Runtz, 1990; Janus et al., 1987; Wells et al., 1997) and a generalized fear of adult women (Briere & Runtz, 1990; Gill & Tutty, 1999). Their consuming apprehension of socially engaging with peers promotes hypervigilance, avoidance, and social introversion (Dubowitz et al., 1993; Forbey, Ben-Porath, & Davis, 2000). Fear of male companions urges their withdrawal from engaging in activities that advance socialization and development, such as physical education, sports, Boy Scouts, and school dances; their fear of female peers prompts daydreams about dating and relating with girls rather than interacting with them (Pescosolido, 1989). These various forms or outcomes of social withdrawal, as well as tendencies for some to behave aggressively around peers, ultimately foster and sustain physical and emotional distance.

Relational Effects Among Adult Males

Among adult males sexually abused as boys, feelings of uncertainty about themselves in relationships, fears around the confrontive and aggressive behaviors of self and others, struggles and conflicts between trust and mistrust, discomfort around authority figures, and conflictual peer interactions frequently characterize their relational experiences (Gill & Tutty, 1999; Lisak, 1994a; Woods & Dean, 1985). Compared to nonabused males, men abused as boys are more likely to experience difficulty in initiating and maintaining friendships (Robin et al., 1997), more likely to have a history of conflictual relationships with family and authority figures (Hunter, 1991), and more likely to be removed, isolated, or distant from their families (Ray, 1996). They alienate themselves from others (Hunter, 1991) and are alienated by others (Woods & Dean, 1985).

The relational statuses of "single, never married" and/or "separated" or "divorced" are more prevalent among adult males with histories of CSA than nonabused males (Nelson et al., 2002; Ray, 1996; Robin et al., 1997). Males abused by adult females are significantly less likely to be married than adult males with histories of male perpetrated abuse (Duncan & Williams, 1998). Female-perpetrated abuse often engenders, within the male, a sense of help-lessness in his anticipation of future encounters with women (Lisak, 1994a). Male-perpetrated abuse frequently incites a sense of emasculation, inferiority, and shame (Dimock, 1988; Hunter, 1991). Social anxiety (Nelson et al., 2002) and feelings of intimidation around women (Burgess et al., 1987; Gill & Tutty, 1999) and men (Gilgun & Reiser, 1990; Pescosolido, 1989) are equally preva-lent. Both currently and historically, males with histories of CSA are signifi-cantly less likely to marry or to be in significant long-term relationships than nonabused adult men and women (Gold et al., 1997; Nutall & Jackson, 1994).

Among adult men sexually abused as boys, there is a tendency to sexual-ize relationships and to experience difficulty in initiating and maintaining rela-tionships based on mutual support and trust (Dimock, 1988). Many use sex as a strategy to avoid emotionally intimate relationships (Gill & Tutty, 1999). Adult gay males with a history of CSA experience greater conflict and discom-fort with their emotional and sexual attraction to other men than do nonabused gay males. Additionally, they are more likely than their nonabused counter-parts to have a sexual relationship with a woman and/or to live with a woman with whom they share a sexual relationship but not a marriage. However, compared to nonabused men, gay males with histories of CSA place greater importance on a sexually monogamous relationship (Bartholow et al., 1994).

Adult males abused as boys experience difficulty in maintaining a sense of relational stability with significant others. To cite an example, adult males score significantly higher in all areas than nonabused counterparts in terms of relational discord, defined as having affairs, the partner having affairs, abuse within relationships, and recurring conflicts over time (Lisak & Luster, 1994). A predominating relational pattern emerges; it typically begins with intense in-volvement, transitions to conflict and abrupt withdrawal, and ends with isola-tion from others, only to begin again (Dimock, 1988). Emotionally, when compared to nonabused males, adult males with histories of CSA are more likely to evidence an insecure attachment style with romantic partners; behav-iorally, they are more likely to insult or hit their partners in the midst of conflict (Styron & Janoff-Bulman, 1997).

Finally, there is a tendency for some males abused as boys to become involved with other adults in relationships that mirror the abuse dynamics they experienced as children (Dimock, 1988). For instance, adult males with histo-ries of CSA are more likely than nonabused males to have problems around relationship violence, that is, experiencing the violence of a partner (Duncan

& Williams, 1998; Olson, 1990) and/or participating in physical violence (Duncan & Williams 1998; Janus et al., 1987; Krug, 1988; Lisak & Luster, 1994). The imposed association between intimacy and abuse engenders the anticipatory fear of both (Lisak, 1994a).

Boys and Sexuality Effects

To a greater or lesser degree, the preponderance of studies included herein that examine CSA also assess its impact on at least one dimension of human sexuality. Compared to nonabused children and/or normative samples, pre-school-aged, school-aged, and latency-aged boys with histories of CSA exhibit significantly more hypersexuality and preoccupation with sex, as evidenced by the following: (a) developmentally advanced sexual knowledge; (b) precocious sexual behavior, as indicated by acting seductively, sexually suggestive dress and mannerisms, provocative gestures, and requesting sexual stimulation; (c) sexual behaviors, including compulsive masturbation, sexualized play with toys and dolls, and insertion of objects in the rectum and simulation of intercourse; and (d) other gender-based behavior, such as wishing to be and/ or acting like a girl. Quite often, expressions of developmentally incongruent knowledge and behaviors are conveyed in repetitive play. Some boys become involved in prostitution and pimping (see, e.g., Adams-Tucker, 1985; Burgess et al., 1984; Conte & Schuerman, 1987; Deblinger et al., 1989; Fontenella et al., 2000; Friedrich & Luecke, 1988; Friedrich et al., 1986; Gale et al., 1988; Hibbard & Hartman, 1992; Kiser et al., 1988; Kolko et al., 1988; Mian et al., 1986; Sebold, 1987; Urquiza & Crowley, 1986; Wells et al., 1997; Young et al., 1994). Boys abused prior to the age of 13 by an older person are four times more likely to be homosexually active than those who have no childhood homosexual experience at all (Finkelhor, 1981). Based on a comprehensive review of the literature (Kendall-Tackett, William, & Finkelhor, 1993), sexualized behavior and PTSD were the only two symptoms or diagnoses found more frequently among children with sexual abuse histories relative to nonabused children in clinical samples.

Adolescent Males and Sexuality Effects

Among adolescents, males with histories of CSA are significantly more likely than nonabused peers to experience sexual acting out (Cavaiola & Schiff, 1988), to be concerned about controlling sexual feelings (Hussey et al., 1992), and to overstate and sexualize their interactions with others (Pescosolido, 1989). These teenagers are more likely to masturbate compulsively, more likely to have consensual and voluntary sex at a younger age (Robin et al., 1997), more likely to have sex with both males and females (Bartholow et al., 1994), more likely to have multiple partners (DiIorio et al., 2002; Raj, Silverman, & Amaro, 2000), less likely to use condoms (Brown, Kessel, Lourie, Ford, & Lipsitt, 1997; DiIorio et al., 2002; Luster & Small, 1994; Mason, Zimmerman, & Evans, 1998), and more likely to have engaged in sex resulting in a pregnancy (Chandy et al., 1997; Hibbard et al., 1990; Luster & Small, 1994; Raj et al., 2000). Finally, adolescent males with histories of CSA are up to five times more likely than nonabused males to report a history of sexual coercion postabuse (DiIorio et al., 2002; Lodico, Gruber, & DiClemente, 1996) and eight times more likely than nonabused males and four times more likely than abused females to report a history of prostitution (Burgess et al., 1987; Chandy et al., 1997; DiIorio et al., 2002; Olson, 1990; Zierler, et al., 1991). The impact CSA on sexual risk behaviors appears to be greater for boys than girls (Raj et al., 2000).

Adults Males and Sexuality Effects

To be sure, CSA has a negative impact on the sexual functioning of adult males (Woods & Dean, 1985). Adult males with histories of CSA are more likely than nonabused males to have problems around sex (Dubowitz et al., 1993; Urquiza & Crowley, 1986), including diminished satisfaction with sexuality in general and a greater presence of sexual problems. Sexual dysfunctions and disturbances are well into the clinical range (Roesler & McKenzie, 1994; Stein, Golding, Siegel, Burnam, & Sorenson, 1988). As a group, adult males abused during childhood experience a statistically significant increase in nonorganic sexual dysfunctions as compared to nonabused males (Johnson & Shrier, 1987). Other sex problems include nausea and stomach cramping when engaging in sexual activity and feelings of panic and terror when contemplating or reflecting on sexual activity (Gill & Tutty, 1999).

Adult males with histories of CSA are more likely than nonabused males to have problems around hypersexuality and sexual compulsivity (Bartholow et al, 1994; Bruckner & Johnson, 1987; Johnson & Shrier, 1985; Olson, 1990). Abused as boys, adult males are more likely than nonabused males to engage in sexual activities with strangers or casual acquaintances, to change sexual partners frequently, to have multiple concurrent sexual partners, to have unprotected anal intercourse, and to engage in receptive anal intercourse with steady partners (see, e.g., Bartholow et al., 1994; DiIorio et al., 2002; Paul et al., 2001; Zierler et al., 1991). Problems of this kind are indicated by preoccupation with sexual thoughts, compulsive masturbation, sexual acts with other men at bookstores and restrooms. Such activities are often experienced as ego-alien and tend to engender feelings of shame, guilt, and remorse (Dimock, 1988). Additionally, adolescent and adult males abused as children are more likely than nonabused males to engage in sex work or to receive payment for sex in the form of money, drugs, food, and/or shelter (Bartholow et al., 1994; DiIorio et al., 2002; Lowman, 1987; Strathdee et al., 1996; Zierler et al., 1991). In many instances, the primary goal of sex is the partner's pleasure and orgasm with little or no regard for their own (Gill & Tutty, 1999).

Along with sexual behavior, adult males with histories of CSA employ more sexual fantasies than nonabused men. These fantasies involve consenting intercourse, forcing someone to have intercourse, being physically forced to have intercourse, participating in an orgy, and having sex with a stranger (Briere et al., 1994). Many fantasies encompass sexually abusive elements. Although masturbation and sexual fantasies hold primary focus (Lisak, 1994b), comparable fantasies utilized during sex with others are often a means to create the illusion of participation while maintaining a sense of detachment (Gill & Tutty, 1999).

A substantial majority of adult males abused as boys attribute their own sexuality as the primary "cause" of the abuse (Spiegel, 1997a). Some men have great difficulty in considering, identifying, and protecting their sexual boundaries. Sexual activity, later in life, often rekindles anxiety coupled with feelings of guilt and helplessness (Johnson & Shrier, 1987). In response, there may be an absolute and outright rejection of sexuality (Lisak, 1994a) or avoidance of sexual relations and activity for extended periods of time (Bruckner & Johnson, 1987; Gill & Tutty, 1999; Johnson & Shrier, 1985).

Homophobia

Regardless of perpetrator gender (Duncan & Williams, 1998; Spiegel, 1997b), boys, adolescent males, and adult males with histories of CSA commonly experience a sense of homophobia, as designated by a fear of gays, lesbians, and homosexuals, a fear of becoming homosexual and hostility directed toward gay people and institutions (Lisak, 1994a). Some experience a fear of becoming homosexual if they were abused by a male (Pierce & Pierce, 1985). That same fear is prominent among boys abused by female perpetrators, but in this context, for failing to maintain the gender directives of initiation and desire (Spiegel, 1997a).

Sexually Transmitted Diseases

Sexually transmitted diseases (STDs) are included among the specific findings associated with CSA (Mian et al., 1986; Roane, 1992), particularly among children. One study reported an STD rate of 11% among sexually abused children, boys and girls (McLeer et al., 1998). In general, the prevalence rate of all STDs among boys with sexual abuse histories is approximately 5% (Ingram, Everett, Lyna White, & Rockwell, 1992) with a range of 3% to 20%, depending on sampling procedures and sample size (Ingram et al., 1992; Lindsay & Embree, 1992; Rimsza & Niggemann, 1982; Tilelli, Turek, & Jaffe, 1980). Across studies, prevalence rates of STDs in prepubertal children tend to converge around 4%, whereas STD rates among postpubertal children approximate 14% (Botash, 2000).

Gonorrhea is the most frequently diagnosed STD among children who have been sexually abused (Desenclos, Garrity, & Wroten, 1992). Concerning children who acquired HIV disease as a result of CSA, a considerable minority (approximately 33%) were coinfected with gonorrhea and syphilis (Gellert et al., 1993). The preponderance of boys with STDs are younger than 5 (Spencer & Dunklee, 1986). Among late adolescent and adult males with histories of CSA, the frequency of positive syphilis serology is significantly greater than that of nonabused males (Bartholow et al., 1994).

HIV Disease

As a mode of HIV transmission, CSA is most likely underestimated, given that its occurrence is difficult to detect without testing (Hammerschlag, 1998). In one study, among 96 children between the ages of 2 and 15 and all with HIV disease, a limited minority (15%) had documented histories of CSA (Gutman, St. Claire, & Weedy, 1991). In another study, a history of CSA was identified as the mostly likely source of transmission for a majority (68%) of HIV-positive children evaluated for childhood sexual abuse (Gellert et al., 1993). Within the general population, it is estimated that the crude rate of HIV infection among children with histories of CSA is 5 per 1,000 (Gellert et al., 1993). In evaluating reports by state and local health departments to the national HIV/AIDS surveillance system, it was found that 26% children with HIV disease had histories of CSA (Lindegren et al., 1998). The mean age at HIV diagnosis tends to be greater for sexually abused children—9.5 years—than for children with HIV disease attributable to blood transfusion (5.5 years) and perinatal transmission (1.8 years) (Lindegren et al., 1998). Children with HIV disease frequently live in home environments characterized by frequent separations, absent biological parents, substance abuse, domestic violence, disabilities, and caretaker illness (Gutman, Herman-Giddens, & McKinney, 1993; Lindegren et al., 1998; Rimsza, 1993)—characteristics also associated with the family environments of sexually abused children.

Adolescent and adult males with histories of CSA, in contrast to nonabused peers, exhibit significantly less knowledge about HIV, less condom self-efficacy (or the perceived cognitive and emotional capacity to use condoms under difficult or incompatible circumstances), less impulse control, and less frequent procurement and use of condoms, as well as significantly higher rates of sexually transmitted diseases (Brown et al., 1997; Brown et al., 2000). Adult males with histories of CSA have at least a twofold increase in the occurrence of HIV disease than nonabused males (Bartholow et al., 1994; Zierler et al., 1991).

Common effects of CSA, such as chronic depression, substance abuse, sexual compulsivity, and subsequent sexual abuse, tend to act as barriers to HIV education and intervention (Allers, Benjack, White, & Rousey, 1993). A history of CSA is significantly associated with the HIV risk behaviors of receptive and unprotected anal intercourse, unprotected sex with multiple partners, choosing a known and identified risk-taking partner, engaging in prostitution, and continuation of these behaviors as young males transition from adolescence through young adulthood (Bartholow et al., 1994; Carballo-Dieguez & Dolezal, 1995; Cunningham, Stiffman, Doré, & Earls, 1994).

A history of CSA correlates with an impaired sense of self-efficacy as well as deficient sexual decision-making skills and HIV preventive communication skills. CSA effects that may promote one's risk of HIV transmission include a lack of anxiety regarding AIDS transmission, high rates of self-mutilation involving the sharing of cutting instruments, high prevalence of drug use, high rates of sex with multiple or high risk partners, and inconsistent condom use (Brown et al., 1997).

Behavioral Problems

The two most common behavioral disorders among boys with histories of CSA are conduct disorder and oppositional-defiant disorder (Friedrich & Luecke, 1988; Livingston et al., 1993). A recent trend indicates that sexually abused boys score significantly higher than nonabused boys for both internalizing and externalizing behaviors (Bagley et al., 1994; De Bellis, Keshavan, et al., 1999; Dubowitz et al., 1993; Friedrich et al., 1986; Hibbard & Hartman, 1992; Mian et al., 1986; National Research Council, 1993). Generally speaking, common behavioral problems include noncompliance, acting out, demanding attention, disruptive behaviors, and antisocial behaviors (Adams-Tucker, 1985; Conte & Schuerman, 1987; Gomes-Schwartz et al., 1985; Hibbard & Hartman, 1992; Mian et al., 1986; Sansonnet-Hayden et al., 1987).

Boys and adolescent males with histories of CSA exhibit a greater deficit in socially-valued behaviors post-abuse than nonabused males (Burgess et al., 1987; Young et al., 1994). They also display an increase in hypermasculine risk-taking behaviors, including jumping from roofs, weaving bicycles through traffic, picking fights with "tough kids," and holding onto the bumpers of moving cars (Burgess et al., 1984). Other behavioral effects include hyperactivity (Dubowitz et al., 1993; Friedrich et al., 1986), firesetting (Burgess et al., 1984; Sebold, 1987), and unexplained and frequent "accidents" (Cavaiola & Schiff, 1988; Pescosolido, 1989).

Aggression Among Boys

Subsequent to abuse and its disclosure, aggression is a common effect (Conte & Schuerman, 1987; Friedrich et al., 1986). Compared to nonabused peers and abused girls, boys with histories of CSA are significantly more likely to be unresponsive to authority, more resistant to social mandates around personal control (Gale et al., 1988), and more likely to direct anger and aggression toward parents and other children (Burgess et al., 1984; Kiser et al., 1988). They are also more likely to exhibit argumentativeness, fighting, hitting, biting, spitting, impulsivity, temper outbursts, attacking behaviors, controlling behaviors, destructive behaviors, and animal cruelty (Brodsky et al., 2001; Dubowitz et al., 1993; Fontenella et al., 2000; Friedrich et al., 1986; Gomes-Schwartz et al., 1985; Grilo et al., 1999; Hibbard & Hartman, 1992; Young et al., 1994).

Aggression Among Adolescent Males

Adolescent males with histories of CSA are significantly more likely than non-abused teen males to experience difficulty with aggression (Burgess et al., 1987; Garnefski & Diekstra, 1997; Hibbard et al., 1990), anger outbursts directed toward others (Burgess et al., 1987), and disregard for familial, social, and legal rules and policies (Gale et al., 1988). More specifically, they are significantly more inclined than nonabused adolescents to fight with friends, participate in group fighting, and engage in other forms of physical violence (Burgess et al., 1987; Chandy et al., 1997). In addition, they are more apt to steal, break, and/or destroy property and to participate in animal cruelty (Burgess et al., 1987; McClellan, Adams, Douglas, McCurry, & Storck, 1995). Also, adolescent males with histories of CSA are significantly more likely than nonabused peers to experience homicidal ideation and to carry a weapon (Cavaiola & Schiff, 1988; Nagy et al., 1994).

Aggression Among Adult Males

Adult males with histories of CSA evidence a greater tendency than nonabused males to have problems with aggression, anger management, and rage control (Brodsky et al., 2001; Collings, 1995; Olson, 1990). In fact, anger is one of the most common effects of CSA (Stein et al., 1988). Adult men abused as boys are more likely to feel resentment and anger, to experience a desire to hurt others, to take tension out on others, and to steal, break, and/or destroy property (see, e.g., Hunter, 1991; Rew et al., 1991; Robin et al., 1997; Urquiza & Crowley, 1986). More often than not, adult males abused as boys are fearful of aggression and anger—of discovering its existence, of suppressing it, of its violent fantasies, and of losing control (Lisak, 1994a).

Regression

Regression, that is, the transitory loss of previously acquired developmental skills such as toilet training, information processing, and language, as well as other developmental disturbances, has been explored in a few studies. Common indicators include infantile behavior, social skill deficits, and impediments toward the development of coping skills and intellectual, physical, and social maturity (see, e.g., Fontenella et al., 2000; Gomes-Schwartz, Horowitz & Sauzier, 1985; Pescosolido, 1989; Sebold, 1987; Spencer & Dunklee, 1986).

Running Away

Adolescent males with histories of CSA are significantly more likely than non-abused adolescents to run away from home (Burgess et al., 1987; Cavaiola & Schiff, 1988; Chandy et al., 1997; Hibbard et al., 1990; Robin et al., 1997). The mean age at which boys runaway for the first time ranges between years 13 and 14 (Janus et al., 1987; Tyler et al., 2001). The substantial majority (75%) of adolescent males with histories of CSA who run away report doing so an average of 10 times (Tyler et al., 2001). A history of CSA significantly and positively correlates with running away, homelessness, affiliating with deviant peers, substance abuse, suicidal ideation, engaging in survival sex, and experiencing subsequent sexual abuse on the streets (Kipke, Unger, O'Connor, Palmer, & LaFrance, 1997; Rew, Taylor-Seehafer, & Fitzgerald, 2001; Rotheram-Borus et al., 1992; Tyler et al., 2001). A limited minority (11%) of runaway males with histories of CSA trade sex in order to survive (Tyler et al., 2001). Finally, relative to all other forms of child abuse and neglect, a history of CSA is significantly associated with running away among children with and without disabilities (Sullivan & Knutson, 2000b).

Sleep Disturbances

Disturbances in sleep frequently manifest in males with histories of CSA, both prior to and after disclosure, and extend across the life span. Sleep disturbances include nightmares, night terrors, difficulty falling asleep, sleep walking, waking up frequently, fear before falling asleep and fear upon awakening. (see, for example, Adams-Tucker, 1985; Briere et al., 1988; Burgess et al., 1984; Dubowitz et al., 1993; Fontenella et al., 2000; Glod, Teicher, Hartman, & Harakal, 1997; Hibbard & Hartman, 1992; Hibbard et al., 1990; Kiser et al., 1988; McClellan et al., 1995; Mian et al., 1986; Spencer & Dunklee, 1986; Wells et al., 1997). When compared to nonabused and/or depressed children, boys with histories of CSA are twice as likely to exhibit greater levels of sleep latency, nocturnal activity, and lower levels of sleep efficiency. Further, abused children discharge significantly greater amounts of their total daily activity throughout the night (Glod et al., 1997).

Self-Blame

Self-blame appears to be a universal effect of childhood sexual abuse (Lisak, 1994a; Spiegel, 1995; Woods & Dean, 1985). More specifically, the vast majority (approximately 89%) of males with histories of CSA blame themselves for failing to prevent the abuse, for not stopping it, for feeling pleasure, for their physiological reactions, and for possessing an attribute that "caused" it in the first place. Boys, adolescent males, and adult males experience a number of core value conflicts as evidenced by struggles around reconciling the occurrence of abuse and their role and responsibility in it, self-blame and perpetrator responsibility, family loyalty in exchange for personal autonomy, gender integrity against personal honesty, and blaming the perpetrator versus the nonoffending caretaker (see, e.g., Adams-Tucker, 1985; Lisak, 1994a, 1994b; Spiegel, 1995; Woods & Dean, 1985).

Feelings

Boys, adolescent males, and adult males with histories of CSA show a greater tendency to experience aversive emotions than nonabused males (Burgess et al., 1987; Hibbard et al., 1990; Janus et al., 1987). Fear, guilt, and a sense of dishonorment are among the most common feeling states experienced by boys and adolescents at the time of the abuse and by adult males long thereafter (Mendel, 1995: Stein et al., 1988; Woods & Dean, 1985). Abuse-specific fear, over time, generalizes within and across various life contexts. Guilt is associated with a male's perceived failure to prevent the abuse as well as his physiological reaction. A sense of dishonorment stems from a male's perceived violations of gender role expectations.

Additionally, males with histories of CSA experience a number of other feelings and/or feeling states, both during and after the abuse. The following represent the most commonly cited in the literature: shock, terror, betrayal, sense of transparency, nervousness, self-reproach, sadness, despair, numbness, hypervigilance, suspiciousness, shame, revulsion, helplessness, diminished sense of self-efficacy, a sense of isolation, and loneliness (see, e.g., Brown & Anderson, 1991; Burgess et al., 1984, 1987; Hibbard et al., 1990; Janus, Burgess, & McCormack, 1987; Lisak, 1994a; Mendel, 1995; Pescosolido, 1989; Rew et al., 1991; Spiegel, 1995).

Somatic Complaints

It is not uncommon for males with histories of CSA to report physical symptoms attributable to psychological and emotional distress rather than physical pathology. A narrow majority (59%) of males with histories of CSA manifest at least one physical symptom that cannot be explained in medical terms (Livingston et al., 1993). Boys, adolescent males, and adult males are more likely than nonabused male counterparts to experience somatization (Briere, Evans, Runtz, & Wall, 1988; Burgess et al., 1984; Dubowitz et al., 1993; Friedrich et al., 1986; Ryan et al., 2000; Spencer & Dunklee, 1986). In some instances, somatization leads to hypochondriasis (Hunter, 1991). Adults with histories of CSA, in contrast to nonabused controls, are more somatic and hypochrondriacal, expressing greater convictions around illness and disease. In fact, among adult males with abuse histories, reports of somatization, pain, injuries, chronic complaints, and doctor dissatisfaction are significantly more common when compared to nonabused counterparts (Disorbio & Bruns, 1998). Further, they report more doctor visits, more hospital admissions and more surgeries (Salmon & Calderbank, 1996).

Criminal Behaviors

Criminal behaviors are significantly more common among males with histories of CSA than nonabused males. They are more likely to report an involvement in stealing, destruction of property and vandalism, trouble with the law, an arrest history, appearances in juvenile court, appearances in adult court, and a history of incarceration (see, e.g., Burgess et al., 1987; Cavaiola & Schiff, 1988; Chandy et al., 1997; Garnefski & Diekstra, 1997; Hibbard et al., 1990; Janus et al., 1987; Olson, 1990; Robin et al., 1997). Children abused before the age of 12 are significantly more likely than their nonabused peers to be arrested as an adolescent for criminal behavior (Widom, 1995; Widom & Ames, 1994). This sustains through adulthood, as adults with histories of CSA are significantly more likely to be arrested for criminal activity relative to nonabused contemporaries (Widom, 1995). In a long-term cohort study, it was found that adults sexually abused as children, in contrast to adults without such histories, are 4.7 times more likely to be arrested for a sex crime and 10.2 times more likely to be arrested for prostitution. However, it must be noted that none of these arrests involved child molestation or abuse (Widom & Ames, 1994).

Miscellaneous Effects

Males with histories of CSA, irrespective of age, are less likely than nonabused males and abused females to have a viable sense of general well-being (Janus et al., 1987; Rew et al., 1991). They are significantly more likely than both comparison groups to have difficulties with finances and personal debts (Olson, 1990; Robin et al., 1997) and to evade or manipulate the truth (Robin et al., 1997). Other common but miscellaneous effects include a loss of spirituality (Rosetti, 1995), compulsive hygiene (Pescosolido, 1989; Sebold, 1987; Spiegel, 1997b), clinging behaviors (Mian et al., 1986), and problems associated with initiative and independence (Kiser et al., 1988).

Risk of Death

Children with reports of CSA evidence rates of subsequent death at a count of 7.6 per 10,000. The overall risk of death among children with histories of CSA is nearly three times that of their nonabused peers (Sabotta & Davis, 1992).

Coping

In many instances, children do not have access to typical means of protection via their parents; in lieu of such external resources, they develop internal strategies to cope with CSA, including denial, regression, withdrawal, and identification with the aggressor (Kiser et al., 1988), among others. Avoidance appears to be the most common coping response among boys with histories of CSA (Sigmon et al., 1996).

Sexually abused males differ significantly from nonabused males in manifesting avoidant feelings, such as trying to forget the sexual abuse, blocking out feelings around the sexual abuse, and avoiding people who remind them about the sexual abuse (Janus et al., 1987). Emotional expressiveness is the least common coping response (Sigmon et al., 1996), often inhibited by the ego defenses of acting out, psychic numbing, projection, and dissociation (Adams-Tucker, 1985; Kiser et al., 1988) along with significant daydreaming and fantasizing (Burgess et al., 1984). Denial, another common coping strategy among males with histories of CSA, is indicated by a reluctance to talk about the abuse and not wanting to be identified in any way with the abuse (Kiser et al., 1988) And sexualization, as a defense mechanism, manifests in children's reenactment behaviors and in posttraumatic play (Adams-Tucker, 1985).

In general, four main coping patterns emerge to the foreground: (a) integration of the event whereby the child masters anxiety about the abuse, believing the adult was not only wrong but also responsible for initiating and maintaining the abusive relationship; (b) avoidance of the event, whereby anxiety associated with the dynamics and effects of the abuse remains segregated both consciously and/or unconsciously; provided the boy is not under stress, life appears manageable as if the abuse never occurred; (c) repetition of the symptoms, wherein posttraumatic stress disorder becomes chronic; and (d) identification with the perpetrator, whereby the child introjects some characteristics of anxiety generated by the abuse and assimilates it by way of impersonating the perpetrator (Burgess et al., 1984).

Abuse Reactivity

Across studies, the proportions of CSA perpetrators with histories of CSA are not high enough to validate the socially constructed and popularly held "abused to abuser" paradigm (Bera, 1994; O'Brien, 1991). While studies with small samples tend to render high rates of sexual abuse perpetration among children—50% (Sansonnet-Hayden et al., 1987)—investigations employing larger samples are more likely to yield rates between 20% and 30% (Freund, Watson, & Dickey, 1990; Hanson, 1990; Hanson & Slater, 1988; Murphy & Smith, 1996). Still, the CSA field lacks consensus as to what may be categorized as developmentally expected sexual behavior and what constitutes abuse reactivity (Hall et al., 1998), and at what age or developmental stage abuse reactivity becomes a juvenile sexual offense.

Among children with sexual behavior problems severe enough to prompt state intervention, a substantial to vast majority (80% to 95%) of boys have documented histories of CSA (Friedrich & Luecke, 1988; Gray et al., 1999;

Ryan, 1995) and a narrow to vast majority (56% to 86%) experience multiple forms of abuse, including sexual, physical, emotional, and neglect (Friedrich & Luecke, 1988; Gray et al., 1999; Ray & English, 1995; Ryan, 1995). Of children with sexual behavior problems, more girls than boys disclose a history of abuse (Hall et al., 1998).

Regarding children younger than 7 years of age, those with sexual abuse histories are significantly more likely to engage in developmentally inappropriate sexual activity, including the placement of objects in the rectum and attempted intercourse with other children (Gale et al., 1988). As for sexually aggressive behaviors perpetrated against others, sexual touching and sexually inappropriate actions, including the use of sexually aggressive language and peeping, are more common than forced intercourse of any kind. Among children and adolescents with histories of CSA in sexual abuse treatment, only a limited minority (2%) perpetrated against others (Conte & Schuerman, 1987). A gender breakdown was not included in the report. In another study, a limited minority (8%) of boys with abuse histories repeated a similar act on another child, such as urinating on a classmate, inserting an object vaginally, or sodomizing a younger sibling (Burgess et al., 1984). And a limited minority (18%) of sexually abused boys involved with child protection teams recapitulated their abuse experience in one way or another (Roane, 1992). It appears that abused boys evidence significantly more sexualized behavior than abused females (Estes & Tidwell, 2002).

Concerning adolescents, a history of CSA is significantly more likely to be reported among sibling-incest perpetrators than nonsibling offenders (Worling, 1995). In other words, a narrow majority to majority—52% (Smith & Israel, 1987) and 63% (Worling, 1995)—of the sibling perpetrators have histories of CSA while a considerable minority (36%) of the nonsibling offenders report such childhood trauma. The evidence also suggests a significantly stronger relationship between a history of CSA and subsequent perpetration for girls than boys (McCarty, 1986; Knopp & Lackey, 1987; Johnson, 1991, all cited in Ray & English, 1995). Still, abused adolescents of both genders, when compared to their nonabused peers, are twice as likely to force sexual contact on a friend or a date and five times more likely to force and be forced into sexual activity (Lodico et al., 1996). Among mentally ill youth with histories of CSA, boys are significantly more likely to evidence offending behaviors whereas boys and girls are equally likely to exhibit sexually reactive behaviors (McClellan et al., 1997).

Still, the degree to which a history of CSA influences one's perpetration against children remains unknown. The empirical knowledge base, at this point in time, cannot endorse a strong or consistent association between a history of CSA and sexual perpetration against children. The evidence does suggest that while most sexual abuse perpetrators have not been subjected to CSA, the experience of CSA may be a risk factor in the perpetration against children (Hanson & Slater, 1988; Weeks & Widom, 1998; Widom, 1995). As a side note, the number of treatment programs for abuse reactive children and adolescents in the United States decreased from more than 1,000 in 1994 to less than 340 in 2000 (Paradise, 2001).

Sense of Legitimacy

Males of all age groups experience an incessant struggle to acknowledge their history of their abuse and its effects (Lisak, 1994a). Consequently, many males abused as boys experience difficulty in verbally expressing their accounts of the abuse (Kiser et al., 1988).

DIFFERENCES BETWEEN MALES AND FEMALES WITH HISTORIES OF CSA

A number of studies investigating CSA effects by gender report significant differences between males and females in terms of both dynamic and effects (Kendall-Tackett et al., 1993; Roane, 1992). However, in many studies employing subjects from each genders, researchers tend to use a symptom checklist that may not be sensitive to highlighting differences between males and females with histories of CSA (Gonsiorek, 1994). Differences are not highlighted here to suggest in any way that the abuse of one gender is more severe than the abuse of the other gender. Differences are important to note, however, in terms of research conceptualization, instrument development, child protection investigations, prevention programs, assessment guidelines, treatment goals and objectives, intervention selection, evaluation procedures, and social policy. Finally, and most consequentially, highlighting similarities and differences validates the authentic experiences of childhood sexual abuse—its dynamics and effects—as reported by males and females subjected to this form of childhood trauma.

At this point in time, the knowledge base, as indicated by the nearly five hundred research reports highlighted in this chapter, reveals the following differences. To begin, the likelihood of a perpetrator abusing a boy is five times greater than that of a girl. In other words, perpetrators of males tend to subject more boys to CSA and to abuse them more frequently. Relative to sexually abused females, males with histories of CSA are significantly more likely to: experience more severe forms of abuse; be physically abused by their perpetrator; be physically abused by someone other than their sexual abuse perpetrator; be exposed to pornography; be physically forced into a sexual abuse episode; be subjected to intercourse of any kind, anal penetration with a penis, and anal penetration with objects; be coerced into performing fellatio or cunnilingus on their perpetrator; be coerced into penetrating the perpetrator with their penis or an object; and experience genital violence or mutilation.

In terms of family as well as public perceptions, the male child is significantly more likely than a female child to: be viewed as responsible for his abuse experience; be perceived negatively upon disclosure; and to be viewed as gay, deviant, and a potential perpetrator.

When compared to the sexual abuse of females, the sexual abuse of males is significantly less likely to: be considered as a possibility; be acknowledged by an adult; be reported to a state agency; be reported by a source known to the boy; come to the attention of a child protection agency; be substantiated by a state agency. Consequently, the male child is significantly less likely to: be removed from the home if the perpetrator is a family member; be placed in protective custody; receive crisis intervention services and counseling; be involved in court action against the perpetrator; and to participate in therapy of any kind.

Relative to a sexually abused female, a sexually abused male is significantly less likely to: characterize the perpetrator-child interactions as sexual abuse; disclose the abuse at the time of its occurrence or during his lifetime; experience protection from the family if the abuse is disclosed; find support from his parents and siblings if the abuse is disclosed; experience parental concern about abuse-related effects, with the exception of worries around sexual orientation and homosexuality.

Regarding effects, sexually abused males are significantly more likely than sexually abused females to: manifest severe effects across multiple domains; manifest biological, neurological, physical, psychological, emotional, and behavioral problems within the clinical range; evidence inconclusive medical findings; experience such problems with a greater frequency; evidence smaller brain structures and brain volumes; experience higher levels of anxiety and greater frequencies of phobic symptoms; experience depression and suicidal ideation; consider suicide as a coping strategy; attempt suicide; be charged with a sexual offense in response to a sexual abuse reenactment; experience psychopathological co-morbidity; evidence higher rates of premorbid obesity; report greater frequencies of homosexual and asexual orientations; experience encopresis; evidence a negative sense of sexual self-esteem; experience academic problems, such as a decline in grades, poor test scores, inability to concentrate, and grade repetition; meet the criteria for attention-deficit hyperactivity disorder; be placed in remedial classes; overestimate their academic competence in order to compensate for perceptions of low self-worth; evidence sexualized behavior as a child even though the knowledge base suggests a stronger relationship between history of CSA and subsequent perpetrator for girls; be involved in prostitution; engage in sex that results in a pregnancy; evidence risky sexual behaviors; experience difficulties with aggression toward parents and peers; experience difficulties with personal finances; underestimate their workplace abilities and potential; and manipulate the truth about their abuse history.

And, continuing with effects, when compared to sexually abused females,

males with histories of CSA are significantly less likely to: receive a diagnosis of posttraumatic stress disorder; experience full or partial amnesia for their history of CSA; report the recovering of sexual abuse memories; and hold a viable sense of general well-being.

RISK AND PROTECTIVE FACTORS

The prevalence of child abuse and neglect, including childhood sexual abuse, increases from 3% when no apparent risk factors are present to 24% under conditions in which four or more risk factors are present (Brown, Cohen, Johnson, & Salzinger, 1998). The following risk and protective factors are presented within ecosystemic categories. Within the self-domain, a boy's risk of sexual abuse increases if and/or when: (a) He has strong unmet needs for constructive parental attention, affection, and care; (b) he has low self-esteem and low self-confidence; (c) he has a disability, any type of disability (see later discussion); and (d) he was previously subjected to CSA.

Relative to the microdomain or the family environment, a boy's risk of sexual abuse increases if and/or when: (a) His conception was unwanted; (b) his mother is very young; (c) he lives with a single mom; (d) his mother is employed outside the home; (e) one or both of his natural parents are deceased, absent from, or live outside his place of residence; (f) he lives with two nonbiological parents or caretakers; (g) he lives in a high-density household; (h) his parents or caretakers evidence dysfunctional marital relations; (i) the communication in the household is indirect and secretive; (j) he perceives a significant level of family conflict; (k) he is the child of a stepparent; (l) he is subjected to harsh punishment within the home; (m) one parent is seriously ill; (n) his mother evidences maternal sociopathy; (o) he is separated from a parent for extended periods of time; (p) he, as a young child, has little or no supervision around activities of daily living, such as bathing and dressing; and (q) his parents are not available, accessible, or competent as psychosocial resources for him.

With respect to the mesodomain, or community context, a boy's risk of sexual abuse increases if and/or when: (a) His parents are not involved in religious or spiritual activities within their community; (b) He has little or no supervision outside the home; (c) he tends to unquestionably trust and comply with adult authority outside the home; and (d) he and other children are exploited in order to meet the needs of caretaking adults, including relatives, neighbors, mentors, coaches, teachers, baby-sitters, and priests. Concerning the exodomain, or institutional policies and practices that directly impact a child, a boy's risk of sexual abuse increases if and/or when: (a) Groups and institutions negate and invalidate the sexual abuse of children, in general, and the sexual abuse of boys, in particular; (b) institutions fail to provide sexuality education and/or CSA prevention programs; (c) the city or county legal system has a record of minimizing the need to adjudicate and punish sex offenders; and (d) he is placed in foster or residential care as an intervention to protect him from further abuse within the home of origin (see, e.g., Benedict & Zautra, 1993; Berliner & Conte, 1990; Boney-McCoy & Finkelhor, 1995a; Brown et al., 1998; Burkhardt & Rotatori, 1995; Dubé & Hebert, 1988; Fergusson, Linskey, & Horwood, 1996a, 1996b; Finkelhor et al., 1990; Hobbs, Hobbs, & Wynne, 1999; Janoff-Bulman & Frieze, 1983; Moisan et al., 1997; Robin et al., 1997; Sobsey, Randall, & Parrila, 1997; Wurtele & Miller-Perrin, 1992).

Factors that may contribute to a boy's manifestation and severity of CSA effects include: (a) the duration of abuse; (b) the frequency of abuse; (c) penetration; (d) use of force; (e) use of weapons; (f) the boy's sexual arousal and ejaculation; (j) the coercive methods used to conceal the abuse; (h) the relational bond and dynamics between the boy and his perpetrator; (i) cognitive appraisals of self before, during, and after the abuse; (j) the degree of dissociation manifested during and after the abuse; (k) the amplification and duration of emotional states sustained during, and after the abuse; (l) cognitive appraisals of others and the world before, during and after the abuse; (m) the type of adaptive strategies employed to cope with the abuse; (n) the responses of others to the boy and his disclosure of abuse; (o) the degree of stress emanating from abuse-related events, such as child protection interviews, out-of-home placements, and legal proceedings; and (p) a protracted stress response (Beitchman, Zucker, Hood, daCosta, & Akman, 1991; Beitchman et al., 1992; Holmes & Slap, 1998; Kendall-Tackett, Williams, & Finkelhor, 1993; Pescosolido, 1989; Romano & DeLuca, 2001; Spiegel, 1997a, 1997b).

A Special Note on Children with Disabilities

Children with disabilities are significantly more likely than their nondisabled peers to be subjected to multiple forms of abuse, multiple episodes, and multiple perpetrators. Children with disabilities are 3.14 times more likely to be sexually abused than their nondisabled peers (Sullivan & Knutson, 2000a). Moreover, disabilities are risk factors for abuse, and abuse may engender a number of disabilities.

Boys are almost twice as likely as girls to experience developmental (cognitive and language) delays (Fontanella, Harrington, & Zuravin, 2000), mental retardation (Roane, 1992), and disabilities of any kind (Sobsey et al., 1997). In general, the prevalence of CSA among males with disabilities is greater than the prevalence of CSA among boys without disabilities (Sobsey et al., 1997). Compared to nondisabled and nonabused children, boys with mental retardation have four times the risk of sexual abuse, boys with speech and language impairments have three times the risk of sexual abuse, boys with behavior disorders have 5.5 times the risk for sexual abuse, boys with health-related disabilities have twice the risk of sexual abuse, boys with learning disabilities are twice as likely to be abused, and boys with orthopedic disabilities are twice as likely to be abused (Sullivan & Knutson, 2000a, 2000b). In the 6 to 11 age range, more males with disabilities are sexually abused than females with disabilities (Sobsey et al., 1997). All in all, children with disabilities, any type of disability, are more likely to experience CSA than children without disabilities (Sobsey et al., 1997).

That being so, children with disabilities may confront a number of dilemmas vis-à-vis disclosure. For example, their ability to visually identify the perpetrator, cognitively perceive the activities as abuse, or vocally or manually disclose its occurrence may be impaired. Further, subjection to CSA may exacerbate the stigma and vulnerability associated with their disability, making it less likely for them to disclose episodes of abuse. Finally, when compared to the disclosures of nondisabled peers, the disclosures of children with disabilities and histories of CSA may be viewed as less credible, given the information-processing styles and primary modes of communication coinciding with the various disabilities (Goldman, 1994; Sobsey et al., 1997; Sullivan & Knutson, 2000a, 2000b).

Protective Factors

Resilience or protective factors are conceptualized as the characteristics and the processes that foster successful adaptation in the face of challenging and threatening risk factors and existent circumstances (Masten, Best, & Garmezy, 1990; Rutter, 1987) such as CSA. Although this area of research, like many others associated with the sexual abuse of males, remains in an early developmental stage, a few studies have highlighted a number of protective factors against the development of adjustment difficulties—not against the occurrence of CSA. Tentatively, it appears that a minority (20% to 25%) of males with histories of CSA will not manifest severe sexual abuse effects (Finkelhor, 1990; Lynskey & Fergusson, 1997). Protective factors within the self domain include, for the boy: (a) above average intelligence or cognitive abilities; (b) developmentally accordant emotional functioning; (c) accessible knowledge about appropriate and inappropriate sexual behavior; (d) the capacity for secure and constructive attachments; (e) an internal locus of control; (f) the capacity to verbally or otherwise communicate internal states (e.g., thoughts, beliefs, curiosities, confusions, sensations, feelings, fears, physiological manifestations, etc.); (g) the ability to empathize with the internal states of others; (h) positive self-regard; (i) physical dexterity; (j) a sense of optimism; (k) a sense of faith and spirituality; (l) positive self-esteem; (m) ego resilience; (n) command of ego functions; (o) the attributes of persistence and assertiveness; (p) external attribution of abuse responsibility; and (q) the ability to relax and remain calm under pressure (see, e.g., Block & Block, 1980; Browne & Finkelhor, 1986; Cicchetti, Rogosch, & Holt, 1993; Egeland, Carlson, & Sroufe, 1993; Egeland &

Jacobvitz, 1988; Faust, Runyon, & Kenny, 1995; Heller, Larrieu, D'Imperio, & Boris, 1999; Herrenkohl, Herrenkohl, & Egolf, 1994; Lynskey & Fergusson, 1997; Rutter, 1987; Toth & Cicchetti, 1996).

Within the microsystem, protective factors include, for example: (a) the presence of maternal and paternal protection; (b) maternal care; (c) the expression of attention and affection from at least one parent or caretaker; (d) a sense of security within the home; (e) viable family relations; (f) clear and direct communication; (g) consistent and available supervision; (h) mutual respect for privacy and boundaries; (i) the teaching and modeling of practical problem solving; (j) economic consistency and security; (k) an enriching school experience; (l) positive peer attachments; and (m) extrafamilial support from teachers, ministers, and mentors. Microsystem protective factors vis-à-vis the sexually abusive relationship also entail the absence of the following: (a) physical restraint and/or violence during the sexually abusive episodes; (b) a family history of drug abuse, alcohol abuse, physical abuse, and sexual abuse; and (c) delinquent or substance-abusing peers (see, e.g., Block & Block, 1980; Browne & Finkelhor, 1986; Cicchetti et al., 1993; Egeland et al., 1993; Egeland & Jacobvitz, 1988; Faust et al., 1995; Heller et al., 1999; Herrenkohl et al., 1994; Lynskey & Fergusson, 1997; Rutter, 1987; Toth & Cicchetti, 1996). Such protective factors may mutually and reciprocally influence one another. For example, various cognitive abilities may contribute to academic achievement, which, in turn, may enhance self-efficacy, self-concept, and ultimately resilience (Cicchetti et al., 1993).

SUMMARY

A knowledge base of increasingly sophisticated empirical research on the sexual abuse of males is beginning to emerge. Numerous and diverse dynamics and effects have been identified across a range of research definitions, methodologies, and samples. However, it is critical to note that among the vast number of dynamics and effects highlighted herein, CSA remains a correlate rather than a linear outcome of dynamics or a casual agent of the effects. Investigators are only beginning to identify the numerous predisposing and mediating variables that may increase or decrease risk of CSA and that may ameliorate or exacerbate its multidimensional effects. Thus, at this point in time, it is premature to answer questions such as:

1. Did subjection to CSA "cause" a particular behavior?
2. Did the behavior in question predispose the boy to CSA?
3. Are CSA dynamics secondary and CSA effects tertiary to micro or macro system variables that create facilitating conditions for CSA?
4. Are the relationships among facilitating conditions, abuse dynamics and abuse effects temporal, causal, or coincidental (Simpson & Miller, 2002)?

The frank act of CSA, like many other ecological phenomena, and particularly more so given its personal and social concealment and invalidation, cannot be experimentally manipulated. Consequently, researchers, clinicians, preventionists, and policymakers evidence greater success in theoretically, rather than empirically, deciphering the dynamics and effects of childhood sexual abuse.

The issues, caveats, and difficulties associated with research around the sexual abuse of females are equally relevant to the sexual abuse of males. The National Resource Center on Child Sexual Abuse (Lipshires, 1994), as well as a number of researchers (Briere, 1992; Holmes & Slap, 1998; Kendall-Tackett et al., 1993), note that, due to the lack of standardization within some studies and the lack of consistency across studies in relation to conceptualizations, definitions, sampling procedures, research methods, and statistical procedures, stable statistics have yet to emerge. Investigators typically confront: (a) difficulty obtaining samples; (b) small samples; (c) bias as a result of recruitment in clinical settings; (d) overrepresentation of gay subjects; (e) underrepresentation of minority subjects; (f) overuse of university samples; (g) sample sizes that lack the power necessary to support multivariate and other more sophisticated statistical procedures; and (h) reliance on self-selection. To be sure, such issues inhibit generalizability and the use of state-of-the-art methodologies. In addition, problems regarding retrospective reporting, selective memory, and abuse corroboration impact research processes and outcomes. However, investigators must continue to push forward despite these challenges and obstacles.

The studies highlighted herein are diverse, in terms of the methodological and analytic strategies employed, and in their strengths and weaknesses. The majority employed some form of control or comparison group; a minority utilized none at all. Some of the studies used widely accepted measures, whereas others generated their own without conducting pilot or psychometric analyses. Additionally, the measures employed varied in type, including both parent and child reports, current and retrospective reports, patient and clinician reports, standardized and nonstandardized instruments, and generic and abuse-related instruments. Many investigators had to rely on samples of convenience; however, a few were able to utilize more rigorous sampling procedures. Finally, although all investigators employed some systematic form of data analysis, only a few had samples large enough, variables suitable enough, data disperse enough, and methods sophisticated enough to conduct multivariate analyses without violating major assumptions and power requisites. Thus, at this stage of knowledge development, the majority of effects highlighted in this chapter must be viewed as nonspecific correlates, rather than linear indicators, of childhood sexual abuse and the sexual abuse of males.

Finally, it is critical to note strengths as well. The sexual abuse of males knowledge base holds discerning conceptual frameworks (e.g., Burgess et al., 1984, 1987), population-specific reports reflective of the realities of CSA (e.g., Dimock, 1988), population-sensitive measures (e.g., Briere et al., 1988), methodologically rigorous sampling (e.g., Stein et al., 1988; Urquiza & Crowley, 1986) and comparison strategies (e.g., Cavaiola & Schiff, 1988; Gomes-Schwartz et al., 1985), state-of-the-art multivariate procedures (e.g., Conte & Schuerman, 1987; Spiegel, 1995), and highly honed analytic discussions (e.g., Finkelhor, 1981), among others. If investigators continue to build on these strengths, the knowledge bases of CSA in general and of the sexual abuse of males in particular will be rich indeed.

THE DEVELOPMENT OF THE SAM MODEL

In Response to Suggestions from the Literature

In 1986, Finkelhor suggested the development of a theoretical "framework based on the links between the experience of sexual abuse and the sequelae that have been widely noted [in the literature, thus] advancing our understanding of sexual abuse and mitigating the effects of these experiences on its victims" (p. 198). He also asserted that new theories serve to foster both intellectual excitement and interventive action—"two developments the field could desperately use" (Finkelhor, 1984, p. 221). Further, Finkelhor (personal communication, 1998) suggested that although the identification and documentation of child abuse effects remains far from complete, model building is both a necessary and critical step toward advancing our knowledge and interventive efforts.

Origins of the SAM Model

Responding to both the recent upsurge of studies and Finkelhor's call for theory development and model building, the SAM model of dynamics and effects was developed. The SAM model, presented in chapter 3, responds to the paucity of scholarly inquiry into this area and the critical need for understanding from a gender perspective.

The initial stage of model development progressed as follows. A critical review of the effects around the sexual abuse of males rendered a list of findings; a subsequent review of the dynamics associated with the sexual abuse of males generated another list. Still, these findings have not yet been classified and ordered into a framework that suggests the ways in which the dynamics and contextual characteristics around the sexual abuse of boys might foster the observed effects. The list of findings became a foundational element of the SAM model.

Next, several focus groups were conducted, composed of the following cohorts: boys with histories of childhood sexual abuse, adolescent males with histories of childhood sexual abuse, adult males abused as boys, and professionals working in the field of childhood sexual abuse. For the first three cohorts, their experiences were noted as to the dynamics and effects experienced upon confronting CSA. For the latter cohort, the presentation of effects in therapy was the primary focus. At this point, the foundational elements of the literature and the stories of males with histories of CSA were integrated to form model hypotheses and a substantial list of dynamics and effects.

A subsequent stage of this research endeavor included intensive, life-history interviews of 51 informants conducted for an average of 6 hours per participant over three or more sessions. Initially, data were generated from a semistructured interview protocol that focused on informants' current situation, family of origin, early history, description of childhood environment, a detailed history of the sexually abusive relationship, coping strategies, responses of others, and assessment of the effects.

For purposes of this discovery-oriented phase, childhood sexual abuse was conceptualized as (a) any sexualized activity (b) imposed on a male child under the age of 18 (c) that occurred within a relationship where it was deemed exploitive (by the boy) by virtue of an age difference, power differential, or physical, social, or developmental differences and (d) that occurred as a result of perceived threat or force. A second phase focused on a similar interview schedule with 50 male and female perpetrators of male sexual abuse. Data from phases 1 and 2 were combined to produce an initial model.

Components of the model and, finally, the model as a whole were then assessed. A public notice, stating the name, objectives, and affiliation of the study, was placed in a national newspaper. Interested males were asked to call an 800 phone number for further information or to schedule an interview appointment. Interviews lasted approximately 45 minutes, as a number of scales and qualitative questions were presented. Participants received no compensation for their contributions. More than 1,100 individuals, from 48 states, offered to participate. Various multivariate techniques, such as exploratory and confirmatory factor analysis, discriminant analysis, and multivariate analysis of variance, were employed. Subsequently, covariance structure modeling in pilot form was employed to test the validity, reliability, and efficacy of the model (Spiegel, 1997a, 1997b). Research findings from the national pilot study support the SAM model, as evidenced by its goodness-of-fit with the data, individual and collective reliabilities of the empirical indicators, and the significance of the paths among the latent variables.

Utility and Application of the SAM Model

Given this knowledge, frontline service providers can use the SAM model to design micro, meso, and macro level protocols. Whatever the mode, the practitioner can evaluate the psychosocial context of the abuse across the seven categories. By assessing the contextual dynamics, the worker can begin to postulate potential effects. Interventions, then, can be designed that both acknowledge the context from the boy's perspective and ameliorate the effects.

Clinicians can also assist caretakers, educators, and policymakers in under-standing sexual abuse from the perspective of male children so that family and social interactions, sexual abuse prevention programs, and social policies can effectively reflect the realities of childhood sexual abuse while deflecting its myths. Academicians may use this model to help students acquire knowledge and skill necessary to treat males with histories of CSA. And researchers may employ the SAM model as a conceptual framework for future studies, perhaps as a basis for developing and piloting biopsychosocial assessment protocols or formulating and validating a structural equation model based on emerging research.

ENDNOTE

This chapter highlighted the evolving literature concerning the sexual abuse of males and briefly illustrated the developmental processes employed to generate and validate the SAM model of dynamics and effects. Chapter 3 presents the assumptions undergirding the model. Chapter 4 introduces the model itself. Chapter 5, the last in Part I, applies the SAM model to seven demographically diverse cases.

CHAPTER THREE

Assumptions of the SAM Model

IN RECENT YEARS, the sexual abuse of males has received purposeful attention. Consequently, its knowledge base, although still embryonic, continues to develop. It holds a relatively small yet growing number of empirical studies, clinical reports, and reviews of the literature. There exists a need for a conceptual and empirical model that integrates data, articulates motive forces and emergent consequences associated with this psychosocial problem, and, most importantly, gives voice to males with histories of childhood sexual abuse (CSA). This chapter presents the assumptions undergirding The *sexual abuse of males (SAM) model of dynamics and effects*. Many of the assumptions have as their wellspring the rich and now classic literature of decades past.

ASSUMPTIONS

The SAM model represents a common denominator of the most frequently observed dynamics and effects associated with the sexual abuse of males. It is a systems model, encompassing self, micro, meso, and macro ecologies (Garbarino, 1981). Causation is viewed as multiple and multidirectional—not only among members of the systems but between the systems and the environment as well.

The self-system embodies the sexually abused male's cognitive, intrapsychic, affective, behavioral, and biophysical subsystems, to mention a few, as well as interrelations between and among these elements. The microsystem encompasses the primary environments in which an individual has direct interaction with both significant and nonsignificant others, including, but not limited to, home, school, work, peer group, church, and community institutions (Garbarino, 1977, 1981). In this context, the microsystem also represents the sexually abusive relationship, accentuating the roles, boundaries, and activities of the boy and his perpetrator(s). It may also include relationships between sexually abused males and significant others, for example, nonoffending caretakers, teachers to whom they disclose, or other boys in a sex ring.

The mesosystem points to similarities and differences, and congruencies and incongruities, across microsystems—for instance, between a sexually abused male and his perpetrator and between a sexually abused male and his family. Such relationships between microsystems convey the interactions and interrelations between and among two or more microenvironments in which the developing child actively participates (Bronfenbrenner, 1977).

Exosystems are environments that are external to an individual's microsystem, yet wield power and influence over them. More specifically, exosystems comprise settings in which a child does not participate but ones wherein important decisions are made affecting him or her and, often, the caretakers and others who interact directly with the child (Belsky, 1980). Examples include a parent's workplace, the mass media, school districts, and local, county, state, and federal agencies of government.

Finally, the macrosystem, albeit "invisible," holds social "blueprints"—that is, sociocultural beliefs, expectations, and directives (Belsky, 1980; Bronfenbrenner, 1977). Rather than specific and tangible environments impacting the life of a child, the macrosystem maintains the prescriptions, protocols, and prototypes embedded within a culture and its subcultures that compel the manifestation of sociocultural ideology through custom and practice in day-to-day life. In the context of the sexual abuse of males, these include socially constructed assumptions and hypotheses particular to gender, sexuality, and victimization, and the manner in which such suppositions guide and inform cultural norms and institutional practices.

Social constructions abound in and emerge from the macro level of the ecosystems perspective. Viewed as universal "truths," social constructions, such as masculinity and femininity, permeate within and across individuals, families, neighborhoods, communities, groups, and institutions (Deaux & Major, 1987; Duncan, Peterson, & Winter, 1997; Pleck, 1987). They are socially inherited from generations past—a bequest of ways and means telling us who we are, who we are not to be, who others are, and what value they hold. In essence, they tell us the "what, how, and why" of appropriate and inappropriate thoughts, feelings, and behaviors. Firmly established within social constructions lie the sanctions and penalties for compliance and noncompliance.

Socially constructed phenomena are initiated and maintained by sociocultural dynamics (Bem, 1981) and, as such, serve as the "curriculum" for a myriad socialization processes, from gender to race and ethnicity, from religion to workplace, from peer relations to dating relations, all along an individual's life span. Within the mesosystem, social constructions imbue and undergird social policy, political and religious doctrine, media and advertisement, workplace protocols, and criminal codes involving incest and sexual abuse, to mention a few. At the micro level, individuals, families and groups encounter, often unknowingly, social constructions compassing children's stories, textbooks, music, movies, and even diagnostic and statistical manuals. At the self level, social constructions serve as internalized schemas or templates, helping us to anticipate, seek, and assimilate schema-congruent information and to use such data to judge self and others.

In keeping with the ecosystems perspective, the SAM model is also biopsychosocial in nature, (i.e., encompassing both internal and external factors) and interactional (i.e., encompassing both dynamics and effects). It focuses on the socially prescribed and psychologically compiled meaning permeating both childhood sexual abuse as a social phenomenon and as a personal life event. In favor of a multidimensional understanding of initial and long-term effects that result from CSA, we must first look at how people learn, adapt, and develop independently of childhood trauma.

THE SELF-SYSTEM INDEPENDENT OF ABUSE

A self, or ontogenetic, system, is viewed as a person in relation to the social environment (Belsky, 1980). This human system embodies a number of distinct yet interrelated subsystems and processes, including, but not limited to, the cognitive/perceptual (e.g., memory encoding and retrieval, the ascription of meaning to people, places, and events), intrapsychic (e.g., personality integration, defensive functioning, regulatory functioning), and biophysical (e.g., nervous system functioning, the development of secondary sex characteristics). This section addresses the following self domains: sense of self, self and social schemas, defensive functioning, memory, and nervous-system functioning.

Sense of Self

Developing a sense of self is both instinctive and essential for all children (Cole & Putnam, 1992; Kohut, 1977). From the moment of birth, children actively strive to interact with and organize their experiential world (Schore, 2001; Sullivan, 1968). Knowledge about the self, and of self in relation to others and the world, emerges from the numerous interactions that manifest within and across a child's microsystems (Bandura, 1986; Erikson, 1963; Fairbairn, 1994; Kernberg, 1980; Piaget & Inhelder, 1969).

Knowledge of this kind is endowed with and biased by all of the enduring familial, social, and cultural constructions that define and sustain human behavior in the social environment. Such knowledge-in-action helps children with the tasks of assimilating information from and about their microenvironments. In this way, they learn about their own roles, tasks, and boundaries, and discover ways in which to receive and elicit responses from others (Bowlby, 1990, 1982; Harter, 1983). In other words, the child's tasks are to (a) develop an autonomous awareness of self in relation to the social environment, (b) evolve a sense of self with respect to rules and regulations of the social environment, (c) acquire experience and skill in self-regulation coping, and (d) develop a viable interpersonal skill base. These activities, taken in their entirety, are fundamental to helping children develop an independent and agentic sense of self (Cole & Putnam, 1992).

Sense of self, then, is conceptualized as a progressive construction, generating for developing children, three subsenses: (a) a sense of who they are (i.e., a sense of being); (b) a sense of how they fit into their environment (i.e., a sense of knowing); and (c) a sense of what they can expect from themselves, others, and the world in which they live (i.e., a sense of becoming) (Goldstein, 1982). A child's senses of being, knowing, and becoming derive from information directly gleaned from experience with others. Social interaction not only provides the child with self-knowledge and an awareness as to how the child fits into their various microsystems; social interaction is the wellspring from which the self begins to emerge and evolve over time. It is, indeed, a cornerstone of the self.

To illustrate, transactions between children and significant others become internalized and function as emerging relational schemas or working models (Bowlby, 1988; Brower & Nurius, 1993; Siegel, 2001). A child's working model of others is a function of his or her perceptions and feelings as to the availability and responsivity of primary caretakers; a working model of self emerges from the child's perceptions and feelings of how acceptable, valuable, and deserving he or she is in the eyes of the caretakers. Such organized cognitive structures guide and inform how the child will develop and sustain subsequent relationships with others. Relational models are critical in helping children organize and efficiently access all of their knowledge about the self, others, and the environment (Hastie, 1980). Without it, children and adults alike would be unable to differentiate between crucial and superficial information, would have no sense of boundaries between personal needs and those of others, and would be quickly overwhelmed with the sheer amount of stimuli available to them and the demands placed upon them. Ultimately, a sense of self guides decisions around what information is important and what can or cannot be done in response to particular information. It also indicates how interactions within and across microsystems might change as a result (Brower & Nurius, 1993). Further, a sense of self helps individuals to adapt to numerous microenvironments, to change as necessary, and to maintain continuity between both intrapersonal and social domains (Guidano & Liotti, 1985).

Additionally, so as to uphold a continuous and structured sense of personal identity, it is equally important to understand and be able to predict, at least to a certain extent, matters of the social environment (Lauer & Handel, 1983). During childhood, adolescence, and adulthood, not only does this help one to understand his or her own roles and niches within various systems, but without this understanding, he or she would likely perceive and consequently experience the world as unpredictable, unsafe, and, for some, unimaginable. Because it is intolerable, as well as impossible, for most to maintain a state of constant watchfulness and preparedness for the unexpected, many continuously seek ways in which to further their understanding of external events in order to make them predictable and, as a result, to perceive and experience them as safer.

It is important to realize, however, that the development of self is a fluid and dynamic process; building and employing knowledge of self together with knowledge of others and the world is both continuous (Flavell, 1985) and interactive (Goldstein, 1995). For example, this self-knowledge generates value-based evaluations or, in other words, self-esteem (Kohut, 1977); self-esteem, high or low, differentially impacts self-efficacy, or one's ability to generate behavioral options and, accordingly, their expectations about executing them successfully; self-efficacy, in turn, influences an individual's perceptions and anticipated outcomes around their coping with future situations and stressors (Bandura, 1982).

Self and social development are inextricably linked (Cole & Putnam, 1992), mutually and reciprocally influencing and reinforcing one another. The ultimate outcome is a viably operational, agentic, and integrated sense of self within the context of meaningful interpersonal relationships and within the world of work—in essence, an evolving sense of striving to live, living, and a sense of having lived a worthwhile and productive life (Erikson, 1963). Thus, the development of the self, as a process, delineates the circularity and interactivity of human behavior in the social environment.

To be sure, the dynamic interplay of subsystems is an important element in the self-system's functional capacity. Three such subsystems are the cognitive perceptual, the intrapsychic, and the biophysical. The first encompasses information processing, namely, schematic development and imposition; the second includes, but is not limited to, ego defense functioning; and the third, but no less important, involves physiologic functioning, particularly in terms of the autonomic nervous system. Although the cognitive-perceptual system allows individuals to regulate and to monitor the information they hold, give, and receive (Piaget & Inhelder, 1969; Brower & Nurius, 1993), the intrapsychic system, acting as a buffer, affords them time or a temporary suspension of full responsivity, in order to balance new information with current and historic ideas and beliefs (A. Freud, 1936; Goldstein, 1995), and the biophysical system acts as a check and balance operation during times of stress (Perry, 2000).

Cognitive-Perceptual Subsystem

Unlike a machine, which is only able to respond to a problem with information input in the present, the self, as a human system, is both able to, and restrained by a capacity to, remember and draw from experiences both recent and remote. However, because the self is capable of receiving so much information, it is essential to develop schemas in order to structure these data, to facilitate access to them, and to provide a sense of consistency across time and microenvironments (Kendall & Hollon, 1981).

Schemas, thus, are internalized frameworks of understanding; they help one to collapse a vast amount of data into categories (Beck, 1976). When individuals are presented with new information, schemas guide them in choosing what information is important and in figuring out whether they have had previous experience with anything similar. Further, these cognitive frameworks overtly or covertly point to the consequences of action. In essence, schemas tell people who they are, what they know, and what to do.

Not only does this increase one's efficiency in responding to new data, but it also allows for a continuity of data processing whereby new information is constantly added to and built on preexisting knowledge. This process, called assimilation, is not, however, the only way in which we are capable of processing data (Flavell, 1985).

In addition to the human ability to assimilate new information, one is also capable of accommodating to new information. During assimilation, a child may be able to absorb new facts by way of adding them to foregoing schemas. During accommodation, this child would actually change his or her schemas, as necessary, to bring the self in line with information that either contradicts previously held beliefs but cannot be disputed, or that does not align with any of their preexisting experiences (Janoff-Bulman, 1992; Piaget & Inhelder, 1969). The accommodation of schemas to discrepant information allows one to reestablish an ordered sense of the world. Be that as it may, when children accommodate to new information, they are essentially changing themselves, by way of their views and beliefs, for the sake of decreasing the conflict between themselves and their micro- and macroenvironments and with a view to recreating their image of the world as a consistent and predictable place in which to live.

In day-to-day interactions, assimilation is far more frequent than accommodation (Horowitz, 1986), in part because encountering exceedingly discrepant information is not a common occurrence. It is also due to the fact that, because accommodation is so taxing and highly disruptive to one's sense of self, many will generally go to great lengths to find ways of disregarding, or at least of diminishing, the importance of such data. When children and adults cannot negate or assimilate information, both are changed by the experience of accommodating to it. Not only does this change affect one, or many, of our schemas regarding the world at large, but it can also alter schemas regarding our views of the self.

Finally, when schemas change, they most often do so by content rather than by title (Kendall & Hollon, 1981). In other words, when an important trust has been violated, the schema for trust may still be referenced by the same words and contexts, but the content has changed. "Trusting people is safe" changes to "trusting people is dangerous." As a result of these schematic alterations, the individual will now have an entirely new understanding of both the world and of his or her role in it. Consequently, a fracture develops between who the person is in the present and who the person was in the past.

INTRAPSYCHIC SUBSYSTEM

Ego functions are the means by which an individual perceives, experiences, responds to, and adapts to the social environment (Goldstein, 1995). Ego functions, such as defense operations, reality testing, affect regulation, moderation of the stimulus barrier, object relations, and integrative functioning, hold a biopsychsocial imperative toward not only survival, but mastery and competence as well (A. Freud, 1936). Regardless of biological, psychological, or sociological impingement, the individual strives toward self-actualization (Rank, 1952; Sullivan, 1953). The ego and its functions—unconscious and dynamic—seek to maintain and, if necessary, reestablish a homeostatic state.

Throughout life, as individuals process, assimilate, and accommodate to an endless stream of incoming information and stimuli, they need an occasional "break"—a time in which to adjust to both external data and their internal responses to it. Ego defense strategies offer more than time; when presented with information that cannot be integrated easily and quickly, defenses provide necessary time while simultaneously allowing one to maintain functionality (A. Freud, 1965).

Defenses are intended to be temporary (Bowlby, 1984; A. Freud, 1936; Kohut, 1984), circumscribed by time and context. As information becomes integrated into preexisting schemas—self schemata, object schemata, relational schemata, and world schemata—defenses allow one to retain a pretense of his or her previous reality until such a time as the new information can be organized and utilized effectively. This respite is both useful and essential in helping one to preserve a continuous sense of self over time and across microsystems. Because defenses operate outside of conscious awareness, someone cannot use them deliberately in order to cope with an anxiety-producing circumstance. Defenses are designed to promote survival, not to be an escape from pain.

Examples of defense mechanisms include: (a) somatization, or the conversion of anxiety into psychobiological symptomology; (b) isolation, or the separation of a distressing thought, behavior, or event from its emanating affect; (c) dissociation, or the temporary alteration of one's perception and experience of self and/or environment; (d) regression, or the return to a prior developmental phase, level of functioning, or type of behavior in order to avoid anxiety generated in the present; (e) suppression, or the mental avoidance of conflictual cognitive and affective content; (f) repression, or the exclusion of thoughts, feelings, and, in some, cases, entire experiences, from awareness, including information they may have at one point reached consciousness and information that may never have done so; (g) projection, or the attribution of unacknowledged or unrecognized thoughts, feelings, and behaviors onto others; (h) introjection, or the internalization of characteristics, typically emotions, associated with an object whereby the emotions correspondent to that object are directed toward the self, thereupon preserving the image of the object; (i) denial, or the negation of one's perceptions of reality, for example, seeing an event take place or hearing about it but psychologically disclaiming what was witnessed or heard; and (j) acting out, or directly expressing an unconscious conflict or memory, often without much forethought, words, or regard for negative consequences; (k) identification, or the internalization of various aspects of another person, typically threatening and evocative characteristics such as violence and aggression, and consequently acting as if they authentically belong to the self (Blanck & Blanck, 1974; A. Freud, 1936; Krystal, 1988; Vaillant, 1992; Wallerstein, 1983).

Without defenses, each time significantly new data are presented to children, for example, their thoughts and feelings would be thrown into a state of chaos, disrupting their sense of self and interfering with their ability to function in the most constructive and adaptive way. With defenses, when new data are presented to children, such strategies permit them to continue working with previously established ways of interacting with the world. That is, the defensive delay helps children to maintain functionality while giving them the time necessary to integrate the new material without becoming unduly overwhelmed by it. Once this is accomplished, the defenses are no longer necessary, and the child is able to work with the sum total of the information—the new integrated with the old.

BIOPHYSICAL SUBSYSTEM

Biophysical development is the process most closely associated with the self-system's capacity for survival (Lovallo & Sollers, 2000). The main goal of the nervous systems is to monitor and maintain a homeostatic internal environment and to monitor and respond to the external environment. Moment to moment, a myriad of stimuli infiltrate the nervous system through sensory channels. Sensory input is received in many forms, including light, sound, taste, touch, smell, blood levels, and hormonal changes. Each is converted into signals and transmitted to the brain or spinal cord. Within the sensory centers, signals are integrated and responses generated. A response, as a series of signals, is transmitted to organs throughout the body, which, in turn, convert the signal into another action, for example, motoric movement, decelerated heart rate, or chemical discharge. Thus, all sensory input is assessed in pursuit of rendering a viable response. However, the vast majority of stimuli are determined to be relatively inconsequential at any particular moment.

Of course, the nervous system is instrumental to adaptation. This vital complex is composed of two main divisions: the voluntary and the involuntary subsystems. The voluntary nervous system controls body movement, specifically the head, torso, arms, hands, legs, and feet. It comprises the brain and spinal cord; impulses arising from the brain travel along units of nerves, each terminating in the muscle it controls. The involuntary, or autonomic, nervous system directs activities of the body unconsciously. It contains all the neurons, or nerve cells, separate and apart from the brainstem and spinal cord. More intricate than its counterpart, the autonomic nervous system consists of two domains: the sympathetic and the parasympathetic. The sympathetic subsystem, activated by hormones, strengthens the self-system against conditions it might experience or encounter, such as hypothermia, dehydration, physical attack, or, in fact, any form of stress. It is central to the fight–flight–freeze response. Its parasympathetic counterpart, activated by hormones as well, holds the sympathetic system in check through relaxation. Each subsystem operates contrary to the other, impacting the same organs but oppositionally in order to maintain equilibrium (Goldstein, 2000; Kollack-Walker, Day, & Akil, 2000)

The autonomic nervous system reacts and responds to internal and external stimuli that hold the potential to threaten survival. A set of similarly related physiological changes emerges, thereby enhancing one's ability to respond to perceived danger. This system increases the flow of breath, blood, blood sugar, and neurotransmitter secretions in order to increase, respectively, the body's oxygen supply, physical energy, visual and sensory acuity, and speed of reactivity. During times of fear and terror, the autonomic nervous system may react too vigorously, triggering any number of effects, such as heart palpitations, free-floating anxiety, depression, speech difficulties, derealization, and temporary paralysis (Schore, 2001; Siegel, 1995; van der Kolk & Fisler, 1995). The parasympathetic system strives to reverse these effects.

BASICS OF THE BRAIN

The human brain is an intricate organ constituting in excess of one hundred billion neurons and one trillion glial cells. Each neuron, or nerve cell, has up to 100,000 or more dendrites, branchlike extensions of the cell body that receive information from other cells and one axon, or extensions that divide in many directions along their length, transmitting information to other cells along the way. Every neuron holds unique structural dynamics that permit it to communicate, that is, to obtain, process, store, and transmit data generated by any of its counterparts within the brain.

Glial cells are specialized in that they nourish, support, insulate, and protect neurons. Unlike neurons, glial have the capacity to divide and reproduce. They inhabit the brain space between and among neurons and provide a protective covering over each and every cell body, including its axon and dendrites. *Glia*, in Greek, means "glue." In essence, glial cells maintain the physical integrity of the brain. They dwell between the neurons, feeding them, covering their cell bodies, axons, and dendrites, and forming protective scaffolding along their neuronal pathways. Both neurons and glial cells hold the same genetic material, and both express a unique pattern of gene activation that is a reflection of the cell's history and current environment (Child Trauma Academy, 2002).

The point of convergence between two neurons is the synapse. More often than not, synapses can be found at the intersections of axons and dendrites. The space between two neurons is the synaptic cleft. These gaps constitute the locations in which data are communicated from one neuron to another. Neurons communicate by way of electrical activity; electrical impulses release chemicals, or neurotransmitters, which, in turn, flow across the synaptic cleft, transferring a signal from one side of the gap to the other. The neurotransmitters, as chemical messengers, bind to receptors on the target cell's membrane, causing ion channels on that cell to open and transmitting a message to that cell's membrane. Neurotransmitters act to excite the next cell, by depolarizing it, or act to inhibit the target cell, by hyperpolarizing it. Both inhibitory and excitatory synapses and neurotransmitters work to modulate the vast array of activity within the brain. In any given millisecond, one-way chains of synapses unite neurons in multitudinous and elaborate formations, each working to generate one minute aspect of human behavior and with many enlisted for specific tasks. In simple terms, every synaptic chain, each in its own way, generates a distinct effect, for example, the blink of an eye, a beat of the heart, or the expansion of a lung. And vast networks of synaptic chains work hand-in-hand to yield an elaborate circuitry of human behavior, for example, driving a car, reciting multiplication tables, or baking a birthday cake.

These neurons and synaptic networks are methodically arranged into systems directed to sense, process, store, receive, and respond to external information—visual, auditory, olfactory, gustatory, and tactile-kinesthetic—and to internal information—hunger, position, oxygen depletion, and temperature. All experience is filtered through the sensory receptors. The reception of sensory data successively commences a cascade of cellular and molecular processes that modify neuronal neurochemistry and cytoarchitechture, which, progressively, alters brain structure and function (Perry, 2000).

The various interacting and interrelated systems of the brain are organized in a precise hierarchical manner, from the bottom up, beginning with the brainstem, or the most primal, to the cortex, or the most advanced (Perry, Pollard, Blakley, Baker, & Vigilante, 1996). Thus, the more simple or regulatory functions, such as the regulation of heart rate, body temperature, or lung respiration, are mediated by the brainstem and midbrain located in the lower regions, and the most complex functions, such as abstract thinking and language, are mediated by the brain's cortical structures (Perry, 1999). The vast majority of the brain is divided into hemispheres, left and right. The hemispheres are connected with bands of nerve fibers known as the corpus callosum. The corpus callosum is essentially a bridge between the two hemispheres, transferring information between the two sides of the brain. As a side note, the corpus callosum tends to be smaller among males relative to females.

The various regional systems of the brain—the brainstem, the diencephalon, the limbic, and the neocortex—store information that is germane to the functioning of each particular domain. These different regions organize during development, and once the brain is mature, they change in a use-dependent manner. The more a particular neurobiological system is activated, the more that state, and functions associated with that state, will build in, thereby producing an internal depiction of the experience congruent with the neural activation (Perry, 2000). Actualized examples of this process include learning how to drive a car, memorizing multiplication tables, and responding with fear to an abuse-related trigger. In other words, the more habitually a particular pattern of neural activation transpires, "the more indelible the internal representation—the more indelible the memory" (p. 5). When confronted with unanticipated, severe, and/or prolonged stress, the body releases endogenous stress hormones that fortify the strength and indelibility of memory representations and memory consolidation.

The Brainstem

The brainstem is located at the top of the spinal cord. Sometimes referenced as the reptilian brain, it regulates functions necessary for survival, including heart rate, respiration, and digestion, and states necessary for arousal, such as wakefulness and vigilance. The brainstem is also the brain's first way station for sensory input. In order for an infant to survive beyond birth, its brainstem must be operative and mature.

In addition to comprising the medulla and pons, the brainstem also contains a number of ascending arousal-related neural systems, including the locus caeruleus (LC) and ventral tegmental nucleus (VTN). The LC encompasses a small area of the brainstem; it embodies norepinephrine neurons. Among many capacities, it monitors and filters information transmitted by way of the senses. Additionally, the LC acts as the key brain hub for anxiety and fear; as a "central relay station," it receives nerve data from and transmits nerve data to all regions of the brain, swiftly and globally activating neuronal functioning (Bremner et al., 1999, p. 106). The LC and VTN, as brainstem catecholamine systems, play an important role in the stress and startle response, as they regulate attention, arousal, vigilance, affect, and locomotion (Perry, 1999; Bremner, Krystal, Southwick, & Charney, 1996a, 1996b). Thus, both are critically involved in recruiting, launching, and sustaining the body's psychobiological response to threat and fear.

The Diencephalon

The diencephalon, or midbrain, encompasses a number of vital substructures, including the thalamus and hypothalamus. The thalamus encompasses a relatively large region of the brain and, as such, contains numerous nuclei. As the gateway to the cerebral or sensory cortex, the thalamic nuclei must process all sensory information, with the exception of olfactory input, before such data can proceed onto more sophisticated and interpretative processing (Perry, 2001). The thalamus factors considerably in relaying somatosensory data within and without the corporeal environment to the amygdala (Fanselow & Gale, 2000). In this way, it plays a critical role in both states of awareness and sensorimotor responsivity and functioning.

The hypothalamus, while comparatively small, is critical to optimum functioning of the brain and the body. The hypothalamus synchronizes the sympathetic component of the autonomic nervous system and, accordingly, critically serves in the operation of the fight-or-flight response set, monitoring alterations in the stress reaction—heartbeat, increased dilation of bronchi, increased oxygenation, blood pressure, and the changes rendered by the release of excitatory and inhibitory neurotransmitters. The thalamus and hypothalamus, as well as the pituitary, are central to survival vis-à-vis the person/environment interface.

The Limbic System

Of all the regions of the brain, the limbic system is viewed as the central nervous system domain that not only regulates and maintains the emotions and behaviors necessary for survival but also is centrally involved with the storage and retrieval of memory (van der Kolk, 1994). In all states of arousal, from waking to sleeping, and from calm to terror, signals from the sensory receptors systematically project to the thalamus from where they are disbursed to the cortex, thereby establishing a cognitive reaction, then onto the basal ganglia, whereupon a behavioral chain is established, and advancing to the limbic system wherein an emotional response is established, and all of this in tandem with the imperative to ascertain the emotional significance of the sensory input. It is hypothesized that the processing of sensory data occurs without conscious awareness (LeDoux, 1992) and that only unanticipated, atypical, critical, or potentially hazardous feedback is selectively projected onto the neocortex for subsequent processing.

Two central regions of the limbic system are central to the processing of emotionally laden experiences: the hippocampus and the amygdala. The amygdala is mature and operative at birth; the hippocampus, on the other hand, typically matures between the ages of 2 and 4. Both the hippocampus and the amygdala consist of two lobes, one located in each hemisphere of the brain.

Hippocampus

The hippocampus, a seahorse-shaped structure, is responsible for a number of key activities. It is largely responsible for the processing of conscious and explicit learning and memory (Squire & Kandel, 2000). The hippocampus, adjacent to the amygdala, connects nerve fibers associated with visual, auditory, tactile, and olfactory information with the limbic system. As it receives nerve-cell input from the various regions of the sensory-cortical complex, the hippocampus plays an important role in both short-term and long-term memory, particularly with respect to the consolidation and storage of contextual information such as time, place, and positional and spatial relationships. The hippocampus is concerned with facts; hippocampal processing helps to answer questions concerning what happened, when, where, and in what sequence, thereby offering a contextualized timeline of personal history.

Memories generated during the first 4 years of a child's life may be difficult to retrieve, given the slow maturation of the hippocampus. This developmental process is associated with the occurrence of infantile amnesia (Brown et al., 1998). Memories associated with the first 4 years of life hold qualities of an experience, but not its context. As the hippocampus matures, it is conceptualized as a "cognitive map" because it holds a significant role with respect to explicit or declarative memory, particularly in terms of consolidating diverse contextual elements of an experience such as conversations, interactions, and environmental details, all within a particular time and space (Joseph, 1999; van der Kolk, 1994). The hippocampus, in tandem with the adjacent cortex region of the brain, assembles contextual data from the various sensory cortices into a single memory on retrieval (Bremner et al., 1999).

The hippocampus is also associated with autonomic functioning and emotionality, particularly in terms of anxiety and fear (Bremner et al., 1999). Stress hormones and stress-related neurotransmitter systems, such as those found within the locus ceruleus and other brainstem nuclei, target the hippocampus (Perry, 1997; van der Kolk, 1996). The hippocampus is also implicated in the formation of a conditioned fear response triggered by a fear-inducing environmental event (Bremner et al., 1999). During such times, the body secretes stress-induced cortiosteroids, enkephalins, and norepinephrine (Joseph, 1999). However, such exposure to protracted or intermittent iterations of environmental stress and autonomic arousal may injure the hippocampus, potentially leading to atrophy. Although the hippocampus holds the intrinsic capacity to regenerate neurons, repeated exposure to stress inhibits hippocampal functioning thereby diminishing its ability toward regeneration (Sass et al., 1990).

Amygdala

The amygdala is conceptualized as an "emotional computer" (LeDoux, 1992). As such, it receives and assesses the significance of input form the sensory processing domains of the brainstem, diencephalon, hippocampus, and cortex. In other words, the amygdala represents another relay station, receiving sensory data from the environment and determining its emotional value. Next, it transmits the evaluated information to regions of the brainstem that regulate autonomic and behavioral responses. This network permits input to exit the sensory receptive system, allows the amygdala to assign feelings of import to the sensory input, and allows the neocortex to infuse the input with personal meaning (LeDoux, 1992; van der Kolk, 1996). If, however, the amygdala appraises the sensory input as novel or dangerous, it also activates arousal centers within the brain, including the autonomic nervous system, which, in turn, initiates the discharge of epinephrine and norepinephrine, thereby preparing one for fight or flight.

The amygdala synthesizes internal representations of the external environment with emotions generated by interactions across microenvironments. Whatever mental representations are present during the amygdala's appraisal-arousal processing will become associated, in memory, with the feelings generated during that particular experience. In other words, memory processes mediated by the amygdala fortify the emotional valence of memories. In fact, it is within these limbic areas that the patterns of neuronal activity associated with threat, and mediated by the monoamine neurotransmitters systems of the reticular activating system, become an emotion (Perry, 1997, 1999; Perry & Pollard, 1998). Given the potency of the amygdala, memories, particularly ones associated with trauma, are less vulnerable to distortion and forgetfulness (LeDoux, 1994). The amygdala is also a component of the basal ganglia.

The Basal Ganglia

Deep within the cerebrum, surrounding the limbic system, are the basal ganglia. These clusters of nuclei are linked with virtually every region of the cortex. It follows that the basal ganglia, then, are involved with the uniform integration of sensations, thoughts, feelings, and behaviors. Exposure to traumatic events may "reset" the basal ganglia from a baseline of relative calm to states of hypervigilance and fear. If the basal ganglia respond more forcefully than necessary, one may become easily overwhelmed by stressors and ultimately freeze, cognitively, emotionally, and behaviorally, when subjected to distressing events.

The Cerebrum and Cortex

The cerebrum, also referenced as gray matter, comprises the most evolutionary advanced area of the brain. Although it represents only one quarter of the brain's total volume, it encompasses approximately three-quarters of the 10 billion neurons that comprise the brain. Generally speaking, the cerebrum mediates higher level activities such as planning, associating, and fine-tuning the data received from other regions of the brain. The cerebrum encompasses the centers for sight, sound, smell and touch, intelligence, and memory. It also houses the cortex.

The cortex spans the right and left hemispheres of the brain, with four distinct lobes on either side, each with distinct capacities: the frontal lobes, the temporal lobes, the parietal lobes, and the occipital lobes. The frontal lobes regulate abilities under the rubric of cognitive flexibility, such as problem solving, decision making, goal setting, cooperation, and will. The frontal lobe encompasses four functional areas: (a) the primary motor cortex and (b) the premotor cortex, both associated with voluntary movements vis-à-vis the musculoskeletal system, (c) the prefrontal cortex, involved with critical thinking, reflective thinking, insight, the capacity to sense and express emotions, empathic understanding and responsivity, and personality, and (d) Broca's area, a substructure critical to the production of speech and written language.

The temporal lobes have a dominant and nondominant side. The dominant side is associated with three main functions, one concerned with the auditory cortex, or hearing and language, another with the generation of emotional and visceral responses as well as emotional stability, and the third with complex aspects of learning and memory retrieval. The nondominant side assists in the identification of facial expressions and the deciphering of vocal intonations. The parietal lobes are generally associated with the reception and processing of sensory information, namely, proprioception, or the kinesthetic sense of self in space and time, and audtion, or the comprehension of language. The latter is, in part, a function of Wernicke's area. Finally, the occipital lobe encompasses the primary visual cortex and the visual association cortex, both involved with the processing of visual information.

Special attention must be given to the prefrontal cortex as it relates to childhood trauma. The medial prefrontal cortex regulates emotional responses, most specifically, fear. It helps to engage one's sense of motivation and drive, at times driving motoric behavior by sheer will. The orbitofrontal cortex, for example, holds a significant role in the fear response and its extinction. When functioning properly, it restrains arousal and other impulsive reactions to environmental stimuli. However, prolonged stress can suppress orbitofrontal cortical functioning.

Although many areas of the cortex are concurred with cognitive, emotional, sensory, and motoric aspects of human behavior, the association areas, including the dorsolateral cortex, have a different function, that of integrating representations from various parts of the brain. Essentially, the association areas synthesize seemingly disparate data—the facts associated with an experience, the sequence of events, the contextual details, sights seen, words spoken, internal sensations, external impressions, thoughts, feelings, and behaviors—into a temporal, unified, and meaningful story. The executive and analytic functions associated with the dorsolateral prefrontal cortex permit one to place a singular fact, such as subjection to CSA, and weave it into the biological, psychological, and sociological contexts in which it occurred. CSA engenders multiple memories; those with an intense emotional valence will eventually be stored in the cortex (Charney, Deutch, Krystal, Southwick, & Davis, 1993). Upon memory formation, the subcortical traces of the conditioned fear response remain indelible. In fact, emotional memories may last infinitely within the cortex (LeDoux, Romanski, & Xagoraris, 1991).

MEMORY

Unlike a snapshot or a reel of film, memory is not a precise reproduction. In simple terms, memory as a process allows us to: (a) "selectively represent (in one or more memory systems) information that uniquely characterizes a discrete experience"; (b) "retain that information in an organized way within existing memory frameworks"; and (c) "reproduce some or all aspects of that information at some future point in time under certain conditions" (Brown, Scheflin & Hammond, 1998, p. 66).

Thus, each and every instance of recall involves a reconstruction, rather than a reproduction, of events and, as such, holds the potential to distort or modify various aspects of memory. Our ability to retrieve memories, in both the short term and long term, is, for the most part, accurate, but it is by no means foolproof. Although the vast majority of inaccuracies in retrieved memory are minor, be they omissions or commissions, significant errors can at times occur (Roth & Friedman, 1998).

The Development of Memory

The development of memory, like other human phenomena, follows an epigenetic course; that is to say, one form or type of memory builds on preceding forms (Bretherton, 1993). Two parallel yet independent and distinct memory systems—a behavioral memory system and narrative autobiographical memory system—develop across time (Pillemer & White, 1989), with the behavioral preceding the autobiographical. From the moment of birth, infants dynamically experience their microenvironments (Siegel, 2001) by way of their sensory receptors, which, in turn, facilitate perceptual, emotional, motoric, and somatosensory learning and memory (Terr, 1991).

During early childhood, the behavioral memory system, in the form of procedural memories, evolves from the interaction between an infant's sensory stimuli and the behavioral responses of his or her caretakers. As the caretakers attune to the infant's states, and subtle shifts between them, all the while accentuating the positive states of pleasure and minimizing the negative states of distress, the infant "feels felt" (Siegel, 1996, cited in Lott, 1998, p. 2). In this way, the caretakers function as affect regulators or, metaphorically, as an auxiliary cortex for the infant's underdeveloped brain. Neurologically, these child–caretakers interactions, as a form of psychobiological attunement, represent the direct and reciprocal communication to and from the right brains of the caretaker and the child. This unconscious demonstration and processing of relational experience evolves into a template for the infant's developing neural circuitry, particularly so within the orbitofrontal cortex (Schore, 2001).

Thus, in the midst of recurrent transactions with caretakers and collaterals, behavioral (i.e., implicit and procedural) memories form as the infant's brain processes these experiences, with the amygdala and other limbic regions processing emotional memory, the basal ganglia and motor cortex responsible for behavioral memory, and the perceptual cortexes handling perceptual memory (Wheeler, Stuss, & Tolving; 1997; Schore, 2001). The database of the procedural memory system includes the attachment and caretaking patterns emerging from the child's microrelationships, for example, the ways in which a parent replies to a child's bonding signals, a child-care worker reacts to a child's hunger cues, and a sibling acknowledges a child's expression of discomfort. Behavioral memories actualize by way of mental imagery and behavioral enactment (Pillemer & White, 1989).

The infant's brain also holds the capacity to discern similarities and differences among sensory receptors, between experiences and across microenvironments. Further, these transactions, now perceptible by comparison, comprise the base from which the infant's mind is able to generate summated or generalized representations, which, in turn, form the basis of mental models or schemata—about the self, about others, and about love, safety, care, and relationships—that categorically help the mind to reflect on past experiences, interpret present experiences, and envision future ones (Siegel, 2001).

A number of memory-related developmental milestones occur in relatively quick succession. During the first year, the child acquires an evolving base of implicit learning, comprised of recurrent transactional patterns encoded ardently in the brain. However, at this stage, the child has no sense of self across time (Wheeler et al., 1997). These sensation–response patterns begin to elicit words and phrases as the child develops language, linguistic, and communication capacities (Crittenden, 1992). Epigenetically, during the second year, the child reaches another milestone, one that progresses across the life span—the cognizance and communication of words and language (Siegel, 2001). Almost simultaneously, as the child learns about and strives to make sense of the world, he or she develops schematic representations of self, of familiar others, and of daily activities. The evolving sense of self, of language, of the physical world, and of time and space comprise four of the many elements central to the establishment of explicit autobiographical memory. Although behavioral responses influenced procedural memory, verbal responses now hold a more focal importance.

Semantic memory enables a child to render propositional representations of self and the environment. These symbols of external or internal phenomena can be communicated by word or by action and can be assessed as "true" or "false" (Siegel, 2001). More specifically, the toddler attempts to understand his or her microenvironments by way of developing schemas for familiar interactions and events and assimilating new information into these evolving and variant memory structures (Brown et al., 1998). The semantic database includes what a child learns about himself or herself (e.g., "boy," "girl," "I am good," "I am bad"), about the microenvironment (e.g., "home is safe," "school is scary," "mother is nice," "friends are fun"), and about the world (e.g., "safe," "unsafe," "predictable," "unbelievable"). Thus, as they amplify and particularize, the schemata, or internal working models, evidence two constituent parts, with the first en-compassing data regarding the understanding, experience, and expectations of others, the environment, and the world, and the second encompassing corresponding representations of himself or herself in relation to others, the environment, and the world. For example, if a boy's perception and experience of others is that of apathy, inconsistency, and mistreatment, then he, in turn, learns to perceive and experience himself as inconsequential, inept at eliciting and receiving attention and care, and, ultimately, discardable (Bowlby, 1980).

Toddlers, typically those between the ages of 2 and 3, encode, store, and retrieve relatively completely and accurately (Pillemer & White, 1989). As the child's memory system evolves from behavioral to semantic, with the latter holding primacy over the former, childhood amnesia occurs even though the earlier experiences remain within the behavioral memory system. Between the third and fourth year, the verbal or semantic memory system rapidly evolves into a highly systematized complex of biology, psychology, and sociology. The child now holds the capacity to engage in conversation—to combine his or her knowledge of self and knowledge of the world and dialogue with caretakers and collaterals (Siegel, 2001). Even though, in general, a child's recollections tend to be incomplete, they also tend to be precise (Brown et al., 1998). When the child is presented with opportunities to engage with others in conversations before, during, and after a particular event, doing so advances the organization, integration, and facilitation of the child's memory for that event (Bauer, Kroupina, Schwade, Dropik, & Wewerka, 1998), and doing so on a consistent basis fosters the child's ability to retrieve detailed memories of life events long thereafter (Wheeler et al., 1997).

During the child's fifth and sixth years, the child's verbal memory system advances into a more socially constructed and socially communal autobio-graphical system. At this point, memory rehearsal is much more likely to occur, as the child observes, shares, and elaborates on personal experiences. With the development of skills around concrete operational thinking, the child, upon and throughout the latency years, develops greater capacity for memory of specific events as well as general events. The expressions of episodic memory at this stage tend to be significantly more comprehensive and enumerate than those expressed by younger children (Brown et al., 1998).

In sum, semantic memory builds on behavioral memory (Brower & Nurius, 1993) and, ultimately, episodic memory builds on its predecessors, encoding in diverse ways and relying on the sensory channels as well as cognition and affect. Unlike its predecessors, episodic memories are retrieved as a set of sequential incidents in narrative form (Crittenden, 1992).

The Process of Memory

Memory, as a process, involves three stages: (a) sensory attention and encod-ing; (b) organization and consolidation; and (c) storage and retrieval (Squire &

Kandel, 2000). Sensory attention and encoding involve the creation of memory, that is, the original input and production of a memory trace by way of symbolic codification (Siegel, 2001). Because memory is circumscribed by perception (Freyd, 1996), the degree to which an experience is attended by the senses is the degree to which the experience, by way of sensory receptors, will be registered (Siegel, 1997).

Experience, or human behavior in the social environment, filters through the senses via two primary systems: the exertoceptive and the interoceptive The exertosensory receptors—vision, olfaction, audition, gustation, and tactility—comprise sensory mechanisms that sense and respond to stimuli emanating from the external environment. The interosensory system—propioception (or the sensation of internal body states such as heart rate, levels of oxygen and carbon dioxide, and muscular tension) and vestibularation (or the internal sense of balance and gravitational pull)—comprises mechanisms that assess activities within the internal environment (Rothschild, 2000). The primary objective of both systems is to maintain constant surveillance within the body and across microenvironments in order to sustain life and well-being. They accomplish this by responding to internal and/or external cues that signal nerve cells, which, in turn, ignite a neural circuitry of activity within the brain and central nervous system (Siegel, 2001).

In the midst of this cavalcade of neuronal dynamism, the brain strives to create an internal representation of the external world (Perry, Pollard, Blakley, Baker, & Vigilante, 1995). Within milliseconds, the brain determines the features of incoming electric signals as they progress along distinct and apportioned pathways, for example, one for perceptual data, another for emotional data, and another still for physiological data (Bremner, 2002). Along this process, the original input will be encoded into a transitory iconic trace and, if processed subsequently, into a short-term memory trace, and quite possibly into a long-term trace (Tulving & Craik, 2000). Depending on one's developmental stage and current circumstance, memories may be encoded visually, verbally, or behaviorally. Regardless of developmental stage or form of memory, the more frequently a certain neural pattern activates, the more indelible is the memory (Perry et al., 1995; Schore, 1994; Siegel, 2001).

Storage, or the organization and consolidation of data, is the intermediate step in the memory process, occurring over several weeks or more, during which time the memory is stabilized, thereby establishing its relative permanence (Brown & Craik, 2000). The internal representation of the external experience is an engram, or, neurologically, the aggregate set of cellular and molecular changes within the brain that now constitute a multisensorial record of the experience. An engram encompasses two primary aspects of the experience: the explicit and the implicit. The explicit memory system encodes and stores factual knowledge—words, definitions, names, faces, descriptions, instructions, and autobiographical episodes. Operationally, it is a conscious process dependent on oral or written language as well as other systems of printed, voiced, and physicalized language. Mediated by the hippocampus, explicit memory places facts and events within their proper contexts of time and place, thereby allowing one, in the present, to reflect on the past and anticipate the future. In essence, explicit memory allows one to narrate one's life. Implicit memory encodes and stores reflexive information—emotional learning, automatic procedures, motor skills, conditioned responses, and habituated behavior. It involves an unconscious process mediated by the amygdala. Implicit memory includes sensory, somatic, emotional, and behavioral forms of memory (Terr, 1991).

As a process, memory storage can be conceptualized as "the change in probability of activating a particular neural network pattern in the future" (Siegel, 1999, p. 25). Events with a great emotional valence, in contrast to more neutral events, tend to be retained over longer periods of time (LeDoux, 1992). Storage also refers to the undetermined span of time between the encoding of an event and its recall, should that occur (Tulving & Craik, 2000).

Retrieval is conceptualized as the process by which individuals procure/access and remember the engram or stored data (Tulving & Craik, 2000). It involves the integration of various forms of information—sensory, semantic, and procedural, for example—that have been disbursed across different regions of the brain and reconstruction of the disparate data into a consonant aggregation (Squire & Kandel, 2000). Retrieval, that is, its content and process, are functions of the context in which retrieval occurs, the retrieval strategy employed, the subject's concurrent state of consciousness and/or emotional stimulation, and the nature of impinging social influences at the time of retrieval (Tulving & Pearlstone, 1966). Thus, retrieval, or the act of remembering, involves more than the reactivation of a stored engram. More precisely, it is the construction of a new, multisensorial record of experience backed by a new cascade of neurological activity. The brain does not, and possibly cannot, create an engram, or neural imprint, for every element of every experience. Rather, current events, as they unfold, are compared and contrasted with the stored multisensorial records of past experiences; if they are distinguishable enough from the existing engrams, neural mechanisms within the brain will activate to encode and store a new memory reflecting the discerned differences (Perry, 1997, 1999). Thus, depending on the cue, context, state, and interaction, the retrieved sensory and somatic content may differ from what was actually stored (Squire & Kandel, 2000). Remembering, then, comprises aspects of the original engram, aspects of memory of similar events, and aspects of the current context of retrieval (Siegel, 2001). In essence, the historic engram and the current retrieval cues, in unison, produce the memory. In other words, memory, as process and outcome, is reconstructive in nature rather than a bona fide moment-to-moment, blow-by-blow, word-for-word duplication of the past.

Simply put, encoding, in this context, involves the conversion of information into a code, just as storage represents the retention of encoded data;

retrieval is the act of transferring the memory from storage into consciousness (Alpert et al., 1996; Bremner et al., 1999).

Forms of Memory

There are two primary forms of memory: explicit and implicit. Explicit memory, also referenced as declarative, encodes, consolidates, and stores consciously accessible facts, both semantic, based on general knowledge of self and the environment, and episodic, generated by autobiographical conditions, situations, and subject matter acquired during a lifetime of experiential learning (Squire & Kandel, 2000). Thus, explicit-semantic memory represents the ability to consciously recall information in the form of verbal propositions and mental imagery (Tulving & Craik, 2000), whereas explicit-episodic memory personifies the ability to consciously recall the self in relation to events of the past, to be cognizant of one's self, identity, and surroundings in the present and to project the self into an imagined future (Siegel, 2001; Wheeler et al., 1997). In terms of explicit-semantic memory, there tends to be general agreement among members of a particular group, such as one's race, gender, or social class, in their conceptualization and comprehension of commonly experienced psychosocial occurrences, characteristics, or phenomena—for example, tailgate parties, hypermasculinity, and dating. Explicit-episodic memory, on the other hand, is idiosyncratic in nature, involving the inner directed thoughts, feelings, and sensations associated with psychosocial roles and functions, such as familial responsibilities, professional experiences, and daily rituals. Explicit-semantic and explicit-episodic memory systems are interactional; for example, semantic memory is utilized to give words and meaning to episodic memory (Brower & Nurius, 1993). Examples of explicit-semantic memory include the facts of a child abuse case or the words to a favorite song. Examples of its explicit-episodic counterpart include recollections of your first day of high school when the principal fell into the orchestra pit, the adoption of your first child after three interrupted attempts, and the evening you introduced your fiancée to your family at your cousin's Edie's wedding in Shadyside, Pennsylvania.

Implicit memory, also known as procedural or nondeclarative memory, comprises information about or knowledge of a phenomenon without conscious recall or verbal components (Pillemer & White, 1989). Implicit memory emerges from experience but is expressed as a change in behavior, not as a recollection (Schacter, 1995). Unlike explicit memory, implicit memory is unconscious; in other words, it involves remembering without awareness of doing so. With explicit memory comes the sense that something is being recalled; with implicit memory, a sense of recollection is absent (Siegel, 2001). Implicit memory is evidenced by the personification of attitudes, skills, and routines in which the knowledge is "second nature" or firmly fixed. Examples of actions operating under implicit memory include riding a bike, changing a diaper, operating a tractor, and playing the violin.

The process of memory, of remembering, is not unitary in nature. As can be seen, memory is truly a systemic process. More accurately, it involves a complex network of processes across various cortical and subcortical regions of the brain (Bremner et al., 1999). Consequently, the memory of a singular event is not encoded, stored, or retrieved in a lone and exclusive region of the brain, nor is a memory processed as or into an intact and autonomous collective of thoughts, sensations, feelings, and behaviors (Tulving & Schacter, 1990). Rather, the divergent sensory receptors transmit data to various regions of the brain and body in order to encode and store the experience, in essence deconstructing the event into a myriad of experiential elements distributed across a network of different areas of the brain. Recollection of the event entails synaptic communication within the neurological network, which, in turn, links the various representational elements of the experience into a memory. Thus, memory is actually a reconstruction of the historic engram within the context of current retrieval cues and states (Siegel, 2001).

Different regions of the brain mediate different functions associated with memory. The hippocampus, amygdala, and contiguous cortical regions, as well as other brain structures and networks, significantly impact the process and content of memory. For example, implicit memory depends on brain structures that are intact at birth and remain so throughout the life span. Explicit memory, on the other hand, emerges subsequently, as it is mediated by brain structures that typically mature a few years after birth (Pillemer & White, 1989; Siegel, 2001).

Implicit memory is a function of a network of brain mechanisms that do not necessitate conscious processing during the stages of encoding and retrieval. It does, however, require processing in the sensory cortices for perceptual memory, the amygdala and other limbic substructures for emotional memory, the somatosensory cortex, orbitofrontal cortex, and anterior cingulate for somatosensory or body memory, and the basal ganglia and motor cortex for behavioral memory. Explicit memory, semantic and episodic, demonstrates the epigenetic course of development as it relies on the maturation of the brain's medial temporal lobe, hippocampus, and frontal cortical regions to encode, store, and retrieve (Schacter, 1996).

The numerous and distinct regions of the brain transact, one with the other and more, in the mediation of memory function (Bremner et al., 1999). The various systems of the brain consist of intricate networks of neurons or nerve cells. Chemically and structurally, these neurons in one system transform in response to input or signals from other regions of the brain, body systems, and the environment. Neurobiological changes permit the storage of information; this storage capacity is the basis for all categories of memory, including sensory, cognitive, affective, motoric, and behavioral (Schore, 2001).

The brain processes information in a use-dependent manner. The degree to which a neurobiological system is set in motion is the degree to which a particular state and affiliated functions become inherent. Examples with differing degree include delivering a speech, driving through a torrential downpour, or getting ready for a first date. Because particular states of arousal, such as terror or relaxation, actuate different neurotransmitters and neuropeptides, the memories stored under such circumstances are a function of that particular state of arousal and the corresponding neural systems. Accordingly, state-dependent learning, hyperarousal, and intrusive memories exemplify this process (Perry et al., 1995). Thus, multiple neurotransmitter and neuropeptide systems are associated with the stress response so frequently found among males with histories of CSA. Chronic abuse and, consequently, chronic stress not only alter the chemistry and structure of the transmitters and peptides but can also lead to long-term behavioral and memory disturbances

SEX, GENDER, AND SCHEMAS

Sex and gender. These terms are often used synonymously, when, in fact, both have distinct meaning. Sex pertains to one's genetic and anatomical composition (Diamond & Karlen, 1980). It is biological, innate. Gender is not.

Gender refers to the state of being male or female (Crooks & Baur, 1993). Gender role is an aggregation of socially prescribed attitudinal and behavioral expectations associated with masculinity and femininity (Bem, 1981). Children learn these mutually exclusive roles through the process of gender role socialization, or the ways in which individuals, families, groups, and other social institutions teach a child to think and act in ways congruent with his or her gender role (Denney & Quadagno, 1992). Gender identity involves an individual's psychological sense of maleness or femaleness vis-à-vis the gender roles prescribed by society, and the integration of this sense into the rest of the personality (Money, 1987). Gender, and its concomitants, then, have more to do with social learning than with biology. Psychosocial meanings around these constructs are initiated in childhood and maintained across the life span by way of the socialization process.

Parents and primary caretakers, as agents of socialization, treat boys differently from girls from early infancy (Sedney, 1987); teachers (Rodgers, 1987) and peers (Kohlberg, 1966), as well as textbooks (Britton & Lumpkin, 1984) and television programs (Kimball, 1986; Tavris & Wade, 1984), reinforce gender-based behaviors in children. Gender constructions, like many of their counterparts, become, for children and adults, an instructional guide. As Bem cogently stated: "No other dichotomy in human experience appears to have as many entities linked to it as does the distinction between male and female" (1981, p. 232). Children not only learn the two gender schemas and convey a clear and stable sense of gender identity by age 3½ (Money & Wiedeking, 1980), but also learn to assess their fitness and appropriateness as a human being in accordance with them.

Systematically, and seemingly "innately," a child learns to superimpose gender schematic constructions on the self. From the vast array of human

behavior, boys and girls, men and women alike, select only that socially prescribed subset congruent with their own gender and, accordingly, only those
socially sanctioned, for inclusion into the self-concept (Bem, 1981).

Bem (1981) further stated:

> The child also learns to evaluate his or her adequacy as a person according
> to the gender schema, to match his or her preferences, attitudes, behaviors,
> and personal attributes against the prototypes stored within it. The gender
> schema becomes a prescriptive standard or guide, and self-esteem becomes
> its hostage. Here, then, enters an internalized motivational factor that prompts
> an individual to regulate his or her behavior so that it conforms to cultural
> definitions of femaleness and maleness. Thus do cultural myths become
> self-fulfilling prophecies. (p. 233)

Children are hereby rewarded for role-congruent behavior, and punished
for behavior deemed inappropriate for their assigned gender (Hyde, 2000).
Not only are gender roles imposed on children by society, but children also
strive to learn, internalize, and personify them as well.

In American society, despite the fact that it is a melting pot of cultures and
ethnicites from around the world, there is consensus about traits for males
(Pleck, 1981; Pollack, 1999) and traits for females (Duncan & Williams, 1998;
Gilligan, 1982). Undergirding this unanimity are separate and distinct social
blueprints, or schemas, that are systematically and systemically enjoined and
socially prescribed, one set for each gender.

Schemas are essentially correlational statements that reciprocally relate a
particular person, group, place, event, or thing with certain characteristics
(Janoff-Bulman, 1992). They typically have two dimensions—declarative and
procedural. For example, a declarative schema holds "knowledge" and inferences about the individual, others, and the world (Kendall & Hollon, 1981).
This schematic categorization process is innately involved in the development
and operation of social mythology. To illustrate, a sexual abuse schema might
hold the following "knowledge": (a) Girls are the predominant victims of sexual
abuse (Broussard et al., 1991; Russell, 1986), and (b) father–daughter incest is
the predominant form of sexual abuse (Eisenberg et al., 1987; Herman, 1981).
This sexual abuse schema, by virtue of its "knowledge," holds the following
inferences: (a) Girls are not abused outside the family; (b) girls are not abused
by females; and (c) boys are rarely sexually abused.

The procedural component of gender schemas shows how seemingly relevant information is employed to render a behavioral response that is aligned
with prevailing social constructions (Kendall & Hollon, 1981). In other words,
what I know (i.e., declarative schema) tells me what to do (i.e., procedural
schema). For instance, behaviors that are valued in males converge into a
socially circumscribed "masculinity" category, directing males to be or become
strong, forceful, muscular, athletic, potent, vigorous, hardy, and rugged. Thus,
a key expectation for males in American culture is that they be powerful and

ready for anything—thereby possessing the characteristics that behaviorally indicate masculinity (Lisak, 1995). Examples of such schematic beliefs are "Male children are dominant, competitive, aggressive, and tough" and "Boys are strong and able to take care of themselves."

Gender schemata reflect and maintain a double standard (Bem, 1981). They prompt individuals to process information on the basis of assigned gender roles and, consequently, evaluate male behavior and female behavior according to different precepts. This upholds and sustains the dichotomization and social allocation of human behavior, including the sexual abuse of children. Given the command of gender to influence the way in which events are processed, it follows that socially constructed conceptions of gender influence the processing of extreme events, such as CSA (Saxe & Wolfe, 1999).

The experience of sexual abuse is highly dissonant with gender role directives. Childhood sexual abuse conjures feelings of powerlessness, helplessness, and submission; gender role socialization requires a boy to be powerful, self-reliant, and resolute. Thus, when a boy is sexually abused, he is thrust into a confrontation between two compelling, interactive, and yet disparate psychosocial processes: the realities of CSA, and the mythology of masculinity (Lisak, 1995).

Whether mythical or real, masculinity defines what femininity is not. In plain words, certain traits and experiences are socially allocated to males and others to females. The male perpetrator/female victim paradigm is a cogent example. It is the foundation from which the vast majority of legislation, research, treatment, and popular writings have emerged. The male perpetrator/female victim paradigm, with its mutually exclusive and dichotomous categories, must give way to a model that recognizes male traumatization and female perpetration. The stark reality of CSA is that neither gender is exempt from either role.

Diagnosis

The impact of childhood sexual abuse is difficult to determine, let alone elucidate, at this point in time (De Bellis, 2001). As CSA occurs, a myriad of biological, psychological, interpersonal, familial, and social variables coalesce, ascending and receding along its own etiologic course, some excitatory, others inhibitory, all contributing to the abuse experience in aggregate. From an ecosystems perspective, consider the multifarious factors that impinge on a boy before, during, and after his exposure to incest or any other form of CSA. For example, in the context of self-system dynamics, his genetic predisposition, exposure to prior trauma, and cognitive appraisals, among others, may intercede with microdynamics, such as family dysfunction, parental alcoholism, and social support. Simultaneously, self-system and microsystem dynamics commix with mesosystem dynamics, including congruities and discrepancies in terms of sex education, gender role expectations, and attachment configurations across microenvironments. Exo factors, such as lack of adequate training for mandated reporters in the identification, assessment, and treatment of the sexual abuse of males, and macrodynamics, such as socially constructed and culturally consigned gender-based reactions to human events, contribute to the totality of the abuse experience. It follows, then, that multivariate dynamics elicit multivariate effects.

CSA, like the vast majority of biopsychosocial phenomena, does not have an uncompounded or unmediated linear relationship with any singular effect. Rather, childhood trauma, including sexual abuse, represents a critical etiologic dynamic that generates a number of effects, immediately or long after the first abusive episode (Terr, 1991). In time, disparate effects can potentially progress into an array of symptom constellations that may or may not meet the requirements for any number of definable diagnostic conditions. Manic depression, sexual compulsivity, and posttraumatic stress disorder are but three of many correlates and potential outcomes of CSA (Kendall-Tackett et al., 1993).

At the outset, it is important to note that posttraumatic stress disorder (PTSD), as classified by the *Diagnostic and Statistical Manual–IV* (American Psychiatric Association, 1994), is a diagnostic category as well as a dichotomous variable. As such, it only depicts the presence or absence of and the temporal dimensions of a cluster of symptoms. Such a discrete categorization does not elucidate the breadth of symptomology across neurological, physiological, psychological, cognitive, affective, emotional, social, and spiritual domains. Nor does it capture the depth of effects along a continuum of absent, partial, or full, for example. The inherited liability in exclusively conceptualizing childhood sexual abuse as a PTSD classification is that the more serious effects and/or effects that do not neatly fall under PTSD's three requisite categories may be overlooked (Finkelhor, 1987, 1990). For example, PTSD, as a phenomenon, does not contribute to the understanding or validation of CSA effects such as encopresis, gender-related cognitive dissonance, confusion around sexual orientation, and loss of spirituality. Thus, as a biopsychosocial phenomenon, PTSD remains too narrow if and when employed as the exclusive conceptual framework for diagnostic, interventive, and empirical efforts (Finkelhor, 1990; van der Kolk, Pelcovitz, Roth, et al., 1996).

Finally, studies within the fields of childhood sexual abuse and the psychobiology of stress indicate that, although children subjected to CSA evidence dysregulation within and among various biological stress response systems and, consequently, manifest symptoms of PTSD, anxiety, depression, dissociative disorders, and the like, the majority of children do not meet such mutually exclusive and differential diagnoses (see, e.g., Ackerman et al., 1998; Brown et al., 2000; Forbey et al., 2000; Kilpatrick & Saunders, 1997; McLeer et al., 1998; Mulder et al., 1998; Ruggiero et al., 2000; Widom, 1999). Outside of theoretical exercise, there exist no "catch-all" diagnoses for individuals with histories of CSA. Indeed, such individuals tend to manifest a variety of effects and symptoms distributed across an array of corporeal and social domains. Accordingly, such a dispersion of effects and symptomology does not yield a "goodness of fit" with established diagnostic categories or, for that matter, with any one explanatory model. Given the nature of childhood sexual abuse, with its diverse biopsychosocial dynamics and effects, perhaps a working "diagnostic category" can be conceptualized as "an environmentally induced complex developmental" (De Bellis, 2001, p. 540) syndrome, as it captures the stressor, stress response, and manifesting symptomology without confining such to a particular disorder and, conversely, without superimposing a disorder on the complex of effects.

SUMMARY

This chapter presented a number of foundational elements undergirding human behavior in the social environment in general and the sexual abuse of males in particular. Assimilation and accommodation, the utilization of schemas and defenses, memory development and retrieval, the workings of the nervous systems, operations of the brain, and gender-role socialization are part of the natural, daily ways in which we, as humans, organize and understand the world. In the event of male sexual abuse, they alternately protect the child and prevent him from integrating this new reality into a uniform and congruent sense of self. Given his understanding of the greater social context in which he lives, and his perceptions of its expectations of him, when sexual abuse occurs and alters his schemas of "reality," SAM is left unable to prepare for disclosure, only to defend against it.

CHAPTER FOUR

THE SAM MODEL
OF DYNAMICS AND EFFECTS

THE SEXUAL ABUSE OF MALES (SAM) model of dynamics and effects evolved in a stepwise manner. A critical review of the effects around the sexual abuse of males rendered a list of findings; a subsequent review of the contextual dynamics provided another list of associated results (Spiegel, 1997a, 1997b). Next, these data were analyzed to determine the essential factors that comprise the model, along with the model's ability to discriminate between boys abused by males, boys abused by females, and boys without histories of childhood sexual abuse (Spiegel, 1996). Finally, a national structural equation modeling study was conducted to validate the proposed conceptual framework (Spiegel, 1997).

The SAM model is composed of seven categories that focus on precipitating events, abusive episodes, their aftermath, and the sociocultural context in which these events occur. Further, the model addresses the biopsychosocial adaptive processes of the boy. Adaptation requires versatility and elasticity; the child must continually adapt to the environment in order to survive.

The categories of the SAM model are as follows: (a) subjection; (b) sexual abuse; (c) concealment; (d) invalidation; (e) reconciliation; (f) compensation; and (g) the cycle continues. In short, *subjection* is the process of predisposing a boy to sexual abuse by means of subtle or blatant interactions that lead to boundary diffusion and role confusion. *Sexual abuse* most typically involves a progression from noncontact to contact behaviors. *Concealment* is the pervasive secrecy that surrounds sexual abuse, both as a social phenomenon and as a personal life event. *Invalidation* is the process of distorting reality by means of intrapersonal defense strategies and numbing tactics and social imposition and denial. *Reconciliation* is the process of submitting to the violations associated with the sexual abuse of boys by assuming responsibility for it. *Compensation* is the process of counteracting or neutralizing the internal conflict associated with sexual abuse by means of cognitive and/or behavioral restructuring. And, *the cycle (of effects) continues* until a male's history of childhood sexual abuse (CSA) is disclosed, validated, and ameliorated.

Caveats

Two caveats are in order. First, a model is merely a systematic way of describing patterns. Therefore, the SAM model does not capture the full extent to which males subjected to CSA experience its dynamics and effects. Hence, it is not a syndrome profile; profiles invariably exclude in the service of parsimony. Second, and more importantly, the intention of the SAM model is to attest to, and to validate, the realities of sexually abused males whose lives are often shrouded in silence. Childhood sexual abuse is profound regardless of gender. Arbitrary and unnatural distinctions serve only to disserve. However, differences in the sexually abusive experience do exist, and the vehicle for such dissimilarity is the socialization process and its consequences—namely, our socially constructed understanding of abuse and gender. Thus, differences may be, in part, a function of the personal, familial, institutional, and social perceptions of and the responses to the sexual abuse of boys in contrast to the perceptions of and reactions to the sexual abuse of girls. Throughout time, this socialization process has influenced the minimization, if not denial, of and around the sexual abuse of males.

Case Examples

This chapter, by way of the SAM model, introduces seven males with histories of CSA. They presented in detail throughout the book, most comprehensively in chapter 4. All describe their past histories of sexual abuse retrospectively. Following are brief descriptions of the selected case examples.

Nicholas is a 7-year-old biracial male of African-American and Euro-American descent. Sexually abused by his mother and her boyfriend, he was eventually referred to treatment after several encounters with a department of social services. Kip is a 16-year-old Caucasian male who was beaten and raped by an ex-convict. A physician noted penile mutilation, a CSA effect among males, and, as part of the treatment plan, directed him to an outpatient sexual abuse therapy program. Palo is Native American; at 20, he is currently separated from his wife. Palo was sexually abused by his father, uncle, cousin, and neighbor, all the while striving to protect his younger siblings from the perpetrators. Matt is a 34-year-old Caucasian male. He was sexually abused by his mother. Compulsive sexual behavior, a series of related arrests, and a succession of failed treatment attempts led him to seek psychotherapeutic services one more time. Victor, incestuously abused by his father for several years, is 43 years old and of Puerto Rican descent. A divorced father of three children, he recently marked an 8-year anniversary with another man. Jake is a 52-year-old Caucasian male with a history of CSA perpetrated by a priest. After years of struggle with binge drinking, Jake, with the encouragement of his wife and three grown children, entered a drug treatment program. Lastly, Ty is a 61-year-old African-American male. He was abused by a male relative and a gang. Their words, generated within clinical sessions or during research interviews, are used throughout to highlight the model's content.

THE SAM MODEL OF DYNAMICS AND EFFECTS

Subjection

It really pisses me off to think about it now. In fact, it's disgusting. My father would be passed out on the floor in an alcoholic stupor and my mother would say things like, "Matt, why did I ever marry that man? Does that look like a man who can make a woman happy? Women have needs, too. We need to be loved and held and touched. When you grow up, I hope that you treat women differently. I know you will, honey. We don't want someone to get on top of us just to grunt and groan. We have needs, too. Remember what mother is teaching you." (Matt, interview with author, October 22, 1994)

Subjection is the process of predisposing a boy to sexual abuse by means of subtle or blatant interactions that lead to boundary diffusion and role confusion (Gill & Tutty, 1999; Hall et al., 1998; Ray & English, 1995). Abused children and abuse perpetrators alike attest to a "grooming" phase that precedes frank sexual abuse (Berliner & Conte, 1990). Typically an evolutionary process (Sgroi et al., 1982), the dynamics of CSA involve intrusion; the boy is in the perpetrator's control and at the mercy of his or her distorted perceptions (Burgess et al., 1987; Summit, 1983). The basis of such distorted perceptions most often can be generalized into two distinct categories: that of the fixated and that of the regressed perpetrator (Groth, Hobson, & Gary, 1982).

At the self-domain of the ecosystems perspective, the fixated or preferential perpetrator, with an erotic and relational orientation toward children, identifies closely with youth and equalizes the discrepancies by matching his or her behavior with a boy's developmental and/or chronological level (Groth et al., 1982). Fixation refers to the temporary or abiding arrestment of biopsychosocial development attributable to unresolved formational tasks and events that persist underneath the organization of succeeding stages of maturation (Groth & Birnbaum, 1978). Highly fixated perpetrators are those whose thoughts, desires, and sexual fantasies focus centrally on children for protracted periods of time (Knight & Prentsky, 1993). Dynamically, the perpetrator perceives and understands himself or herself to be the boy's emotional, psychological, and relational peer, whereas the boy's experience is that of interacting with an adult (Pescosolido, 1989). Additionally, the fixated perpetrator's pedophiliac interests tend to begin during adolescence, with no apparent precipitating stressor. The abusive behavior is persistent, compulsive, and premeditated. Developmentally immature and socially inept, such perpetrators harbor self-perceptions akin to those found among children. Relative to regressed perpetrators, fixated or preferential offenders are more rare and, as a rule, emotionally and sexually prefer children to adults (Jenny et al., 1994). Their greatest area of differentiation, independent of sexual orientation, may be that of social competence (Knight & Prentsky, 1993).

The regressed or situational perpetrator, with a primary sexual orientation toward adults, often replaces conflictual peer relationships through involvement with boys (Groth et al., 1982). Regression is conceptualized as the temporary or abiding manifestation of primitive behavior following the actualization of more sophisticated and age-congruent modes of interaction, regardless of whether the immature behavior actually materialized in the perpetrator's early development (Groth & Birnbaum, 1978). Thus, regressed perpetrators revert to a less mature psychological state, wherein the views of self, children, and sexual relations are palpably different from the prior state of consciousness. Given the transitory dynamic underlying regression, the regressed perpetrator's interest in children tends to be episodic, often accelerated by a detectable stressor, perhaps in the workplace, perhaps at home. In terms of social competence, perpetrators who fare well in this area are likely to evidence a number of the following: (a) employment consistency; (b) a stable history of marriage or cohabitation; (c) the continuous parenting of a child; (d) active participation in an adult-oriented organization; and (e) a stable friendship with a peer (Knight & Prentsky, 1993). Frequently, the sexual abuse of a child runs concurrent with adult sexual relations. Relative to a highly fixated offender, the regressed but socially competent perpetrator tends to have a more traditional lifestyle (Groth et al., 1982).

Psychologically and behaviorally, just as the fixated perpetrator becomes a "child," the regressed perpetrator perceives and experiences the child as a pseudo-adult. The majority of perpetrators, however, may personify attributes of both fixation and regression (Conte, 1990). However, fixated or preferential perpetrators who target toddlers or very young school-age children are less apt to discriminate between boys and girls. In contrast, sexual offenders with orientations toward older children are more inclined to perpetrate decisively against either boys or girls (Jenny et al., 1994).

Female and male perpetrators, in an attempt to master their own histories of childhood trauma, may reenact personally relevant dynamics of CSA with the unconscious intention of undoing or ameliorating the pain, shame, guilt, blame, and humiliation generated by their traumatic pasts (Wurtele & Miller-Perrin, 1992). Additionally, through the years, they may have used aspects of their abusive histories in masturbation fantasies or may have conjured sexual fantasies associating coercion and care, sex and violence, or, perhaps, love and pain, thereby habituating a particular arousal response (Lambie et al., 2002; Proulx et al., 1996; Ryan & Lane, 1997). On average, perpetrators begin abusing during adolescence, around age 15, and, through the years, incestuous perpetrators subject an average of 1.7 children to CSA while extrafamilial perpetrators subject an average of 150 boys and approximately 20 girls to CSA (Abel et al., 1987). Female perpetrators are similar to male perpetrators in terms of the number of children they abuse, the proportions of incestual mother and father offenders they encompass, and the frequency and degree of force employed (Faller, 1987). Finally, female perpetrators are inclined to abuse equivalent numbers of boys and girls or to show a preference toward female children (Faller, 1987, 1995; Fehrenbach & Monastersky, 1988; Mayer, 1992; Rudin et al., 1995; Travin et al., 1990).

It is not uncommon for intrafamilial and extrafamilial perpetrators to harbor a sense of inferiority within the self and around interactions with adult peers; with chronic feelings of vulnerability, humiliation, powerlessness, anger, inadequacy, and loneliness, they fear exposure and rejection (Proulx et al., 1996). Threat-sensitive and easily stressed around others, they tend to contend with these relational deficits by evading social interactions whenever possible (Smith & Saunders, 1995) and by engaging in sex more frequently to cope with their negative feeling states (Cortoni & Marshall, 2001). In fact, the majority of perpetrators report that stress emanating from home and work and distress associated with psychological, interpersonal, and sexual problems frequently precipitates another abusive episode or the engagement of yet another child into a sexually abusive relationship (Elliott, Browne, & Kilcoyne, 1995; Proulx et al., 1996).

In essence, problematic situations in the workplace and intimacy deficits in the home engender negative emotional states, which, in turn, provoke a need to relieve such states. CSA perpetrators retreat into fantasy when confronted with stress. Detached from reality, they cognitively deconstruct their current situations and sexual intentions (Ward et al., 1995). In this state, immediate, concrete, and positive consequences, for example, relief from anxiety and the potential for sexual pleasure, overrun more abstract contemplations about the immorality and illegality of their actions and corresponding long-term consequences (Marshall et al., 2000). Sexual activity, alone or with children, is a perpetrator's global response to a multitude of stressors (Cortoni & Marshall, 2001). The primary reasons for failing to employ more adaptive strategies to coping with a negative mood include the lack of will, anticipation of failure, and absorption in the emotional state (McKibben, Proulx, & Lussier, 2001). While preparing for the abuse, facilitative behaviors or states, such as the misuse and abuse of drugs and alcohol, the use of pornographic materials, recurring fantasies about prior encounters with children, the presence of psychosis, and incompetent regulation of impulses, for example, may be in operation and serve to biologically, psychologically, and socially disinhibit the perpetrator (Elliott et al., 1995; Finkelhor, 1984; Wurtele & Perrin-Miller, 1992).

Perpetrators often possess an uncanny penchant for identifying and selecting vulnerable children—children with unmet emotional needs, who seem to be insecure; boys ostracized from family and peers; children hungry for acceptance, care, and affection; prepubescent boys and girls who appear to lack secondary sex characteristics; boys who they believe to have traits commonly associated with the other gender; and postpubescent girls and boys who appear to be older, more developed, and, therefore, from the perpetrator's perspective, more inclined to view the sexual interaction as mutual and recip-rocal (Budin & Johnson, 1989; Conte et al., 1989; Elliott et al., 1995; Harry, 1989, in Doll et al., 1992). Maternal, paternal, and sibling perpetrators, of course, have ready access within the home (Elliott & Peterson, 1993; Faller, 1995; Worling, 1995). Whatever the case, through social learning, perpetrators ob-serve and learn that children can be used for sexual gratification (Baker, Tabacoff, Tornusciolo, & Eisenstadt, 2001; Ryan, 1995).

The vast majority of nonincestual perpetrators offend against one child at a time (Elliott et al., 1995); however, over the years, the sum total frequently exceeds 100. In fact, perpetrators abuse boys with an incidence that is five times greater than the molestation of young girls (Abel et al., 1987). Perpetra-tors tend to frequent places where children would be expected to go—after-school games, shopping malls, video arcades, amusement parks, playgrounds, public parks and beaches, carnivals, and swimming pools. Depending on the age of the boy and the context of subjection, many perpetrators will endeavor to establish rapport with his family members (Elliott et al., 1995; Roane, 1992), not only to gain access but to incrementally contrive the illusion of trust and normalcy. Perpetrators outside of the immediate family circle offer to baby-sit, mentor, or coach—teaching the boy when to hit the baseball, how to recite his multiplication tables, where to fish, what life is all about. They stalk for an empty niche and seek to fill it. In some cases, older siblings, abused within or outside the family, are used by perpetrators to recruit younger siblings and peers (Burgess et al., 1987; Elliott et al., 1995).

Many sexual offenders cognitively construct and, moreover, believe dis-torted rationales that permit and condone their sexual involvement with chil-dren. Common rationalizations include:

1. "My husband doesn't want me. You don't want me to be lonely, right?"
2. "I want you to learn things the right way so that's why I'm teaching you."
3. "Your erection says it all. Don't ever try to put this on me."
4. "Everyone knows you're a fag but they don't say nothing to your face. At least I'm honest and letting you know that you want this kind of sex."
5. "You're my son. I love you."
6. "You want me to do this to you, I can tell."
7. "I look out for you, take care of you, break my back for you. The least you can do is give me love and affection, too."
8. "This doesn't hurt. Just relax. Besides, you won't remember any of this. Trust me."
9. "You're very mature for your age. Better me than someone from the street."
10. "If you do what I tell you, no one will find out."

Although patterns of distortion are common to all perpetrators, the particulars vary according to contextual dynamics—the perpetrator's age, personality, degree of fixation, level of social competency, and relational status with the boy, and the boy's age and gender presentation, for example.

Within the microdomain, and, in particular, the family system, many perpetrators have a history of family aggression and violence (Hanson & Bussière, 1998), often in association with alcohol abuse (Spencer & Dunklee, 1986) and criminal behavior (U.S. Department of Justice, 1996). The abusive family culture normalizes unusual sleeping arrangements, nudity, overt sexual behavior, pornography, and other acts and utterances that may unduly stimulate children and, in turn, give "license" for their maltreatment (Finkelhor, 1986; Hall et al., 2002).

Parents in abusive families often inhibit the separation and individuation processes of their children; children are not to be seen, not to be heard, and furthermore, not to stand out in any way, so as to steer unwanted attention away from the family. Parents with histories of CSA may simultaneously intermesh with the child and create distance within the marital dyad. A mother's history of CSA may exacerbate her emotional reliance on her son to such a degree that she is both ineffective and unavailable when it comes to fulfilling her needs for intimacy, companionship, and support within her current adult relationships (Alexander, Teti, & Anderson, 2000). One parent, in an attempt to defend against the escalating conflict within the marital dyad, may initiate a triangulation dynamic by turning to SAM, or a sibling, for his or her sexual and emotional fulfillment. SAM, once an outsider vis-à-vis the parental dyad, and rightfully so, is made an insider by virtue of incestual relations, whereby the nonoffending parent is relegated to the position of outsider.

In the mesodomain, contradictions abound. On the one hand, various mainstream media and advertising show the erotic portrayal of children; on the other hand, children are often taught that sex is dirty, secretive, and private (Wurtele & Miller-Perrin, 1992). Undoubtedly, this conveys a mixed and confusing message. What's more, the vast majority of perpetrators are known to the children they abuse (Feiring et al., 1999; Kisiel & Lyons, 2001; McLeer et al., 1998) and yet, a major emphasis in child protection strategies is that of "stranger-danger" (Levesque, 1994)—a confounding message, once again.

Within the exodomain, social policies regarding and state statutes concerning CSA present a number of gender-based and child-based biases. To illustrate, some statutes hold as a requisite penile penetration; others overtly or covertly suggest an age of consent (Struve, 1990). In some cases, the burden of proof is on the child to show that force, beyond that required for penetration, was necessary and therefore sufficient to render compliance. Further, there is a reluctance on the part of the legal and judicial systems to adjudicate and punish perpetrators (Wurtele & Miller-Perrin, 1992). For example, of CSA cases accepted by a district attorney's office, the vast majority do not go to trial (Cross et al., 1995; Faller & Henry, 2000; Gray, 1993; Gray et al., 1999). In mnay instances, perpetrators are not charged with a sexual offense. Rather a limited minority result in criminal court conviction (Bradley & Wood, 1996; Gray et al.,

1999). If and when a perpetrator is convicted, the charges are frequently dropped or a plea bargain to a lesser, nonsexual charge is filed. Even when a jail term is requisitioned, most are suspended at some point in time (Cheit & Goldschmidt, 1997; Cullen et al., 2000; Gray et al., 1999). If a boy is 12 or older, the chance of a case resulting in a conviction is significantly less likely than if he were 11 or younger (Isquith et al., 1993). Even when cases are substantiated by child protective services, a substantial majority are not criminally adjudicated (Tjaden & Thoennes, 1992). The situation is even more alarming as it relates to female perpetrators. The vast majority of female offenders were not prosecuted for sexual offenses against children, even after they coerced boys into vaginal and anal intercourse, penetrative and/or receptive (Faller, 1995; Fehrenbach & Monastersky, 1988).

Continuing with exodynamics, the vast majority of prevention and intervention programs emanate from the male perpetrator/female victim paradigm (Spiegel, 1995; Struve, 1990), leaving boys more confused, less understood, and with little or no recourse to prevent further abuse. It's no wonder that girls view CSA prevention programs as more informative, interesting, helpful, and applicable than boys do (Finkelhor & Dziuba-Leatherman, 1995). Unfortunately, little is known about how prevention agendas and curricula, as a matter of course, actually operate and fulfill programmatic objectives in their communities (Plummer, 2001). Finally, the lack of or biased presentation of sexuality education within schools, community centers and places of worship limits knowledge acquisition and skill building for children, adults, and families alike (Krivacska, 1990).

With regard to the macrodomain, there exists (albeit not fully recognized) the social allocation of sexual dominance, initiation, and power to males and a denial of such to females; the social allocation of emotionality and caretaking to females is, in turn, denied to males. Further, the macrosystem also upholds the social construction of children as parental property and the ideology of family sanctity, characterized by a respect for privacy, parental authority, and noninterference (Allen, 1990; Lew, 1990).

This discussion does not represent a "profile" of a perpetrator, nor does it fully characterize the abusive family in America today. In fact, the breadth, depth, and dispersion of demographic, historic, personality, and systemic attributes among perpetrators and abusive families are not easily captured by prototypic profiles (Murphy & Peters, 1992; Smith & Saunders, 1995). Hence, this presentation merely conveys characteristics that have shown an association with perpetrators of CSA and families in which abuse occurs.

Regardless of perpetrator category and impinging factors, sexual offenders equally distort reality, impose roles, and lie to boys about love, safety, and trust. As a result of these distortions, impositions, and lies, the boy experiences boundary diffusion and role confusion. With the former, he must adapt to the violation of private, intimate, and personal boundaries (DeJong et al., 1983; Janus et al., 1987; Reinhart, 1987). Much of this predispositional activity takes place in both public and private bathrooms. It might include invasive observation, exhibitionism, bathing with a parent, the administration of enemas for nonmedical reasons, and the use of sexually explicit language with an eye to taunt or entice (Spiegel, 1998b). Female perpetrators, and more so if they're in a caretaking role, subject a boy to CSA under the pretense of "normalized behavior"—"accidental" exposures, inspecting his body, inserting suppositories—all contrived to stimulate themselves and the boy (Dimock, cited in Lipshires, 1994, p. 4).

Boundaries can be diffused in other ways as well. Some boys are manipulated with drugs or alcohol (Cavaiola & Schiff, 1988; Mendel, 1995), through either direct or deceptive means. Before an abusive episode, drugs and alcohol are frequently employed by the perpetrator as a way to prepare and control the boy; after an abusive episode, drugs and alcohol are utilized to benumb his traumatic memories and effects of CSA (Burgess et al., 1987). Other boys must adapt to physical violations, as it is not uncommon for them to be subjected to aggressive behavior prior to sexual abuse (Friedrich & Luecke, 1988; Gale et al., 1988; Leverich et al., 2002).

The boy is also manipulated into a state of role confusion (Dimock, 1988) as he is thrust into gender-discordant and developmentally advanced roles. For a boy, regardless of age, gender-discordant labels include "sissy," "faggot," and "Daddy's little girl." Further, male and female perpetrators alike may coerce SAM into wearing clothing designed for girls, and most often under duress (Lawson, 1993; Spiegel, 1997b). Five-year-old Nicholas stated: "His big man penis goin' inside me hurt bad. But the worst hurt was when he kept calling me a 'girl' and makin' me wear my Mama's nightie. That means I'm a big mistake." Developmentally advanced roles, such as "Mommy's little man," confidant regarding sexual issues, peer, lover, and protector, are inappropriate and confusing independent of the boy's age or level of maturity (Spiegel, 1995). Matt stated: "In any given day, she [his mother] would tell me how inept my father was sexually, make me do my homework, mix her martinis, send me off to Boy Scouts or catechism and then make me have sex with her at night. I remember saying to myself, 'It's only a movie, only a movie.' I thought I would go insane."

With respect to any strategy involving gender or developmental discordancy, the target of attack is SAM's sense of gender integrity. Perpetrators who are motivated by, or who are attempting to reclaim, power and control often try to impair the worth of a boy's sense of gender identity in order to render him vulnerable. Other perpetrators, stimulated by the fantasy of equality and the illusion of love, strive to enhance and amplify his sense of gender identity. Thus, an underlying dynamic of intimidation exploits SAM's need to feel validated and accepted as a male child. Regardless of method, a boy manipulated and falsified in this way develops a distorted role perception of himself (Adams-Tucker, 1985; Hunter, 1991; Lisak, 1994a) and of others (Ben-Porath & Davis, 2000; Janus et al., 1987; Lew, 1990; Urquiza & Crowley, 1986). Subjection, then,

not only fosters boundary diffusion and role confusion but vulnerability, isolation, and dependency as well—rendering the boy under the perpetrator's control.
Does the perpetrator realize that the recurrent violations of physical, psychological, emotional, spiritual, familial, and social boundaries incite disarray within
SAM's evolving sense of self (Putnam & Trickett, 1993)? SAM guesses not.

Sexual Abuse

> He would stumble in drunk. I often prayed that he would never come
> home. But he did. I would pretend to be asleep. He would come into my
> room drunk and fall onto my bed. I was always pretending to be asleep. I
> never knew if he was going to beat the shit out of me or hug me. God, he
> smelled so bad. He would say, "Son, I love you so much. You make me so
> proud." "Bullshit," I wanted to scream back. "You're a fucking liar!" And he
> would grab my face and kiss my cheek and then my lips. He seemed to stay
> there forever. I would hold my breath until he let go. God, I hated that. But
> it didn't stop. It just kept getting worse. I was his boy. Then I became his
> cocksucker. Finally, he made me his wife. (Victor, interview with author,
> November 30, 1994)

Sexual abuse is far from an uncommon in the United States today. It is
estimated that 16% of males—or roughly 1 of every 6—are sexually abused
prior to the age of 18 (Finkelhor et al., 1990; Kellogg & Hoffman, 1995; Rosetti,
1995; Urquiza & Capra, 1990). Contrary to social mythology, the vast majority
of these boys are abused by perpetrators known to them (Feiring et al., 1999;
Fondacaro et al., 1999; Fromuth & Burkhart, 1989; Kisiel & Lyons, 2001; Kolko
et al., 1988; Reinhart, 1987). Additionally, between one-third and two-thirds of
males abused by one perpetrator will subsequently confront abuse by others
(Harrison et al., 1997; Hunter, 1991; Robin et al., 1997). Indeed, childhood
sexual abuse, as an interpersonal form of violence, has a tendency to be chronic
and more severe than traumas occurring outside of a relationship (De Bellis,
2001).

When compared to the sexual abuse of girls, SAM is more likely to experience physical abuse in tandem with sexual abuse (Cavaiola & Schiff, 1988;
Kelly et al., 2002; MacMillan et al., 2001; Sansonnet-Hayden et al., 1987) and is
more likely to be abused with force (Doll et al., 1992; Gold et al., 1997; Pierce
& Pierce, 1985).

Childhood sexual abuse often involves a progression from noncontact
types of behavior, such as sexualized talk, verbal abuse of a sexual nature,
invasive observation, and exhibitionism, to contact behaviors such as inappropriate kissing, fondling, and intercourse (Berliner & Conte, 1990; Sgroi et al.,
1982). It can also be acute, with little or no progression, as is often the case
with rape. More often than not, CSA typically originates with what is perceived
to be, and what is experienced as, expressions of care and affection. More
often than not, a progression begins within the context of familiar physical

activities. For example, bathing a boy, examining a bruise or rash, teaching him how to swing a bat, hugging him, tickling him, tucking him into bed, and snuggling with him provide opportunities for physical contact (Berliner & Conte, 1995). As subjection transitions into sexual abuse, perpetrators steadily and shrewdly test the boy's reactions to escalating increments of sexualized talk, sexual materials, and sexual touch (Elliott et al., 1995). At first, SAM does not realize that he is the object of coercion, manipulation, and deception; behaviors and activities like these seem incidental or accidental; he does not discern their sexual nature, the intention of the perpetrator, or the progression of abuse (Berliner & Conte, 1990).

Why would he? In anticipating the likelihood of life events, boys perceive the following as more conceivable and probable than CSA: (a) a sports injury; (b) a serious injury from bike riding; (c) failing a subject in school; (d) a car accident fatality; (e) nuclear war within the United States; (f) drowning while swimming; (g) a gunshot wound; (h) being kidnapped; and (i) getting AIDS. Interestingly, in the United States, the fatality rate from automobile accidents is 19.9/100,000 and the death rate from drowning is 2.2/100,000. The reported rate of sexual abuse is 630/100,000 (Dziuba-Leatherman & Finkelhor, 1994). As Victor stated: "I imagined getting hit in the head with a baseball. I imagined what it might be like to get killed by a hurricane. I even imagined fighting and dying for my country in World War III. But never in my worst nightmare did I imagine that I would be incested by my father." In a like way, parents view their own children as less vulnerable to perpetrators and CSA than children from other families (Collins, 1996). Perhaps they are in error, understandably so, but misled nonetheless.

Among boys, contact behaviors are more common than noncontact behaviors and penetrating sexual acts are more common than nonpenetrating acts (Allard-Dansereau et al., 1997; McLeer et al., 1998; Paul et al., 2001). These contact behaviors and penetrative acts include kissing, fondling, masturbation, fellatio, cunnilingus, anilingus, frottage, penetration of the vagina with a finger or object, penetration of the anus with a finger or object, penile penetration of the vagina, penile penetration of the anus, and sexual relations with other children, adults, or animals (see, e.g., Kelly et al., 2002; Paul et al., 2001; Sigmon et al., 1995). For SAM, coercive receptive rectal intercourse is the primary offense perpetrated against him (Gully et al., 2000; Holmes, 1997; Huston, 1995; Wells et al., 1997; Woods & Dean, 1985). It is important to note, however, that abuse also extends beyond activities done to the boy. A substantial majority of boys are coerced into performing sexual acts on their perpetrators (Gold et al., 1997; Moisan et al., 1997), including vaginal and anal penetration (Kelly et al., 2002; Paul et al., 2001; Richardson et al., 1993; Sigmon et al., 1996). In fact, vaginal intercourse is the modal abusive act involving boys and their female perpetrators (Duncan & Williams, 1998; Lisak & Luster, 1994; Mendel, 1995). Hence, the male child is commonly required not only to submit to actions done to him, but to perform actions on others as well.

Whatever the sexual act or context, it is erroneous and capricious to suggest that penetration is more severe than fondling, that contact abuse is more harmful than noncontact abuse, or that male perpetration is any more or less corrupt than female perpetration, especially when viewed theoretically and out of context. For example, Kip was anally penetrated while a knife was held to his head; Matt was incestuously abused by his mother, no material weapons involved; and Palo was forced to pose for pornographic pictures that were distributed to adult males. CSA, in all its variations, forces the child to confront, and adapt to, interpersonal violations, a dispossession of will, isolation, and loss of agency. But a question, as voiced in social, clinical, and legal circles remains: Is it traumatic?

CSA is startling; it often occurs with little, if any, notice, and, particularly for boys, without anticipation (Finkelhor & Dziuba-Leatherman, 1995). Indeed, confrontation with the unknown, especially for a child, holds little promise for adaptation by way of forethought (McCann & Pearlman, 1990). Antithetically, CSA imposes immediate threats that engender momentous fear and horror (Brown & Anderson, 1991; Burgess et al., 1984, 1987; Hibbard et al., 1990). Thus, when abuse occurs, SAM instinctively responds by entering what Krystal (1978) termed the "traumatic state." Trauma here is defined as the "overwhelming of the normal self preservative functions in the face of inevitable danger. The recognition of the existence of unavoidable danger and the surrender to it mark the onset of the traumatic state" (p. 76).

"For children, sexually traumatic events may include developmentally inappropriate sexual experiences without threatened or actual violence or injury" (American Psychiatric Association, 1994). However, threats and acts of violence are common perpetrator strategies (Friedrich & Luecke, 1988) used to commence and conceal the sexually abusive relationship. Actual force is more commonly brought to bear against males than females (Gold et al., 1998; Pierce & Pierce, 1985) and is executed in the majority of sexually abusive relationships involving boys (Finkelhor, 1981; Gully et al., 2000; Ratner et al., in press; Roesler & McKenzie, 1994; Wolfe et al., 1994). Thus, in the face of CSA, children are markedly without defense, as they confront abject terror, fear of the unknown, and helplessness. Sexual abuse, as a traumatic event, arouses neurological (De Bellis et al., 2001), physiological (Perry & Pollard, 1998), psychological (Calam et al., 1998), cognitive (Siegel, 1996), emotional (van der Kolk & Fisler, 1995), behavioral (Grilo et al., 1999), and spiritual (Rossetti, 1995) states of distress upon its occurrence and upon its recollection. To be sure, CSA obstructs SAM's anticipated developmental path, intruding on his frames of reference as a child, as a male, of love, of the world, and of God (Pearlman & Saakvitne, 1995). In essence, a boy's physical, psychological, emotional, spiritual, and gender integrity are threatened and, in some cases, irreparably harmed. Thus, childhood sexual abuse is traumatic given its sweeping potentiality for damage—upon its occurrence and well into adulthood (Courtois, 1999).

PSYCHOBIOLOGY OF THE STRESS RESPONSE

The constellation of human reactions to stress and trauma appears to be universal in that the central nervous system's adaptive and patterned responses are consistent across individuals and across threatening and overwhelming stimuli (van der Kolk & Saporta, 1993). In other words, "while there are an infinite number of stressors that can cause a subjective sense of overwhelming stress and distress in a child, there are finite ways that the brain and the body (i.e., biological stress systems) can respond to those stressors" (De Bellis, 2001, p. 540).

The contour of stress envelops a number of biological, psychological, and sociological transpirations. For example, a perpetrator subjects SAM to CSA; CSA, as a biopsychosocial stressor or stimulus, not only invades his boyhood body but galvanizes a reaction within his brain, sometimes referenced as primary appraisal (Kollack-Walker, Day, & Akil, 2000). During this time, SAM unconsciously codifies the stressor's depth of threat and degree of endangerment, comparing and contrasting it with previous experience. Instantaneously, SAM unconsciously predicts his ability to cope with and, if possible, control the mounting frenzy of CSA. This stress perception, in turn, activates the stress response. Within milliseconds, psychobiological systems within his body evoke the discharge of neurotransmitters and hormones that operate as the brain's messengers throughout his central nervous system (Bremner, 2002; Dhabhar, 2000; Yehuda, 2000). His boyhood body is simply striving to accommodate the perpetrator's advances and reestablish biological, psychological, and social equilibrium. SAM's stress response can be acute, persisting from a few minutes to a few hours, or chronic, occurring daily, for hours at a time.

Theoretically and experientially, SAM's stress response can be conceptualized along a stressor–arousal continuum (Perry, 1999, 2001). For example, each sexually abusive episode has a beginning, middle, and end. As a sexually abusive episode ensues, particularly the initial or more violent ones, SAM's internal state may transform from calm to vigilant, from alarm to fear, and ultimately advance on to terror, depending on the nature of the abuse and his biopsychosocial response constellation. SAM's brain conducts, instructs, and regulates this complex total-body response. As threat increases, SAM traverses along the arousal continuum. Acute or chronic stress reaches traumatic dimensions as his stimulus barrier is breached (A. Freud, 1967). When this occurs, CSA, as a traumatic event, besets SAM's neuronal homeostasis (Perry & Pollard, 1998), shatters his cognitive assumptions about self, others, the world, and his future (Janoff-Bulman, 1989), conditions his emotional networks of fear (LeDoux, 1995), sensitizes and habituates his psychobiobehavioral responses (Schore, 2001), and interferes with his systems of implicit and explicit memory (Siegel, 1999). Thus, SAM embodies the stress response as it manifests and permeates within and across his neurological, psychological, physiological, cognitive, affective, behavioral, and interpersonal domains of functioning and responsivity.

The Arousal Continuum

The arousal continuum, spanning from calm to terror, is undergirded by a progressive stream of activities within the body (Perry, 2001; Perry & Polland, 1998). Upon exposure to a traumatic stressor, like childhood sexual abuse, SAM's body initiates a number of neurobiological and physiological operations, spontaneously and, at times, simultaneously (Yehuda, 2000), all with an eye toward preservation and the reestablishment of a homeostatic state. To begin, SAM is likely to evidence beveled and irregular fluctuations in stress-responsive neurotransmitters, the endogenous chemicals released at the synapse of a neuron with the objective of conveying a signal from one nerve cell to another, and stepwise fluctuations in neuropeptides, the linear sequences of proteins functioning as neurotransmitters. These stress-induced hormones, acting as chemical messengers of and within the central nervous system, include catecholamines, such as norepinephrine, epinephrine, and dopamine, corticotropin-releasing factor (CRF), adrenocorticotropic hormone (ACTH), glucocorticoids, acetylcholine, serotonin, and opioids (Bremner et al., 1999). Indeed, within this neural network of transmitted activity, SAM's brain and central nervous system cogently evidence a biopsychosocial imperative toward survival, in defiance of the predatorial invasion of his body and in defense of his birthright to life-affirming respect and care.

The arousal continuum, or stress response, is mediated by the brain's limbic system (van der Kolk, Burbridge, & Suzuki, 1997). The objective is twofold: to estimate the nature and degree of threat, and to coordinate neurological, psychological, and behavioral responses within an ecosystemic context (Harvey, 1996). The limbic system, complex in nature, comprises a number of substructures including the amygdala and the hippocampus. However, given the hierarchical nature of the brain, SAM's stress-response constellation emanates from the blunt but vital lower region, the brainstem, progressing on to the complex and highly honed neocortex (Perry, 1999, 2001).

THE BRAIN'S RESPONSE TO THREAT

In simple terms, the brain develops sequentially into a hierarchical structure, from the brainstem to the cortex, with the simplest and most reflexive activities, such as body temperature and blood pressure, regulated by the brainstem; sleep, arousal, and motoric behavior modulated by the diencephalon; more sophisticated activities, for instance, emotional reactivity, attachment, and explicit and implicit memory functions, processed by the limbic system; and the most complex activities, including abstract thought, concrete operations, and analytic interpretation, mediated by the neocortex.

The Brainstem as First Processing Point

Sensory information, for example, the perpetrator's footsteps, the smell of his body, the sound of her voice, the sight of his penis, the taste of her saliva, and the sensation of penetration, register in the sensory processing receptors of SAM's body (LeDoux, 1994). These first-order sensations, cued and occurring within the abusive space, are transformed into sensory neurons. As "data," they enter his brainstem, an initial processing point, wherein they are immediately appraised against an amalgam of experience, that is, SAM's previously stored patterns of neural activity (Perry, 2001). When sensory input registers as unanticipated or novel, or as a mnemonic reminiscent of a prior traumatic or overwhelming event, the brainstem signals an initial yet undiscerning phase of an alarm response, which, in turn, activates the central and peripheral nervous systems. Within this more primitive region of the brain, the reticular activating system, composed of the locus caeruleus, noradrenergic neurons, serotonergic neurons, dopaminergic neurons, and other excitatory and inhibitory neural systems, regulates the activity level of the entire nervous system (Perry & Pollard, 1998). It is acutely involved in the excitation and inhibition of kinesthetic sensations, including pain. However, this reticular formation, together with the locus caeruleus, does not fully myelineate until early adolescence (Perry, 1997, 2001).

The locus coeruleus is conceptualized as the "trauma center" of the brain (Krystal et al., 1989) due to its possession and regulation of the preponderance of SAM's noradrenergic nerve cells. Not only does it receive sensory data of all types, it also responds to the vast majority of stressful stimuli, consequently impacting multiple areas of the central nervous system (Sutherland & Davidson, 1999). In this way, the locus caeruleus functions as another checkpoint with the task of ascertaining the emotional significance of incoming sensory data, and all within a matter of milliseconds. If SAM perceives and appraises internal or external stimuli as threatening, the locus caeruleus, along with the ventral tegmental nucleus, releases catecholamines throughout his body, further orchestrating the arousal response (De Bellis & Putnam, 1994). SAM is now hypervigilant. As a cautioning monitor, the locus caeruleus–norepinephrine system, once mobilized, sharpens SAM's sensory field, empowering him to focus more acutely, barring irrelevant, neutral, or distracting information that might otherwise assail the central nervous system. Thus, only the particulars within SAM's immediate microenvironment deemed critical remain fixed in his sensory field, as all other seemingly nonrelevant details recede outside the frank act of CSA.

At this juncture, SAM has little subjective perception, let alone consciousness of these psychobiological machinations. Even though he is alert and primed for fight-or-flight-or-freeze, discernment is crude, interpretations shallow, and reflexivity swift (Perry, 1999). However, it is at a subsequent checkpoint—the diencephalon and, in particular, the thalamus—that SAM begins to palpably sense anxiety's upward slope.

The Diencephalon as Second Processing Point

Next, and with headlong velocity, the sensory information proceeds to the diencephalon. The diencephalon anatomically comprises the uppermost region of the brainstem (Perry, 2000). As a bridge between the body and the brain, the diencephalon plays a key role in the formation of memory. It includes the thalamus, hypothalamus, and the pituitary gland. The thalamus functions prominently within the factual memory network. As the gateway to the cerebral or sensory cortex, the thalamic nuclei process all sensory information, with the exception of olfactory input, before the data proceed onto more sophisticated and interpretative courses of action. The thalamus factors considerably in relaying somatosensory data within and beyond the corporeal environment to the amygdala (Fanselow & Gale, 2000). In this way, it plays a critical role in both states of awareness and sensorimotor responsivity. The hypothalamus synchronizes the sympathetic component of the autonomic nervous system and, that being so, centrally serves in the operation of the fight-or-flight response set, monitoring alterations along the arousal continuum—SAM's heartbeat, increased dilation of bronchi, elevated oxygenation and blood pressure, and changes rendered by the release of excitatory and inhibitory neurotransmitters (see later section). The pituitary gland is conceptualized as the master of the endocrine system as it secretes hormones that modulate the discharge of additional hormones, thereby directly and indirectly impacting every major gland of the body (Antoni, 2000).

In terms of SAM's sensory data, all exterosensory information, excepting the olfactory, enters the thalamus while the hypothalamus and pituitary stand watch over the body, mutually and reciprocally commanding the stress-responsive hypothalamo–pituitary–adrenal (HPA) axis and regulating other functions in order to ensure the best possible compromise between environmental stimuli and corporeal resources. Once processed, the data, emotionally laden with fear, trepidation, and the unknown, bisects along two separate neuronal trajectories—one reflexive, the other integrative—both involving the limbic system and, most notably, the amygdala.

The Limbic System as Third Processing Point

The limbic system is centrally located between the diencephalon and the neocortex. By now, its amygdala is superabundant with sensory data from SAM's body and the abuse environment. In fact, the amygdala can be conceptualized as an axial hub for emotional processing given its anatomical connectivity with a number of key brain substructures (LeDoux, 1992, 1994). It imbues experience with emotional meaning and, more specifically, it acts as the registrar and generator of fear.

SAM's sensory information travels along two major pathways—one from the thalamus and another from the neocortex—with both entering the limbic system by way of the amygdala (LeDoux, 1992, 1996). The data transmitted from the thalamus are blunt, unrefined, and fragmentary, as they are processed sensorially and preliminarily; SAM hears the stairs creak and panics, assuming it's the perpetrator. The same data, transformed within and transmitted by the neocortex, are, by contrast, sharp, detailed and coherent, as they are processed cognitively and comprehensively; SAM, listening more acutely, remembers that the perpetrator is at work and, because it is midafternoon, his sister has come home from school and it is she who is climbing the stairs. Thus, the thalamo-amygdala transmission route is direct, composed of mono-synaptic linkages. The thalamo-cortico-amygdala pathway is monosynaptic, longer by several links, and consequently slower in its projection time to the amygdala (Öhman, 2000).

Here's an example. It's Saturday night. Mountain laurel permeates the last house on River Ridge Road. With fits and starts, SAM strives to sleep, but rest lies beyond approach. Fearing another episode of sexual abuse, he feigns sleep, hoping against hope that his father stays out all night, at least until his mother returns from her third shift at the nursing home. The clock ticks. The faucet leaks. Drip. Drip. Toss. Turn. Bang! The back door slams shut!

Sensations of sound dispatch swiftly through SAM's auditory receptors onto the relay nuclei of the thalamus, translocating primarily into the central and lateral nuclei of the amygdala. Sensing danger, the amygdala triggers a conditioned fear response; SAM's mind floods with fear. Norepinephrine surges—SAM jumps. Dopamine rushes—SAM freezes. Nowhere to run. Only submission. SAM's afraid he might swallow his heart, it is beating so loud.

Unbeknownst to SAM, the sensory data reach the cortical regions of his brain. Soon, he remembers that it is Friday night, not Saturday after all. Oh, yeah, his parents are in Atlantic City for the weekend. He left the door un-latched so Bull, his German shepherd, could come and go throughout the night. With trepidation, a sense of hopefulness, and a decelerating heart, SAM slowly descends the stairs, only to find Bull lying near the door. He's not sure why, but he begins to cry. A reprieve, if not a blessing.

As indicated, by way of the shorter route, the amygdala mobilizes for action an immediate defense strategy. No contemplation—SAM simply reacts. This reflexive thalamo-amygdala maneuver occurs in advance of the thalamo-cortico-amygdala pathway's comprehensive analysis that actually determines the legitimacy of the threat (LeDoux, 1992, 1996). Time is on SAM's side. More specifically, the thalamo-amygdala pathway affords SAM the opportunity to respond, albeit unconsciously and in service of self-protection, before he ascertains the degree of threat associated with his impending encounter with

CSA; independent of will, he is simply defending against the unanticipated, the overwhelming, the unknown. If he found himself in confrontation with danger, at least potentially, he could respond long before he became cognizant of the specifics that confirmed or refuted it. There are consequences, however, as a conditioned fear-generated response pattern emerges without delay after this unconscious analysis. Simply and cogently, SAM's experience of the central and peripheral elements of his first sexually abusive episode— the perpetrator's stature, the dark at the top of the stairs, the light glinting through the slats of a shack, the sound of shoes against wooden steps, the scent of sweat overlaid with perfume, the slamming of a door, among infinite others—inculcate him with fear.

By way of the longer route, the crude autonomic modifications transmit back to the cortex and, as a result, the emotionality of the situation at hand, in this case SAM's experience of CSA, may now begin to be interpreted: "I'm not dreaming, he is putting his snake in my bum" or "I hear footsteps. Oh, God, she's coming to get me again. Wait. Wait. Where can I hide? Oh, good, it's only Grandma." Generally speaking, given the more accurate cognitively processed representation of threat generated by the neocortex, it may be important that cortically analyzed data prevail over those proceeding from the shorter, more reflexive thalamo-amygdala pathway (LeDoux, 1992, 1994). Moreover, because CSA tends to be an unanticipated life event, especially for boys (Finkelhor & Dziuba-Leatherman, 1995), subjection to it necessitates higher order processing within the central nervous system as abuse exposure is incongruent with his catalogue of life experience (Kollack-Walker et al., 2000) and gender-based expectancies (Lisak, 1995). For example, the registration of threat within the context of CSA is not necessarily immediate but rather a matter of time delay. Sexual abuse dynamics, such as the perpetrator's cunning subterfuge around his or her intentions, the slow and deliberate evolution of the subjection period, and the incremental transformation of falsely benign grooming or preparatory activities into incalculably virulent sexual abuse, serve to potentially suspend SAM's recognition of threat and danger.

In any case, on the perception of threat, and by way of both transmission routes, the amygdala, in quick procession, determines its emotional significance, ascertains the degree to which a more definitive stress response is necessary, and, if so required, signals a distinct alarm (LeDoux, 1992). In doing so, the amygdala, as conductor of this highly honed interconnective network, activates a cavalcade of intracellular events within SAM's body that comprise a neurally orchestrated "circuitry of fear" (Yehuda, 2000, p. 15). Specifically, the amygdala projects sensory information into the areas of the brainstem and diencephalon, including the lateral hypothalamus, that regulate autonomic, behavioral, and humoral response systems (Yehuda, 2000), including sympathetically regulated reactions such as heart rate acceleration and skin conductance, and parasympathetically dominated responses, such as heart rate deceleration (Öhman, 2000). Additionally, neural pathways from the amygdala to the hypothalamus signal the activation of the HPA axis (see later discussion) just as neural pathways from the amygdala to the locus caeruleus signal the noradrenergic, dopaminergic, and cholingeric systems of the forebrain. Further, neural pathways from the amygdala to the brain stem regulate SAM's fear-initiated motoric responses such as fight, flight, and freeze (Perry, 1999, 2001). And the amygdala projects the same sensory data into regions of the neocortex that regulate problem solving, judgment, and language, to mention a few. Thus, within a few thousandths of a second, the amygdala sets into motion a number of responses.

Further, the hippocampus, a seahorse-shaped substructure adjacent to the amygdala, connects nerve fibers associated with visual, auditory, tactile, and olfactory information with the limbic system. As it receives nerve-cell input from the various regions of the sensory-cortical complex, the hippocampus plays an important role in both short-term and long-term memory, particularly with respect to the consolidation of contextual information such as time, place, spatial relationships, body positions, words uttered, words heard, and other factual details of the sexually abusive relationship and the expression of its effects (Joseph, 1999). Essentially, SAM's ability to discern the perpetrator's initial subjection strategies as novel, his capacity to collate covert patterns of manipulation over time, and his ability to integrate disparate sensory elements of the abuse experience into a multidimensional composite are functions of the hippocampus, and all are indispensable when it comes to leaning, adaptation, and survival (Bremner et al., 1999).

The Cortex as Fourth Processing Point

The brain's cortex is the unifying mechanism of the stress response as it fundamentally and ultimately formulates and coordinates the prioritization, selection, and execution of voluntary actions and operations (Watts, 2000). The cortical regions of the medial temporal lobe system—the entorhinal, perihinal, and parahippocampal cortices—adjoin the hippocampus and are vital to the efficient functioning of memory (Zola, 1998). Associations between patterns of neuronal activity and specific sensory stimuli occur in all regions of the brain. However, more complex associations—those requiring the synthesis of numerous sensations across multiple sensory receptors—involve more complex brain regions, such as the amygdala and hippocampus. The most complex associations depend on the cortical domains and substructures of the brain (Perry, 1999). Together, the amygdala, hippocampus, and adjacent cortex concurrently link information from multiple sensory receptors and cortices and, in doing so, transform the disengaged sensory elements into a single memory upon retrieval (van der Kolk et al., 1997).

By way of illustration, during an episode of CSA, SAM visually experiences the perpetrator's bodily attitude and outward behavior as well as particulars of the environment in which the abuse occurs; he auditorily encounters the noise of cunnilingus and reverberation of bed springs; he olfactorially confronts the odor of feces and the pungency of alcohol or smoke-tinged breath; he tactilely sustains the choking sensations and rectal pain from forced penetration; gustatorially, he detects the tang of semen and the waxiness of lipstick. All of these sensorial experiences are stored within their correspond-ing sensorial domains of the sensory cortex. When another abuse episode occurs, or when SAM chances on a cue associated with his history of CSA, the hippocampus and adjoining cortex stimulate the sensory-specific cortical do-mains. Systematically, and by the agency of his brain, the multicellular and disparate elements integrate within their appropriate spatiotemporal context, thereby generating a cohesive, polysensory memory of CSA.

What does all of this mean for SAM within the biopsychosocial context of childhood sexual abuse? From the spinal cord to the brainstem, onto the diencephalon, the limbic system, and the cortex, SAM's sensory data ignite myriad neural activity, from the reflexive to the analytic, and everything in between.

The perpetrator's glare. SAM's wince. The smell of bourbon seeping from pores. The sound of bluejays chirping. The taste of uninvited flesh. The boy witnesses the invasion of his body, hearing the words, "I love you," as pain sears through his rectum. Exertosensory and interosensory data begin their voyage, from the sensory filter to the thalamus to the limbic system. Fear registers as an impulse in SAM's amygdala. The anterior hypothalamus gener-ates the sympathetic arousal of the autonomic nervous system. The sympa-thetic nervous system regulates hormone secretion and prepares SAM's body for action by way of nerve chains originating in the cerebral cortex and pro-jecting throughout the body. Upon activation of the sympathetic nervous sys-tem, the amygdala triggers the adrenal medulla into action. During the fight-or-flight response, adrenaline, the chief sympathetic neurotransmitter, discharges epinephrine and norepinephrine at the nerve endings, thereby in-ducing manifestations of hyperalertness, increases in respiration, perspiration, metabolism, and, perhaps, fear and confusion, too. Aroused by this sensory and sympathetic stimulation, the parasympathetic nervous system strives to circumscribe the body's reactivity. However, as subjection to CSA threatens SAM's homeostatic state, his hypothalamus, pituitary gland, and adrenal gland, or HPA axis, recruit neural pathways, rallying his heart, his lungs, his skin, and his respiratory, circulatory, immune, and metabolic systems, some suppress-ing, others unleashing, all in due order, with the aim of coping with, adapting to, and outlasting the immediate trauma. The catecholamines signal the hip-pocampus, tightly binding the ensuing memories for the long term while sup-pressing the frontal regions of the brain, thereby relieving the ensuing memories in the short term. With a keen balance of power, the complementary nervous systems automatically and unconsciously regulate and adjust SAM's body to the impending danger, permitting the frontal cortex to willfully and consciously pursue sensory data in service of interpreting, calculating, problem solving, and making it through, one moment to the next. The hypothalamus and the pituitary power up the brainstem, the diencephalon, the limbic system, and the cortex, galvanizing the sympathetic nervous system once again to spur his body into high gear. Blood flows, priming SAM's brain, coaching his muscles, and preparing his lungs for the perpetrator's attack. Pupils dilate. Nostrils flare. Heart races. The scalp tightens. Muscles contract. Mouth dries. But SAM can't run. Digestion ceases; stomach churns. Limbs tremor. Head buzzes. Senses heighten. But SAM can't hide. Immune-boosting troops traverse to the front lines to fight and ameliorate potential infection or injury. Vision may narrow, hearing may amplify. Hands tingle. Lungs spasm. He sweats and trembles. SAM feels "pins and needles" throughout his body. Bowels discharge. Stomach heaves. Fear of vomiting. Of going crazy. Of reality. Of the unknown. Norepinephrine—charge onward! Epinephrine—retreat! Cortisol marshals the body. Serotonin inhibits. Dopamine exerts control. Acetycholine strengthens movement. Glutamate enhances long-term memory. GABA relaxes the body. Opioids camouflage his pain. Inhibition! Excitation! Fight! Flight! Freeze! Persevere—and that's exactly what he does, no matter what.

SAM's ego, as a psychic mechanism, now overwhelmed, falters in its capacity to synthesize, integrate, and gain mastery over the stimuli (A. Freud, 1967; Krystal, 1988). As one or two senses, audition and tactile-kinesthesis, for example, avoid and dodge the stimuli, the others, such as vision and taste, confront and contain the sexually abusive experience. His neurotransmitters continue to fastidiously convey messages from one nerve cell to the next with a view toward his survival.

Thus, sexual abuse violates SAM's sense of agency, obstructs his sense of self-determination (Lisak, 1995; Spiegel, 1997), and overloads his usual ways and means of information processing (Hartman & Burgess, 1993; van der Kolk et al., 1997). SAM's sensorimotor circuits—vision, audition, olfaction, taste, and tactile-kinesthesis—typically open and available for information processing, tend to overload from new, unwanted, unanticipated, and bewildering stimuli. The stimulus barrier of a child, with a developing threshold, now encountering the bewildering stimuli of sexual abuse, inhibits, if not obliterates, capacities toward self-regulation (Krystal, 1988). But his body works to survive.

NEUROTRANSMITTERS AND THE STRESS RESPONSE

As can be seen, the registration of trauma transpires within and across the range of sensory modalities, igniting any number of neurophysiological responses. Upon exposure to an intense and novel stressor (and a boy's subjection to incest or sexual abuse certainly satisfies the conditions of such), SAM's body musters a stress-generated allostatic response (McEwen, 2002a). This constellation of allostatic responsivity encompasses activation of the sympathetic nervous system, the hypothalamic–pituitary–adrenal (HPA) axis, and the cardiovascular, metabolic, and immune systems. Such systemic and axial mobilization prompts the release of epinephrine and norepinephrine as well as other endogenous stress-responsive neurohormones, including corticotropin-releasing factor (CRF), adrenocorticotropic hormone (ACTH), and glucocorticoids, cortisol, serotonin, dopamine, glutamate and gamma-aminobutyric acid (GABA), acetycholine, and various endogenous opioids (Bremner et al., 1999; De Bellis, 2001; LeDoux, 1994). Some of these neurotransmitters have an excitatory action, others have inhibitory properties, and all with the purpose of initiating and maintaining homeostasis. Dysregulation of various neural transmitters and neuronal peptide systems is found among individuals across the trauma spectrum (De Bellis, 2001; van der Kolk et al., 1997) and across the life span, not just among those who meet the sharply defined and divisional criteria for posttraumatic stress disorder. Following is a brief presentation of the neurotransmitters implicated in SAM's responses to CSA.

Catecholamines

Fear-enhanced startle is a function of and impacted by a number of neurotransmitters and the release of endogenous stress-responsive hormones, including, among others, the catecholamines—epinephrine and norepinephrine (van der Kolk, 1996) and dopamine (see later discussion). Both epinephrine and norepinephrine are excitatory in nature; epinephrine prepares the body for flight; norepinephrine prepares the body for fight (Lundberg, 2000).

Epinephrine, also referenced as adrenaline, is generated by the adrenal medulla; regulated by sympathetic nerves, its route constitutes the most vital, albeit circuitous, pathway of sympathetic activation (Pollard, 2000). Epinephrine figures prominently in SAM's neurophysiological responses to biological, psychological, and social stressors. As such, it engenders effects similar to those evoked by direct sympathetic activation, invigorating SAM's body into a state of preparation for physical and mental activity, and without delay. The difference, however, is that the neurotransmitted effects diffuse more slowly (Pollard, 2000). Finally, epinephrine not only enhances the performance of the heart, but also imprints images and sensations indelibly in his brain, especially those extorted by traumatic experiences such as childhood sexual abuse, and much more so than ordinary memories (Bremner et al., 1999; Chu et al., 1999; McGaugh, 1992).

Norepinephrine is the major neurotransmitter of the sympathetic nervous system. Discharged by the locus caeruleus, it is distributed through multiple regions of the central nervous system. More specifically, it disperses within the neocortex and limbic systems, where it helps to activate the neuroendocrine response to stressful stimuli, regulating blood pressure, modulating emotions and moods, adjusting perceptions of pain, consolidating memory, and managing the "fight" response (Hamner & Arana, 2000; van der Kolk, 1996).

As a class of catecholaminergic neurotransmitters, epinephrine and norepinephrine reach abnormally high levels in children confronting biopsychosocial stressors (De Bellis, 2001; Krystal et al., 1989) such as CSA, and they play a key role in making traumatic memories more resistant and persistent than ordinary memories (LeDoux, 1994; Perry, 1999). Metaphorically, the catecholamines are like glue or inerasable ink, firmly fixing or deeply inscribing memories into the brain. Low to moderate doses of catecholamines, in response to acute stress, tend to enhance memory, while extraordinarily high doses of catecholamines tend to impede memory formation. Acute and protracted effects of dysregulation within the adrenergic and noradrenergic systems, evoked by recurrent bouts of epinephrine secretion as well as persistent and excessive levels of norepinephrine, include increased blood pressure and heart rate, hypervigilance, exaggerated physiological responsivity to abuse-related cues, flashbacks, spontaneous abreactions, anxiety, panic attacks, generalized autonomic hyperarousal, agitation, and difficulty around falling and staying asleep, as well as immune suppression (Bremner et al., 1999; De Bellis, 2001; Pollard, 2000; Southwick, Yehuda, & Wang, 1998; Sutherland & Davidson, 1999). Symptoms like these are mediated by the relationship between the catecholamines, the limbic system and the hypothalamic–pituitary–adrenal axis (De Bellis, 2001).

The HPA Axis

Acute stress also involves the hypothalamo–pituitary–adrenal (HPA) axis. Although the stress response arouses multiple and diverse, yet highly synchronized, cellular transformations, the HPA axis is more sensitive and, perhaps, more pivotal to the stress response continuum than its other stress-responsive counterparts (Sutherland & Davidson, 1999). The hypothalamus regulates the sympathetic component of the autonomic nervous system and the hormonal section of the endocrine systems. Accordingly, it plays a key role in the fight-or-flight response. It also regulates the vegetative functions of the body, including blood pressure, respiration, hunger, sexual functioning, and the wake/sleep cycle. The pituitary, as the master gland of the endocrine system, commands the primary endocrine response to stress, working in conjunction with the hypothalamus' autonomic regulation. The adrenal glands include two vital substructures of the endocrine system, the adrenal medulla, the secretor of epinephrine and norepinephrine and the adrenal cortex, the secretor of corticosteroids. All three substructures of the HPA axis, the hypothalamus, the pituitary, and the adrenal glands, synchronize their efforts to restore SAM to a homeostatic state after an episode of CSA.

During times of stress, the locus caeruleus activates the HPA axis by way of its indirect networking through the limbic system (De Bellis, 2001). Subsequently, neurotransmitters within the anterior hypothalamus actuate the anterior pituitary gland to discharge corticotropin-releasing factor (CRF). CRF stimulates the HPA axis which compels the release of adrenocorticotropic hormone (ACTH) from the pituitary. Instantaneously, ACTH arouses the adrenal cortex, prompting secretion of glucocorticoids, namely cortisol, into the bloodstream. Cortisol cues the release of amino acids (Chu et al., 1999). These neurobiological activities, in tandem, systematically intensify SAM's state of arousal and behavioral responsivity. However, protracted exposure to stress may engender, within SAM, neurological and physiological disequilibrium and dysregulation.

The pituitary is conceptualized as the "master endocrine gland" because it has feedback loops with endocrine glands throughout SAM's body. When cortisol increases beyond its homeostatic setpoint, the hypothalamus restricts the secretion of CRF. Consequently, the pituitary gland constrains the discharge of ACTH and the adrenal cortex suppresses the release of cortisol, thereby evidencing a self-regulating system (Krystal et al., 1989). This essential network, with an enhanced negative glucocorticoid feedback loop of cortisol (Yehuda, 2000), reestablishes the homeostatic state by regulating the level of cortisol flow within the bloodstream.

Children with histories of CSA tend to produce low levels of ACTH, a condition known as ACTH blunting (De Bellis, Baum, et al., 1999; De Bellis, Hall, et al., 2001). Over time, they transition from a state of being hypercortisolemic, or generating too much cortisol, to being hypocortisolemic, or discharging too little cortisol. When this occurs, the established negative feedback loop offsets and, as a result, the hypothalamus continues to secrete CRF. Given the reciprocally operative neuroendocrine and neurotransmitter effects ensuing from the chronic nature of CSA-generated stress on the HPA axis (De Bellis, 2001; Yehuda, 2000), a primed system like this tends over time to excessively respond to subsequent stressors, such as actual and recurrent episodes of CSA as well as the anticipatory fear of the next episode or of disclosure.

In general, males tend to have greater glucocorticoid responses to stress than females (Kirschbaum, Wust, & Hellhammer, 1992). Effects of HPA axis dysregulation include a hyper-responsivity to stressors and exaggerated biological and behavioral responses to internal and external stimuli associated with the experience of CSA (Sutherland & Davidson, 1999) and autoimmune dysfunction (De Bellis, 2001). Further, elevated levels of glucocorticoids may generate damage within the bilateral hippocampal region, which, in turn, may promote diminished memory and attention, concentration, and learning problems (Edwards, Harkins, Wright, & Menn, 1990).

The Dopaminergic Neuronal System

Within the class of catecholamines, dopamine, as an inhibitory neurotransmitter, modulates the activities of other neurotransmitters. In fact, SAM's stress response activates virtually every neuron that has dopamine as its neurotransmitter and, by that means, figures prominently in the regulation of mood, emotion, cardiovascular regulation, mental stasis, hypnotic activities, voluntary movements and reactivity, not to mention survival (see, e.g., Bremner et al., 1999; Spiegel, 1995; Stanwood & Zigmond, 2000). Irregular elevations of dopamine are found in individuals across the trauma spectrum (van der Kolk, 1996; van der Kolk & Saporta, 1993). When discharged in response to a biopsychosocial stressor, dopamine inhibits excessive muscular activity, permitting SAM to maintain a sense of command over his motoric functioning. This catecholaminergic neurotransmitter also plays a key role in hypnotic activities (Spiegel, 1995). Effects associated with dysregulation of the dopaminergic neuronal system include an inability to concentrate, emotional numbing, a sense of detachment from others and/or the environment, decreased interest in familiar activities, depression, lethargy, and problems with working memory, particularly with lower levels of this neurotransmitter, and agitation, hypervigilance, excessive application of significance to life events, fear, paranoia, and obsessive-compulsive behavior with higher levels (Sutherland & Davidson, 1999). Given dopamine's extensive reach, abnormalities within this neuronal system may, over time, contribute significantly to neurological and psychological disorders (Stanwood & Zigmond, 2000).

The Serotonergic System

Serotonin is another inhibitory neurotransmitter within the brain and central nervous system; it holds a regulatory role in mood and states of consciousness. Appropriate levels of serotonin promote SAM's ability to survey his microenvironments and to respond to cues in a manner congruent with the situation at hand as opposed to overreacting to internal stimuli extraneous to current conditions (van der Kolk, 1996). In essence, serotonin pacifies his brain and body. Akin to the dopaminergic system, dysregulatory effects of the serotonergic system, typically indicated by depleted levels of this neurochemical, include difficulties with concentration and short-term memory, aggression, impulsivity, insomnia, exacerbation of intrusive memories and cognitions, obsessive-compulsive behaviors, destructive behaviors, and suicidality (De Bellis, 2001; Sutherland & Davidson, 1999). Excessive levels of serotonin are implicated in depression, hypersomnia, an inability to focus, lack of motivation, and a sense of meaninglessness.

The Glutamatergic and GABA Pathways

Glutamate and gamma-aminobutyric acid (GABA), neurotransmitters of amino acids, hold key roles in the process of registering factual memory. Glutamatergic input is excitatory in nature; as a mediator of sensory input to the brain, it is extensively involved in the dynamics of consciousness and memory, forging the neuronal links necessary for learning and long-term memory storage (Nutt, 2000). Additionally, it plays a key role in the efficient functioning of the hippocampus. GABAgeric input, on the other hand, is inhibitory by nature, shaping the activities of other neurotransmitting systems by curtailing the firing rate or electrical activity of corresponding neurons (Lambert, 2000).

These two neurotransmitters balance each other; the repercussions of acute or protracted stress are mediated by the inhibiting effects of the GABA system permitting the excitatory activity of the glutamate system to facilitate the tracing of factual memory (Nutt, 2000). However, the spelling GABAgeric system is more than a balancing mechanism against glutamatergic and other excitatory activity; it also significantly contributes to SAM's ability to process person/ environment information, particularly in the realm of spatiotemporal integration (Lambert, 2000).

Dysregulation of the GABAgeric pathway, as evidenced by decreasing levels of this amino acid, may promote an excessive firing of neurons, akin to chain lightning, thereby causing affective shifts, unexplained panic, anxiety, seizures, and difficulties around sleep. Steep levels, on the other hand, may impede cognitive functioning and contribute to states of depression, apathy, and passivity (Mathew et al., 2001). Given glutamate's vital role in the efficient functioning of the hippocampus, dysregulation of the glutamatergic pathway may also render a heightened awareness of and hyperresponsivity to internal and external stressors, a greater proclivity toward generating "flashbulb" memories, and a greater propensity toward recalling "facts" of a situation absent of space and time. Motor disorders and the release of endogenous anxiety-generating benzodiazepines in response to the emergence of traumatic memories may manifest as well.

Acetycholine

Acetycholine is one of two autonomic nervous system neurotransmitters. Moreover, it involves the most extensive neurotransmission in SAM's body, and vitally so between nerve cells and the musculature. As an abusive episode ensues and even after it recesses, the parasympathetic nervous system strives to attenuate and stabilize the body's internal activity by way of discharging acetycholine. A key excitatory neurotransmitter within and among vital brain regions, acetycholine is responsible for functions such as learning, memory, and motoric behavior and for maintenance of attention, motivation, and vigilance. During a state of hyperarousal, wherein stress is prolonged or whereby SAM perceives escape to be more intolerable or unreasonable than succumbing to the abuse, the amygdala arouses the peripheral nervous system, engendering a state of tonic immobility or freeze (Rothschild, 2000). Dysregulation of the acetycholinic system is evidenced by affective instability, identity confusion, feelings of emptiness, erratic interpersonal relationship behaviors (Koenigsberg & Siever, 2000) and, in some cases, spasms, tremors, and paralysis.

Endogenous Opioids

Fear and stress also incite the secretion of endogenous opioids, a collection of inhibitory neuropeptides that constrain a number of synaptic transmissions activated by the occurrence of pain. Endogenous opioids have the capacity to engender stress-induced analgesia (SIA), thereby countering the effects of no-radrenergic-supported hyperarousal (Sutherland & Davidson, 1999). During an episode of sexual abuse, stress-induced analgesia inhibits SAM from pain recognition and, in consequence, reduces stress and heightens his protective and defensive capacities (Russell & Douglas, 2000; van der Kolk, 1994). In essence, SIA promotes a state of hushed serenity in SAM as endogenous opioids suppress the potentially excessive actions of neurons slated to respond to CSA in a more excitatory way. If avoidance of or escape from CSA is perceived as futile, then CSA, as a biopsychosocial stressor, may conjure not only stress-induced analgesia, but learned helplessness as well (Russell & Douglas, 2000), a state akin to tonic immobility (Rothschild, 2000).

In the central nervous system, endogenous opioids foster inhibitory action in the amygdala, a group of nuclei within the limbic system, with a central role in elucidating memory with emotional meaning. Even decades after the cessation of traumatic experiences, SAM may continue to generate opioid-mediated analgesia, equivalent to 8 mg of exogenous morphine, in reaction to stimuli reminiscent of the original trauma (van der Kolk, 1996). Thus, stress-induced analgesia is not only conditioned to traumatic cues but, over time, can become conditioned to remotely analogous yet formerly neutral ones. Dysregulation of the opioid system is evidenced by a baseline of opiate depletion with intermittent upsurges of opiate levels in response to trauma-related stimuli. Opioid dysregulation maintains numbing and avoidance symptomology (Charney et al., 1993). Consequently, endorphinergic activity may underlie SAM's compulsion to reenact dynamics undergirding and effects roused by the experience of CSA (van der Kolk, 1989). As a boy, SAM learns that sexual abuse induces pain and that pain evokes the calming, if not euphoric, effects of endogenous opioid discharge. Years later, he may discover that re-creations of the abuse experience, as well as any number of self-injurious behaviors such as cutting, biting, burning, breaking bones, hair pulling, and head banging, hold the capacity to trigger the same or similar response.

Effects Associated With Neurotransmitter Dysregulation

These multiple neurotransmitter and neuropeptide systems mutually regulate one another in the initiation and maintenance of the stress response (Bremner et al., 1999) and substantially impact physical and cognitive development as well as emotional and behavioral regulation (De Bellis, 2001). For example, the synchronic neurotransmitted discharge of catecholamines and corticosteroids prompt and fortify coping behaviors. However, within the corporeal context of accelerated arousal and low levels of glucocorticoids, such a tripartite combination may, in fact, yield indistinguishable fight-or-flight responses, thereby diminishing SAM's adaptive capacity toward survival (van der Kolk, 1994). Also, catecholaminergic interaction with the serotonergic system has the potential to exacerbate mood and anxiety symptomology. As a case in point, given the mutual relationship between the noradrenergic and serotonergic systems, children with reexperiencing symptomology may be at greater risk for comorbid major depression and aggression (De Bellis, 2001).

When the allostatic response is circumscribed by a time-limited exposure to and termination of a stressor, "adaptation predominates over adverse consequences" (McEwen, 2000a, p. 146). Dynamically, CSA is not so amenable to circumscription. In reality, SAM is likely to experience multiple episodes of abuse by one perpetrator (Feiring et al., 1999; Gully et al., 2000; Kellogg & Hoffman, 1995), often lasting for a period of 3 to 5 years (Briere et al., 1994; Fischer & McDonald, 1998; Gellert et al., 1993), and subsequent abuse by another perpetrator (Boney-McCoy & Finkelhor, 1995a; Kelly et al., 2002; Ryan et al., 2000). Since he rarely discloses to anyone, the trauma remains within (Gries et al., 1996; Lynch et al., 1993; Ray, 1996). Given the potency of protracted stress, SAM is likely to evidence a dispersion of neurochemical effects, such as increased catecholaminic functioning and increased opioid responsivity to stimuli reminiscent of the sexually abusive relationship, downregulation of adrenergic and glucorticoid receptors, suppression of the HPA axis, erratic alterations in cortisol levels, ACTH blunting, CRF elevations, and decreased serotonergic activity, among other inhibitory and excitatory malfunctions (De Bellis, Baum, et al., 1999a; De Bellis, Hall, Boring, Frustaci, & Moritz, 2001; Bremner et al., 1999).

As dynamics, these neurochemical alterations give rise to a number of physiological effects including, but not limited to, disordered circadian rhythms, accelerated startle response, as evidenced by a decreasing threshold for and increasing amplification of stressor reactivity, exaggerated sympathetic arousal in response to stimuli associated with (and stimuli independent of) the sexually abusive experience, disturbances in the sleep/wake cycle, and elevations or decrements in heart rate, respiratory rate, and blood pressure, depending on whether the individual is more prone to hyperarousal or dissociation (Chu et al., 1999; Schore, 2001; Yehuda, 2000).

Because risk and danger linger on, SAM's subjection, not only to CSA but also to elevated levels of stress-induced chemicals, can contribute significantly to any number of physiological, psychological, behavioral, and social effects. With acute stress, neurophysiological activation is typically swift and revertible; with prolonged, frequent, and/or intense stress, sustained neurophysiological activation inhibits the efficacy of the stress response, engenders desensitization, and, moreover, alters the brain (Perry et al., 1995; van der Kolk et al., 1997).

Back to the Sexually Abusive Episode

To be sure, CSA is relentless. Perpetrators, by definition, are unyielding. While perpetrators maintain their threatening stance, SAM's physiological responses become fixed as they continue to resist the onset of dread, exposure, and frenzy. The young boy is transfixed—in and of the moment—a moment all too stimulating, yet he strives to fight.

Throughout this volatile process, SAM's self-determination, will, and boundaries are extorted, and he is forced to pay with his limited psychic and physical economies (Rieker & Carmen, 1986). He is overwhelmed as sexual abuse impales normal self-preservative functions. The boy's inner core, the synthetic-integrative center in which perception, sensation, intention, and action coalesce, is overwrought (Herman, 1992; Krystal, 1988; Krystal et al., 1989).

Ironically, in such a crisis state, SAM may simultaneously be surprised at feeling so calm and yet also feel compelled to take action. In doing so, he may think as though he is acting rationally. However, due, in part, to this fear–adrenaline–fear cycle, he is actually reacting, not acting; his decisions are determined solely on the basis of trying to shield what is happening—both the facts from others and the meanings from himself. Additionally, SAM may experience a sense of disbelief at how well he appears to be coping, yet what he's assessing is behavior in isolation—action independent of affect. Unfortunately, such a separation of thought from feeling, and of feeling from behavior, is strongly and socially condoned, especially for males, and thus sustains this coping pattern.

In the event of such trauma, not only are the boy's senses of self-integration and safety disrupted but his very senses of gender identity and sexual orientation are undermined as well. Indeed, SAM experiences sexual identity confusion and stigmatization irrespective of the gender of his perpetrator (Richardson et al., 1993). When the perpetrator is male, the boy perceives himself as a participant in homosexual behavior (Dimock, 1988; Mendel, 1995), thereby rendering him gay (Finkelhor, 1986). When the perpetrator is female, the boy perceives himself as emasculated (Spiegel, 1995; Woods & Dean, 1985), because he did not fulfill the socially constructed gender role demands of initiation and desire (Duncan & Williams, 1998). Under both scenarios, the perpetrator, male or female, is in the dominant role with SAM relegated to the submissive role. Either way, his perceptions (and the perceptions of many others) are functions of sociocultural biases, one prejudicially homophobic and the other dispositioned against viewing sexual interactions between an adult female and young male as abusive (Richardson et al., 1993). Thus, SAM simply internalizes these socially constructed views that comprise the macrosystem of his person/environment ecology.

Three males describe their experience. Palo stated: "It was like a giant wave coming over me. I was drowning. I couldn't move. I didn't fight back. I didn't fight back! That means I'm a queer, right?" Jake revealed: "I couldn't focus my eyes. I couldn't feel my body. But my ears. They kept hearing things so loud. His grunts. The sucking sounds. Everything in me was dead but my ears." And Matt noted: "I felt empty, like—like I was a puppet. Like she had her hands inside me, and made me say the things I did, and do the things I did, because that wasn't me. I didn't know who 'me' was anymore. I didn't know how to be a boy anymore."

When moderate levels of catecholamines and other stress hormones are circulating, memory traces are deeply imprinted (Bower & Sivers, 1998; Cahill, 1997; Roozendaal, Quirarte, & McGaugh, 1997). In states of high sympathetic nervous system arousal, the semantic and episodic encoding of memory is inactivated, and the central nervous system reverts to sensation-based forms of memory that prevail during the first years of life (Herman, 1992; Siegel, 1996; LeDoux, 1994).

SAM, as a whole person, fractionates into shards—shards of sensations, knowledge, feelings, images, visual memories, auditory memories, olfactory memories, gustatory memories, and kinesthetic memories—thereby creating an array of altered states of consciousness and sensations of heightened reality (Herman, 1992; Krystal, 1978; van der Kolk et al., 1997). SAM's traumatic memories appear lifeless, no words to speak, with no voice to speak them. CSA fractionates unity among the senses; what the eyes saw the ears could not hear and what the nose smelled the body could not feel. CSA fractionates thought from feeling, fact from meaning, meaning from experience, and experience from context. CSA fractionates the continuity of time, demarcating SAM into preabuse, abuse, and postabuse selves. The whole, once greater than the sum of its parts, shatters into shards.

Relief, or its illusion, may momentarily succeed the first abusive episode, but soon SAM's self-preservative instincts hold a watchful and immutable vigil, ever scanning for the return of the perpetrator and further abuse, or any associations with it. Once thought detaches from feeling, meaning from memory and history from currency, SAM feels, and is, different, lost, changed. Only remnants remain of a sense of self once unconsciously experienced as intact—but now broken.

Does SAM know that CSA effects predominate from his first moment of subjection, during and between sexually abusive episodes, and, in many cases, long after cessation of the abuse? Some effects emerge from the shock of recognition; others surface after the first episode of abuse abates and SAM experiences a sense of "relief"; others still arise as such recognition converges with developmental milestones and life events such as the onset of puberty, dating, marriage, partnership, participation in sexual expressions of choice, the birth of a child, and so on.

Surely, as sexual abuse occurs, the boy is bewildered. Time is rendered motionless. Agency is obstructed. And there is an unwilling suspension of belief. Of what happened. Of what is happening. And of what may happen still.

CONCEALMENT

I tried to protect my brothers from my father and uncles. I mean, it got to the point that I realized that something was really wrong with the baths and strip poker. One night I heard my brother screaming in the basement so I ran down to see what was happening. My uncle was trying to force his dick into my brother's mouth. I grabbed him and told my brother to run. My uncle pinned me down and threatened to kill me if I ever said anything to anyone. Then he made me do it to him. Even today, some ask, "Why didn't I do more?" (Palo, interview with author, November 8, 1994)

Concealment is the pervasive secrecy that surrounds childhood sexual abuse, both as a social phenomenon and as a personal life event. It is typically enforced by the perpetrator, reinforced by social mythology, and complied with by the boy. The social concealment around the sexual abuse of males thus creates a barrier to intentional disclosure. To be sure, CSA is a bona fide biopsychosocial stressor as it occurs to SAM, within an interpersonal relationship and surrounded by a social context that constructs its course. What does SAM have to conceal?

Childhood sexual abuse, as a rule, occurs episodically and continually rather than as a singular event (Doll et al., 1992; Finkelhor et al., 1990; Kisiel & Lyons, 2001). The initial episode of CSA launches an overwhelming state of psychic and physiological hyperarousal (Chu, 1998; Krystal, 1988; Perry, 2001). Hyperarousal—a compelling, tenacious, and unyielding experience of fear— fear of CSA once it has occurred, fear of its accidental or purposeful disclosure, fear of its initial and long-term effects, and fear of its biological, psychological, sociological, and spiritual implications long after the last episode. Regardless of the frequency and duration of CSA, and even in cases involving one incident, the fear of recurrence maintains a persistent and inveterate state of hyperarousal. Nicholas stated: "I know that Saturday and Sunday was always abuse days. But on Monday and Tuesday and Wednesday and Thursday and Friday sometimes it was and sometimes it wasn't. If I told on him, he would come and kill me. So every day when I come home from school, I hided in the broom closet or underneath the porch, with Mittens, my cat. I wasn't a very good hider though. He always kept finding me." Kip revealed: "Fuck, man, I had nowhere to go, nowhere to hide. He knew where I lived, he knew where I went to school. He threatened to tell. The pain of the rape and the fear of the knife at my head lasted maybe, what, fifteen minutes? The fear of it happening again or someone finding out still lives right here [pointing to his head]. My body can't forget. That's the real abuse."

SAM rarely knows when and if CSA will next transpire; it happened once, and it can happen again. Regardless of whether the episode count is one or numberless, the fact remains that concealment is endowed to last a lifetime and beyond. More often than not, it does.

Between sexually abusive episodes, and even long after the last, fear reigns supreme (Gill & Tutty, 1999; Mendel, 1995; Robin et al., 1997). Common fears include the following: (a) fear of feelings; (b) fear of body sensations; (c) fear of losing control; (d) fear of becoming ill; (e) fear of going crazy; (f) fear of dying; (g) fear of attention; (h) fear of discovery; (i) fear of being around girls; (j) fear of being around other boys; (k) fear of gym class; (l) fear of showering in front of others; (m) fear of bathrooms; (n) fear of thinking about sex; (o) fear of developing secondary sex characteristics; (p) fear of sex; (q) fear of masturbating; (r) fear of erections; (s) fear of being viewed as deviant and gay; (t) fear of contaminating others; (u) fear that the old self is forever lost; and (v) fear of what the future might bring (see, e.g., Carballo-Dieguez & Dolezal, 1995; Hibbard & Hartman, 1992; McLeer et al., 1998; Robin et al., 1997; Spiegel, 1998). Reinforcing this web of fear are traumatic memories.

Qualities of Traumatic Memories

Just as memory, in general, is not unitary in nature, it follows that traumatic memories, as a subset, likewise represent a heterogeneous and complex phenomena (Hopper & van der Kolk, 2001). "On the one hand, traumatized people remember too much; on the other hand, they remember too little . . . memories intrude when they are not wanted . . . yet the memories may not be accessible when they are wanted" (Herman, 1995, p. 7). Dynamically, traumatic memories tend to emerge progressively, beginning with sensations. Characteristically, they are invariable, state-dependent, and timeless, too.

SENSATIONS

Traumatic memories of CSA represent fractionated shards of the abuse experience wherein the sensory, affective, and motoric features—visual images of the perpetrator, the scent of sexual violation, the sounds of penetration, the taste of seminal fluid, the bodily demonstration of retching between thighs, oscillations of shame, guilt, confusion, and degradation, muscle contractions, and the like—override the declarative or semantic elements (Terr, 1993; van der Kolk & Fisler, 1995; van der Kolk & van der Hart, 1995). As SAM encounters CSA, and experiences its vast array of biological, physiological, psychological, sociological, and spiritual dynamics and effects, he confronts this acute and protracted onslaught with "speechless terror" (van der Kolk, 1996, p. 286), unable to comprehend, let alone arrest, the experience with words. Encoded and consolidated on sensory, affective, and motoric levels, traumatic memories impede verbal comprehension and articulation (LeDoux, 1994; Siegel, 1995; Terr, 1991). This supports the assumption of two independent systems of memory wherein cognitive, affective, and behavioral subsystems operate under the domain of unconscious execution and the verbal subsystem operates under the domain of conscious control (LeDoux, 1996; Pillemer & White, 1989; van der Kolk & Fisler, 1995).

Typically, traumatic CSA impedes explicit or declarative memory, or the conscious recollection of the facts—the who, what, where, and when—surrounding the abuse experience (Krystal et al., 1995; Siegel, 1996; van der Kolk, 1996). However, SAM's implicit or nondeclarative memories—the anxiety, fear, guilt, and shame, or the conditioned emotional responses, fellating a penis without choking, detaching from his body, feigning sleep, in other words, the skills and habits acquired during the abuse and sphincter pain, the perpetrator's scent, or the breathlessness from the density of an adult, among other sensorimotor sensations—remain unaffected. Therefore, SAM's facts of CSA remain detached from their meanings, an assertion consonant with the principles of independent systems of memory.

Functionally, memories of the trauma tend to, at least initially, emerge sensorially (van der Kolk & Fisler, 1995), not in a bundle, but one by one. Jake stated: "It's not like I totally forgot what happened to me. Deep down inside I knew. But I worked so hard not to think about it and after a few years, I discovered that drinking and making up stories in my head about being someone else kept it down. When I couldn't run away from it anymore, it didn't come back in one fell swoop. Bits and pieces—smells, they were the worst. Whenever my wife wanted to have sex with me, I smelled, uh, shit. I felt crazy but that's what happened. And then I would feel cramping. I was in my fifties but felt like a little boy. Then I started hearing his words. She would be saying, 'Jake, I love you' and in my head I would be hearing, 'Love is supposed to hurt, altar boy. Take it like a man.' A couple of times she found me sleeping in the closet. That's where I used to hide from him, Father Simon, in the rectory. It's hard to explain something like that to your wife, to yourself even. It made it really hard to run, to keep it down. But even with all those pictures in my head, the sounds, the smells, I couldn't speak. I just couldn't say the words—not while it was happening, not the day after and not even thirty-five years after it happened the first time."

TRAUMATIC MEMORIES ARE INVARIABLE

Given the profound, developmentally discordant, and vehemently transgressive nature of CSA, swathed in shame, eclipsed by silence, and resistant to logic, the mechanisms for encoding and storing the sexually abusive experience, or traumatic memories, may be different from the mechanisms employed for processing ordinary or nontraumatic memories (LeDoux, 1994; McGaugh, 1992; Perry, 1999). For example, ordinary memories, or memories amenable to narrativization, are semantic and symbolic. They tend to be spatially, temporally, and sensorially integrated; that is, such memories comprise elements of both the facts of an experience and their corresponding meanings. Additionally, memories amenable to narration are, by definition, congruent with SAM's extant cognitive schemas (Horowitz, 2001). In fact, semantic or declarative memory is a function of operational and primed mental schemata; as soon as an experience or a set of details are assimilated into existing schemata, the sensory data are unretrievable as isolated, immutable entities. Further, depending on personal needs and/or environmental conditions, narrative memory as well as nontraumatic schemata can be intentionally condensed or expanded. Moreover, narrative memory can be consciously summoned forth at will whereas, on the contrary, traumatic memories cannot, as they are unconsciously conditioned by fear (see, e.g., Armony & LeDoux, 1997; Chu et al., 1999; Crabtree, 1992; van der Kolk & Fisler, 1995).

Although the emotionally laden shards of the sexually abusive experience float in the foreground, some contextual details of the event subsist in the background. Relative to nontraumatic memory, traumatic memories are indelible (LeDoux, 1992), less malleable (Perry, 1999), less amenable to suggestion or distortion (Squire, 1995), formidable and constant (Bower, 1994), unconscious (Chu, 1998), devoid of spatial and temporal context (Krystal et al., 1995), cued by internal or external stimuli remindful of the sexually abusive experience (Hartman & Burgess, 1993), and fixed in time (van der Kolk & Fisler, 1995).

In terms of limbic system processing, explicit memories—conscious, semantic, episodic, and autobiographical—are mediated by the hippocampus whereas implicit memories—unconscious, procedural, and traumatic—are mediated by the amygdala (Bremner et al., 1999; LeDoux, 1994; van der Kolk & Saporta, 1993). The hippocampus is sensitive to prolonged stress; the amygdala is not. Consequently, given the association between the hippocampus and explicit memory, the facts of the sexually abusive experience may ebb at times while their isolated meanings continue to flow. Palo revealed: "I felt like I was in a big dust storm. I couldn't tell the difference between Tuesday and Friday or the reservation from school. They all seemed the same to me. I was like this robot that knew I was supposed to go here or go there but I always felt disconnected. I felt alive inside with all of these feelings swimming around in me—I don't know if I can explain this—but I also felt dead to the world. The feelings in my body and the pictures in my mind never seemed to match with what was really going on. I felt disconnected on the inside, like I didn't know who Palo was anymore and I felt disconnected to the world, like I didn't belong to it anymore."

TRAUMATIC MEMORIES ARE STATE DEPENDENT

Memory, or the process of creating an internal representation of an external experience, is a function of neuronal activity—its pattern, power, and periodicity—generated by way of sensing, encoding, consolidating, and storing signals (Perry et al., 1995; Schore, 2001; Siegel, 1996). State-dependent learning refers to the way in which traumatic memories, by definition, are acquired during a heightened states of arousal, typically tinged with terror, and encoded, not semantically, but sensorially, affectively or motorically (Hartman & Burgess, 1993; Terr, 1991; van der Kolk et al., 1997). It follows, then, that traumatic memories abide beyond approach under conditions contrary to the sexually abusive experience. Yet they may be readily reached when SAM's current state of consciousness echoes the dynamics and effects associated with his history of CSA.

The intrusion of heretofore defended memories of CSA are typically triggered by any number of relevant but seemingly unrelated stimuli across SAM's microenvironments. If SAM's exposure to a CSA episode evoked a state of physiological arousal by way of an altered neurochemical state, for example, rapid heart rate, breathlessness, hypervigilance, and stress-induced analgesia, the contemporaneous manifestation of such, irrespective of the original context, may spur the reassembling of disparate elements of the sexually abusive experience. More simply, the central and peripheral particulars of the sexually abusive experience—SAM's "there-and-then" sensorial, neurological, mental, emotional, physiological, and behavioral activities—or, in other words, his memories, emerge in the "here and now" when a state of consciousness, akin to the past, materializes in the present.

Victor stated: "The day after the first night my father incested me, I was pitching in a league playoff game. On the mound, I was fine. Every single inning, I was fine. When I took my last trip to the plate, I saw my father in the stands. He never came to my games, but here he was, standing and eating a hot dog like nothing happened the night before. He reminded me of the night before and that made me mad. I was there to play ball, not to be his whore. I lost it. I was shaking so hard, I could barely get into the stance. I smelled him, I heard him and I couldn't even think about the ball. That's how it was, whenever he was out of my mind, the whole thing was out of my mind. Whenever I thought about him or saw his truck or smelled someone smoking a cherry cigar, I felt like I was back in his bed."

TRAUMATIC MEMORIES ARE TIMELESS

It is further hypothesized that traumatic memories customarily remain intact and invulnerable to other life circumstances (van der Kolk et al., 1997). They may emerge in response to intrapersonal, interpersonal, and/or circumstantial triggers, within and across microenvironments, irrespective of the intervening time between subjection to abuse or abuse cessation and the present (Butler & Spiegel, 1997; van der Kolk & Fisler, 1995). The discharge of endogenous hormones during the sexually abusive experience impacts memory consolidation. In fact, the secretion of endogenous stress hormones strengthens the memory consolidation process. Decades beyond the abuse, SAM may still experience visual and somatic sensations, even after transposing his abuse experience into a personal narrative (van der Kolk & Fisler, 1995). Thus, memories of traumatic, stressful, and/or emotionally charged events are often timeless and frameless, floating freely in the unconscious (Chu, Matthews, Frey, & Ganzel, 1996). Nicholas reported: "I think my foster Mama and Daddy think I'm crazy. They are very nice to me. But when foster Daddy comes to tuck me in at night, I think he is going to turn into Terry and my stomach hurts and I have to run to the bathroom cause I'm 'fraid that I'm gonna poop my pants and I don't want foster Mama and foster Daddy to make me go back to Terry if I poop in the bed. I'm not trying to be bad. Tell them not to be mad."

HOW TRAUMATIC MEMORIES MANIFEST

Traumatic memories manifest in a number of ways, but primarily in the form of intrusive symptomology, including, but not limited to, flashbacks, nightmares, night terrors, sensory, affective, and/or motoric reexperiencing and behavioral enactments of abuse-related dynamics and effects (Herman, 1992; Krystal et al., 1995; Terr, 1991). Upon emergence, traumatic memories may persist for a few seconds or several hours (Butler & Spiegel, 1997). They are not only recalled, but reexperienced as if aspects of the abusive episodes are recurring again, in the present moment (van der Kolk & Fisler, 1995). Further, they impact behavior outside of conscious awareness (van der Kolk & Saporta, 1993). Two examples follow.

In one instance, Victor revealed: "For the longest time, I kept my secret of incest away from Kevin. I guess he didn't need words though. One morning he said to me, 'Victor, I don't know what this means, but I think I know why your wrists are always sore.' My wrists hurt but I didn't know why. He said, 'Since we've been sleeping together, I've noticed something. I wake up several times during the night because I hear you moaning and feel you thrashing. I usually just go back to sleep, but this morning I looked to see what was really going on, and your hands were clutching the bars on the headboard, white-knuckling them. Your body was stiff, Victor, like a two by four. And your feet were stuck between the bars of the footboard, almost like you were paralyzed, or tied down or something. Like you were having a nightmare and wanted to get away from something but couldn't.' I didn't know what to say. I felt so exposed. My father used to tie my hands and feet to the bed. And rape me that way." In a similar vein, Palo revealed: "I just thought it was a quirk, my not wanting to be in a bathtub. And I hardly ever had to because I always lived in a place with a shower stall. Gyms have stalls and dorms have stalls so there was never a problem. But when I stayed with ———'s family for the first time, there was no stall, only a bathtub, and I had to bathe. I didn't really understand my aversion until I walked in the bathroom and saw the setup. I'm standing in the bathroom thinking why am I acting so weird, so detached. 'It's only a bathroom, Palo, get a grip.' I looked in the mirror and had that detached feeling, like I didn't know who was looking back at me. I'm there to meet my girlfriend's family and here I was having a panic attack in their bathroom. It was Friday and I knew I would be there till Sunday. I tried not sweating, tried washing at the sink on Saturday but knew I would have to take a bath on Sunday. I woke up real early, trying to get in there before anyone else woke up. I filled the tub. I still didn't know what I was making such a big deal about. Or why. I just felt afraid. I sat in the tub and started to shake. I was shaking, I was crying and thought I was going out of my mind. As soon as someone knocked on the door and asked if everything was all right, I remembered. That's where my father first penetrated me. It's strange—the mind. How can anyone be afraid of a bathtub? Who ever thought you can have a panic attack by getting into one?"

HYPERAROUSAL

Given the context of CSA and associated fears, what might SAM experience in a state of hyperarousal? Between sexually abusive episodes, and, at times, long after cessation of the sexually abusive relationship, intrusive thoughts, feelings, and behaviors appear and recur, with the force of a thunderbolt, out of the blue.

To begin, SAM startles easily. Touch can traject him. Brightness can astound him. Bathtubs, priests in Franciscan robes, and foster Daddies who care can alarm him. He's hypervigilant to both internal and external stimuli. "Is it me? Is it him? What is going on here? I know something bad is gonna happen!"

Whether on the football field or in a Sunday school classroom, riding a bike or driving a truck, holding his infant or being held by a partner, intrusive cognitive, emotional, sensory, and kinesthetic images strike without notice and without apparent reason. In his world, SAM may experience choking sensations during a third-grade spelling bee, or hear the perpetrator's derogatory insults—pig, fag, whore, she-boy, no-boy—while attempting to hit a softball. How disconcerting it must be to sense hands groping his body at the very time he's delivering a report at a weekly staff meeting, all the while recognizing that no one in the room is near enough to be doing so. He may detect the taste of semen on the tongue during his wedding rehearsal, or watch mental images of the abuse, as if on a silent reel, while washing the car with his children. Concealment surely reaches far beyond the abusive episodes.

Then there is the painful and ceaseless introspection. "Who knows? When will they find out? Can they tell I'm holding a secret? What will they think of me? Why is this happening to me? When will it be over? How can I make it stop? Am I gay? Will I become a perpetrator? Will I ever know what it's like to be normal again? Can you hear me, God? Can you see me, God? Are you punishing me, God? Why is that girl looking at me?"

Emotions overwhelm. Guilt shrieks. Shame blames. SAM feels naked, exposed, wishing for invisibility. Self-disgust envelops him. Confused by bouts of implosive and, at times, explosive rage, along with ruminations about when, why, and how, it's no wonder SAM feels crazy, out of context, without control, bizarre, agitated, frustrated, and paralyzed with fear and panic. He longs for peace.

Restless during the day, and exhausted by night, SAM's hyperaroused state can emerge during sleep. Repetitive dreams, in which aspects of SAM's CSA experience rerun without much modification (Terr, 1991; van der Kolk, 1987), recur time and again. He awakens from night terrors with soundless screams. Such dreams engender fear; fear gives rise to insomnia; insomnia depletes already diminishing resources; diminishing resources usher a sense of despair. Uncontrollable motoric discharges throughout the night, along with intermittent bouts of sleepwalking, impede his need for safe and restful sleep.

This heightened sense of arousal may appear to occur instantaneously, or it may build over time (Krystal et al., 1995). In either case, because fear of further abuse and fear of its discovery are fundamental effects, they remain unabated and act as barriers against the cessation of SAM's state of hyperarousal. Indeed, such fears are its wellspring. Accordingly, the initial state of hyperarousal, initiated by the occurrence of CSA and maintained by fears of its recurrence and the implications of its disclosure, habituates, developing a pattern of regularity within the central nervous system (CNS) (Perry, 1997). In essence, CSA reconditions the CNS (Herman, 1992).

Subjected to this type of chronic stress, the perpetuance and force of the autonomic arousal propel SAM instantly and abruptly from stimulus to response (Krystal, 1978, 1988; van der Kolk, 1987). Once demarcated and sequential, SAM's emergency psychological reactions of anxiety and physiological preparedness overlap (Herman, 1992), apparently unbroken, as if stimulus and response are one in the same. That being so, mediating factors such as the opportunity to differentiate between actual and perceived danger and the opportunity to generate response alternatives—in other words, the time and capacity to assess the biopsychosocial situation with a sense of confidence, composure, and relative objectivity—are bypassed. Consequently, the mutual relationship between the recognition of danger and the fight/flight response gives way to an increasingly generalized and seemingly automatic stress response.

Dynamically, this creates imbalance and disequilibrium as the sympathetic nervous system now commands its parasympathetic counterpart, rather than each component checking the other. Optimal functioning of the body requires that all domains of the central nervous system operate with a sense of coordination and balance; CSA generates evasion and strife, thereby obliterating homeostatic equipoise.

Although memories of and encounters with people, places, and things remindful of the initial episode of abuse trigger fear, eventually even non-aligned and unaffiliated people, places, and things, separate and apart from the abusive experience, begin to evoke similar responses simply by association (Chu, 1998; LeDoux, 1994; van der Kolk, 1996). That is to say, after SAM acclimates to the initial abuse stimuli, in time, additional stimuli, once neutral, rouse the same or similar fear response when coupled with memories of the abuse.

If SAM was, for example, abused by a woman wearing red lipstick or by a man with a full red beard, seeing others with resembling characteristics could conjure the fear response. As this fear response habituates to various stimuli across a number of microenvironments, contexts, and relationships, even minor stimuli begin to compel hyperaroused thoughts, feelings, and behaviors congruent with sudden states of danger, thereby generalizing the fear response as well (Bremner et al., 1999; Krystal, 1988; van der Kolk, 1987).

Shards of memory—sometimes impressionistic, sometimes vividly realistic in detail, and often with a psychophysiological potency reminiscent of the historic episodes of CSA. Like a decimal fraction, in which the same figure repeats indefinitely, memory shards emerge. Despite the iterative nature of intrusion, SAM repeatedly reacts in a congruent way, with fear, with recoil, and with dread, as if each emergence is new, as if each shard is an ambush.

Roles, activities, and relationships across SAM's microdomains all hold the possibility of triggering memory shards. As his fear escalates, and as triggers generalize, how can he convince himself, with any degree of confidence, that a remnant of the abuse will not encroach on him as he strives to bury the abuse out of existence? The cogency and potency of the central nervous system's autonomic response—initiated during the sexually abusive experience, and maintained thereafter by incessant fears of its recurrence, disclosure, the responses of loved ones and peers, and implications of what it now means to harbor the self-image of a sexually abused male—make it most difficult for SAM to separate the abuse from the abused. Even after his removal from the abusive relationship and environment, and even after the final episode, the psychophysiological responsivity cycle maintains itself, as it is fast, seemingly fixed, and resolute. And all it needs is fear, including the deathless fear of discovery.

Is SAM aware that adults rarely ask (Burgess et al., 1984; Homles et al., 1997; Mills, 1993), that boys rarely tell (Finkelhor et al., 1990; Gordon, 1990; Mian et al., 1986)? Disclosure at this stage, or at any other life stage, is disproportionately low for males (Rew et al., 1991; Roesler & McKenzie, 1994; Salter, 1992), indicative of the sociocultural disregard for sexually abused boys.

Suspicion without disclosure or confirmation is the most common form of social service acknowledgment, once a sexually abused boy has entered the child protection system (Dersch & Munsch, 1999; Haskett et al., 1995; National Center on Child Abuse and Neglect, 1994). Discovery tends to be accidental, and by unsuspecting outsiders (Nagel et al., 1997; Reinhart, 1987; Sorenson & Snow, 1991). Retrospectively, adult males often state that, as boys, they provided clues about their abuse history, but rarely were they overt and rarely were they received as intended (Dimock, 1988; Lew, 1990; Spiegel, 1995).

The sexually abusive relationship, as a microcosm of the greater social environment, reflects and makes operational the mythology around the sexual abuse of males. Following are some of the more common myths:

1. Sexual abuse does not happen to boys.
2. If sexual abuse does occur then you must have wanted it.
3. If the perpetrator is male, then you must be gay.
4. If it happened with a female, then it really wasn't abuse.
5. Sexually abused boys are unable to take care of themselves (Spiegel, 1995).

The social view of the male perpetrator/male child dyad as homosexual and the female perpetrator/male child dyad as heterosexual conceals the fact that childhood sexual abuse is a violent crime.

Such social mythology then becomes the regulating rule across the self, micro, meso, and exo ecologies. It guides and informs social responses, or lack thereof, to the sexual abuse of males, it supports the claims and counter-charges typical of perpetrators, and it becomes an internalized part of the abused child's identity. Abuse mythology also impacts the ways in which sexually abused boys' needs are accounted for in criminal codes, social service investigations, graduate and continuing education programs, prevention efforts, and the like. In other words, it outlines the appropriate patterns of response to the abuse not only for the child himself but also for the perpetrator, and for any person or institution to whom the child discloses (see, e.g., Bartholow et al., 1994; Ratner et al., in press).

Despite the fact that some may dispute the validity of these social myths, they are the path of least resistance and often maintained without question. They are familiar and, more importantly, they are supported by the greater social environment. To be sure, abuse mythology is instrumental in determining the meaning around the sexual abuse of males (Lisak, 1995; Struve, 1990)—and how it is going to be constructed, comprehended, addressed, and, unfortunately, internalized (albeit not particularly in that order).

Until recently, the prevalence, dynamics, and effects of CSA have been concealed from social consciousness. To illustrate, a boy is up to 10 times more likely to be abused by a recognized adult (National Center on Child Abuse and Neglect, 1994; Robin et al., 1997; Wells et al., 1997), yet far too many primary prevention programs are based on the notion of "stranger danger" (Levesque, 1994). The conception of "stranger" perpetration as a prevalent form of CSA is mythical. Although such programs may prevent abuse by strangers, there are few, if any, community resources that help children acquire the knowledge and skill to potentially avert sexual abuse within and across their microenvironments, including home, school, and church. Further, some prevention programs are founded on the male perpetrator/female victim paradigm, leaving boys disinterested in the knowledge and skill that could potentially be acquired and that could ultimately help them prevent CSA (Finkelhor & Dziuba-Leatherman, 1995). To date, there is no evidence to show that prevention programs achieve the ultimate goal of preventing CSA (Finkelhor, Asdigian, & Dziuba-Leatherman, 1995; Krivacska, 1990). Moreover, children's perceptions of their risk of stranger-perpetrated sexual abuse increase on exposure to primary prevention programs (Jacobs, Hashima, & Kenning, 1995). One male perpetrator stated: "Children never considered me a stranger if I dressed all right and seemed nice. Stereotyping people as bad, mean strangers makes kids more at risk from people like us" (Elliott et al., 1995, p. 590). In a similar vein, a female perpetrator stated: "Children don't know what a stranger is. Once I tell them a name, any name, and compliment how they look or how strong or pretty they are, I am no longer a stranger" (Spiegel, 1997).

Additionally, if acts of sexual abuse are reported at all, a boy is more likely to be taken to a police station or through the criminal justice system and not to child protection teams or treatment centers (Dersch & Munsch, 1999). Perhaps that is why boys, and particularly young boys, are less likely than girls to be placed in protective custody (Fontanella et al., 2000; Gordon, 1990; Pierce & Pierce, 1985). Moreover, the male perpetrator/female victim paradigm has given form to the law and to treatment. As a case in point, some states employ the term "rape" only within the context of forced vaginal intercourse (National Center for Victims of Crime, 1995a, 1995b). Forcible rape, as defined by the Federal Bureau of Investigation (1999), reads "the carnal knowledge of a female forcibly and against her will. Assaults or attempts to commit rape by force or threat of force are also included; however, statutory rape without force and other sex offenses are excluded" (p. 25). Additionally, the vast majority of sexual abuse treatment programs, empirical investigations, and education materials are founded upon the male perpetrator/female victim paradigm (Lisak, 1995; Mendel, 1995; Struve, 1990), making it even more unlikely for males with histories of CSA to disclose, with so little to gain and, perhaps, so much to lose (Crowder, 1995). Further, the denial of female perpetration is intricately, and perhaps invisibly, interwoven into the very systems designed and operating to protect children. One judge stated: "Women don't do things like this." Similarly, a prison warden said: "Public sentiment did not allow for such charges [female perpetration] to be brought to trial" (Lipshires, 1994, p. 2).

Indeed, within both public and professional realms, two macrosystem dynamics impinge on perceptions of and responses to the sexual abuse of males. The discrepancies between the gender role expectations females and the ability to apprehend women as perpetrators (Allen; 1991; Hetherton & Beardsall, 1988), coupled with the consonance between the gender role expectations of males and the inability to perceive them as anything but perpetrators (Lew, 1990; Spiegel, 1997b), create cognitive dissonance and resistance when contemplating the sexual abuse of males and extensively reinforce the social mythology and concealment around it. Frankly, social mythology initiates and maintains the feminization of victimization and the masculinization of perpetration—and it does so invasively and fraudulently.

As a result of social mythology, many boys remain naive and unprepared to confront such violations and have to depend on the perpetrator to label the interaction and identify attributions. The perpetrator, who wants the abuse to remain unacknowledged, is fully supported by social mythology, which, by its very nature, undermines and denigrates the boy. Thus, SAM is left facing a unified front between his abuser and his environment—making the disclosure of his perception of reality to anyone both doubtful and, often, dangerous.

Ironically, the perpetrator, who is the provocateur of the boy's distress in the first place, now becomes the teacher, modeling for the boy everything that he needs to know in order to keep the reality of the abuse concealed. This is accomplished both through the perpetrator's words (e.g., "Don't tell," to which the boy responds "Okay, I can do that") and through the perpetrator's actions—misdeeds that include everything from easy lies to evade any possibility of suspicion (Berliner & Conte, 1990) to the use of threats and physical violence (Furniss, 1991; Kaufman et al., 1996; U.S. Department of Justice, 1997), even to the point of attempted or actual murder (Elliott et al., 1995). Further, the perpetrator functions pivotally as SAM's self-object, mirroring and confirming for the boy his absence of masculinity and/or presence of deviancy (Schwartz, 1994). As SAM looks in the "mirror," he sees a boy who once was, a boy who has failed, a boy whose culture even views him as responsible for the abuse, a deviant, a misfit (Gill & Tutty, 1999; Lamb & Edgar-Smith, 1994; Ray & English, 1996; Richey-Suttles & Remer, 1997; Spencer & Tan, 1999).

Even though the perpetrator is often verbally and physically (as well as sexually) abusive (Gold et al., 1997; Melchert & Parker, 1997; Mendel, 1995), he or she is, more often than not, the only other person in the child's life who knows about the sexually abusive relationship and, as such, becomes an icon of hope for the child. Unfortunately and paradoxically, the needs of the child—to have his experience of the abuse validated—and the needs of his perpetrator—to keep the boy from feeling validated enough (and therefore safe enough) to reveal the abuse—are mutually exclusive.

In order to make certain that SAM continues to perceive concealment as absolutely vital to his survival, perpetrators rely on threats, physical and/or psychological aggression, expressions of anger and rage, blaming the boy, manipulation, threatening the loss of a loved one, and other high-pressure methods of enforcement (Berliner & Conte, 1990; Burgess et al., 1987; Conte & Schuerman, 1987; Elliott et al., 1995; Janus et al. 1987; Kiser et al., 1988). By way of example, Ty was coerced into concealment with accusations and humiliation: "Who the hell is going to believe you? You liked it and you wanted it. If you do tell, then everyone will know that you're nothing but a faggot!" Nicholas received a number of threats from his perpetrator: "Say one word and your dog is dead," "If you tell, I will kill myself," and "I will kill you," among others. Ironically, perpetrators state that their single greatest deterrent from abusing is hearing SAM threaten to disclose the abuse (Berliner & Conte, 1990). Still, males are significantly more likely than females to conceal the abuse from everyone, at the time of its occurrence and long thereafter as well (Finkelhor et al., 1990; Gordon, 1990; Gries et al., 1996; Keary & Fitzpatrick, 1994; Lamb & Edgar-Smith, 1994; Lynch et al., 1993; Ray, 1996).

Children, of course, conceal the abuse for a multitude of reasons. For instance, SAM may not have the capacity, knowledge, or language to label and describe the abusive episodes. As a preschooler, his concrete thought processes (Waterman, 1986a), in addition to the delayed development of his hippocampus (Joseph, 1999; Siegel, 1999), may prevent him from verbalizing details of the abuse. If and when he does, the expressed facts may lack cohesion as well as the spatial and temporal contexts in which the abuse occurred (Fontanella et al., 2000; Kolko et al., 1988; Reinhart, 1987). Younger children are more easily pressured into secrecy due to the perpetrator's illusion of care (DeJong et al., 1983). For older children with relational deficits, the abuse may be viewed as a small price to pay for the perpetrator's attention. If children tell, they're apt to lose that as well. Indeed, males with abuse histories who feel responsible and/or possess some positive feelings for or concerns about the perpetrator are even more reluctant to disclose the abuse experience to anyone (Kellogg & Hoffman, 1997). Additionally, the perpetrator may convince SAM that his silence will ultimately protect his parents from knowledge of their son's perverse behavior (Berliner & Conte, 1990). SAM is quick to oblige.

Furthermore, confusion regarding his physiological responses may foster concealment (Pescosolido, 1989). Without question, many sexually abused boys experience a seemingly incompatible sense of betrayal by their bodies. The social construction of gender and male role expectations is the vantage point from which males with histories of CSA tend to view themselves and consequently assess themselves as failures in masculinity and manhood, as evidenced by their inability to prevent the abuse and, not only that, but their incompetence in controlling their physiological responses, too (Gill & Tutty, 1997). In their view, CSA disqualifies them as males—at least ordinary, healthy, and harmless males. Understanding the physiology of the penis and its sensitivity to internal and external manipulation is of no consequence. In fact, this sense of betrayal is so powerful that it unequivocally disputes any responsibility on the part of the perpetrator.

Children with supportive caretakers, that is, adults who are at least willing to consider the possibility that their child was abused and to do so without manipulating, pressuring, or punishing the child in any way, are significantly more likely to disclose their histories of CSA than children of unsupportive caretakers; the rate of disclosure among the former is more than 3.5 times greater than that of the latter (Lawson & Chaffin, 1992). Nevertheless, boys, adolescents, and adult males with histories of CSA experience an overwhelming fear of disclosing the abuse to others. The greatest deterrent to SAM's disclosure is his fear of negative consequences, including, but not limited to, his: (a) fear of being perceived as gay, (b) fear of being perceived as "feminine," (c) fear of being perceived as a potential perpetrator, (d) fear of disbelief, (e) fear of being blamed, (f) fear of being viewed as abnormal or deviant,

(g) fear of any repercussions experienced by the family such as turmoil, shame, separation, and divorce, (h) fear of negative repercussions experienced by the perpetrator, since he or she may be loved and respected by many, (i) fear of being placed in foster care, with or without siblings, (j) feelings of shame and guilt (guilt for experiencing pleasure, shame for failing to prevent the abuse from occurring), (k) fear of the attitudes of others, (l) fear of familial and peer rejection, and (m) fear that the perpetrator's threats will become a reality (Bagley et al., 1994; Carballo-Dieguez & Dolezal, 1995; Gordon, 1990; Kiser, et al., 1988; Robin et al., 1997; Sebold, 1987; Sorenson & Snow, 1991; Spiegel, 1997; Woods & Dean, 1985). Unfortunately, his fears are not unfounded; disclosures of CSA, more often than not, give rise to insensitive responses and negative consequences for the boy (Lamb & Edgar-Smith, 1994).

Finally, enforcers of concealment reach far beyond the sexually abusive relationship. These include gender-biased statutes, services founded on the male perpetrator/female victim paradigm, an empirical and popular literature base wherein the terms "children" and "girls" vis-à-vis CSA are used synonymously, gender stereotypes, homophobia, and sociocultural views of motherhood. Thus, intrapsychic, interpersonal, and social factors create barriers around the sexually abusive relationship, serve as verdicts of guilt, and reinforce the boy's responsibility for his abuse.

Alone, harboring secrets of his abuse experience, and lonely, isolating from others in order to protect them from learning his truth, SAM is orphaned from potential holding environments of positive self (Schwartz, 1994). Childhood sexual abuse transgressed his confidence in the integrity of adults; it dishonored his name, his innocence, his potential; it retracted his birthright to love and care. That sexual abuse occurred is the first harm. That SAM lives in a country and culture replete with socially constructed gender dictates banning his ability to recognize, let alone acknowledge and report, his subjection to CSA is the second harm. And that others around him forsake their duty to protect, to intervene, to listen, to validate, and consequently to offer hope for healing is the third harm. Thus, the trauma stems not merely from the act of CSA, but from the roots of its intimately related and resounding silence. Why is it, then, that adults rarely ask, and that boys rarely tell? SAM knows firsthand.

INVALIDATION

> When the health teacher said that girls are victims and that men are perpetrators, I knew right then and there that either what happened to me wasn't real or that I didn't have a place in this world because I didn't fit her facts. So, if I want to be real, or if I want to belong, I have to lie to live. (Kip, interview with author, June 17, 1999)

Invalidation is the process of distorting reality. At the self level, this is achieved by way of biased information processing and the overuse of defensive strategies (Courtois, 1999; Hartman & Burgess, 1993; Horowitz, 2001). At all ecosystem levels, this is accomplished through strict adherence to dichotomized gender role directives (Duncan & Williams, 1998). Such intrapersonal, interpersonal, and social processes preserve the mythology surrounding the sexual abuse of males.

Sexual abuse is not a socially sequestered phenomenon. It occurs within a context that is a function of, or mediated by, schemata around gender and abuse (Lisak, 1995). The male perpetrator/female victim paradigm, a cultural lens reflective of gender socialization, allocates one role to males and the other to females. The implications of such social mythology harbor enduring consequences. To be sure, the following equation pervades all levels of the sexually abused boy's ecosystemic context: If males cannot be victims, then victims cannot be males (Lew, 1990). In accordance with the rules and regulations of society, male gender identity is deemed adequate only when a male projects and lives by the socially constructed doctrine of masculinity (Schwartz, 1994).

Young males strive to fulfill our culture's version of the masculinity credo (Lisak, 1995). It requires them to be powerful, independent, courageous, masterful, aggressive, dominant, and competent. The experience of CSA obliterates a young male's sense of autonomy and self-determination; he is overpowered and overwhelmed. He feels powerless, dependent, fearful, incompetent, submissive, subordinate, and inefficacious. Essentially, SAM is thrust into internal states that are the antithesis of all he is striving to be. Given this sociocultural milieu, what happens, then, when a boy strives to cope with his experience of childhood sexual abuse? His fundamental burden and goal is to forge ahead in service of survival, willing to do whatever it takes to get through the experience alive. Because of this, however, identifying and comprehending the extent and meaning of the abuse is discordant, not only with psychological survival (Rieker & Carmen, 1986), but with social perceptions of maleness as well (Gill & Tutty, 1999).

Such perceptions, or myths, are illusory correlations, growing out of unidimensional, stereotypical thinking and consequently restricting the expression of many potential male gender roles. Deviations are not welcome. Essential, then, to the understanding of the sexual abuse of males is an awareness of, and empathy for, both sexual abuse as an event and the aftereffects of sexual abuse induced by the socially constructed notions of masculinity, sexuality, and victimization.

Given his preexisting knowledge of these social regulations regarding sexual abuse, SAM is left, after the abuse occurs, with the certainty that these myths are false, but also with the realization that, in order to belong, he is required to act as though the myths are real. To do this, the boy must juxtapose reality with mythology, treating myth as fact and his reality as myth.

As SAM learns, and terrifyingly so, just how different his reality is from social mythology, he also confronts this disturbing notion: If what he authentically believes about sexual abuse is so blatantly wrong, then it is also quite possible that everything else he has learned, which makes the world a safe, stable, and predictable environment for him, might be counterfeit as well. The fear this evokes is instrumental in his decision to accept and believe the myths as facts and to doubt his authentic impressions and reactions. If he is truly wrong, then the world can remain a secure place for him to live and grow. However, if he is mistakenly right, then everyone and everything around him—his friends, his family, his safety, and his very survival—become suspect. With a newfound urgency to avoid another avalanche of shattered assumptions about himself, his gender, sexuality, abuse, love, and life, SAM must learn how to live the facade.

Quietly, SAM begins to view his experience of sexual abuse increasingly as a paradox. On the one hand, it occurred, and may still be occurring; on the other hand, social contradictions around its very existence abound. Quietly, too, he defies the rendered discrepancies with dissociation and denial. Invalidation, for many, is inevitable. With silent force, the social myth that "this doesn't happen to boys" becomes, for SAM, "this didn't happen to me" (Rieker & Carmen, 1986).

For SAM, during and after the sexual abuse, survival is, of course, the ultimate goal. Sexual abuse is not simply a matter of bodily or boundary invasion. To be sure, SAM confronts offenses against all intrapersonal subsystems, including the biological, physiological, cognitive, affective, behavioral, anatomical, sexual, and spiritual. SAM is forced to respond in any way he can, without the luxury and means to stop, assess the situation, generate options, identify positive and negative consequences, select the most viable plan, and take a premeditated action. He has to survive. As a child, SAM's internal resources, such as his problem-solving abilities and his comprehension of the complexity of interpersonal relations, are limited, fragile, and tentative—in other words, under development. Additionally, external resources, such as parental empathy, peer support, public service announcements, primary prevention curricula, and treatment programs focusing specifically and factually on the sexual abuse of males, are virtually nonexistent.

Due to these limitations, SAM is required to make sense of the abuse utilizing the only resources he has at his disposal: his internal knowledge of the world, the information he receives from his perpetrator(s), and whatever he can glean from his surrounding environment. This act of cognitive processing involves a balanced interaction between both assimilation and accommodation (Horowitz, 2001; Janoff-Bulman, 1992; Piaget & Inhelder, 1969). Assimilation is the reception and integration of self or environmental data into an existing schema; accommodation renders a change in the schema in order to incorporate new and usually dissonant data (Flavell, 1985). Information or experiences that are only slightly inconsistent or moderately discordant will be assimilated into a preexisting schema, whereas, on the contrary, momentous and dramatically inharmonious information or experiences will necessitate accommodation or schematic change (Janoff-Bullman, 1989). Further, the amygdala relies on and functions in accordance with stored information necessary to assess the gravity of the sensory stimuli it receives (LeDoux, 1996). However, given the very nature of childhood sexual abuse, with dynamics and effects beyond the realm of "normal" or anticipated experience (Finkelhor & Dziuba-Leatherman, 1995), SAM's amygdala has few, if any, internalized experiences to draw on, let alone use as a framework for measuring threat and, consequently, as a springboard for preventive action (Perry, 2001).

Because sexual abuse, as an event, does not provide a "good fit" with a male's stereotypical, and current, gender schema, it cannot be easily assimilated into preexisting frameworks; alternatively, a boy must accommodate this experience, or change his self-schema, in order to incorporate this new data (Janoff-Bullman, 1989). How can SAM integrate the experience of childhood sexual abuse and all that it means biologically, psychologically, and sociologically with his prior assumptions about gender, about love, about sex, about life? Matt stated: "I just couldn't believe that mothers would do this to their sons. I didn't want to believe that it was happening to me. If I saw my mother as 'crazy' or 'guilty'—pointed the finger at her in any way—she would have been hospitalized or would have gone to jail. Either way, if she was out of the picture, then we would have been orphans. I couldn't have done that to my brothers. So, it just seemed better for me and everyone else to, first and foremost, keep it a secret and second, believe that it was somehow my fault. I became the guilty one, the offender, the sexual deviant. To make my world normal, including her, I had to be the fall guy. I was the perpetrator. She was the victim of her son." When a boy integrates the various elements comprising his history of abuse, the most fundamental assumptions about the self change, sometimes instantaneously. Thus, Matt's "male" schema was overridden by his new "sexually abused male" schema, with the latter comprising all that the former is not. Ty revealed: "I was homeless a time or two. Five, I think. I know deep down inside me I could keep a job and I could pay my rent and such but I just didn't want to go outside. Inside my house or in a shelter I knew I was a loser. But when I would step outside and go to work or pass the neighbors or ride the subway or eat at a diner, the world knew I was a loser, too. People just want to take advantage of you, treat you like you don't have a heart." For Ty, his assumptions about the goodwill of others and safety in the world were shattered as well.

Conformably, and simultaneously, the boy must conceal, minimize, deny, that is, perceptually distort his reality to provide a made-to-order fit with the prevailing social mythology. This accommodation brings with it a great sense of internal imbalance as SAM severely restricts the expression of his authentic responses in order to align with stereotypica, gender role expectations. Despite his ability to adapt to these socially imposed expectations, he remains traumatically affected and influenced by an event that has already altered his life in many ways.

His self-schemas have changed; he is no longer the boy he thought himself to be. His schemas around others have changed; he can no longer count on love and care without a counterassault of deception and pain. His schemas regarding the world have changed; it is no longer a safe and nurturing place in which to explore, learn, and grow. And his schemas concerning the future have changed; he will forever carry the stigma of childhood sexual abuse. Where does he go from here? Needless to say, invalidation strategies are mobilized (Adams-Tucker, 1985; Briere et al., 1988; Herman, 1992; Krystal, 1978, 1988; van der Kolk, 1987). Invalidation is one of the most hazardous coping strategies SAM can employ (Spaccarelli, 1994).

Invalidation Strategies

Evading another abusive episode, dodging disclosure, camouflaging the budding effects—these are activities of daily living for SAM. His only refuge of safety, his only shelter from the truth, lies within. SAM discovers temporary relief from the dynamics and effects of CSA, not by alloplastic adaptation, whereby he can alter his microenvironments to oblige his wants and needs, thereby stopping the abuse or preventing its occurrence in the first place, but by autoplastic adaptation, wherein SAM changes and modifies himself, psychically and internally, as a means of complying with the demands of external reality (Goldstein, 1984). Yes, the sexually abused boy's greatest resource is an ability to alter his states of consciousness. Invalidation strategies exemplify the ego's struggle to distort, in some form or fashion, the fact that sexual abuse occurred, and to numb the cognitive and emotional meanings this childhood story holds for SAM.

Invalidation strategies encompass a broad range of conscious and unconscious as well as a number of intrapsychic, psychoemotional, sensorimotor, and behavioral actions. Psychic invalidation tends to be global, rather than circumscribable, impacting a wide range of mental and psychic activities including attention, learning capacities, memory, autonomous perception and action, motor functions, the ability to anticipate and assess consequences, problem solving, imagination, emotional regulation, impulse control, judgment, stimulus thresholding, perceptions of, the ability to differentiate between, and responses to internal and external stimuli, defensive functioning, stimulus synthesis, personality integration, and self-preservation instincts.

Altered states of consciousness are core elements of the traumatic response (Herman, 1992), particularly alterations in and perceptions of the self, one's microenvironments, and perceptions of one's interactions with others. Psychic invalidation is the intended destination; the paths leading to it are numerous.

Defenses

Between abusive episodes, and/or following the cessation of the sexually abusive relationship, intrusive repetition of conflictual and overwhelming thoughts, memories, sensations, feelings, and motoric discharges fill the body (Hartman & Burgess, 1993; Terr, 1991). Consequently, defense strategies become essential, as they can maintain functionality while buffering the impact of sexual abuse, including the psychic, cognitive, affective, behavioral, physiological, interpersonal, and social responses to it.

Defenses are meant to be temporary, to serve a particular purpose in a particular situation (Brenner, 1986). For example, following an abusive episode, responsibilities such as getting ready for school or joining the family for dinner will require immediate attention, yet thoughts like "I really am a sick whore" or "Why did I make this happen" intrude as powerful emotions of rage, shame, guilt, and fear begin to surface. Inevitably, defenses are summoned. Once activated, defense strategies, functioning to buffer intolerable thoughts and feelings against conscious awareness, distort, alter, and give a false appearance to reality in a way that fosters a most willing suspension of belief.

For the sexually abused male, defense strategies become necessary, not only to shield him from the full impact of physical and interpersonal violation, but to conceal the abuse as well. Concealment, mandated by the perpetrator and supported by social mythology, is executed by the sexually abused male 24 hours a day, 7 days a week, for weeks, months, and years. Because males cannot be victims, and victims cannot be males (Lew, 1990), to reveal the reality of abuse is to risk being viewed as feminine, deviant, and gay (Gill & Tutty, 1999; Spiegel, 1997b). Accordingly, any person, place, or thing that has the potential to uncover it must be viewed as the enemy. Thus, defense strategies, once temporary, are now enduring, forming an ever-present constellation of barriers to the truth. As this constellation becomes entrenched, it constructs and seeks to maintain a new reality, a new self.

Essentially, the defensive maneuvers, indispensable for confronting, enduring, and, in fact, surviving the abuse, assume the position of cornerstone in the construction of a new self. This constructed self is impelled toward the goals of concealment, invalidation, reconciliation, and compensation. Truth and reality are rendered null and void; myth and deception exercise authority.

Given that defenses, as a function of the ego, enhance biopsychosocial adaptation, any number of them can be activated, depending on the context. There is, however, a configuration, recurrently erected by SAM, as a matter of course. This constellation of defenses typically includes denial, isolation, suppression, and dissociation.

DENIAL, ISOLATION, AND SUPPRESSION

Denial acts as a gatekeeper to SAM's sensory channels. SAM sees, hears, tastes, smells, and feels the abuse, but negates, distorts, blocks, or otherwise denies the sensations. Thus, denial, as a defense mechanism, affords SAM the opportunity to invalidate, in varying degrees, certain aspects of the abuse experience. It functions as an organizing filter, directing the acknowledgment and integration of distorted perceptions (Vaillant, 1992). As Matt, abused at 15, stated: "I saw it with my eyes. I smelled the sex. I heard her grunts. I tasted her sweat. I felt the horror of it all. But it wasn't abuse. It was my mother." Denial, however, is not foolproof; affect, associated with the abuse, can and will trespass beyond the defensive barrier.

Accordingly, SAM willfully strives to shield himself from simultaneously experiencing abuse-related thoughts and feelings. Through the defense of isolation, SAM is conscious of the cognitive aspects of the abuse, as if viewing, in silence, a series of snapshots in his mind. During this process, corresponding affect is compartmentalized. Kip, an adolescent male, put this in perspective: "It's not like a real movie. A real movie has people talking, sounds and music. The sex movie—the movie in my head—is quiet. No words. No music. No feelings. No pain."

Summoning courage and creativity, the boy disowns the abuse through suppression and repression (Kiser et al., 1988). During repression, thoughts and feelings, once conscious, are now kept from awareness. With suppression, thoughts and feelings are consciously controlled or inhibited (Vaillant, 1992). Therefore, a sexually abused boy might remember details of his abuse but detach from his emotional responses. Others block memories but experience the emotions associated with the abuse. Still others block cognitive and affective memories, experiencing only the kinesthetic, in various parts of the body. Victor reported: "When I would wake up in the middle of the night, my feet lodged in the footboard, my hands anchored to the headboard, head to toe paralysis, I knew my body was trying to speak for the silent images of the incest that never left my mind unless I was playing ball."

While suppression provides a sense of relief as it disengages affect from internal and external data, it also fosters a sense of doubt around the validity and significance of SAM's history of abuse. Further, as suppression does not affect the data, only their corresponding affect, SAM is, and always has been, aware of his abusive history (although he may not have labeled it as such), but has difficulty linking it to initial effects, aftereffects, and current functioning. Whatever the mode, such protection can only be rendered by invalidation, and may last for years, decades, and, in some cases, entire lives.

DISSOCIATION

Ego functions, such as judgment, object relations, stimulus regulation, and reality testing, as well as the mental processes of thought, feeling, memory, and identity function as an integrated whole. Dissociation, in short form, is the structured separation of ego functions and mental processes (Spiegel & Cardena, 1991). Palo stated: "I was taking a final exam in psychology class. I was prepared. I knew the material. I was hitting each question and felt really good. I felt confident. Then I read question '33.' A question about family violence. I looked at the question and my exam book and this wave just came over me. I thought I was going to faint. The room seemed so strange. I felt too big for the desk. As I tried writing the answer, my hand seemed like it was attached to someone else, like it wasn't mine. I sat there just trying to talk to myself, letting me know that I wasn't going crazy. It was like the dream you have when you're screaming on the inside but nothing comes out. You're just like a stone, a volcanic stone."

The driving force behind defensive strategies is protection from pain. With dissociation, SAM's psyche derives safety in a way his body cannot. It involves intermittent transformations of the ego's integrative function of consciousness and identity. Dissociation has a broad range, from highway hypnosis, to splitting and sleepwalking, on to derealization and depersonalization, and finally to the development of altered and multiple identities (American Psychiatric Association, 1994; Goldstein, 1984; Putnam & Trickett, 1993). From these examples, it can be seen that dissociative processes are qualitatively different, with an escalating slope in the direction of psychopathology (Waller, Putnam, & Carlson, 1996). Dissociation, perhaps the most common unconscious form of invalidation response, emerges as SAM's overcharged ego strains to mediate daunting external stimuli and bewildering internal stimuli. What is SAM's most pressing mission toward survival? Objective: the creation or, at least the bearing, of intrapersonal and interpersonal functionality—whatever it takes—as there is little time to consider costs and implications, time only to survive the moment, to get through to the next.

Dissociation, as a psychobiological operation, disunites the synthetic and integrative network of sensory and communication channels between and among thoughts, feelings, behaviors, knowledge, sensations, and memories (Krystal, 1978, 1988; Spiegel & Cardena, 1991). Strategic, protective, and self-preservative, it, as well as other invalidation responses, generates a shift in and modification of consciousness (Herman, 1992). At the same time, dissociation relieves SAM and his ego by detaching, not often wholly but more so fractionally, from the full sensory experience (Davies & Frawley, 1994; Moore & Fine, 1990)—in essence, from the facts and meanings associated with childhood sexual abuse. The ego apportions itself into a detached, observational self and into a detached, experiential self (Krystal, 1978; Sarlin, 1962). Consequently, initial attempts at recollection or narration fragment into shards. Jake revealed the following: "During the abuse and even as late as last year, what's that—thirty-seven years after the abuse, I was aware of the part of me that *did* and the part of me that *watched me doing*. The part of me that *did* was too scared to speak; the part of me that *watched* was mute, deaf I guess, but I was still aware. Whenever I tried to tell my wife about the abuse, I couldn't speak. I cried. I shook. I saw in my mind what happened to me. But I couldn't say the words. My mind and body were trying but my voicebox could not. It was the same exact feeling when Father Simon was on top of me. I felt him. I felt it. But I just couldn't speak."

Dissociation numbs and narrows, compresses and constricts, squeezes and strangulates aspects of the sexually abusive experience because they are too unusual and stimulating—too strident, sharp, repugnant, too offensively violent—to be processed and recorded by more conventional means. Defensive strategies, although available to a child, are neither developed sufficiently nor resolute enough to fully and functionally control the biological, psychological, and sociological stimulation triggered by CSA; more often than not, they are maladaptive and rigid (Daldin, 1988). Consequently, various elements of the experience—the tactility of anal pain, the sensation of trickling blood, the sounds of forced friction, the sight of a caretaker's utter indifference to SAM's well-being, the scent of urine, semen, feces, breath, the taste of another, the recognition of betrayal under the guise of care, the tangibility of losing one's identity in a life-altering moment, the perception that life, as one knows it, will never be the same, the shock of recognition of one's erection and ejaculation, and the guilt, the pleasure, the shame, the fear, and the wish to be dreaming, the wish to be another boy, any boy, anyone at all but who he is at that moment—fraction off, manifesting into detached ego states that alternate in consciousness. Each state harbors its own thoughts, feelings, behaviors, sensations, and memories; as one state descends from consciousness, another ascends, bringing with it a different view of self and of the world, with or without a view of the abuse. The view is not full, but fractionated.

Victor, abused by his father, describes this process: "I hated my bedroom. I knew it was my bedroom, right? I saw my bed, my baseball awards, my books, but it was like they weren't mine, like I had never seen them before. And it wasn't just my room. It was my hands, too, my body. When I was on the field, throwing the baseball, I saw my hand around it, my arm throwing it, but it's like it wasn't mine. Like my body didn't belong to me. I mean, it was fine when he was doing it to me, because it was like I wasn't there. But in the morning, when I had to go to school, or on the diamond, when I had to give it my all, I wanted to feel like I knew who I was. And I didn't. Sometimes I still don't."

Dissociation, Hyperarousal, and Memory Retrieval

Within and across human development, childhood sexual abuse, the sexual abuse of males, memory, and traumatic memory knowledge bases, hypothetical agreement prevails over scientific consensus with respect to mechanisms that operationalize trauma-specific amnesia and subsequent memory retrieval (Brown et al., 1998). Still, there are a number of hypotheses that may demonstrate the ways in which traumatic memories lapse from consciousness. These include state-dependent learning, repression, and dissociation.

THE STATE-DEPENDENT PSYCHOBIOLOGY OF HYPERAROUSAL AND DISSOCIATION

There appear to be two configurations of the trauma response associated with CSA, one fundamentally characterized by hyperarousal and the other primarily dissociative in nature, and both representing particular, but not necessarily disunited, pathways to chronic stress-related symptomology (Bremner, 1999). As sexual abuse effects, hyperarousal and dissociation are essentially state-dependent memories cued by stimuli perceived to be associated with abuse episodes. If SAM's immediate response to CSA is hyperarousal, such a reaction involves dramatic accelerations of circulating stress-responsive chemicals from the adrenergic and noradrenergic systems as well as the HPA axis (Perry, 2001; Yehuda, 2000). In keeping with hyperarousal as well as the fight-or-flight response, the neurobiology of dissociation entails catecholaminic discharge, particularly of epinephrine. Thus, both response sets entail mediation by the brainstem and activation of the central nervous system. Unlike hyperarousal, dissociation also involves the dopaminergic and the opioid systems. At some point along the stress-response continuum, dopaminergic systems may activate, modulating mood and affect by way of detached calm (Perry et al., 1995) and, at the same time, the opioid systems may activate, obstructing the sensation of pain, diminishing the amplitude of alarm, and altering SAM's sense of person, place, and time—in essence, his reality (van der Kolk, 1996). Additionally, the endogenous opioid systems modulate the dissociative responses of surrender and freeze.

Ultimately, if SAM's subjection to CSA predisposes him to a frequent or elongated startle response set, he may exhibit the distinct patterned neurobiology of hyperarousal. Alternatively, if SAM dissociates along the stress-response continuum, and remains in such a state for extended periods of time, he is likely to manifest a sensitized neurobiology congruent with this protective brain/mind/body strategy. Sequentially, dissociation typically succeeds hyperarousal, manifesting more precisely in response to it (Perry & Pollard, 1998). Children tend to react to CSA with gradient combinations of arousal and dissociation and often with one predominating the other. If the neurobiology of these response sets protracts beyond the initial threat or, given the chronic nature of CSA, excessively actuates within and between abusive episodes, the result is structural and functional dysregulation at the cellular level between and among the neurobiological systems undergirding the stress response (Perry, 1997, 2001). Any conditions that serve to maintain the stress response—concealing the abuse, fearing its recurrence, anticipating the execution of the perpetrator's threats, worrying about disclosure and the reactions of others, not to mention the frank experience of CSA itself—also promote and sustain the restoration of the psychobiological states of hyperarousal and dissociation. Furthermore, if SAM recurrently experiences hyperarousal or a dissociative state by way of reexposure to contextualized stimuli within the sexually abusive relationship, for example, the nonoffending caretaker's departure from the home, leaving him without protection, or exposure to generalized stimuli reminiscent of the abusive experience—for instance, spotting any priest in a Franciscan robe or walking down the basement stairs of any locale—he exacerbates these already sensitized psychobiologic states.

With habituated hyperarousal or protracted dissociation or, in fact, a recurrent cycling of the two, more and more corporeal and environmental stimuli become conditioned by them, producing a burgeoning pool of stressors which, in turn, serve to generalize the response sets once confined to the sexually abusive relationship. Thus, if particular memories originate under particular conditions, state-dependent learning suggests that memory retrieval is most likely to occur upon the reactivation of dynamics and effects correlated with the original state (Squire & Kandel, 2000). Palo's misunderstood fear of bathtubs and his catharsis when he found it necessary to bathe in one is a cogent example of state-dependent learning and memory retrieval. He went on to say: "Sitting in that bathtub, feeling the hot water slowly rise and envelop my body, that was enough to bring it all together. I was detached to begin with because I was afraid to sit in the tub and didn't want to do it. It was that feeling of looking in the mirror and not recognizing the reflection, but still knowing it is you. When I sat in the tub, and felt the water, my memories of the abuse were different than ever before. This time, I saw the pictures in my mind, I felt the feelings in my heart, I felt the pain in my abdomen, just like it was happening all over again."

REPRESSION AND DISSOCIATION

Repression represents the unconsciously driven unawareness of external events, such as childhood sexual abuse, and internal material, such as authentic thoughts and feelings regarding the abuse experience (Vaillant, 1992). Some authors tend to use dissociation and repression as if one was synonymous with the other. They are, in fact, two distinct concepts. Dissociation does not involve "forgetting," but rather, an temporary inability to retrieve the encoded memory (Yates & Nasby, 1993). However, repression, as an intrapsychic anticathexis against CSA, lacks the necessary and sufficient power to explain amnesia beyond a singular episode. At this point in time, dissociation holds the most likely explanation for partial and complete amnesia (Chu et al., 1996). With respect to traumatic dissociation or dissociative amnesia, "specific memories are inaccessible because they are associated with a highly charged negatively toned affective component. Dissociation is not forgetting. In dissociation, the item is encoded but cannot be retrieved" (Yates & Nasby, 1993, p. 309).

Depersonalization and Derealization

"Dissociation," as a psychic phenomenon, is broad, both in form and content; thus, *dissociation*, as a term, is a misnomer when employed as if it relates to a unitary psychic function. This ego defense mechanism also includes depersonalization and derealization as well as the containment of traumatic memories within distinct ego states (van der Kolk & Fisler, 1995) although not every individual will experience dissociation in a homogenous manner.

Depersonalization involves alterations in self-perception (Moore & Fine, 1990; Sarlin, 1962). Identity, as one knows it to be, becomes palpably changed, as if lost or absent. More specifically, SAM's sense of self divides into two distinct and demarcated selves—a disengaged yet observing self and a detached yet participating self. The chasm between the two feels vast, highlighted by the fact that SAM's sense of, and connection with, the observing self are greater than those of its counterpart.

A sense of self-alienation predominates; SAM feels as if he is outside himself, silently observing his mental, motoric, physiologic, and often involuntary processes—blinking, swallowing, gesturing, thinking. He recognizes his hand, but it appears to belong to someone else. Senses dull, to a point of his feeling skeletal, invisible, robotic, and, in some cases, dead. When looking in the mirror, SAM acknowledges a reflection but his relationship to it is lost. He knows that he is SAM, that he is not "invisible"; thus, reality testing remains intact. However, with such manifest detachment and feelings of unreality, his fear of going and growing crazy permeates this altered state of consciousness. Anxiety and panic evoke these states, and anxiety and panic emanate from them as well. Depersonalization can be episodic or continuous, with a frequency continuum from seconds to years (Sarlin, 1962).

Palo, a 21-year-old Native American male, abused by his father and uncles, described depersonalization in this way: "I'm afraid to look in the mirror. I'm afraid to see my reflection anymore. So I walk with my head down, which goes against all I was taught about honor. When I do see my reflection or when I do have to shave or comb my hair, what I see back is not who I used to be. It's like a stranger looking at me. I know his name—I mean my name— is Palo. And that's only because I haven't forgotten my name."

Like depersonalization, derealization involves a sense of estrangement, with detached observing and participating selves, and feelings of unreality, but in this case, in relation to the surrounding environment (Moore & Fine, 1990; Sarlin, 1962). SAM's microenvironments—his living room, his bathtub, the street on which he lives, his workplace, the corner store—both familiar and unfamiliar, appear somehow different, foreign and unlike they ever used to be. SAM's world, once recognized, perhaps taken for granted, looms distant. His attachments to, and the meanings of, people, places, and things now seem outwardly unreal, lost, strange—yet enigmatically familiar. Jake, a 45-year-old father of three, explained: "Do you know how crazy it is for me to have to tell myself:

'I'm at my desk at work now.' 'I'm in my living-room chair watching the Jets now.' 'I'm at the friggin' Sizzler now eating dinner with my family now.' I have to keep reminding myself where I am, what I'm doing or supposed to be doing, because if I don't, I feel lost, like I don't really know who my wife is, or even where I am, anymore."

Dissociation, depersonalization, and derealization are altered states of consciousness and core elements of the traumatic response (Herman, 1992). Psychodynamic alterations modify perceptions of the self, of one's microenvironments and perceptions of one's interactions with others. They impact the senses, too.

Sensory anesthesia and sensory elaboration, in a combination of forms, typify altered states (Krystal, 1988). Vision may be illusional; three-dimensional objects, such as the sofa, cars along the street, a favorite bat and ball, appear two-dimensional, cartoonish at times. Space seems to change, as if one's field of vision narrows, with periphery lost. Objects seem duller, brighter, larger, smaller than before, and able to move even though stationary. When walking on a flat surface, an interosensory impression arises, that of riding on a swiftly moving elevator, making it feel as if the road or floor is in flux. Time may be altered; milliseconds read like minutes.

Audition may be distorted, too, with sounds, near or far, solo or choral, appearing louder, harsher, and in some cases muted or absent altogether. Likewise, olfaction can be impacted, as one scent permeates all others, or as another scent, unanticipated and out of context, infiltrates the space, or where SAM's sense of smell diminishes or seemingly disappears. Sensory anesthesia also applies to touch and other bodily impressions, as SAM often experiences sensations akin to "pins and needles" and numbness or detachment of body parts from his psychological sense of identity. His sense of taste may alter just like the others. With sensations distorted, some in the foreground, others in the background, and with a sense of detachment from self, others, and microenvironments, feelings of unreality and personality disintegration soon follow.

Childhood sexual abuse wields a mighty force in its ability to induce dissociative reactions. Although some may have the capacity to willfully, wantingly, and reflexively detach, others do not. They soon discover, however, similar results by way of different means, namely through body numbing, the use, misuse, and abuse of drugs, alcohol, and food, and sexual acting out, among others.

Body Numbing

SAM attempts to psychically and physiologically numb or inhibit regulatory body functions and corporeal states (Spiegel, 1997). As a result of CSA, SAM feels shameful, dirty. Bowel movements only serve to exacerbate such feelings. He strains to control his bowels, sometimes for weeks at a time, in order

to avoid this normal and necessary body function. He will purposefully constipate, freeing himself from elimination worries on a daily basis, and after some
time will ingest laxatives, most likely when privacy is assured. After elimination, SAM painstakingly scours and sanitizes himself, at times with hot water
bottles, hoses, and any instrument that will flush him clean.

Similarly, in an attempt to inhibit the growth of his penis and testicles, he
may bind them, tie them, prick them, anything to strangulate sensations aroused
by and through them. The epigenetic development of secondary sex characteristics holds, for SAM, the capacity for evoking feelings of guilt, humiliation,
and shame (Pescosolido, 1989; Spiegel, 1997). The broadening of his shoulders, the widening of his chest, and the growth of facial, pubic, and body hair
are, for example, ego-dystonic; that is, such characteristics collide with his
feelings of emasculation and inferiority, thereby exacerbating conflict derived
from the abuse, and particularly so between his perceptions of self as an
abused male and his perceptions of gender role expectations.

Compulsive Behavior

Males with histories of CSA are significantly more likely than nonabused males
to engage in a number of self-destructive behaviors, including bingeing, purging, drinking, drugging, frequent and unprotected sex with unknown partners,
sadomasochistic role playing, and excessive exercising, among others
(Hernandez, 1995). How might obsessive, compulsive, and risk-taking behavior alleviate the stress and diminish the anxiety associated with the hyperaroused
or dissociative state? Childhood sexual abuse and the ensuing traumatic response may generate durable and persisting alterations in the regulation of
endogenous opioids (Herman, 1992). Such naturally occurring physiological
chemicals as beta-endorphins, metenkephalins, and dynorphin peptides resemble the molecular structure of, and have the same reactions as, opiates
within the central nervous system (Grunberg & Baum, 1985). They manage the
electrochemical interactions within the brain (van der Kolk, 1987). Further,
reexposure to the traumatic and sexually abusive stimuli may arouse an endogenous opiate reaction, because such natural chemicals are secreted in response to stress (Bloom, 1983; van der Kolk & Fisler, 1995), and, accordingly,
generate effects similar to the applying, snorting, injecting, ingesting, or
freebasing of exogenous opiates.

Individuals who have been subjected to severe, prolonged interpersonal
and/or environmental stress, such as CSA, evidence inordinate increases in
both catecholaminergic and endogenous opioid responses to subsequent stress,
including further episodes of abuse, exposure to abuse-related reminders, and
confrontation with life events independent of the abuse. This endogenous
opioid reactivity holds the potential to render cycles of dependence and withdrawal, comparable to that engendered by the use of exogenous opioids. This
helps to explain, particularly in terms of SAM's psychobiology, the relationship

between childhood trauma, as a dynamic, and subsequent self-destructive behavior, as an effect (van der Kolk, 1989; van der Kolk & Fisler, 1995).

Exogenous opiates and endogenous opioids share several psychoactive properties and effects: (a) analgesic action; (b) antidepressant action; (c) tranquilizing action; (d) reduction in responsiveness to stressful stimuli; (e) adjustment and regulation of stress responses such as habituated fear; (f) a sense of euphoria; (g) a sense of relaxation and weightlessness, as if one is floating through air; (h) a decrease in paranoia; and (i) diminished feelings of inadequacy (Bloom, 1983; Grunberg & Baum, 1985; Kaplan & Sadock, 1998, 1999). Such tranquilizing and antidepressant properties rouse relief for many males with histories of childhood sexual abuse. Moreover, the manipulation of endogenous opiates may be more compelling, as they are much more potent than their exogenous counterparts (Grunberg & Baum, 1985; van der Kolk, 1987).

How might this apply to SAM and his state of hyperarousal? When SAM senses an onslaught of pain, numbing becomes omnipotent—his locus of control and, momentarily, his locus of life. In a hyperaroused state, SAM may feel desperate for remission: He could be frantic, frenzied, wild with agitation, impulsive, without deliberation, hasty, incautious, and rash. And agitation grows. Numbing and invalidation, of some form, and right now, emerges as the only immediate, available, and viable remedy. Thoughts of alleviating the pain dominate, distract, and engross his mind. The anticipation of numbing, which may be very different from the actuality of numbing, absorbs his full attention. SAM transfixes on a bountiful outcome, soon entering a trancelike state where only one factor exists—relief.

With numbing perceived as a panacea for pain, the strategies for achieving medicinal effects are considered—drugs, alcohol, sexual acting out, gambling, bingeing, self-mutilation—but without precaution and forethought as to meaning, consequences, and implications. Stress-induced trance states, like exogenous opiates, generate a dissociative phase in which the recognition and sensation of pain severs from the emotional meaning it holds (Herman, 1992). Guilt, shame, sorrow, and regret, current or anticipatory, seem to simply break away, at least for a time.

Typically, SAM follows a prescribed order of preparatory rites, thereby enhancing the trance. These include his special routines and rituals that precede acting out. This systematic drill incorporates a number of mechanical and habitual actions that prevent a break in focus and maintain a state of preoccupation, anticipation, and arousal. SAM doesn't have to think, doesn't have to feel, only has to do what he needs to do to get where he needs to go in order to paralyze, at least temporarily, the facts and meanings of CSA that infiltrate his psychological and sociological space.

SAM is about to put himself at risk, thereby exacerbating, one would think, his stress response. However, endogenous opioid release could provide an explanation for his feelings of composure and tranquillity upon reexposure to traumatic stress (van der Kolk, 1987). Matt described this process, as it related to his sexual compulsions: "It's better than a six pack, better than the buzz from champagne. I'm never more focused, never more committed to what I'm doing, than when I'm getting ready to act out. It's like having tunnel vision, and I'm driving in the tunnel, and nothing can get in my way, not work, not obligations of any kind. All I can think about is getting there. Nothing can numb me like acting out. Nothing at all."

Next, SAM performs the compulsive behavior. He might reenact an aspect of a sexually abusive episode with a stranger at a truck stop, public park, or X-rated movie theatre. He might inebriate with drugs or alcohol. Perhaps he will run to the local grocery store, buy a cart full of food, race home, and voraciously eat behind closed doors. Then again, he might self-injure by sticking a pencil or screwdriver into his penis, or self-mutilate by slitting his testicles or thighs with a razor blade. Such behaviors are so compelling, for in their enactment, SAM experiences decompression and euphoria—a sense of control. Now, as opposed to then, he is the one deciding who to put at risk and when and how to abuse (Davies & Frawley, 1994). At this stage of the process, compulsive behaviors and activities are difficult to control or stop, for the positive consequences are immediate and tangible. Moreover, these behaviors and activities, with self-medicinal properties, are perceived as the remedial and readily available treatment for hyperarousal, unwanted memories, associated pain, and emotional dysregulation. They have the power to invalidate—to inactivate and nullify, at least for the time being—the facts, and especially the meanings, of SAM's sexual abuse history.

However, as with any prophylactic remedy, the effects wane. Euphoria ceases. And recognition of the act, with its negative consequences and implications, looms large. SAM now may feel guilt for taking time away from family or work, shame for degrading his body, sexually or otherwise, and humiliation for transgressing against his personal code of ethics and conduct, and for inviting others, even strangers, to participate in this self-destructive process as well. What began with a sense of desperation now culminates with a sense of despair. Additionally, although endogenous opiate secretion in response to traumatic stress may foster a transitory sense of competence and control, this altered state may be followed by withdrawal symptoms manifested in the form of sleep disturbances, hyperactivity, and explosive outbursts of aggression (van der Kolk, 1989).

Thus, SAM escapes pain only to find more. And the circuit begins again, maybe with different strategies, but certainly with more and more of the substance or activity employed in order to maintain the same level of emotional relief (Carnes, 1983; Spiegel, 1997b). In the end, reexposure to traumatic stress, or the reenactment of it, may yield a transient reprieve from distress; however, with it comes a perpetuation of the addictive cycle, which, in turn, leads to further loss of psychophysiological control (van der Kolk, 1987, 1989). Still and all, when it comes to invalidation strategies, the immediate consequences are more compelling than the long-term consequences, and the positive consequences are more tangible than their negative counterparts.

Positive Consequences of Invalidation Strategies

The object of SAM's intention and efforts, of course, is invalidation—the most positive consequence of all. Often the numbing response is immediate. Even when delayed, the anticipation of the protective or analgesic reaction, and the comfort it brings, soothes the process of getting there. Interestingly, the array of invalidation strategies—dissociation and other defenses, addictive behaviors such as drinking and drugging, compulsive behaviors, including bingeing, purging, sexual acting out, inordinate exercising, and gambling and risk-taking behaviors, among them stealing and speeding—render similar effects, namely distance from and alterations in reality (Harrison et al., 1997; van der Kolk, Perry, & Herman, 1991).

Invalidation strategies tend to silence the chatterbox in SAM's mind. Ceaseless introspection and painful rumination give way to an endeavored, albeit fleeting, sense of calm. In this state, SAM finds the freedom to adopt an "I don't care" stance and posture, even though a veneer like this fends off the underlying truth, "I'm afraid to care anymore because it hurts so much." Furthermore, depending on the type of invalidation strategy consciously or unconsciously employed, SAM may strive for and experience the following positive consequences:

1. The automatization of certain behaviors, allowing him to "go through the motions" while remaining cognitively, emotionally, and/or physiologically detached.
2. A temporary solution to seemingly irreconcilable conflicts, or at least a buffered reprieve from them.
3. A retreat from daily confrontations with abuse-generated effects, including fear of the next episode and fear of disclosure, as well as guilt, shame, and a degenerating sense of identity.
4. The compartmentalization of the abuse experience, allowing him, as much as possible, to keep it separate and apart from the immediacies of his life, including school assignments, work responsibilities, family obligations, social engagements, and organizational commitments.
5. The cathartic discharge of certain feelings, usually potent or somehow threatening, that would otherwise remain suppressed or detached under more typical states of consciousness (Putnam & Trickett, 1993).

Adaptive defenses shield SAM from anxiety while concurrently promoting some semblance of productivity and functionality; likewise, maladaptive defenses shield SAM from anxiety, but often at the expense of optimal functioning (Goldstein, 1984). Sometimes the cost of adaptation, that is, dissociating, detaching, numbing, drinking, drugging, eating, or acting out in one way or another, is maladaptation.

Negative Consequences of Invalidation Strategies

Negative consequences of invalidation strategies abound, yet pale in comparison to the cogency of the anticipated abolishing response. To begin, invalidation, intermittent or otherwise, preserves the memory shards fractionated off from ordinary consciousness, and consequently impedes the integration necessary for healing (Herman, 1992; Krystal, 1988). Defenses act as yeoman of the guard, inhibiting memory, distorting perceptions, and protecting SAM from anxiety, no matter what the cost. Further, unconsciously motivated and risky invalidatory behaviors, such as purging, sexual acting out, excessive drinking, and the like, frequently ensue while SAM is in a dissociative state, when he already feels detached from himself or the environment, out of control and likely to do something against his will and better judgment (Putnam, 1997). Dissociation places SAM in a double bind: He may not be aware of his dissociative state unless it is observed and mentioned by others and yet, others may not know that SAM is dissociating, since only he can positively ascertain whether he feels detached or unreal (Friedrich et al., 2001)—a stranger to himself or the world, at least at that moment in time.

Because invalidation strategies, as defense modalities, distort reality and delay emotional reaction by way of severing thought from feeling and meaning from context, SAM is unable to discern the truth for himself, let alone express his authentic thoughts and feelings to caring others. Invalidation renders emotions unfamiliar; over time, SAM finds it difficult to identify feeling states. He may be able to point to the physiological or tactile-kinesthetic indicators of emotions—clenched jaw, tense muscles, upset stomach, nervous laughter, inability to sit still—but not be able to perceive or single out the underlying emotion or even such sensory states as sleepiness, hunger, and pain. Numbness and discomfort become his two overriding feeling states, with each sensory, affective, or physiologic manifestation allocated to one or the other.

Because numbing constricts emotions, distorts sensations, and alters consciousness, SAM feels as if he is in a movie, as if he is a robot, as if he is watching himself from outside himself, with a sensation suggesting that what he is observing or what he is experiencing is not really happening. The sensation of being enveloped by a movable and upright screened partition, seemingly palpable but ironically invisible, prevents him from fully engaging with others, as if he is in a bad dream, wishing to wake, yet knowing he is already so. He is an alien in once familiar places, now strange and peculiar, a world once memorized but no longer his to know.

Such psychological and sensory alterations, bewildering as they may be, paradoxically coexist with the sensation of being a shell of a person and with feelings of emptiness, detachment, and indifference. Yet SAM knows that something is vitally wrong; he fears that he is going crazy or that he may soon die. He experiences a conspicuous dullness, muted emotions, apathetic thinking, an unresponsiveness to others, inactivity. Goals and aspirations, once able to invigorate, now remain frozen in time.

Further, like a kaleidoscope, critical components of identity, such as body image, gender image, self-esteem, self-worth, and self-efficacy, shift dramatically in form and content as states of consciousness shift dramatically, thereby hindering opportunities toward identity consolidation and constancy. Because the development of self and the consolidation of identity are state-dependent processes, the misuse and overuse of invalidation strategies ultimately exacerbate disruptions in the stability of identity—disruptions initially generated by the abuse itself. Invalidation strategies, including dissociation, (a) render extreme affective and segregated states with distortions of identity; (b) impede the retrieval and consequently the recollection of autobiographical memory, vital to a personal sense of continuity; (c) interfere with the self-capacities of impulse, affect, and behavior regulation; and (d) create social situations that impact negatively and, at times, destructively, on the self (Putnam & Trickett, 1993).

Thus another paradox: Invalidation and psychic shutdown generate a welcome sense of relief vis-à-vis the traumatic response. But with time, they also conjure a sense of shallow living, as SAM's thoughts, feelings, and behaviors, in fact, his day-to-day interactions, become increasingly measured and mechanical, driven by his tenacious cleaving to whatever it takes to get him through to sleep.

Continuing with negative consequences, invalidation strategies invite and propagate opportunities for the psychosomatic expression of underlying repressed and suppressed abuse-related phenomena. Rashes, headaches, stomach pains, and elimination problems, as well as other manifestations, circuitously bypass and distract SAM from conflicts brewing below his level of consciousness. Although compulsive behaviors, such as sexual acting out, kleptomania, obsessive shopping, excessive exercise, and pathological gambling, serve as distracters from life demands and as a temporary balm for anxiety, SAM must also confront a number of negatives, including feeling out of control, the time-consuming nature of compulsive activities, his neglect of other life responsibilities, the betrayal of others, and the shame, remorse, and mood shifts engendered by the compulsions, lasting, in some cases, for days (Black, Kehrberg, Flumerfelt, & Schlosser, 1997).

Invalidation strategies delimit adaptive opportunities toward self-soothing, self-caring, and ultimately self-efficacy. Both SAM's progressive withdrawal into the self, with the intention of numbing, and his progressive use of external stimuli, such as drugs, alcohol, and compulsive behaviors, all with the intention of numbing, increase his dependence on such measures. Consequently, invalidation strategies thwart the accrual of more adaptive responses and, in essence, push SAM forward on his foreboding course of self-destruction and maladaptivity.

SAM may become terrified of anything adjacently or remotely associated with CSA, because he fears the emotions evoked by such an encounter. Although invalidation strategies tend to ameliorate panic, at least temporarily, they also promote self-absorption, escalate fear of future stressors, and arrest peer relations. They also defer possibilities toward the integration of history with currency, of cognition with affect, and of the fractionated aspects of the sexually abusive experience.

When SAM recognizes the consequences of psychic invalidation, particularly the feeling of lifelessness, his sense of helplessness, and his dread of acceptance and surrender, he may initiate an activity—self-mutilation, an aggressive outburst, anything—in order to jump start his life, to assert a sense of mastery over the fear of self-abandonment, the fear of emptiness and the fear of becoming less than he already experiences himself to be. In the long run, SAM's fear of surrender to the traumatic state is more devastating than the abuse itself (Krystal, 1978, 1988).

Infused with wishes to be so, SAM's invalidation strategies, including dissociation, are not foolproof. Indeed, sexual abuse is more than a mere rival, for dissociation is penetrable. While dissociation provides degrees of suppression, proportions of detachment, fractions or shards of the sexually abusive experience break through the protective and preservative barrier. They upsurge as cognitive ruminations, emotions detached from context, startle responses, intrusive imagery and sensations, visual, auditory, olfactory, gustatory, and tactile-kinesthetic memories, sleep disturbances, nightmares and night terrors, repetitive and reenacting behaviors, and regressive actions, to mention a few. Ultimately, invalidation strategies, as a means of "self-medication," impede the development of self, interrupt the acquisition of healthy coping skills, interfere with personal relationships, hinder the concentration necessary for academic and workplace functioning, and delay integration of the truth (Chu, 1998; Harrison et al., 1997).

In summary, invalidation strategies and detached states of consciousness may provide an emotional analgesic, but what a price to pay for temporary relief. Such responses and states also bring constriction of liveliness, narrowing of reflective and analytic thought, deferment of emotional responsivity, restriction of desire and motivation, and confinement of action and interaction across microrelationships and environments. CSA maintains itself in memory; no matter how hard SAM tries, it cannot be fully forgotten.

So no one will ask. Don't tell if they do. Don't think. Don't feel. Invalidation, for many, is inevitable. All invalidatory maneuvers are in service of survival; all involve the rewriting of one's life context and history—a reconstruction of the self (Rieker & Carmen, 1986).

RECONCILIATION

They were calling me "cocksucker" and "faggot" before I even knew what they meant, but I knew from the tone that they were degrading and shameful names. Those words cut me deep; they told me that I was not as good as other boys, that something deep inside me was so ugly and wrong that it showed on the outside. (Ty, interview with author, December 7, 1994)

Reconciliation is the process of submitting to the violations associated with childhood sexual abuse by assuming responsibility for it. A sexually abused boy must do this because he is unable to either fully escape the realities of abuse, or fully defend against its consequences. This is SAM's dilemma—an impasse—difficult, if not impossible, to reconcile, especially in the presence of traumatic memories.

The Brain and Traumatic Memory

To be sure, subjection to CSA, and its subsequent concealment, invalidation, reconciliation, and compensation are biopsychosocial stressors. The excitatory and inhibitory stress-responsive chemicals transmitted within SAM by way of his psychobiological response system may also enhance or impede the encoding, consolidation, and retrieval of his memories associated with CSA. Low levels of stress have a neutral impact on memory. Moderate levels of stress enhance the memory process. However, high levels of acute or protracted stress tend to impair memory function and other brain activity (Bremner et al., 1999; Roozendaal et al., 1997; Siegel, 2001).

The four major regions of the brain—the brainstem, the diencephalon, the limbic system, and the cortex—store memories consonant with the functions they regulate (Perry, 1999). Vis-à-vis the experience of childhood sexual abuse, the cortex retains, for example, facts of the abuse, the perpetrator's face, what he did, how she did it, in essence, cognitive memory. The limbic system is responsible for the emotional valence of the experience, that is, the meaning imbuing the facts, or emotional memory. The diencephalon stores behaviors, or motor-vestibular memories, such as performing fellatio, cunnilingus, and intercourse. Finally, the brainstem "remembers" the physiological states engendered by SAM's subjection to CSA, such as hypervigilance, fear, and terror.

During states of arousal, and after data are processed in the neocortex via the thalamo-cortico-amygdala pathway, the neocortex transmits the various sensory stimuli—the color of the walls in the bedroom (from the visual cortex), sounds of the neighbor's birthday celebration as SAM experiences penetration for the first time (from the auditory cortex)—to the transition region located between the neocortex and the hippocampus. This transitional region, including the entorhinal cortex, integrates the disparate sensory data into a more coherent and multidimensional representation of the sexually abusive experience. The transitional cortex transmits these once isolated sensations but now cohesive representations to the hippocampus, a sensitive substructure intimately related to the amygdala and pivotal to the efficient functioning of the limbic system (LeDoux, 1992).

Among the various regions of the brain, the limbic system is most associated with the processing of memory (van der Kolk, 1996). The hippocampus is responsible for laying down memory traces or engrams of the facts affiliated with SAM's history of CSA. Further, this limbic system component is central in circumscribing episodes of abuse with a beginning, middle, and end, thereby positioning CSA memory traces in their proper perspectives of place, space, position, and time. During the encoding process, the hippocampus centralizes associative patterns between and among historic and current events, and during the retrieval process, the hippocampus synthesizes disparate sensory elements into a composite memory, thereby facilitating and accelerating the processes undergirding the operation of explicit memory (Brinton & Berger, 2000; Squire & Zola, 1998). The amygdala, too, plays an active role during traumatic sexual abuse and in the act of remembering it. Although the hippocampus is presumed to process the facts—words spoken, words heard, the stealthy acts of CSA in time and space—the role of the amygdala is to imbue the facts of CSA with contextualized emotionally charged meaning. Thus, by means of the amygdeloid-hippocampal relationship within the limbic system, memory is processed. Essentially, sensory data enters the amygdala; the amygdala assesses their emotional significance and transmits its evaluation to the hippocampus; the hippocampus synthesizes the data with previous memories of comparable sensory particulars (Damasio, 1994). By that account, the limbic system encompasses the brain region in which memories are processed and the brain region from which memory anomalies may be detected (van der Kolk, & Saporta, 1993).

Under ordinary circumstances, SAM's explicit and implicit memory systems function independently (Squire & Kandel, 2000). As SAM encounters traumatic CSA, however, they operate synchronically (Armony & LeDoux, 1997; Cahill, 1997; LeDoux, 1996; Roozendaal et al., 1997). In other words, subjection to CSA sets into motion both the explicit and implicit memory systems to a degree over and above that required for nontraumatic events. Explicit memory, or the conscious recollection of facts, concepts, and ideas, is, in part, a function of the hippocampal system and corresponding cortical areas of the brain. In contrast, implicit memory, or unconscious memories of emotional states and conditioned traits, is more closely associated with the amygdaloid system (LeDoux, 1996; Siegel, 2001).

Independence does not preclude synchronicity, as both systems function in parallel (LeDoux, 1992). Thus, between abusive episodes, and, in many instances, long after the cessation of the sexually abusive relationship, when exposed directly or indirectly to contextual or generalized stimuli related to the abuse, SAM's explicit and implicit memory systems transact concurrently. Responding to the same stimuli and functioning simultaneously, this dual activation spawns the illusion of a "unified memory function" (p. 202). However, they are independent, as evidenced by the following. During reactivation, as chemicals discharge throughout his entire body, SAM will remember the explicit facts—the perpetrator's position on top, his taunting, her threats—by way of the hippocampal system. At the same time, SAM will remember the implicit meanings—helplessness, shame, intimidation—by way of the amygdaloid system.

However, as the amygdala tends to thrive under acute or protracted stress whereas the hippocampus tends to diminish in capacity (Joseph, 1999), it is also possible that explicit facts detach from their implicit meanings. Such outcomes are personified by virtue of SAM's conditioned fear response. By its very nature, the conditioned fear response, a by-product of the implicit and unconscious emotional memory system, is not a function of conscious explicit memory, and therefore acts independently (Pillemer & White, 1989). Triggered internally or externally, these conditioned fear responses typically take shape during a sexually abusive episode and often exacerbate across time and place. Germinating within SAM's body, they epitomize and personalize trauma's "incubation of fear" (Yehuda, 2000), and are expressed by way of visual, auditory, olfactory, gustatory, and/or tactile-kinesthetic flashbacks and memories (LeDoux, 1994). Thus, SAM's conditioned fear response exemplifies the disengagement of the amygdaloid-hippocampal relationship and, consequently, the implicit–explicit systems of memory and, most concretely, the CSA facts from their meanings. When the implicit meanings emerge, SAM will likely evidence hyperarousal or dissociation and their concomitant neurological, biological, psychological, and physiological manifestations (Perry, 1997, 1999).

With all of this going on—the biology, psychology, and sociology of childhood sexual abuse—questions continue to buffet SAM's bewildered mind: "What is reality, what is truth? What is mythology and what is my imagination? If I can see the pictures in my head but feel numb at the same time, maybe the abuse doesn't mean anything. But then, again, if this didn't really happen, or if it did but it's really not a big deal, where are all of these emotions coming from? Why do I feel dead one day and like I'm going to jump out of my skin the next day? And if it really did happen, whose fault is it anyway? My fault? The perpetrator's fault? Why am I thinking so much how can I make it stop?"

Dichotomous Thinking

How, then, does SAM gain, however illusionary, a sense of control? Dichotomous thinking. Dichotomous thinking, akin to personal and social schematization, is a type of cognitive error (Beck & Emery, 1985); it involves perceiving, dividing, and interpreting people, places, circumstances, events, and just about everything into one of two opposite categories (Mahoney, 1974).

The diversity and dispersion of human behavior in the social environment collapse into dichotomies.

Whereas CSA is an experience that engenders a sense of intrapsychic chaos and physiological depletion, dichotomous thinking, through its imposition on perception, and consequently on affect and behavior, reduces each and every aspect of life into one of two possible denominations. Thoughts and feelings about self and others are all interpreted within this frame. Examples include:

- Perpetrator/victim.
- Friend/enemy.
- Stranger/intimate.
- Dominant/submissive.
- Angel/whore.
- Teacher/student.
- Leader/follower.

- Love/hate.
- Love/sex.
- Love/fear.
- Powerful/powerless.
- Brave/fearful.
- Sensual/prudish.
- Belonging/alienation.

- Light/dark.
- Masculine/feminine.
- Smart/stupid.
- Right/wrong.
- Good/bad.
- Healthy/unhealthy.
- Favorite/outcast.

Dichotomous thinking firmly declares that life is bound by rules (Brown, 1988). Everyone and everything—people, thoughts, actions, places, days, sexual abuse, candy, holidays, and wishes—can be and must be classified as right or wrong, good or bad, the abuser or the abused, and so on. Analogous to splitting (Pearlman & Saakvitne, 1995), dichotomous thinking, too, helps a boy to disavow certain instances of reality in order to prevent any further calamities of childhood (Davies & Frawley, 1994). Psychological representations of the perpetrator, for example, split vertically into compartmentalized images of good and bad, caring and abusive, loving and hating (Adams-Tucker, 1985; Grotstein, 1985). Even though the mental representations are isolated from one another, they remain concurrently extant. For instance, Ty revealed: "Even to this day, it's hard for me to look at Rodney as a perpetrator, even though he did all those bad things to me, even got someone to shit on me. In my mind and in my heart, Rodney is the one who loved me. Maybe he just didn't know how or such, but I bet he tried." Just as aspects of the object can be split from one another, self-representations can be compartmentalized as well. For example, Jake disclosed: "When I was with Father Simon in the rectory, in his bedroom, I was 'Satan's Son,' an immoral sexual bastard. When I was his altar boy, I felt so special, so fortunate, to be celebrating the life of Christ. And Father Simon was His representative on earth."

Dichotomies annul the need to acknowledge, let alone cope with or adapt to, ambiguities, uncertainties, and things too indistinct or too complex (Brown, 1988). They abolish the need to reconcile, to synthesize or to do anything about the perplexities, complexities, discrepancies, and contradictions of life. Everything can rounded up or rounded down to its lowest common denominator. Everyone and everything falls only into category "this" or category "that." With dichotomous thinking, life and people are easy to read. With absolutes,

SAM can have with him, at all times, prefabricated responses, since at any given moment, in any given context, there are only two ways to see, two ways to feel, two ways to do. With absolutes, there are no surprises.

For dichotomous thinkers, everything in life shifts from "and" to "or." That love and fear, ignorance and consciousness, empathy and apathy can coexist is beyond the parameters of this intrapersonal strategy. When one compartment opens, the other closes, by function and default. With dichotomous thinking, the only viable and recognizable dimension is "presence" or "absence;" the degree to which love is growing and fear diminishing, the extent to which awareness is developing, and the depth to which empathy can be expressed, is immaterial. With dichotomous thinking, there are no gradations, no phases, no evolution; something is, or is not. Period.

There is, however, a sense of being in a rut, because no matter how hard SAM tries, no matter what he does and no matter how effective dichotomous thinking may seem to be in a particular instant, situation, or context, SAM is spinning his wheels. Why? First, dichotomous categories are, at their very essence, absolutes, and second, absolutes are illusions. They do not capture the dispersion and the diversity of reality, and thus, its shades of gray.

What is the bottom line here? The degree to which SAM tries to impose absolute and illusory categories on himself, his experience, others, and the world is also the degree to which he will feel out of sorts, out of sync, incongruent, anxious, and depressed because, ultimately, reality is not aligning with his socially imposed perceptions of self, others, and the world.

With regard to dichotomous thinking and childhood sexual abuse, there are only two vantage points from which to perceive and respond to, the self, others, the future, and the world—two vantage points that are polar opposites. For example, SAM, in order to create a sense of control in his world, albeit unknowingly and illusionary, may classify each and every person with whom he interacts into the victim category or the perpetrator category. When a person is compartmentalized as "perpetrator," he or she is imbued with the following characteristics: powerful, aggressive, unafraid, and guiltless. In a like way, a person compartmentalized as "victim" is experienced as one who is weak, passive, fearful, and blameful. What a price to pay for the illusion of power, the falseness of balance, the misimpression of control.

Further, dichotomous thinking maintains the reconciliatory tenet that the perpetrator is blameless (though not necessarily innocent) and that SAM is culpable because, from this perspective, one has to be innocent and the other guilty; one has to be good and the other bad, one right, the other wrong. Consequently, SAM fears any mistake he might make. Any "bad" thought, any "wrong" feeling, any miscalculated action that transpires has the potential to call up the category of "loser," "deviant," "sinner," "queer," any of the these and many more to follow. In SAM's psychological and sociological space—his microenvironments—if what the perpetrator says is true and if the social messages are true, then the message he receives is quite clear: "There is nothing wrong with sexual abuse. There is something wrong with me, because I am living it, reacting to it, and because I allowed it to happen in the first place."

Indeed, SAM strives to interpret, rationalize and give reason for everything that is happening to him: Flooding. Numbing. Rage. Nightmares. Sleepwalking. Fear. Guilt. Shame. Feelings of unreality. Fear of the bathroom. Constipation. Stomach problems. Anal bleeding. And on and on. Feeling flawed, isolated, and in need of validation, SAM continues to construct a rationale that is congruent with the social environment. The boy is left with the certainty that social myths are false, but also with the realization that, in order to belong to his gender, to his family, he is required to act as though the myths are real. Fighting for a way out of this paradox, SAM must exchange reality for mythology, truth for illusion, and personal perception for socially imposed propaganda. Thus, with support from social mythology, he constructs a life story that accounts for its existence. Alone, he chooses to resolve this causal ambiguity by assuming responsibility for the abuse.

Here, attribution, and three of its dimensions, namely, locus of control, misattribution, and self-attribution, come into play (Kendall & Hollon, 1981). All three merge to minimize the impact of situational factors such as power differentials and coercive methods (Cavaiola & Schiff, 1988; Mendel, 1995). They also serve to exaggerate the role of the boy's personal qualities (Burgess et al., 1987; Janus et al., 1987) such as his perceived inability to prevent the abuse and perceived inferiority as a result of the abuse. Thus, sexually abused boys make attributions in opposition to circumstantial facts but congruent with their gender schemas.

Locus of control, at first glance, appears to be external in source, given that sexually abused males typically experience the occurrence of abuse as beyond their control. To illustrate, the boy initially asks, "Why is the perpetrator doing this to me?" Next, misattribution emerges as the sexually abused male ascribes effects to the wrong cause. For example, SAM's physiological response renders the perpetrator blameless and himself at fault. Finally, self-attribution operates as internalized, socially generated negative myths and consequences, such as "Even though sexual abuse doesn't happen to boys, it happened to me. Maybe I was supposed to be a girl. Maybe I am a fag. Something is really wrong with me." By way of deduction, SAM construes himself to be worthy of guilt.

Mediated by gender "blueprints," attribution, as a cognitive process for sexually abused males, begins with a locus of externality and ends with a locus of internality, or, as in this case, self-blame. Thus, the question "Why is the perpetrator doing this to me?" becomes "What did I do to make the perpetrator act that way? Is it the way I walk, the way I talk? What?" SAM must rationalize and interpret his history of CSA in a social environment that is replete with illusions (e.g., adults act according to the best interests of a child), contradictions (e.g., sex means he loves me; love hurts my body), gender dichotomies (e.g., boys are perpetrators; girls are victims), and mythology (e.g., abused boys grow up to become perpetrators) around the very life event he is striving to understand.

Sexual abuse does not exist in a vacuum; accordingly, the meaning ascribed to it must be viewed in context. If the boy thinks, feels, or acts in accordance with the reality of abuse, his thoughts, feelings, and behaviors will be incongruent with abuse mythology. Thus, he is placed in a double bind wherein truth is dishonorable and illusion is virtuous. Facing devaluation no matter what side he takes, it is easy to understand why SAM feels tentative, crazy, and out of control.

Further, the sexually abused male does not derive meaning in isolation; rather, this process unduly involves the perceptions, judgments, and attributions that others hold around his abuse (Rieker & Carmen, 1986). Without doubt, perpetrators, family members, and others similarly participate in this reconciliation process. For example, in many instances, sexual abuse is reconstructed as sex education, an act of love, or a common yet ironically private family activity (Berliner & Conte, 1990; Elliott et al., 1995). This mythological view is supported by public perceptions as well, for it is not uncommon for some to view a boy's subjection to CSA as a developmental milestone or even harmless (Broussard et al., 1991; Spencer & Tan, 1999). Parents of sexually abused boys appear to be less concerned about the effects of CSA on their sons than parents of female children with similar experiences or histories (Gill & Tutty, 1997). In fact, individuals close to the boy, including many caretakers, view the boy, regardless of age, as the enticer, "queer," "she-male," seducer, or culprit (Spiegel, 1995).

Unfortunately, children, more often than not, are designated as blameworthy (Back & Lips, 1998; Johnson & Shrier, 1987; Spencer & Tan, 1999). Child protection workers, district attorneys, police officers, and judges and juries alike tend to view the sexual abuse of boys as less traumatic than the sexual abuse of girls (Broussard et al., 1991; Spencer & Tan, 1999). Adult males and females are inclined to perceive older children as more responsible for their abuse than younger children (Back & Lips, 1998; Waterman & Foss-Goodman, 1984) and are more likely to perceive older boys as less masculine than younger boys vis-à-vis the sexually abusive experience. And, in support of social mythology, adult males tend to attribute greater responsibility for the abuse to the boy's characteristics and behavior and, accordingly, less responsibility to his perpetrator (Spencer & Tan, 1999).

Reports alleging the sexual abuse of males tend to be screened out with little or no investigation. Prosecution is more likely when the boy is older than 6 but younger than 12, when the abuse is perceived as severe by child protection, police, and legal officials, when the child is deemed an effective witness, when force was employed during the abuse and when there is substantial evidence to corroborate the boy's testimony (Myers, 1994; Tjaden & Thoennes, 1992). Clearly, the burden of proof is on SAM. Sadly, when it comes to the sexual abuse of males, there already exists reasonable doubt.

Many children, fighting against coercion, violation, and stigmatization—and trying to control their lives—reconcile the abuse by assuming responsibility for it. For the sake of survival, children will attribute the cause of abuse to themselves. SAM unknowingly internalizes the social mythology surrounding the sexual abuse of males; he unconsciously introjects the guilt feelings of the perpetrator; now SAM is to blame and the perpetrator is free to act as if all is well (Daldin, 1988). That notwithstanding, SAM, unintentionally or otherwise, uses self-blame to his advantage. When a sexually abused boy believes, "It's my fault. I am the cause of this," he can also think, "I can do something to change it." This strategy permits him to fight against an overwhelming sense of powerlessness and to develop an illusion of control (Conte & Schuerman, 1987; Lamb, 1986). Besides, if SAM believes that the abuse is the perpetrator's fault, then he experiences an even more staggering sense of powerlessness, as well as the actual or potential loss of love and loved ones (Spiegel, 1997). While, in the immediacy of the abuse experience, perceived internal control may function as a protective factor against the proliferation of internalizing effects (Bolger & Patterson, 2001), over time, abuse-specific internal attributions, in conjunction with engendered shame, play a key role in the manifestation and exacerbation of trauma symptoms and internalizing behaviors (Feiring, Taska, & Chen, 2002). Blaming himself, yet believing he can do something about it; blaming the perpetrator, then feeling helpless and hopeless; for SAM, the choice—if one could call it a choice—is simple.

This unconscious process evolves over time. The sexually abused boy is unaware of such intrapsychic occurrences; he is simply doing what seems natural because it is natural to survive. Survival is instinctual, even in the face of childhood sexual abuse. Sadly, he does not realize that characterological self-blame, that is, or blaming the abuse on his personhood, his characteristics and traits, will continue to shatter his assumptions about self, others, and the world. No, SAM, it's not over yet.

COMPENSATION

On the inside, I felt like a freak of nature. Satan's son. On the outside, I wore a mask: John Doe, Joe Regular, Jake Normal. My greatest achievement, or so I thought, was keeping people from coming too close to see the real me on the inside. (Jake, interview with author, April 5, 2000)

Compensation is the process of counteracting or neutralizing the internal conflict associated with sexual abuse by means of cognitive and/or behavioral restructuring. To offset the shame, humiliation, guilt, and self-blame, males with histories of CSA do whatever they can to make reparation through the development of a compensatory self. In doing so, they strive to make amends for their perceived transgressions. This adaptation occurs not only by concealing, invalidating, and reconciling CSA, but also by revising the reality of the abuse so that the experience itself and the sexually abused boy's genuine thoughts, feelings, and behaviors are nullified to comply with gender-role expectations (Rieker & Carmen, 1986).

The compensatory process involves cognitive dissonance (Festinger, 1964), ensuing from incompatibilities between and among one's day-to-day experiences—or one's beliefs about the self—and one's expectations based on prevailing social directives. In this case, cognitive dissonance is rendered when sexual abuse, an unanticipated event for males given its social allocation to females, occurs. Dissonance manifests as SAM holds knowledge that threatens the ways in which he perceives himself, his gender, and his role in the sexually abusive relationship.

Cognitive dissonance emerges in response to conflicted cognitions and their discrepant behavioral implications. For SAM, one thought registers as "I am a boy," followed by "I was sexually abused" and "But boys aren't supposed to be sexually abused." Yet another thought suggests, "Boys are supposed to be strong, courageous, and competent," whereas another indicates, "I am weak, fearful, and inferior because I was sexually abused."

Due to the disparity between the reality of the sexual abuse of males on the one hand, and socially constructed notions of masculinity and gender on the other hand, males with histories of CSA are likely to experience a variety of conflicts and problems in the cognitive domain of personal beliefs and social prescriptions (Finkelhor & Dziuba-Leatherman, 1995). Discrepancy engenders dissonance; dissonance gives rise to shame and guilt. This internal friction (e.g., "Sexual abuse shouldn't happen to boys but it happened to me") serves as a source of motivation to engage in cognitions or behaviors intended to ameliorate the dissonant repercussions (Marlatt & Gordon, 1985). Thus, such an aroused state impels SAM to act in ways that are consistent with one of the contradictory cognitions, thereby minimizing the negative effects. Eventually, boys take compensatory measures with the intention of undoing and, in some cases, overdoing the initial effects of CSA.

The course of these compensatory measures is dependent on SAM's personal hypotheses, which, in combination, impact his sense of self-efficacy. Personal hypotheses mirror schemas about the self, others, the world, and the relationships among these three domains (Greene & Ephross, 1991). Personal hypotheses, or theories of the self, arise from macro-based social blueprints, that is, social prescriptions about roles and corresponding actions. Acting in socially prescribed ways solicits validation. When conflict ensues from knowledge of the self on the one hand, and social prescriptions on the other hand, the latter typically supersedes the former (Duncan & Williams, 1998). Thus, as Thomas Kuhn (1970) argued, [personal] theories do not succeed by virtue of their truthfulness but rather by the extent of their popular support.

When categorizing personal experiences and meanings, SAM places them into symbolic systems that include evaluative frameworks. These frameworks, in turn, shape his perceptions and expectations and lead to self-fulfilling prophecies. In American culture, when it comes to the male gender, a high premium is placed on self-protection, aggression, and physical competency. Self-worth is often a function of one's abilities to meet, if not surpass, these socially sanctioned prescriptions. The cultural meanings, including the social mythology surrounding the sexual abuse of males, as well as gender role prescriptions, comprise the context in which CSA occurs. These very meanings—that SAM is gay, deviant, sex-crazed—hold steadfast as overly generalized, prejudicial, and negative social schemas.

SAM internalizes the external meaning; his personal theories about the self emerge from and are validated by social categories. For instance, to categorize oneself as a "male" or a "sexually abused male" is to evaluate, according to social precepts, a certain type of individual; one then acts in ways that are socially perceived as typical of such individuals.

Self-efficacy involves a perception of oneself as masterful and competent, as well as the knowledge and skills necessary to actualize desired psychological and behavioral changes. With high self-efficacy, one has a sense of personal power to wield control, at least over choices and behaviors that promote well-being (Bandura, 1990). In other words, behavior is mediated by efficacy expectations, or the belief that one has the ability to carry out an intended behavior pattern (Bandura, 1986). Self-efficacy theory proposes that, when encountering a current situation requiring action, individuals cognitively appraise their prior behaviors from similar situations. Such an assessment renders an efficacy expectation, which, in turn, mediates current behavior. Thus, self-efficacy is a function of the meanings associated with the intended behavior, the skills accessible to execute the behavior, and the degree of perseverance necessary for such execution.

Ty offered the following personal hypotheses: (a) "I was sexually abused. Sexually abused people are sick"; (b) "I was sexually abused. Sexually abused boys are queer"; and (c) "I was sexually abused. I am a shame to my family and to other guys." As one who perceives himself as sick, queer, and shameful, Ty's sense of self-efficacy was greatly diminished, especially when he interacted with peers in physical education class, or when he encountered street gangs in his area. For example, prior to gym class, Ty often remembered how inferior he felt around his peers, especially because his athletic skills were made fun of by students and teachers alike. As an adolescent, when thinking about gym class, Ty anticipated failure, having stumbled and fallen short several times that year. Consequently, he expected to fail again and to be the target of mockery as a result. Further, since self-efficacy involves mastery, Ty was likely to seek experiences that confirmed his personal hypotheses and reflected his sense of self-efficacy, namely, cross-dressing and hustling. He did so in order to validate his sense of self and his perceptions of his place in the world. Thus, he compensated for his perceived lack of masculinity by dramatically exaggerating traits socially allocated to females.

The construct of masculinity, the biopsychosocial definition of manhood, functions as the cornerstone of sexuality. For Ty and other males with histories of CSA, masculinity becomes equated not only with aggression but also with victimization (Lew, 1990). Consequently, they must try to separate the abuse from the abused, the battle of their lives—and not easily won. Consider the following compensatory (and socially constructed) attributes most personified by SAM: hypermasculinity, feminization, and androgyny.

Fighting against a sense of emasculation, SAM might identify with the aggressor by projecting a hypermasculine role (Friedrich & Luecke, 1988; Friedrich et al., 1986; Gartner, 1999). SAM might assume a hypermasculine posture to defend against the chance of being labeled gay, victim, powerless, or any classification that doesn't support current views of masculinity (Spiegel, 1997a). His sense of self is dependent on the notion of how much, how far, how fast, and how hard. As a means of promoting this facade, males with histories of sexual abuse might evidence aggression and temper outbursts (Robin et al., 1997), a desire to hurt others (Rew et al., 1991), cruelty to children and animals (Brodsky et al., 2001), running away (Chandy et al., 1997), criminal behavior (Widom, 1995), and excessive body building (Spiegel, 1995). If SAM falls under this category, he is likely to join organizations such as the Boy Scouts of America or participate in organized athletic teams, because organizations and activities like these in one way foster a sense of belonging and the appearance of "normality" and, in another way, demote close interpersonal connections (Gill & Tutty, 1999).

Although identification with the aggressor has a number of costs, particularly in the arena of negative social reactions, doing so helps SAM to maintain a facade that is congruent with gender role expectations. In this way, he maintains some semblance of equilibrium, allowing him to function as best he can in a manner congruent with society's standards (Daldin, 1988; Duncan & Williams, 1998). Victor disclosed: "As a boy and as a man, my most important job was to be meaner, tougher, bigger and stronger than any man who came into my world. In my father's world, I was his puta. In my world, I had to be on top."

SAM learns to frame others dichotomously—as perpetrators or victims (Lew, 1990). Therefore, one is either aggressive, abusive, and powerful or submissive, withdrawn, and powerless. In an attempt to reject any form of identification with the male perpetrator, SAM may strive to incorporate traits culturally and socially allocated to females. Thus, he internalizes the socially constructed role of victim and, accordingly, feminizes himself (Gill & Tutty, 1999; Krug, 1989). As such, he may be more likely than others to experience an overt fear of male peers (Wells et al., 1997), inhibition around female peers (Briere & Runtz, 1990), fear of physical education class (Pescosolido, 1989), desperate attachments (Dimock, 1988), and a vulnerability to subsequent abuse (Boney-McCoy & Finkelhor, 1995a). This does not suggest a disorder of gender identity. If SAM falls under this category, he most likely accepts and "knows" that he is male but feels like a failure when it comes to masculinity. Additionally, if he equates masculinity with perpetration and femininity with the abused, he, in fear of being perceived as a potential offender, may take great strides to incorporate and present characteristics that are socially prescribed to females. This creates a buffer zone against his own authentic feelings of rage, hostility, and aggression directed toward the perpetrator and allows him to split or compartmentalize self representations of the aggressor and the aggressed. Palo disclosed: "When people say, 'Men are this' or 'Men are that,' I resent being put into a category with other men. To me, men are abusive, violent, smelly, greedy, stupid, and alcoholic. I don't want people to think that I, as a man, am capable of abuse. I don't want to be a woman but I also don't want to be the stereotypical man."

Even though femininzation is likely to evoke a range of gender-based ridicule and derision from others, it's a price SAM is often willing to pay in order to achieve a sense of congruency between his self-concept and his outward appearance and behavior. He's simply striving to make the outside match the inside. Ty reported: "I know I ain't a woman. God didn't birth me that way. But I've always been afraid of men. Afraid they would beat me, hurt me, see me as a mistake. Afraid of women, too. Afraid they would think I was wrong somehow, being a man the wrong way. I know God doesn't make mistakes so I know that I am a man. I'd rather have people call me a 'screaming queen' or a 'nigger queer' than to call me a 'mistake.' So I don't act like all the other men. That's when I would really fail. That would be my biggest mistake."

Repudiating both ends of this continuum, SAM assumes an androgynous or undifferentiated presentation (Richardson et al., 1993). Love, intimacy, and sexuality—even the thought of them—prove far too threatening for more than a few males with histories of CSA. Because, for some, sex and violation are one and the same, any expression of sexuality requires one to take on the role of the abuser or the abused (Lew, 1990; Spiegel, 1997). Rejecting each side of the dichotomy, SAM discards his sexual self. In this way, he might evidence a greater tendency than nonabused males to gain weight so as to distort the V-shaped male figure, hide, invert, or bind his penis, wear large and loose clothing, and isolate from others (Pescosolido, 1989). Males with an undifferentiated sense of gender identity or presentation evidence low mastery across microenvironments, including identity confusion, low self-esteem, problematic social relations, withdrawal from or avoidance of social contact, deficient study and work habits, sexual promiscuity, delinquency, and bizarre behavior (Richardson et al., 1993). Kip said: "I don't hate that I'm a guy. I hate that I have a penis, that my cock got hard during the abuse and nothing nobody says can make me change that hate. I'm not fat because I was born that way. I got fat on purpose because guys who are fat, you can't see their penis. It shrinks. Plus nobody wants to look at you. And that's just fine with me."

Regardless of the three compensatory styles, peer groups and peer activities still pose a great threat to SAM. His sense of vulnerability, real or imagined, evokes a sense of transparency, defenselessness, and fear. This fear of transparency—as if others can see what he is striving to conceal and, as a result, target him for sexual harassment, sexual abuse or gender exploitation—may be particularly acute in the context of athletic activities, physical education classes, locker and shower rooms, and the like (Pescosolido, 1989). The dissonance germinating between SAM's subjection to CSA and his perceived expectations of society with regard to the male gender role arouses unwavering distress. SAM's sense and personification of gender were not only revised by the sexual abuse but actually forged by the dissonance as well (Gill & Tutty, 1997).

Beyond compensatory presentations to the world, hypermasculine, feminized, and undifferentiated males with histories of childhood sexual abuse are equally likely to experience, vis-à-vis the abuse, a fear of reoccurrence and repercussions (Spiegel, 1995), generalized fear (Gomes-Schwartz et al., 1985), role confusion (Hunter, 1991), self-blame (Woods & Dean, 1985), a negative self-concept (Conte & Schuerman, 1987), academic problems (Calam et al., 1998), dissociation (Briere et al., 1988), anxiety (Mendel, 1995), depression (Sirles et al., 1989), intrusion and numbing of trauma-related thoughts and feelings (McLeer et al., 1998), posttraumatic stress disorder (Kiser et al., 1988), suicidal ideation (Sansonnet-Hayden et al., 1987), confusion between sexual and gender identities (Spiegel, 1995), a heightened sense of sexuality (Kolko et al., 1988), shame (Johnson & Shrier, 1987), emasculation (Dimock, 1988), sexual compulsivity (Bartholow et al., 1994), self-injurious behavior (Olson, 1990), drug and alcohol abuse (Stein et al., 1988), conflictual peer and intimate relationships (Janus et al., 1987), and occupational problems (Lisak & Luster, 1994), among others, such as sexual abuse reactivity and sexual abuse effects on the brain.

ABUSE REACTIVITY

The proportions of CSA perpetrators with histories of CSA are not high enough to validate the socially constructed and popularly held "abused to abuser" paradigm (Bera, 1994; O'Brien, 1991). Rates of CSA among adolescent and adult perpetrators tend to coalesce within the range of 20% and 30% (Freund et al., 1990; Hanson, 1990; Hanson & Slater, 1988; Murphy & Smith, 1996). However, the CSA field lacks consensus as to what may be categorized as developmentally expected sexual behavior and what constitutes abuse reactivity among children (Hall et al., 1998) and at what age or developmental stage abuse reactivity becomes a juvenile sexual offense.

Sexual behavior problems secondary to CSA may fall along a continuum of problematic behaviors, that is, from behaviors that are developmentally anticipated and normative to behaviors that are intentional, aggressive, and coercive. More concretely, such behaviors range from cooperative sex play, to compulsive masturbation, sexual preoccupation, sexualized gesturing, expression of adult sexual acts, planning of sexual acts, and continuation of sexual behavior in the presence of adult limit-setting. As children's behaviors escalate along this continuum, a number of personal and social characteristics manifest, too, including negative self-concept, diminished self-esteem, misperceptions and confusion about "right" and "wrong," a sense of hopelessness, constricted affect, and deficits in empathy, as well as manipulation of others, blaming of others, nonsexualized boundary difficulties, and problematical peer interactions (Hall et al., 2002; Pithers et al., 1998). Sexual behavior problems are significantly more likely to occur among abused children who were sexually aroused during an abusive episode and who were subjected to perpetrator sadism as well as physical and emotional abuse (Hall et al., 1998).

A number of factors may contribute to a children's sexual behavior problems in response to CSA. These children, when compared to abused peers without sexual behavior problems, are more likely to have abuse histories characterized by multiple forms of abuse, abuse of longer duration, more severe abuse, and the perpetrator's use of sadism coupled with the experience of sexual arousal. In terms of micro or family dynamics, children with sexual behavior problems are significantly more likely to have a permanently absent father, a mother who experiences chronic stress, and numerous boundary violations within the family (Hall et al., 1998).

Self-system factors may help prevent a boy from reiterating the abuse cycle. For example, abused males that do not perpetuate the abuse cycle, when compared to abused males who have abused others, are significantly less likely to have experienced unqualified pleasure during the abuse and less likely to have fantasized about and/or masturbated while reflecting on the abuse (Lambie et al., 2002). The degree of risk associated with abuse transmission may be mitigated or augmented by the presence or absence of environmental experiences independent of sexual abuse history. Facilitative factors with majority representation include witnessing and/or experiencing domestic violence, rejection by family members, loss of a parental figure, and discontinuity of care (Ryan et al., 1996; Skuse et al., 1998).

Still, the degree to which a history of CSA influences one's perpetration against children remains unknown. The empirical knowledge base, at this point in time, cannot endorse a strong or consistent association between a history of CSA and sexual perpetration against children. The evidence does suggest that while most sexual abuse perpetrators have not been subjected to CSA, the experience of CSA may be one of multiple risk factors in the perpetration against children.

Sexual Abuse Effects Upon the Brain

To be sure, subjection to CSA alters the development of SAM's brain in a number of ways (Teicher et al., 1993), particularly in terms of left-hemispheric abnormalities, hemispheric connectivity, and hemispheric asymmetry. Children and adolescents with histories of CSA evidence asymmetric brain abnormalities, including smaller brain volume in the corpus callosum, a substructure connecting the two hemispheres of the brain responsible for communication between them (De Bellis, 2001; Teicher, 1997, 2000). Reciprocal collaboration of the right and left hemispheres is essential; altered development in this area may prevent the consolidation of traumatic memories and, accordingly, contribute to the preservation of the traumatic state (Bremner, 2002). Due to this lack of hemispheric cooperation and, consequently, symmetrical functioning, memories of CSA may be preferentially stored in the right hemisphere, thereby accounting for both emotional intrusiveness and constrictivity (Rauch et al., 1996; Schiffer, Teicher, & Papanicolaou, 1995). Therefore, left-hemispheric abnormalities in SAM are likely to promote a greater dependence on the right hemisphere (Ito et al., 1993). Further, subjection to CSA, as well as chronic experiences of invalidation, promotes the overpruning or the destruction of synapses within the right orbitofrontal cortex, which, in turn, leaves SAM with difficulties in the regulation of emotion in response to subsequent stress (Schore, 2001). In general, males tend to have smaller corpus callosum areas than females (Allen, Richey, Chai, & Gorski, 1991; de Lacoste, Adesanya, & Woodward, 1990); however, in addition to that, males with histories of CSA evidence more deleterious brain effects, secondary to CSA, than females (De Bellis et al., 1999).

In terms of the memory processes, the left prefrontal cortex holds a key role in autobiographical encoding whereas the right prefrontal cortex is fundamental to autobiographical retrieval (Tulving & Craik, 2000). Authentic narratives, or, in this context, verbal expressions of CSA, that integrate the linear facts with the contextual meanings necessitate the cooperation of and flow between the left and right hemispheres (Bremner et al., 1999; Siegel, 2001). Additionally, abnormalities in hippocampal functioning, resulting from protracted stress, mutate the formation of and interrelationships within SAM's brain, leaving as a consequence potential impediments to his explicit memory and narrative recall. Thus, although emotionally charged memories of CSA are indelible (LeDoux, 1992), albeit distorted and fractionated (van der Kolk, Burbridge, & Suzuki, 1997), they may not be able to be placed in space and time (Bremner & Narayan, 1998). Consequently, limbic system abnormalities obstruct the dynamics and effects of the sexually abusive experience from integrating into a cohesive mnemonic and, moreover, from progressively metabolizing into SAM's history as a relatively neutralized event (van der Kolk, McFarlane, & Weisaeth, 1996).

The left hemisphere is the primary domain of language. Three substructures in particular are germane to the experience and narration of SAM's history of CSA. The angular gyrus is responsible for the idiosyncratic meanings imbuing SAM's subjection to CSA as well as its effects. Broca's area, located in the frontal lobe, is accountable for the expression of language, namely, talking and writing. Wernicke's area, a region of the parietal lobe, is largely liable for language comprehension. All three areas are vital to SAM's imbuing the facts of his CSA history with meaning and communicating his story. Abnormalities, found within the left hemisphere, promote the displacement of cortical activity to the right hemisphere (Ito et al., 1993; Schiffer et al., 1995), advancing the likelihood of emotional intrusion, or the experience of surging affect.

Thus, what could be a harmonic narrative remains a discordant story, indisposed to words, as the fractionated shards of the sexually abusive experience emerge randomly, isolated and out of context. Under these circumstances, SAM's memories of CSA persist with little or no semantic translation, stealthily organized within sensory, somatic, emotional, motoric, and behavioral systems (Rauch et al., 1996), memories in search of a context, a context in search of its facts, facts in search of their meaning, a story in search of an author, and an author in search of his voice. Interestingly, when a fractionated shard emerges, perhaps through a flashback, body memory, or by way of emotional flooding, SAM exhibits an increased activation of the right hemisphere. Simultaneously, he may evidence a notable decline of cerebral blood flow to the left cortical regions as well as Broca's area, a substructure that, when impacted, inhibits the translation of personal life events into speech. In essence, the amygdala overacts, the hippocampus overloads, and the Broca's area does not let a word escape. For this reason, SAM may understand more than he can say. He knows the words, he simply can not speak them aloud (Rauch et al., 1996; van der Kolk & Fisler, 1995).

Damage to the amygdala and hippocampus may also contribute to problems around bilateral hemispheric interaction and connectivity. In response to the immediate stress of CSA or, for that matter, to stimuli subsequently conditioned as a result of CSA, SAM frequently produces excessive levels of endogenous opioids. This neurochemical action may ultimately have an inhibitory impact upon the amygdala's ability to assess the emotional valence of a stimuli and transmit signals to the hippocampus, thereby interrupting memory consolidation and storage (McGaugh, 1992). As for the hippocampus, even though it has the capacity to regenerate neurons, acute or protracted stress holds the potential to diminish such nerve cell regenerativity (Sass et al., 1990). In basic terms, the neurotoxicity of hypercortisolemic states engender damage to the hippocampus (De Bellis & Putnam, 1994). For example, adults with histories of CSA evidence a 12% reduction in the size of the left-hemispheric hippocampi; decreases in volume appear to be a function of abuse duration, with longer duration rendering greater reduction (Bremner et al., 1997). However, what remains inconclusive at this point in time are the temporal and linear dimensions. Is smaller hippocampal volume a function of sexual trauma and, as such, a sexual abuse effect? Or, does a smaller hippocampal volume predispose one to a protracted stress response, thereby making it a dynamic (Southwick et al., 1998; Teicher et al., 1997; van der Kolk et al., 1996)? These, and many other questions, are currently under investigation.

Finally, prolonged stress in the form of frequent secretory doses of catecholamines and coritcosteroids may hyperactivate the amygdala and atrophize the hippocampus (Bremner et al., 1999; Joseph, 1999). These detrimental effects may be functions of the accelerated metabolic loss of neurons, delays in myelination, dysfunction in the neuronal pruning process or through the inhibition of neurogenesis (De Bellis, 2001). Indeed, as so aptly stated, "While experience [such as childhood sexual abuse] may alter the behavior of an adult, experience literally provides the organizing framework for an infant or child" (Perry et al., 1995, p. 272).

DEFENSES AND THE COMPENSATORY SELF

When a boy confronts childhood trauma, a certain coping pattern emerges. CSA fractionates the self; defenses maintain this fractionation. While defense strategies help SAM to allege some semblance of functionality, they exact a high price from him in doing so. Defenses distort reality; they manipulate the memories; they sever SAM's truth and they tell him lies. Defenses create an illusion.

The illusion, then, becomes an ever-present way of coping with life. It, in combination with SAM's altered perceptions of self, others, and the world in relation to CSA, form a newly constructed sense of self. This new self, or compensatory self, not only perceives the world as being a different place, but also perceives one's role and the roles of others as being altered, too. Thus, all of SAM's expectancies regarding how to interact with the environment are transformed to match this new reality. For example, Palo stated: "In my father's and uncles' eyes, I knew I was like a wounded animal. I was no longer a man. From the moment I was abused, I felt changed. I could never look at another man and feel like I was his brother. I could never look at a female without feeling castrated somehow. I felt like everyone knew my secret. I was afraid to be with men. I didn't want them thinking that I thought I was good enough to be in their company. The same thing with women. I didn't want them thinking that I thought I was good enough to be with them. Everyone would see me as a failure—a wounded animal—so in my mind I guess I just psychologically castrated myself. I didn't know what else to do. As long as I could fade into the background, no threat to anyone, I was okay." And Victor revealed: "When I made it to the majors, I fiercely programmed myself to be the man of all men. I was always monitoring the way I talked, the way I walked, the way I hit the ball. I made sure I had women in my hotel room for out of town games. I fought with umpires, got in the face of some of the players, just to prove—not to prove, just to keep anyone from suspecting anything about my past. I told so many lies that it was hard to remember the truth."

Boys typically create a line of demarcation between the self that was, or is, abused, and the compensatory self. In order to maintain the compensatory self, SAM must defend against any message or messenger that may threaten this new structure. And there can be great disparity between the authentic and the compensatory selves; the former is genuine, grounded in reality; the latter is imitative, arising from mythology. Unfortunately, the compensatory self receives more attention, corroboration, and substantiation than the abused self.

Validation of a negative self-concept is just as compelling as the validation for a positive sense of self and a safe place in this world. Since SAM rarely finds validation for the abuse in the social environment, he must create a life space in which the internal matches the external. Ty stated: "People was calling me 'whore' and 'faggot' and 'cocksucker' before the abuse but then even more after. Round about that time, the time of Rodney and the abuse, my Mama told me not to call her 'Mama' anymore. She didn't want me calling her that 'cause she found blood in my drawers and she knew what was up and that I couldn't be her son anymore. Said she didn't know what I was. Said I was a fraud as a boy. She beat me so hard with the toilet plunger and a pipe. I didn't know what to do so I tried to give her what she wanted. I tried to be her daughter." Validation—compromise with great cost. Indeed, SAM lives in a world wherein truth—the truth about the sexual abuse of males—is a refugee.

THE CYCLE CONTINUES

> God will punish me if I lie. Mama will punish me if I tell the truth. Sometimes I feel like a ping-pong ball. (Nicholas, interview with author, February 2, 1992)

By this stage, the boy has lived and learned the milieu of abuse. He has experienced oppression and violation; he has learned that the world is a dangerous and frightening place in which to live. He is raging at himself, his God, at anyone who would allow such abuse to occur. Perhaps others are watching in silence, choosing to minimize, if not deny, his plight. He hears of this happening to girls, but not to boys. He feels exposed, as if everyone knows about the abuse but is refusing to do anything about it. A body, once his, is now host for and harbor of the perpetrator. He has no position, no voice, no experiential foundation from which to battle the intraspsychic, biologic, interpersonal, familial, and social forces and, at the same time, continue to develop a personality, a dream, a life uncorrupted by the dynamics and effects of childhood sexual abuse.

Still, the effects emerge. The intrusive effects—the reexperiencing of aspects of CSA—can traject so suddenly, as if from nowhere, impelling a sense of disintegration within the self, a sense of detachment from the current microenvironment, and in some cases both. Asking "why" is all too overwhelming. And for some, there's amnesia.

Amnesia

Sexual trauma can be conceptualized by type (Terr, 1991). Type I traumas with respect to CSA tend to involve one unanticipated episode, whereas Type II traumas tend to be chronic in nature. Both types, by virtue of their dynamic differences, give rise to different coping strategies and different effects. Characteristically, Type I traumas promote efforts, on the part of SAM, toward the construction of a rationale for the abuse and explanations as to how it could have been prevented as well as some minor misperceptions, perhaps in terms of timing and peripheral particulars. Nevertheless, they yield full, detailed memories of the sexually abusive episode. By contrast, Type II traumas evoke, within SAM, monumental efforts with an aim of shielding the self from psychological conflict, physical pain, and interpersonal distress by means of ego defense strategies such as denial, dissociation, introjection, and projection and by way of psychobiological maneuvers such as stress-induced analgesia and altered states of trance. In Type I traumas, the consciously expressed facts and meanings of the experience tend to come forth in parallel; with Type II traumas, memories tend to fractionate into shards of the experience, as horror, rage, sadness, and fear surface independently and out of context. With the latter, as well as crossover traumas, or massively intense albeit singular episodes of CSA, the chronicity of psychological and biological effects engendered by defensive coping holds the capacity to obstruct the developmental course, induce permeating characterological changes within SAM, and impede the process of memory and narrativization.

Autobiographical memory revolves around an axis of data and experience associated with the self (Wheeler et al., 1997). This memory system encompasses an information base of perceptual and sensory data as well as reflections about such data. They "may be accurate without being literal and may represent the personal meaning of an event at the expense of [complete] accuracy" (Conway, 1992, p. 9). If memory is impacted by CSA, it will be of the autobiographical kind (Siegel, 2001).

Amnesia and delayed recall transpire across a number of traumatic events, but significantly more so for experiences involving interpersonal maltreatment (Elliott, 1997). Traumatic events, such as subjection to CSA, generate "intense fear, helplessness or horror" (American Psychiatric Association, 1994, pp. 427–428). Fear, helplessness, and horror are three of the most common feeling states reported by boys and adolescent and adult males with histories of CSA, both at the time of the abuse and long thereafter (see, e.g., Brown & Anderson, 1991; Burgess et al., 1984, 1987; Hibbard et al., 1990; Janus et al., 1987; Lisak, 1994a; Mendel, 1995; Pescosolido, 1989; Rew et al., 1991; Spiegel, 1995). After cessation of the abuse, or perhaps intermittently through the years of chronic abuse, SAM may vacillate somewhere between the poles of hyperamnesia, or virtual retention, and full amnesia, or virtual disremembering (Courtois, 1999; Terr, 1991; van der Kolk et al., 1997).

When the emotionality generated by SAM's subjection to CSA "reaches the point of being traumatic in intensity . . . in a certain subpopulation of individuals, material that is too intense may not be able to be consciously processed and so may become unconscious and amnesic." Further, "this incomplete processing of emotional and cognitive material may quite possibly be associated with dose-related effects of trauma . . . and may be positively correlated with the use of dissociative or repressive defenses resulting in amnesia for the traumatic event" (Brown et al., 1998, p. 97). The key indicator of dissociative amnesia is SAM's inability to partially or fully recall his history of CSA (Kaplan & Sadock, 1999). Although there are only pockets of consensus regarding the mechanisms by which SAM "forgets," three distinct but theoretically converging pathways emerge to the foreground, one within the brain, another within the mind, and another still within the microenvironments of childhood sexual abuse.

Disremembering and the Brain

Within the brain, the amygdala, hippocampus, and surrounding cortex are implicated in trauma-related problems with memory (van der Kolk et al., 1997). For example, a single expulsion of stress-induced neurohormonal activity tends to enhance memory. However, given the protracted nature of CSA, and ceaseless and untold fears around a recurring episode, SAM's brain may be intermittently and vigorously steeped in chemicals, resulting in the suppression of hippocampal functioning (Bremner et al., 1999), thereupon producing memories, conscious or unconscious, absent of localization in space and time. Without a spatial or temporal context, memories cannot become autobiographical (LeDoux, 1992); rather, they remain wordless, free-floating, and with the capacity to materialize sensorially without apparent reason.

In addition to neurohormonal stress-induced shifts, another mediating factor may constrain the hippocampus from processing explicit memory, namely, divided attention. While in the midst of a sexually abusive episode, feeling threatened, fearful, and insecure, SAM may also experience a constriction of consciousness wherein only certain central sensory details come to the fore (Christianson, 1992). He may adjust his vision to blur the perpetrating activities, riveting his attention to seemingly benign aspects of the environment or, perhaps, turning his attention inward so as to escape. Exemplifying the former, Matt stated, "I couldn't escape her physically, my mother, but I kept counting the slats in the wood paneling of her bedroom. If I messed up, I would start all over again. I messed up a lot." Illustrating the latter, Nicholas reported: "Elmo say the 'magination is good. Preacher Mike say God lives in my heart and my 'magination. I'm glad Big Bird lives in my 'magination. He don't fly on TV, but when Terry—when he put that big snake in my bum, Big Bird flies and he takes me with him. My 'magination is good. Just like God. Just like peanut butter."

As much as dissociative strategies facilitate coping in the moment, in the absence of focal attention, the myriad of elements comprising the sexually abusive experience may not be encoded explicitly, semantically, or episodically, but rather implicitly. Thus, somatically palpable and sensorially resonant aspects of the experience are etched ardently in SAM's memory, in contrast with the fact that the attendant conditions of time and place register more weakly (Herman, 1992). Consequently, SAM may temporarily lose the capacity to piece together the associative linkages necessary for efficient recall and narrativization (Siegel, 2001). More often than not, he is left in a state of deafening silence—without words to describe such a life-defining event. Although he may not possess the words or the wherewithal at that moment in time to speak, let alone provide for himself or any willing listener a chronicle of events, SAM's exposure to CSA will not thwart the emergence of his implicit memories or the memory system responsible for conditioned emotional responses, sensorimotor sensations, and learned unconscious behaviors emanating from a sexually abusive episode (van der Kolk, 1994). However, his explicit memory may be impaired for that certain episode or for any of its contextual details (Siegel, 1999). In other words, he "may 'know' the emotional valence" of the sexually abusive experience, cognizant of his perceptions and sensations, "without being able to articulate the reasons for feeling or behaving in a particular way" (van der Kolk & Fisler, 1995, p. 511). Under these conditions, divided attention and perception may, at some point along the course of memory from attention to long-term storage and retrieval, yield fractionated or disoriented memories (Chu et al., 1996).

Additionally, in spite of their indelible burn within the amygdala (LeDoux, 1992), memories of CSA may be laid down in a fragmentary fashion within the cortex. The fear-laden unconscious memories allied with CSA tend to be stored within the amygdala. However, the cortical region, responsible for interpreting sensory information and mediating the acts of analyzing, reflecting problem solving, and remembering, also tends to suppress activation of the amygdala. This activation/suppression dynamic, on the one hand, produces memories that defy willful recall, yet, on the other hand, these very memories hold the capacity to emerge in a seemingly haphazard manner, particularly when SAM's defenses relent (Bremner, 2002).

Disremembering and the Mind

Within the mind, the action and efficacy of ego defense mechanisms may promote partial or full amnesia upon SAM's exposure to, or even after the termination of, CSA (Terr, 1994). Dissociation and dissociative amnesia appear to be the most common process and outcome associated with the presence or absence of traumatic memories (Briere & Conte, 1993; Chu et al., 1996; Siegel, 1996). Dissociative defense strategies help a child to disengage from stimuli in the microenvironment by internally partitioning and secluding traumatic or overwhelming facts and meanings emanating from the external event (Putnam, 1995). Abuse-generated trauma seemingly ameliorates through dissociative alterations in perceptions (i.e., depersonalization and derealization), alterations in memory (e.g., psychogenic amnesia), or alterations in perceptions and memory, historically and currently, whereby the former self is supplanted by a number of altering states (e.g., dissociative identity disorder) (Chu & Dill, 1990). Dissociation can occur between categories of mental events, for example, good and bad experiences with the same object, between certain events and their affective representation, between events and the meaning of those events, and perhaps even between events and the words that symbolically represent them (Davies & Frawley, 1994). Thus, dissociation, as a spontaneous, primordial countercharge to CSA, entails alterations within and shifts between states of consciousness during the abusive episode and during recollections of it as well (Lewis, Yeager, Swica, Pincas, & Lewis, 1994).

In terms of memory, dissociation can also sever explicit from implicit processing ,thereby lacerating autobiographical memory from any number of elements associated with the sexually abusive experience (Siegel, 1999). For example, dissociation transpires along three stages. Peridissociation occurs during the sexually abusive episode. Primary dissociation involves the unmindful and voluntary segregation of the memory of CSA from consciousness. Secondary dissociation entails the dissection of the abuse memory into disunited entities. In other words, CSA memories fractionate into behavioral, affective, somato-sensory, and knowledge (BASK model of dissociation; Braun & Sachs, 1985) shards of the abuse experience, free-floating with no verbal or declarative memory. Implicit or nondeclarative memory, however, remains unbroken. Apparently, "verbal memories require conscious awareness, but behavioral memories do not" (Terr, 1988, p. 103). In service of survival, dissociation essentially disjoins SAM's conscious facts of CSA from their unconscious biopsychosocial meanings, that is, content from affect (Christianson, 1992). Thus, dissociation may be a facilitating factor in the emergence of partial or complete amnesia for memories generated within and as a result of the sexually abusive experience.

Disremembering and the Social Environment

Within the social context of abuse, an early age of onset, the perpetrator's use of force and violence, perpetrator threats, SAM's experience of penetration, abuse chronicity, subsequent abuse by other perpetrators, and distress about the abuse correlate with partial or complete amnesia (see, e.g., Briere & Conte, 1993; Elliott, 1997; Elliott & Briere, 1995; Feldman-Summers & Pope, 1994; Grassian & Holtzen, 1996). From a social standpoint, concealment factors must be addressed as well. It is likely that SAM will refrain from disclosing the abuse for a number of reasons, including, but not limited to, his fear of being perceived as gay, effeminate, deviant, or a young man on the fast track to perpetration. Further, guilt for experiencing pleasure, shame for failing to prevent the abuse from occurring, fear of rejection by family, peers, and "society," and fear of losing an attachment calculate prominently in the concealment process (see, e.g., Bagley et al., 1994; Carballo-Dieguez & Dolezal, 1995; Gordon, 1990; Sebold, 1987; Sorenson & Snow, 1991; Spiegel, 1997; Woods & Dean, 1985). For these and many other reasons, SAM does not talk.

"Memory talk," or the discussions that occur between children and their caretakers before, during, and after a particular life experience, expedite the organization, integration, and recall of the generated memory (Bauer et al., 1998). Because the vast majority of males with histories of CSA do not disclose as children, SAM, as a boy and as a man, may be denied a vital opportunity to integrate this experience into his narrative history, left only with the vacillating and unprocessed fractionated shards of memory with their potent ability to evoke heightened states of arousal (Fivush, 1998). Sadly, if children are not presented with opportunities to engage in the verbal expression of their abuse histories, independent of their interactions with perpetrators, their memories of the abuse may lack the qualities typically found in recollections of concurrent events that are openly communicated with and validated by caring others (Fivush & Schwarzmueller, 1995). Further, it is not uncommon for adults with histories of CSA to consciously experience fractions of the abusive episodes. However, they simultaneously find themselves ineffective as they strive to narrativize the dynamics and effects, despite their attempts. Already lacking localization in space and time, SAM's traumatic memories emerge in sensorimotor form and therefore cannot be easily translated into the symbolic language necessary for linguistic retrieval (van der Kolk et al., 1997). Like a boat without an anchor, he cannot secure his story of abuse into an autobiographical context.

Continuous Memory and Amnesia

It must be noted that the majority of individuals with histories of CSA acknowledge having continuous memories of the abusive experience and only a minority of individuals with histories of CSA report amnesia for at least one segment of their lives. All in all, two-thirds of individuals with histories of CSA retain continuous and uninterrupted memories of their abuse experience whereas approximately one-fifth manifest full amnesia for their abusive episodes (Elliott & Briere, 1995; Elliott & Fox, 1994; Epstein & Bottoms, 1998; Feldman-Summers & Pope, 1994; Grassian & Holtzen, 1996; Melchert, 1996; Polusny & Follette, 1996; Widom & Morris, 1997). Further, the rate of forgetting among males tends to be lower than that of females (e.g., Epstein & Bottoms, 1998; Grassian & Holtzen, 1996; Melchert, 1996). Perhaps CSA and amnesia are best understood not as a bivariate causal relationship but rather as multivariate, multistaged phenomena, functioning within a network of biological, psychological, relational, and social factors as well as idiosyncratic and universal dynamics, coping strategies, and effects that, as contextual factors of the sexually abusive experience, impinge on each other in a manner that produces a continuum of remembering and forgetting.

Additionally, the "memory for events of impact show a very high accuracy rate over time in terms of total amount of information recalled and in terms of memory for central actions" (Brown et al., 1998, p. 147). Further, the essence of a child's memory of CSA is, as a general rule, factual; however, the specific details may be distorted. Developmentally, visual memory precedes behavioral memory; behavioral memory foreruns verbal memory. Behavioral memories appear early, accurately reflect what happened to the child, and continue indefinitely. Unlike verbal or narrative recall, behavioral memories do not necessitate conscious awareness (Terr, 1988). After the onset of CSA, visual memories activate behavioral reenactments of the abuse. These behaviors trigger additional visual images. Both visual memory and behavioral memory are enduring.

Recall

Strategies intended to protect and preserve SAM from an onslaught of abuse-related facts and meanings—intrapsychic dissociation, cognitive avoidance, emotional suppression, and behavioral elusion—yield an ample defense when they diminish his susceptibility and reactivity to congruous triggers across micro-environments that hold the capacity to summon forth the original memory traces. "However, when recognition cues are sufficient in number, intensity or meaningfulness, they may overwhelm existing avoidance defenses, resulting in the emergence of previously unavailable memories" (Elliott, 1997, p. 812).

Three patterns of CSA recollections emerge to the foreground. The first involves relatively continuous recall of facts in tandem with evolving but delayed meanings. The second pattern exhibits partial amnesia followed by an amalgamation of delayed recall and delayed meanings. The third pattern of CSA recollection encompasses a span of complete amnesia followed by delayed recall of facts and meanings (Harvey & Herman, 1994). Regardless of pattern, continuous or delayed, it is likely that fractionated sensory, affective, and motoric aspects of the sexually abusive experience will emerge as the introductory mode of awareness (van der Kolk & Fisler, 1995). As the shards ascend into consciousness, sensory modalities begin to integrate, and a narrative memory begins to materialize.

In general, the most commonly reported triggers associated with delayed recall of childhood sexual abuse include watching a television show or movie focusing on CSA, a contemporaneous event reminiscent of a historic abuse episode, and biopsychosocial crises. Participation in therapy represents the least commonly reported cue (Brown et al., 1998). Regarding the qualitative differences between the patterns, particularly the first and second, explicit statements denoting fear, terror, and shame are more likely associated with the emergence of delayed recall, whereas sadness, depression, and a sense of loss tend to imbue continuous recollections (Dalenberg, 1996). Further, SAM is likely to experience upon recall state-dependent elements affiliated with the abusive episodes, including the psychobiologies of hyperarousal and dissociation, schemas around masculinity, sexuality, abuse, and blame, and feelings of guilt, shame, fear, and rage. Whether memories are continuous or delayed, intrusion and numbing tend to prevail (Burgess et al., 1995; Elliott & Fox, 1994; Grassian & Holtzen, 1996; Horowitz, 2001; van der Kolk & Fisler, 1995).

The Oscillation of Intrusion and Numbing

Intrusive phenomena seek expression, as they hold the facts and meanings of the sexually abusive experience; numbing phenomena seek expression, as they hold self-preservative intentions to deny, invalidate, and escape the facts and meanings of the sexually abusive experience. At times intersecting, and at times spliced with a periods of relative reprieve from both, these surface and submerge with distinct changes in diametrical phases (van der Kolk, 1989).

How one phase begins as another ends varies from individual to individual. Form is constant; content and recurrency are variable. In other words, while many males with histories of CSA experience the oscillating processes of intrusion and numbing, how they do so varies across the domains of cognition, affect, and action. Thus, sequences of intrusive thoughts, images, and ruminations, along with chaotic emotions and compulsive behaviors, change repeatedly with intermittent denial, dissociation, and any other idiosyncratic actions that are repelling, avoiding, and blocking unwanted manifestations of the abusive experience (Horowitz, 2001; van der Kolk, 1987).

Intrusion and numbing. Phasing in and phasing out. SAM oscillates between extremes of invalidation and compensation, from depersonalization and derealization to a sense of neutrality. Caught in a bout of panic and agitation, he soon finds himself with a loss of reactivity. In the morning he may be internalizing the abuse, going to school with feelings of shame, guilt, and emasculation; that evening, he may be externalizing the abuse, by way of injuring his penis or reenacting an abuse dynamic. While dating, and perhaps in response to a confusing comment from his partner, SAM may leap from blind trust to gross mistrust. Disallowing himself opportunities for intimacy yet wanting to be held and touched, SAM, upon experiencing a kiss, may find that he is at once repelled by the affection. Now quite accustomed to self-deprivation, such lack propels SAM to compulsively seek immediate gratification, perhaps of any kind.

Through trial and error, SAM soon learns that some actions ignite the oscillation process, complete an unwanted phase of it, or jolt him from one phase to the other. Some actions involve self-injury and self-mutilation, with the penis as a familiar target of attack. Others compulsions include drinking, drugging, gambling, sexually acting out, checking the body for signs and symptoms, and inspecting the house for leaky faucets, loose plugs, and the on and off switches of stoves, stereos, clocks, and computers.

Equilibrium is usually hard-found. Moving from one phase to another, from extreme to extreme, often without a sense of why or wherefore, SAM's feelings of bewilderment, mistrust, confusion, helplessness, and fear marshal on. As an initial effect, intrusion dominates the biphasic momentum. Over time, numbing tends to hold command (Herman, 1992). It is in a state of numbing or dissociation that reenactments are most likely to occur.

Reenactments

Reenactments are, in essence, natural strivings to re-create, with the intention of mastering, unresolved conflicts related to childhood trauma (Levy, 1998). Repetition compulsion is a means through which SAM attempts to come to terms with his traumatic memories and his role in what generated them. A reenactment, within the context of CSA, actualizes, through the unconscious, a means to remember, understand, communicate about, and integrate the abuse by reliving it (Pearlman & Saakvitne, 1995).

SAM reenacts the dynamics of the original trauma so that he may conquer the evocative dynamics and overcome any of the myriad of effects, initial and long-term, experienced over the course of his life (Levy, 1998). Helplessness, powerlessness, shame, and inferiority are universal effects in the face of trauma (Lisak & Luster, 1994). As a result, males with histories of CSA, including SAM, will spontaneously seek to reestablish control in order to rebuild a sense of efficacy, even to the point of reliving historic trauma through choices made in the present.

SAM, when he experiences a reenactment of CSA, does so without recognizing his participation in bringing it to fruition (Davies & Frawley, 1994). Although reenactments seem to evolve from conscious choice, they also appear to be involuntary (Herman, 1992). For example, the choice to engage in a sexual encounter may be conscious; the impetus for doing so is most likely unconscious. Consequently, SAM has a difficult time perceiving the relationship between the current incident and his history of CSA. In fact, SAM often views these iterations in behavior and their generated effects as a function of bad timing, bad luck, bad karma, or bad fate, rather than as a function of his own doing. Even though reenactments seem to occur unexpectedly and appear to be unrelated to the abuse, they could not manifest if awareness of the stimulus/response was conscious and clear (van der Kolk, 1989). Matt stated: "My life revolved around acting out. I spent years chasing the feeling I would get from acting out—almost euphoria. But that wasn't always the case. That good feeling happened in the beginning but faded over time yet that didn't stop me. The shame and guilt after acting out didn't stop me. Getting arrested several times couldn't stop me, either. It never occurred to me that the incest with my mother was driving the car. I just thought I was a pervert, sick. It's hard to not think of myself that way now."

As with all life energies, the reenactments are moves toward wholeness, toward creation, and away from destruction, away from fractionation. They involve a process of undoing time, unraveling the subjected dynamics and releasing the unresolved and unsettled effects. However, given the dynamics often replicated—subjection, harassment, aggression, physical violations, sadism, enforced concealment—and the effects reexperienced—shame, emasculation, humiliation, betrayal, rage, fear, powerlessness—the reenactment can be as dangerous and disruptive as the original abuse, if not more so (Levy, 1998).

Thus, reenactments, in this context, are unconscious, seemingly involuntary, persistent, and purposeful. They are, in essence, self-inflicted, allowing SAM an opportunity to transform his history of sexual trauma from passive to active, by controlling the timing, pace, and severity of his self-directed abuse and, paradoxically, generating a sense of power and mastery (Davies & Frawley, 1994). Still, the reenactment of CSA dynamics necessitates, by definition, the entry into high-risk situations mirroring the abuse, which, by their very nature, not only can reproduce the historic abuse but can generate it currently as well. The anticipated outcome, or the guiding objective underlying the compulsion to reenact, is mastery and control. Accordingly, SAM may need to reexperience role confusion in order to regain role constancy, just as he may need to reexperience boundary diffusion so he may come to know boundary integrity. From a cause like this, SAM psychically seeks an emotional balm to heal the hidden wounds.

SAM is undoing the dynamics of his abuse experience and conquering the potency and power of its effects. He is healing from historic trauma and overcoming years of invalidation, reconciliation, and compensation. This is not psychopathology; this is saving one's own life. Although there is potential harm, there is hope, too.

From Fractionation to Integration

Sensitization, in general, pertains to the ways in which an individual learns about the properties of harmful or threatening stimuli (Squire & Kandel, 2000). Repeated exposure to a stimulus, internal or environmental, gives rise to a condition of continuously intensifying and widening magnitudes of response (Saxe & Wolfe, 1999). Sensitization, within the context of CSA, refers to the process by which SAM, given the continual subjection to stress, becomes urgently and immediately reactive, not only to the experience of abuse but also to its effects and to any person, place, or thing that might threaten his abilities to conceal and invalidate it. An intrusive thought, a sense of transparency, feelings of shame and guilt, a frightening nightmare with abusive overtones, going near the place where the abuse transpired, seeing someone with a characteristic similar to the perpetrator's, SAM's erection, washing his own body—anything and everything that reminds him, consciously or unconsciously, of the abuse—activates a constellation of nervous system responses, so explosively, so abruptly, as if assailing SAM with a volcanic blow. It is difficult indeed to be aware of the stimulus when the response emerges so forcefully and with such rapidity.

The effects of the sensitized response parallel the effects of CSA; the fear of recurrence, the fear of discovery, the fear of reactions of others; such inner tumult, products of CSA, and the CNS perpetuate psychological and physiological conflict and become yet another source of hyperarousal. Even when the abuse terminates, the anxiety, panic, and fear abide, erupting by way of SAM's overly sensitized stress response (LeDoux, 1994).

The oscillation process in not futile. The ego's self-preservation instincts hold an innate imperative toward mastery and competence. Although SAM's senses of agency and efficacy have been shattered by the sexually abusive experience, his will, his spirit, and his ego strive for adaptation, integration, and resolution. Just as SAM became sensitized, that is, reactive to his sexually abusive experience through the process of conditioned learning, so too can he unlearn, or become desensitized to, the dynamics and effects of CSA. Thus, sensitization is a reversible phenomenon (Weekes, 1976).

In this way, the oscillations between intrusion and numbing ultimately exemplify SAM's innate endeavor to integrate the abuse into his life story. This graduated, gradual, and controlled process involves:

1. The graduated and controlled exposure to abuse-related content with a delicate balance between approach and avoidance (Courtois, 1999).
2. Verbally encoding and translating implicit aspects of the abuse experience from the visual, sensorial, motoric, and behavioral systems of memory of CSA into words (Siegel, 1995).
3. A cumulative assimilation of the cognitively dissonant and intolerable facts and meanings associated with SAM's history of CSA (Horowitz, 2001).
4. A cumulative accommodation of the ego-dystonic and anxiety-inducing emotions imbuing the facts and meanings (Rachman, 1980; Citco in Briere, 1996a).
5. A stepwise desensitization of the facts and meanings, that is, the thoughts and feelings associated with SAM's history of CSA (Briere, 1996a).

As defenses relax, facts emerge. As facts emerge, meaning follows. As meanings affix, integration occurs. Conceptually, the authentic self, holding the authentic truth, fractionated and unprocessed as it may be, breaks through the imposed layers of abuse, concealment, invalidation, reconciliation, and compensation. This iterative process toward integration occurs slowly, and over time. Until then, however, males with histories of CSA withstand, brave, and defy a number of aftereffects, particularly in the areas of work and relationships.

AFTEREFFECTS IN THE DOMAINS
OF WORK AND RELATIONSHIPS

CSA is an act of violence. It obstructs the path of anticipated human development; it robs the young boy of his birthright to explore and discover his evolving sense of self in the arenas of school, work, and relationships. Typically, one learns to associate sexuality with love. For SAM, this constructive coupling was overthrown and replaced with the destructive fusion of sexuality and violence. This latter connection has undeniable and profound effects on the attitudes, values, and behaviors of males with histories of CSA. Following are common issues confronting SAM.

School Experiences

At the very time when peer groups prove most vital, SAM's fears of exposure and disclosure, of being viewed as deviant, gay, or as a perpetrator, inhibit social development and peer relations. His feeling rejected by family, friends, and acquaintances alike, in addition to his sense of inferiority around other males and his feelings of emasculation around females, often prevents him from forging potentially viable friendships.

    A constructive and nurturing school experience has the potential to buffer the negative effects of CSA by enhancing SAM's sense of self-esteem and self-worth and by promoting a sense of control over his destiny (Herrenkohl et al., 1994). Unfortunately, there are a number of palpable stumbling blocks. To begin, intrusive thoughts and states of hyperarousal make it difficult to focus, let alone learn (Pynoos, Steinberg, & Wraith, 1995; Pynoos, Steinberg, & Aronson, 1997). For SAM, school-related problems and difficulties might include attention deficits, cognitive deficits, a significant and abrupt decline in grades, behavioral problems, problems with teachers and school officials, withdrawal from school and extracurricular activities, delinquency, and truancy. Further, he is more likely than his nonabused peers to experience consequences such as placement into remedial or special education classes even with average or above-average intelligence scores, corporal punishment for misbehavior, the repetition of a grade or course, rejection by classmates, and suspension or expulsion from school (see, e.g., Adams-Tucker, 1985; Dubowitz et al., 1993; Eckenrode et al., 1993; Friedrich & Luecke, 1988; Friedrich et al., 1986; Hibbard et al., 1990; Janus et al., 1987; Lisak & Luster, 1994; Olson, 1990; Perez & Widom, 1994; Robin et al., 1997; Ryan et al., 2000; Straus & Smith, 1990).

    To compensate, SAM may strive to achieve first chair in the orchestra, first string on a sport's team, or first place in a student body election. Victor said: "If I wasn't on the top, Dean's list, MVP, student government president, I was nothing at all." Alternatively, SAM may say little, do little, just white-knuckling his way through. For him, attention of any kind feels like exposure. Palo reported: "I was afraid to raise my hand. I didn't want anyone looking at me. I didn't want to stutter and make things worse. Once, a teacher called my parents in, wondering why I participated so little and yet received the highest scores in the district on achievement tests. I took care of that real quick. The teachers after that were very confused but back then, confusion was safer than knowledge." Or, SAM may simply surrender to the social mythology, wherein he finds proof of his failure as a male. Ty stated: "Once I knew and saw that Mama and Grandmama and Rodney [his perpetrator] and practically everyone in school and church and the county thought of me as a mistake, I stopped trying to be good. I was always apologizing for this or that. One teacher even said to me, 'What is wrong with you? You apologize for the very breath you breathe.' I just gave up. I couldn't even be good at saying 'I'm sorry.'"

College Experiences and Vocational Training

SAM, as a late adolescent and young adult male, strives to complete normative developmental tasks, such as the maturation, differentiation and constancy of identity, and the formation of a personal life philosophy (Erikson, 1963), while simultaneously trying to conceal, invalidate, reconcile, and compensate for his stress responses, anxiety, panic attacks, depression, and dissociation, as well as other CSA effects. Feeling flawed, isolated, and fearful, it's easy to understand why SAM tries twice as hard to be half as good as the next person. Dreading further assaults against an already vulnerable sense of self, when faced with the stress inherent in academic pursuits, SAM may drop out, withdraw from classes, or change majors without much forethought (Lisak & Luster, 1994). When compared to nonabused adult males and abused females, SAM is significantly more likely to evidence lower IQ scores, a lower reading ability, a lower intellectual ability, and lower educational accomplishment (Perez & Widom, 1994). Over the years, these correlates of CSA hold the potential to progressively chip away at his senses of self-esteem, self-worth, and self-efficacy, all the while validating his internal sense of shame. Palo stated: "I knew I was the first one in my family to attend college, but I felt like I was disgracing such an honor because of my past."

Conversely, SAM may take on a double major and participate in numerous organizations, thereby creating a whirlwind of activity in which to hide and keep unwanted reminders of the abuse at bay. More often than not, SAM's drive toward overachievement is a function of his need to compensate for and conceal his history of CSA. Victor said: "College was tough for me. I had a baseball scholarship. In baseball, I knew how to be a man. In the classroom, I didn't know how a real man was supposed to act. So I played the role of a dumb jock except when it came to taking tests and doing homework. I wish I could do it all over again."

Career

Viewing the world in dualities—the abuser and the abused, good and bad, success and failure—SAM brings a fierce dichotomy into the world of work (Lew, 1990). As he tends to possess little, if any, internal value, social indicators of success shoulder great weight. Regardless of his rung on the status ladder, SAM's rationales for workplace success and workplace failure arise from the same place. More often than not, he rationalizes success as a function of luck, and failure as a function of just punishment, all the while fearing what others may discover about him.

Across a number of occupations and workplaces, males with histories of CSA earn approximately 14% less per hour than nonabused counterparts (Macmillan, 2000). In comparison to nonabused male colleagues, SAM in the workplace is more apt to anticipate failure, work compulsively, underachieve, hold a lower level position, experience conflicts with coworkers, supervisors, and administrators, generate an insufficient income, be terminated, and/or be unemployed (see, e.g., Bagley et al., 1994; Gill & Tutty, 1999; Janus et al., 1987; Lisak & Luster, 1994; Olson, 1990). Jake reported: "I'm not sure how I made it so far. I didn't make any choices when it came to career or advancement. I waited until something fell into my lap. I've never been on a job interview. I never bid for a higher position. I just clock in, follow the rules, do what I'm supposed to do and watch the clock. I got promoted—not because I tried to but because circumstances just turned out that way—people abruptly leaving positions, bosses desperately looking for a replacement." Matt said: "After the incest started, I saw sexuality everywhere. There was a big construction site across town. I would walk by after school and see women—well, mostly women but some men—stop and watch the construction workers. Over the months, I heard things like, 'Damn, Daddy, give me some of that' and 'If I could marry a man like that, I would be in heaven.' That's when I decided I would become a construction worker. I've been doing it for twelve years now. When I hear people talking about their life purpose, I just have to walk away." Finally, Ty asserted: "If I took all the hate and disgust I have for me and it got turned into love and belief in me, I would have initials behind my name: MSW [master of science in social work]. That's my dream. That's my dream."

SEXUALITY AND RELATIONSHIPS

Table 4.1 presents abuse effects associated with gender, sex, and sexuality. Subjection to childhood sexual abuse confounds the already complex process of developing a sexual and relational identity (Gilgun & Reiser, 1990). Boundary diffusion and role confusion, two dynamics intrinsic to CSA as well as two effects inherited by SAM, contrive and fortify his working models of interpersonal relationships. The perpetrator, the reactions of others, systemic responses

TABLE 4.1. EFFECTS ASSOCIATED WITH SEX, GENDER, AND SEXUALITY

IMAGE
- Suppressing sexuality
- Feeling like victim
- Feeling like perpetrator
- Shame and guilt about sexuality
- Feelings of sexual inadequacy
- Deliberate "male" presentation
- Deliberate "female" presentation
- Deliberate "androgynous" presentation
- Overemphasis on sexuality

PHYSICALITY
- Preoccupation with body/physique
- Self-mutilation
- Obsessive-compulsive about hygiene
- Distorted physical image
- Disregard for hygiene, appearance
- Eating disorders
- Discomfort with bodily elimination
- Detached from body
- Keeping body "boy" like
- Overweight to hide body
- Shame regarding genitals

CONFUSION
- Confusion regarding sexual orientation
- Confusion regarding gender identity
- Fantasy to be another male during sex
- Fantasy to be female during sex
- Teasing/accosting effeminate males

SEXUALIZATION
- Sexualize social relationships
- Flirtation/seduction to gain attention
- Sex to validate relationship
- Seduction without sex
- Misinterpretation of intimacy
- Sex for self-esteem

COMPULSIONS
- Compulsive masturbation
- Denying consequences of sex
- Sex with strangers
- Obsessing about sex
- Sex as a means to find love
- Desperate prior to acting out
- Despair after acting out
- Promiscuity
- Intoxification
- Dissociation during sex
- Emotional numbing
- Seeking "high" from sex
- Inflicting pain to numb body

FEARS
- Fear of sex
- Fear of intimacy
- Fear of rejection
- Fear of performance
- Fear of emasculation
- Fear of being dominated
- Fear of being passive
- Fear of sexual dysfunction
- Fear of intrusive thoughts
- Fear of losing control
- Fear of sexually abusing others
- Fear of the male gender
- Fear of the female gender

RELATIONAL DYNAMICS
- Mistrust of partner
- Idealization of partner
- Aversion to being touched
- Dependency
- Feeling obliged to have sex
- Abusive partners
- Passive partners
- Needs sex to feel loved

SEXUAL DYNAMICS
- Concurrent sexual relationships
- Successive sexual relationships
- Letting partner get sex from others
- Sexual activity outside orientation
- Using clubs, Internet, organizations for sex
- Humiliating/degrading sex
- Sexual role playing/ritualization
- Celibacy

REENACTMENTS
- Abusive fantasies
- Self-abusive behavior
- Receiving harm/pain
- Causing harm/pain
- Withholding sex
- Sexually exploitive of others

DYSFUNCTIONS
- Arousal dysfunctions
- Lack of sensation
- Premature ejaculation
- Erectile dysfunction
- Retarded ejaculation
- Sexual withdrawal
- Choking response
- Muscle spasms
- Involuntary responses

(or lack thereof) to abuse, disclosure, child protection, and perpetrator adjudication and, ultimately, social mythology generate a number of assumptions and propositions, including those reported by boys and adolescent males in sexual abuse treatment programs:

1. If someone cares about you, then they will betray you.
2. If someone touches you, then they want to have sex with you.
3. If you have sex, you must keep it a secret.
4. Sex hurts.
5. If people find out that you had sex, they will call you names.
6. If you do everything the adult wants you to do, you won't get hurt.
7. If you say "no," then you get punished.
8. If you're a failure as a boy, then you can try to be a girl, you can fake your way as a boy, or you can neuter yourself into nothing.
9. If all you're good for is sex, then you better not try to do anything else.
10. The world doesn't seem to look when boys are sexually abused and doesn't seem to listen when sexually abused boys cry.

These beliefs germinate within the context of CSA when SAM, at age 5, 9, or 13, is gathering data, based on experience, to guide and inform his view of the world. In the abuse context, they are seemingly logical deductions of the trauma, lessons learned about the self, others, love, care, affection, gender, sexuality, and SAM's life journey. However, in the context of caring others, such beliefs serve only to invalidate SAM's authentic truth and obstruct his path to success and contentment in personal development, love, and work. If SAM does not have the chance or ability to cognitively and experientially dispute these faulty assumptions as a boy, he is likely to incorporate them into his view of self, others, and the world. If, as a boy, he has little or no opportunity to ameliorate his feelings of guilt, shame, and self-blame regarding his role in the abuse, he may erroneously label himself as a misfit, gay, deviant, or any other label socially constructed to indicate a sexually abused male's subordinate status (Gill & Tutty, 1999). This can eventuate independent of the perpetrator's gender. It must be remembered that, at least in the United States, sexual abuse occurs and its effects emerge in a culture wherein all things gender-related are wholly divided (Cazenave, 1984; Duncan & Williams, 1998; Pollack, 1990). The childhood perceptions, traits, and states engendered by SAM's subjection to CSA not only shape the brain and fuse into his cognitive assumptions but eventually generalize across the various microenvironments of his life, actualizing as self-fulfilling prophecies.

The Development of a Sexual Self-Concept

As previously stated, when CSA is perpetrated by a female, SAM experiences anxiety and confusion regarding his sexual identity (Ruchkin, Eisemann, &

Hagglof, 1998). When sexually abused by male, the boy perceives himself as a participant in homosexual behavior (Dimock, 1988; Mendel, 1995), thereby rendering him gay (Finkelhor, 1986). Not surprisingly, gay males abused as boys believe their sexual orientation is an effect of the abuse; heterosexual males abused as boys believe that it's only a matter of time before they become gay (Lew, 1990). Kip, abused by a male, revealed: "I hate my penis. It got hard. Never thought about guys before then but, fuck man, when a man has sex with you—who cares if he's raping you—when a man has sex with you and you pop a woody, you are gay. It means nothing that I had a girl-friend, that I wanted to grow up and get married and be a Dad. I got hard. That means gay. Period." Matt, abused by a female, stated: "Deep down, I know I'm straight. But my mother taught me to hate sex. One time in therapy, I told this therapist that the very thought of a vagina gives me the dry heaves. He said, 'Why do you think you're so resistant to being gay?' I was stymied. I didn't know what to say. I remember thinking, 'The thought of a penis does nothing for me, it doesn't disgust me, it doesn't excite me. The thought of a vagina makes me sick. Maybe that does mean I'm gay. Maybe he's right."

The sexual penetration of males is socially condoned within a number of American subcultures and across a number of ethnicities (Blechner, 1998; Co-mas-Diaz, 1995); rather than viewed as homosexual activity (Groth & Burgess, 1980), sexual penetration ultimately validates the penetrator's power, man-hood, and masculinity (Donaldson, 1990, 1993). The sexual perpetration by females is glorified; viewed as heterosexual activity, it is normalized, even though the abused male feels confused, degraded, and shamed in the process.

Although it is the perpetrator, male or female, who sexually assaults SAM, it is his gender-dichotomized culture that commits a type of larceny, essentially "stealing" his personal property, namely, a sense of gender identity and per-sonal integrity. SAM's culture upholds the social mythology surrounding the sexual abuse of males. Judges, juries, parents, teachers, child protection work-ers, police officers, doctors, nurses, psychologists, and social workers—male and female—have been known to minimize, deny, or otherwise invalidate his experience (Davies, 1995; Isquith et al., 1993; Kenny, 2001; Lamb & Edgar-Smith, 1994; Mills, 1993; Spencer & Tan, 1999; Vullimay & Sullivan, 2000; Zellman, 1990). Their failure to act leaves him without services that could potentially ameliorate his abuse effects and, moreover, places him at risk for subsequent abuse (Faller, 1995; Schwartz, 1994; Stroud, 1999).

Upon disclosure, mothers of abused children perceive a number of per-sonality problems in their sons (Friedrich & Luecke, 1988). Fathers may ac-knowledge the abuse but punish the boy (Weihe, 1990). Female perpetrators are socially judged as relatively immune from responsibility (Back & Lips, 1998). Male perpetrators, despite the knowledge base, are socially constructed as strange, deviant, dirty old men (Spiegel, 1997). Professionals are more likely to ask a female about a history of CSA, more likely to believe a female's disclosure, and less likely to conceptualize a link between a male's biopsychosocial problems and a history of CSA and less likely to align with the male patient/client/witness by responding to his disclosure in a manner that invalidates his history of abuse (Holme et al., 1997; Lab et al., 2000). Perceiving the sexual abuse of males as critical and as generating negative effects may call into question the perceiver's sense of gender identity (Hunter, 1991; Smith et al., 1997). In general, the degree to which an observer perceives himself or herself as personally dissimilar to the child is the degree to which he or she will place responsibility on the child (Back & Lips, 1998).

SAM's role as a male child prior to the abuse and his role as sexually abused male during and after the abuse are, in part, a function of social expectations and labeling (Davis, 1986). Cultural norms, gender scripts, environmental circumstances, and personal experiences inform SAM as to who he is and who he can become (Duncan & Williams, 1988; Pollack, 1999). So, into his sense of identity he must incorporate a myriad of negative appraisals. For example, social mythology prescribes that, on the one hand, sexual abuse does not happen or should not happen to boys and, on the other hand, if it does, you are to blame, you must have wanted it, and, consequently, something is wrong with you. Perpetrators, throughout and after the sexually abusive relationship, and even some parents upon disclosure, punish, threaten, and denigrate SAM with a number of names—fag, queer, whore, she-boy, pervert, stud—all of which stigmatize him to the core and deepen his responsibility for the abuse. Ultimately, SAM's erection and, in many cases, ejaculation not only confuse him but often help him to confirm the perceptions and reactions of others, which, in turn, convinces him to conclude that something about him caused something unlawful, sinful, and immoral to happen.

As SAM transforms from boy to adolescent and from adolescent to adult male, he experiences the developmental milestones of puberty, first date, first love, going steady, school or college graduation, career selection, relational commitment, first sexual experience of choice, marriage, partnership, and so on. While he fulfills the developmental tasks of identity formation and consolidation, for example, or while he strives to trust and love another, SAM simultaneously conceals, invalidates, reconciles, and compensates for his sexual abuse history. And he endeavors to actualize both objectives—human development and human sacrifice—within the very culture that sustained the abusive relationship and its mythology. Jake stated: "I never tried dating. I always felt like I was going to be found out. My wife pursued me. I tried to get away many times, gave her many reasons to reject me. But she stayed. I didn't know what love was until I turned fifty, until I came to get help." Needless to say, CSA obstructs the process of developing a positive and life-affirming sense of self, sexual identity, and relational model.

Changes in a boy's self-concept during and following CSA are overwhelmingly negative (Adams-Tucker, 1985), as indicated by a loss in self-esteem, lack of self-confidence, and feelings of guilt and shame (Conte & Schuerman, 1987).

Prevalent concepts of self include that of "misfit," "outsider," "queer," "whore," "vulnerable boy," and "damaged male" (Dimock, 1988; Gill & Tutty, 1999; Janoff-Bulman, 1989; Spiegel, 1997a, 1997b). This internalized sense of disparagement, seeded by the perpetrator and fortified by social mythology and social responses, spawns a number of core beliefs such as "I am unacceptable," "My life is meaningless," and "I am unlovable," and a number of core feelings including inferiority, shame, and dishonorment (Lisak, 1994a).

As psychosexual development progresses, fears around body image and gender-related tasks and expectations increase and intensify (Sebold, 1987). Many adolescent males are ashamed of and frightened by the developmental processes and normative functioning that occur after the abuse (Pescosolido, 1989). Fear and shame in response to the growth and maturation of secondary sex characteristics and confusion between sexual orientation and gender identity are commonplace. Seemingly inescapable fear, shame, and confusion compensatively give rise to one adolescent male's projection of an aggressive masculine identity and another's strident efforts toward presenting a neutral or desexualized self (Richardson et al., 1993). By adulthood, negative self-concepts are the norm among adult males with histories of CSA (Mendel, 1995; Ray, 1996; Woods & Dean, 1985). By now, years of concealing the abuse all the while invalidating its effects, reconciling responsibility, and compensating for the social mythology surrounding it have propelled and overburdened SAM's self-concept and left him with an enduring sense of alienation from self, others, and life tasks, goals, and aspirations (Lisak, 1994a). Indeed, SAM is likely to encounter a number of relational challenges.

Sexualization

SAM may mistakenly perceive a relationship between emotional intimacy and sexual expression, acting as if one cannot occur without the other. For many, the brutality of sexual abuse was camouflaged by the pretense of intimacy. Intimacy became synonymous with seduction, coercion, power, and rage (Gartner, 1999). Consequently, intimacy can be more anxiety-provoking than sex. The fusion of sex and nurturing during the abusive episodes leaves SAM unable to differentiate where affection terminates and where abuse begins. Given the contradictions associated with sexual abuse, he often misinterprets feelings generated from interpersonal relationships. In other words, among adult men sexually abused as boys, there is a tendency to sexualize relationships and to experience difficulty in initiating and maintaining intimate relationships based on mutual support and trust (Dimock, 1988). For example, SAM may feel a fondness for a coworker or excitement over a budding friendship. Interpreting these feelings as sexual, he could eroticize the relationship. Many relationships are laced with sexual feelings, which may trigger inappropriate behavior and thus terminate what could have been a viable source of social support. Conversely, if someone communicates to SAM a sincere interest in pursuing the possibilities of a romantic relationship, fearing intimacy, he may abruptly and defensively do away with contact of any kind.

Matt stated: "Get close, but not too close. If you say you love me, I'll leave a trail of dust. If you act like you don't care, I'll stick around until you do." Palo revealed: "I do it every time, especially with men. It doesn't matter where I am or who I am with—the boss, the landlord, the mailman, or security guard. If a man, almost any man, if he is kind, caring, or even if he just pays a little bit of attention to me, I turn him into a dream partner. Common sense vanishes and I feel like a little boy. My fantasies or daydreams don't involve sex. It's strange. I'm straight. I've always been straight, but when I see an older man like that, something comes over me. I want to ask them questions. I want to be with them. It's almost like I want them to love me. I don't think of myself with them. I imagine them with a wife. I live vicariously through the wife. I envy what she has with him. Does that mean I'm gay?"

Power and Control

A sense of powerlessness is a common aftereffect for SAM (Lew, 1990). Female-perpetrated abuse often engenders, within the male, a sense of helplessness in anticipation of future encounters with women (Lisak, 1994a). Male-perpetrated abuse frequently incites a sense of emasculation, inferiority, and shame (Gill & Tutty, 1999; Hunter, 1991; Kellogg & Hoffman, 1995). Sadly, there is a tendency for some males abused as boys to become involved with other adults in relationships that mirror the abuse dynamics they experienced as children (Davies & Frawley, 1994; Dimock, 1988; Gartner, 1999). Essentially, the power disparity between SAM and his perpetrator in terms of role, status, authority, developmental capacities, psychological maturation, physicality, anatomy, and ability to reason, among others, can infiltrate his internalized models of relationship, incisively directing his interpersonal pursuits. SAM's premature and untimely initiation into sexuality was in the context of dominance and submission, subjugation, and servitude; consequently, his inroads to adult relationships may be unconsciously driven by attempts to reclaim and preserve power over and control of an intimate other (Gartner, 1999).

Even though SAM, as a boy, had no control over the perpetrator's behavior and was, indeed, powerless to prevent it, he may continue to claim responsibility. And if by way of dichotomous thinking or splitting SAM categorizes everyone as the "abuser" or the "abused," he, in unconsciously defending against feelings of powerlessness and inferiority, may take one of two primary routes. SAM may attempt to exert power and control over his interpersonal relationships, sometimes becoming violent (Duncan & Williams, 1998; Janus et al., 1987; Krug, 1989; Lisak & Luster, 1994). With anger and rage, two shades of only a few emotions socially allocated to males (Struve, 1990), SAM is able to feel personally robust and relationally powerful, given the psychobiology undergirding these emotional states. Oppositely, SAM may take on the role of the "abused" (Duncan & Williams, 1998; Olson, 1990). Desperate for love, but feeling desperately flawed and unlovable, he may find an all too willing partner to complete this two-dimensional dyad, confirming his socially imposed beliefs about the self—I am unworthy, unlovable, discardable, and worthless—and, in the process, confront the risk of further abuse and violence.

With trust of self and others a foreign commodity, a predominating relational pattern emerges; it typically begins with intense involvement, transitions to conflict and abrupt withdrawal, and ends with isolation from others, only to begin again (Dimock, 1988). The imposed association between intimacy and abuse engenders the anticipatory fear of both (Lisak, 1994a, 1994b). Indeed, adult males abused as boys experience difficulty in maintaining a sense of relational stability with significant others. Jake stated: "As a Marine, I fiercely intimidated young recruits in order to show my superiors that no one could get past such a tough man as myself. I intimidated my wife and children, too. Please understand. I didn't hit them or beat them. I just couldn't let them in. The Wizard of Oz hid behind a curtain. For most of my life, I hid behind my height, my weight, and my icy cold exterior. If I wasn't 6'4" and if I didn't weigh 250 pounds, I would have been more lost than I already was." Victor disclosed: "When Kevin and I first got together, after my divorce from Teresa, I had so much going on in my head. When we were friends, I felt fine. When I found myself wanting him, I felt queer. When he came on to me, I felt like a little kid. When I came on to him, I felt like I was a rapist. I was falling in love with the man and for the longest time I couldn't let him know. I couldn't allow myself to be vulnerable. I had to be the one in control. I had to be louder, stronger, tougher, and make him the opposite. That lasted until he showed me that I was treating him the way my father had treated me."

Risky Behaviors

SAM may use sex as a strategy to avoid emotionally intimate relationships (Gill & Tutty, 1999). Perhaps he views sex as his life mission; he's an expert at it, it pleases others, and, like the applause of an actor's audience, it brings him immediate verbal and nonverbal feedback. Sex, in SAM's psychological and sociological space, may be his greatest wellspring for self-esteem, self-worth, and self-efficacy. Matt stated: "Sex was the axis of my life. I rarely had physical sex. Most of my time was spent in getting someone to want me. When they said they did, it was over. I just needed to know that somebody wanted me. I wish I could go back today to each and every one and say 'I'm so sorry.'" Alternatively, SAM may consciously or unconsciously use sex as an implement of war in a battle waging toward his own demise. Permeated by shame, self-loathing, and rage—introjects of the perpetrator—he seeks to find the most dangerous situations, the most willing of partners, and the riskiest of activities to validate his hate. Palo revealed: "What can you say about a married man who was about to be a father, a man who had the most precious wife, a man trying to make it through law school, who had so much to live for, a man who almost ruined it all by going to truck stops and biker bars and sex clubs looking for men with guns and knives, men who were willing to penetrate me without a condom, who were willing to tie me up and hold a knife or gun to my face? What can I say? I want to understand. I want it to stop." Or, SAM, so desperate for love, searches far and wide—in the neighborhood, throughout the state, across the country, in bars, at church, on the Internet—for an idealized other, often tinged with attributes of the perpetrator but absent in the self. Ty revealed: "It was like this bottomless pit inside me here that I just had to fill up. Every night after my prayers before I would go sleep, I would dream in my awake mind about the man I wanted to love me. I would feel hope and that would let me sleep. In the day, I would have done anything to get someone to tell me they loved me. And I practically did. I just never got the dream." Irrespective of reason, it's not uncommon for SAM to engage in a seemingly immeasurable succession of sexual encounters.

Abused as boys, adult males are more likely than nonabused males to engage in sexual activities with strangers or casual acquaintances, to change sexual partners frequently, to have multiple concurrent sexual partners, to have unprotected anal intercourse and to engage in receptive anal intercourse with steady partners (see, e.g., Bartholow et al., 1994; DiIorio et al., 2002; Lisak, 1994a; Paul et al., 2001; Zierler et al., 1991). Additionally, adolescent and adult males abused as children are more likely than nonabused males to engage in sex work or to receive payment for sex in the form of money, drugs, food, and/or shelter (Bartholow et al., 1994; DiIorio et al., 2002; Lowman, 1987; Strathdee et al., 1996; Zierler et al., 1991). Such activities are often experienced as ego-alien and tend to engender feelings of shame, guilt, and remorse (Dimock, 1988). In many instances, the primary goal of sex is the partner's pleasure and orgasm with little or no regard for one's own (Gill & Tutty, 1999).

Before, during, and after a sexual encounter, SAM finds himself in a dissociated, depersonalized, or derealized state (Black et al., 1997), feeling detached from his mind, from his body, from his immediate surroundings, or from all three. Males with histories of CSA are astute at compartmentalizing their lives (Gartner, 1999; Lew, 1990). Even though some men learn to devalue themselves socially, interpersonally, and in the workplace, they may place great worth on their sexual potency. A dissociative state provides SAM with an opportunity to experience physical closeness or to feign a connection in the absence of intimacy. Neurologically, it may also contribute to stress-induced analgesia (van der Kolk, 1996). Kip revealed: "You know that doctor who sent me here? Well, once the social workers sent me to him and once he got a look at my penis, he kept asking me how I could hurt myself [with pencils, carpentry nails, and screwdrivers] and not stop doing it because of the pain. Hey, I'm no head doctor, what the fuck do I know? But I do know when your body makes enough pain, your mind makes cocaine. He's a doctor and he didn't understand that part. I hope you do." The compulsion-generated opioid effects, however, flow intermittently and ebb quickly as the obsession progresses.

Confusion Between Sexual Orientation and Gender Identity

Far too frequently, but understandably so, males with histories of CSA confuse gender identity with sexual orientation (Spiegel, 1995, 1997a). Social myths inform individuals, families, groups, and institutions that masculinity is equated with competition, power, and aggression and that, inversely, femininity is correlated with relationship, vulnerability, and compliance. SAM, given his history of abuse, may psychologically align with myths of femininity or may superficially project the myths of masculinity—the former involving the rejection of masculinity and the latter making a mockery of it. Concurrently, he is confronted with the socially constructed double-barreled myth that sexually abused males are gay and that all gay males are effeminate (Duncan & Williams, 1998). These misconceptions, left unchecked, may lead SAM to believe that he is gay when, in actuality, he is not. Furthermore, if he is gay, SAM may relinquish his sense of masculinity. With the label of "homosexual" branded by the perpetrator, family members, peers, or self-imposed, the boy may consequently find himself in circumstances or situations that lead to homosexual activity (Johnson & Shrier, 1987). Palo stated: "In my culture, the one who penetrates, he is in many ways like the warrior—respected, masculine, a leader. The one who is penetrated—a wounded animal. Death will come to it before morning. I had so many perpetrators, as a boy and as a man. I think I was looking for someone to kill me. Will I or anybody ever understand that my father and my uncles and the neighbor told me that I was gay, they treated me like I was less than other males and that out of respect, I believed what the elders told me?"

Isolation

SAM may experience great difficulty in contemplating, identifying, and protecting his sexual boundaries. Sexual activity, later in life, often rekindles anxiety coupled with feelings of guilt and helplessness (Johnson & Shrier, 1987). Further, simply the thought of sex is potent enough to evoke a myriad of perceptions, sensations, and impressions, including flashbacks, dissociation, depersonalization, derealization, images of self involved in bizarre sexual scenarios, perceptions of self as a whore, perpetrator, abused boy, sexual deviant, or she-male, exertosensory and interosensory memories of the abuse, feelings of shame, guilt, disgust, and inferiority, sensations of nausea, stomach cramping and bowel tension, the fear of rejection, and the fear of AIDS. When SAM is actually engaged in sexual activity, these and numerous other manifestations may pervade the experience. Unaware of the ways in which subjection to CSA shaped his thoughts, feelings, and behaviors vis-à-vis erotic desire, intimacy, love, and affection, SAM may call for an absolute and outright rejection of sexuality (Lisak, 1994a) or avoidance of sexual relations and activity for extended periods of time (Bruckner & Johnson, 1987; Gill & Tutty, 1999; Johnson & Shrier, 1985). Kip stated: "All these girls from the project, they was looking for someone to take them to the prom. I was avoiding the prom, just didn't—couldn't go. Just the thought of being a guy with them, of seeing them look so dressed up and pretty with flowers and all of that, I just felt like I would contaminate them with myself if I took them. And just the thought of having to kiss them, or knowing they would be thinking they were out with a guy and a guy is gonna kiss you—I just didn't—couldn't go. I can't even think about being a real guy with them. They would be kissin' poison."

Overresponsibility

As a boy, SAM reconciles the abuse by assuming responsibility for its occurrence, his erection, for conveying a subliminal or overt message that he wanted it to happen, for falling prey to a predator, for making a priest fall from grace or a husband or wife break their vows of fidelity, for concealing the abuse, for safeguarding his parents from the knowledge of his deviancy, for shielding his siblings, cousins, and friends from the perpetrator, for protecting the perpetrator from public humiliation or legal injunctions, and for disgracing his gender. Over time, SAM's sense of responsibility extends to a number of microsystems, for example, the schoolyard, the workplace, church committees, and adult relationships—and to all that would be, could be, and is across the various domains of his life.

With a hyperdeveloped caretaking capacity (Mendel, 1995) driven by a sense of inferiority and abasement, SAM, out of fear of rejection, may assume sole responsibility for the state of the relationship and for his partner's happiness. Quite frequently, SAM's self-esteem is a function of his ability to initiate and maintain his partner's interest, pleasure, commitment, and day-to-day well-being. A partner's shift in mood reads as anger, contentment as boredom, a hug instead of sex as relational demise. Indeed, much of the "relationship" occurs in SAM's mind as he vigilantly evaluates potential indicators of concern, fills in the blanks as to the whys and wherefores, and responds, not so much to the partner's stimulus but more to his cognitive appraisals of events, faulty or otherwise. The partner is often bewildered by SAM's incessant efforts toward self-analysis and interpersonal problem solving in the absence of any apparent relational difficulties. SAM is left careworn and the partner, frustrated and confused. Victor stated: "One night Kevin told me, 'Victor, if you continue to feel accountable for what's not working in my life and try to fix it, you're taking the lessons I need to learn away from me.'"

Dichotomous Relating

CSA trajects SAM into a world of dualities, of mutual exclusivities. Perceptions, affect, and behaviors related to self and others are all interpreted within a dichotomous frame. SAM often has difficulty in discerning trust, the intentions of others, his feelings, their actions. To compensate, SAM focuses on the absolutes—the presence or absence of trust, the acceptance or rejection of his love, one's agreement or disagreement with his point of view. With dichotomous thinking, life and people are easy to read. However, in a world framed by dualities, SAM does not have the opportunity to comprehend, experience and appreciate the evolution of interest, the gradations of trust, and the stepwise processes of romance, commitment, and sexual expression. Nor can he see that love and hate have the capacity to coexist, that happiness and contentment have many hues, and that life, for the most part, occurs between the poles of victory and defeat.

Kip stated: "I thought I was going paranoid. At school, if someone looked at me mean, I thought they wanted to fight. If they looked at me nice, I thought they wanted me for sex. About a month ago, this new kid moved into the projects. He was the first kid I hung out with since this whole thing [violent rape] happened. On the third day, he says he would like to become friends. I was like, 'What the fuck do you mean you would like to become friends? I thought you had my back, man. I thought you was my best friend.' I wish you could tell him I'm sorry."

Sexless Relationship

In many instances, SAM, in spite of his discomfort and, in some cases, aversion, finds it possible to have sex with a potential mate prior to the commitment or marriage, but soon thereafter, the sexual relationship wanes as SAM loses interest and desire. At a time when SAM feels loved, a sense of security, and the hope and promise of a long-sought future, the abuse experience, including memories, meanings, and effects, takes center stage. Although rarely forgotten, the abuse-related material is less a matter of emergence and more a matter of attention and focus. Before, SAM defensively suppressed his mindfulness of the abuse, whereas now, defenses relent in an evolving relational context of safety and trust. Ironically, it is in this burgeoning sanctuary of comfort that his sense of mistrust, vulnerability, and discomfort around sexuality emerges from the shadows of his mind. It is extremely difficult for SAM and his partner to understand that he feels safe enough, secure enough, and ready to not only cope with, but to advance beyond, the abuse. More than likely, sex before this point was enacted in a dissociated state; now, with the freedom to metabolize his traumatic memories, SAM has the opportunity to explore intimacy and sexuality in a context incompatible with the abuse experience. This temporary reprieve from sex is not a sign of disinterest but, in fact, an opportunity to redefine love, affection, and care. Of course, much of this is dependent on SAM's willingness to confront his past, his partner's patience and understanding, and their capacity, as a couple, to stumble and prosper individually and as a team. Jake stated: "It just amazes me. I was never the therapy type. I spent almost forty years trying to hide my story, thinking that if it came out, my life would be over. I never knew that putting my memories into words would be the answer to my prayers. I thank God that my wife stood by me. She deserves a husband, a friend and a partner. I can be all of that now."

Enduring a childhood akin to a war zone, many males with histories of CSA feel damaged. Having lost opportunities to learn care and concern for themselves, some men desperately search for others to bring meaning to their lives. Sadly, this search often produces dependent, unrequited, and abusive relationships, thereby perpetuating guilt, shame, and isolation (Gartner, 1999; Olson, 1990; Styron & Janoff-Bulman, 1997). As one SAM said: "I searched for sex—for love all my life. I was so desperate. Nothing, not even the threat of AIDS could stop me. But when I learned to look within, when I began to heal and learn to love myself, the desperation died."

Aftereffects can be devastating, but they are not insurmountable. The expression "males with histories of childhood sexual abuse" recognizes that SAM endured childhood and adolescence even though he confronted sexual, physical, psychological, emotional, and spiritual violations. He learned to persevere in spite of these violations. Now he can learn to thrive.

SUMMARY

This chapter presented the sexual abuse of males (SAM) model of dynamics and effects. It highlighted a boy's experience of CSA within a biopsychosocial context. Figure 4.1 depicts and summarizes the SAM model. Tables 10.1 and 10.2 highlight common dynamics and effects (pp. 442–3). A boy is subjected to boundary diffusion and role confusion. He is sexually abused. The sexual abuse of boys is concealed intrapsychically, interpersonally, and socially.

Responding to internal pressures (e.g., guilt for experiencing pleasure and guilt for failing to prevent the abuse) and external pressures (e.g., discordance with gender role expectations and perpetrators' distorted perception of attribution), the sexually abused boy invalidates his experience. To gain an illusion of control, the boy reconciles the abuse by assuming responsibility for it. Feeling flawed, sexually abused boys take compensatory measures to separate themselves from the abuse.

Reconciliation helps the boy to restore a sense of equilibrium; however, it also reinforces guilt, shame, and responsibility. At any given time, SAM is invalidating the abuse, attempting to reconcile, or compensating for it, and all the while concealing an event that has changed their lives forever. This cycle will continue until males with histories of CSA have an opportunity to rediscover the truth, and find validation in it.

SUBJECTION
- Perpetrator's Invasion of Sam's Body
- Impales Self-Preservative Functions
- Circuitry of Fear
- Hyperarousal & Dissociation

Female Perpetrator: *"I'm a mistake as a boy."*
Male Perpetrator: *"I must be gay."*

SEXUAL ABUSE
- Perpetrator's Distorted Perceptions
- Boundary Diffusion
- Role Confusion
- Premature & Discordant Sexualization
- Target: Sam's Sense of Gender Integrity

"I don't feel like a boy anymore."

CONCEALMENT
- Pervasive Across Human Ecology
- Gender Socialization Demands Non-Disclosure
- Abuse is Acceptable; Truth is Sinful
- Body Betrayal
- Social Mythology Inhibits Acknowledgement

"This isn't supposed to happen to boys."

COMPENSATION
- Cognitive Dissonance
- Demarcation of Self Before, During and After Abuse
- Theories of Self Based on CSA
- Compensation Measures
- Hypermasculinity, Feminization or Undifferentiation

"I can't let anyone see who I really am."

THE CYCLE CONTINUES
A Story Indisposed to Words

Compensate • Conceal • Invalidate • Reconcile

INVALIDATION
- Habituating Hyperarousal; Protracting Dissociation
- Altered States of Consciousness
- Defensive Constellations
- Distortions of Reality
- Cannot Assimilate; Must Accommodate

"What happened? Was it my imagination? Don't talk. Don't think. Don't feel."

RECONCILIATION
- Dichotomous Thinking/Splitting
- Minimize External Attribution
- Maximize Self-Attribution
- Rationalize & Reason the Abuse
- Search for Empowerment

"It's my fault. I can do something to change."

FIGURE 4.1. SAM response cycle for sexually abused males.

CHAPTER FIVE

APPLICATION OF THE SAM MODEL

CHAPTER 4 PRESENTED the SAM model of dynamics and effects, highlighting the experience of childhood sexual abuse (CSA) from a boy's perspective and within an eco-systems framework. This chapter applies the SAM model to the seven cases introduced in the previous chapter.

SUBJECTION

To predispose; to cause to submit; to bring under control; to expose, subdue, reduce, beat down, break down.

Nicholas

My name is Nicholas. Terry say he love me [1]. Terry, he—he call me bad names. My name is Nicholas, but he tell me my name is Nicole [2]. My name is Nicholas. I am a boy. But Terry told me I was a girl—that I was wrong as a boy and cause I cried like a girl and that my nippies are gonna grow into titties, like my mama. He say my bum is a pussy [3]. He say that he loves me. That's why he put that bag on my bum and keep making water gush inside of me [4]. My mama said that Terry loves me and he's always gonna take care of me when she is at work [5].

CLINICAL NOTES

1. Terry, the perpetrator, was setting the context for constructing a relationship predicated on his distorted perceptions of love, affection, and care. He can be classified as a regressed or situational perpetrator given his primary sexual orientation toward adults.
2. At age five, Nicholas had a highly demarcated sense of gender role and a well-established sense of gender identity. Like many perpetrators, Terry was attempting to disrupt Nicholas's sense of gender identity in order to

render the boy more vulnerable. Strategies employed to shame a boy are critical tools in the perpetrator's arsenal.

3. Terry was psychologically shaping Nicholas through his use of gender reversal injunctions so that the boy would eventually believe that something was innately wrong with him; Nicholas fought back by proclaiming his sense of biological sex and gender identity.

4. This is a common subjection activity, one that confuses a young boy, diminishes his sense of body integrity and associates the love of a caretaker with manipulation, pain, humiliation, and powerlessness.

5. With a unified front between mother and perpetrator, Nicholas's sense of helplessness was on the rise.

Kip

I'm from the projects. Proud of it. Never had a problem with it. Liked the fact that I had to be tough, 'cause if you're not, if you weren't, you were sunk [1]. Being tough [2], that was your ticket into this life; being a wuss, a wimp, that was your ticket out [3].

To stay in, you need tools. A knife. A gun. Whatever. I never really had to use them, but I would have. Too much shit goin' down. One dude, a friend from the projects, he was walking home from school and this gang pounced, brought him down, and with a broken Coke bottle, cut his balls off. His gang, to get back, pounced on this other dude, tied him up, threw him in a big metal trash can, and set the thing on fire. Ticket out.

This kind of stuff was happening to younger dudes, thirteen, fourteen. I was sixteen, so I felt like I could relax down some. Wrong, baby. Here I am, walking home, high on some shit, walking along the river tracks, and out of nowhere, this fuckin' giant, not like my age, but big dude, a man, this animal—POW! He got me. It was my time [4].

He was a dealer—big time. I was a runner for him a few times. I thought he was cool but he was actin' like a crazy fuck. Sure I fuckin' ran. But he caught up with me. Dragged me down to the river. Tied my hands behind my back. Thought he was gonna drown me. But it was worse, man. I was kicking, fighting. He said he wanted my ass. I thought this kind of stuff might happen to my sister, not to me [5]. Thought I was trippin' out. No, this was my ticket out—out of a life that was never gonna be the same again [6].

CLINICAL NOTES

1. Kip viewed himself as a "fighter," one who survived living in an environment rife with economic decay, drive-by shootings, and tension among the races, living in a housing project abounding in drug traffic, prostitution, and violence, and living in a home with his mother's alcoholic binges, her re-

volving male companions, and unpredictable care. At that time, Kip's attachment to his mom could be characterized as disorganized. His internal model of relationship had little to do with mutuality and respect; in fact, it was personified by one of his first session statements: "Don't want somethin', don't need nothin'. Don't depend on anyone or count on them in any way. Take care of you cause nobody, not even your Moms, is gonna love you."

2. Kip's notion of "tough" was highly congruent with social mythology. He acted as if there was something innately dangerous about him. His public presentation of gender role behavior invoked fear in and respect from others, which, in turn, fortified his sense of self-esteem and self-efficacy.

3. In Kip's microenvironments, deviations from socially prescribed and community enforced gender-based expression instigated severe consequences, such as communal taunting, gang beatings, and the coerced stripping of clothes.

4. Given the dynamics of Kip's microenvironments, one of his fundamental expectancies included becoming the target of physical and/or gang violence. This apparent eventuality was socially constructed as a rite of passage or, at the very least, a normalized event internal to the urban male socialization process.

5. However, to be male and to be a target of sexual assault could not coexist, even in the realm of possibility. During an early session, Kip stated: "I thought maybe I could die from a drive-by or get killed by a bus or get pushed from the roof of the project. But raped? I never even knew it was possible."

6. Kip's comment about life never being the same again suggests the ways in which subjection to childhood sexual abuse shattered his schemata related to self, gender, security, and life expectancies.

Palo

It was confusing—beyond confusing—like when you first wake up in the morning and you're not sure if you're sleeping or dreaming. It seemed like no matter where I was in my house, someone was watching me. In the bathroom, my bedroom, everywhere [1]. I thought it was one of my brothers, so I talked to my mom and dad. She said I was imagining things [2]. But it didn't stop. It got worse [3]. When I was in the tub, I would hear the door creak open. When I was getting dressed in my room, I would see a shadow outside the door.

I started to think it was my imagination [4]. Not for long, though, because it started happening at the camp, too. My father and his brothers had a cabin in the mountains. Every summer, all of us, my father, uncles, cousins, brothers, and myself would spend time there. And the same thing happened there away from home. Worse, though. It wasn't my imagination. It was my uncle [5]. I would be in the bathroom, and he would come in to take a leak. But he was in there for something else, too, because he held it too long, shook it too much, wanted me to see it [6]. When I told my father, he laughed it off. Told me to relax [7]. No, it wasn't my imagination. It was real [8].

Things were beginning to make sense to me now. I just happened to be one of the last to know. There were two bedrooms in the cabin. The men stayed in one, the boys in the other. But sometimes during the night, I would hear whimpering coming from the other room, and one of the beds next to mine, one where one of my cousins was sleeping, would be empty [9]. I guess I was afraid to put two and two together [10]. But when my uncle began to linger in the bathroom, when my father began to make excuses so he could jump in the shower with me, when my other uncle would watch me dress and undress, two and two made four [11].

CLINICAL NOTES

1. The intrusive observation of children is a common ploy used by perpetrators; in response, children tend to feel mistrustful of their perceptions, intimidated, vulnerable, and, eventually, easily assailable.
2. Through her words and lack of action, Palo's mother refused to validate his reality, which, in turn, led him to further doubt his own perceptions.
3. Often, subjection activities progress gradually, leading up to the actual sexual abuse, as perpetrators have more than the child's "compliance" to manipulate. For example, perpetrators have to gain the "compliance" of others and shield their progressive activities from those who may interrupt them.
4. Perpetrators commonly challenge a boy's sense of reality. In this case, the goal of Palo's perpetrator(s), which was to render Palo insecure and discomposed, was actualizing as per the lead offender's master plan.
5. The overt factual evidence was beginning to override Palo's attempt to attribute these predispositional activities to imagination or chance. In many instances, the perpetrator and child foster a relationship of mutual denial, but for different reasons. Biologically, psychologically, and sociologically, it is easier to deny or rationalize a perpetrator's subjection strategies than it is to accept and experience their reality in full operation.
6. Palo's uncle was attempting to unnerve the boy with his size and stature, especially in contrast to Palo's developing anatomy. When a boy feels intimidated in the presence of another male, particularly an older adolescent or adult, his gender-related self-esteem and self-efficacy diminish rapidly.
7. By telling him to relax, Palo's father was not only denying his son's discomfort, but was also establishing for Palo the united front between his perpetrator(s) and the nonoffending adults in his life.
8. Palo found a way to substantiate his own perceptions despite being surrounded by people upholding the illusion that nothing unusual was occurring.

9. Perpetrators often attempt to arouse the sexual curiosity of boys by systematically and sequentially exposing them to sexual activities they are engaging in with other children.

10. Palo was struggling to avoid data that were highly discrepant with his previously held beliefs regarding appropriate family roles and activities. He stated: "Elders were to be honored. To dishonor was to transgress against the generations who have passed their wisdom on for hundreds of years."

11. Overwhelmed with environmental evidence, Palo was forced to acknowledge that he could not physically escape because they were in a cabin in the mountains, and that he could not depend on protection from adult family members because they were apparently in collusion with each other. Consequently, he was forced to confront this situation on his own.

Matt

This didn't happen suddenly [1]. It wasn't like that at all. I was the middle of three boys. My Dad came in and out of our lives ever since I was a boy. My oldest brother, he was the smart one, always doing homework and studying. My younger brother was always in some kind of trouble [2]. In some ways, I tried to become the man of the house, doing things my older brother couldn't do, trying to keep the younger one in line, and by working after school and on weekends, and fixing the car [3].

She complimented me a lot, telling me that I was becoming a fine young man. I liked hearing that [4]. Even though my father wasn't really around, I wanted to make him proud. No problem so far, right?

But then it started to change. She started to confide in me, telling me how much she missed my father. I understood that. I missed him, too. Her telling me all the time—it didn't feel right—started getting real personal, too private, and I didn't like that [5]. She told me how much she missed his touch, sleeping with him, feeling him inside of her [6]. Disgusting. It wasn't my business and I didn't want to know. But she—she was my mother [7]. Are you with me?

It got worse. She would call me into her room after my brothers were asleep, half naked most of the time. I would run out of the bedroom because I didn't want my brothers seeing her that way [8]. Crazy. She followed me everywhere. Outside. I didn't want the neighbors to see. In the basement. I felt trapped [9]. The living room. I just wanted to fly away. "You're mommy's big man now," she would say in this creepy sort of way [10]. I didn't know where to turn. She made me drinks—high balls, she called them. "Yeah," I thought, "That'll do" [11].

Her words made me sick, so the drinking helped. "You're big, just like your Dad. You have muscles like him. A body like him. Everything like him, just like I remember" [12]. I promised my dad, once when he was sort of sober, that I would be the man of the house. And the fourth commandment is "Honor thy mother and father." So I did [13].

CLINICAL NOTES

1. This was an indication of the progression involved, from persuasion to intimidation, from innuendo to exploitation, and from noncontact to contact behaviors. In many instances, the subjection strategies employed by male perpetrators and female perpetrators are quite similar in terms of manipulation and coercion.
2. Matt was searching for his niche within the family—his familial role and corresponding activities.
3. He was innocently assuming responsibilities of the father. Perhaps his mother was fostering this as well.
4. Emotional seduction often begins with praise. Perpetrators tend to be astute at targeting areas of vulnerability, particularly those related to gender integrity and a child's affectional and attachment needs. Having already experienced the loss of one object, his father, Matt had to defend against the potential loss of his mother.
5. Matt's role as confidant to his mother was developmentally discordant. Developmental discordancy and role confusion impede the maturational tasks of identity formation and personality integration.
6. This points to conflict arising from a discrepancy between Matt's concept of mother, as nurturer and protector, and her invasive message of "sanctioned" sexuality. Perpetrators intentionally strive to manufacture a sense of disequilibrium within their target child. Matt's mother was successful in doing so.
7. Matt's internalized relational model of "mother," "relationship," and "son" was influenced by the early loss of his father, teachings of the Catholic Church on the commandments and obligation, and overarching social constructions of "mother" as caring and innocent, at all times and in all ways.
8. He was invested in protecting his siblings from their mother, and shielding the mother's behavior from the siblings. It is not uncommon for children to barter with the perpetrator: "If you leave my brothers and sisters alone, you can have me all you want. I'll do whatever you want me to do as long as you don't touch or hurt them."
9. The mother was trapping her son, and intentionally so, thereby leaving him with few apparent options.
10. His developmentally discordant role now had a name.
11. Manipulation through alcohol, a common strategy among perpetrators, substantially contributed to Matt's burgeoning state of vulnerability. Encouraging Matt to drink helped the mother advance toward her objective, and it helped Matt detach from his reality.
12. Subjection began with emotional seduction, evolved into immoral sexualization of the parental relationship, and progressed to the illegal and premature sexualization of Matt.
13. Matt's schematic construct of "mother" did not and could not take into

account her behavior; however, his schematic construct of "father and son" as well as his need to remain connected to his father, even in fantasy, drove him to follow the father's order without reservation. In essence, he rendered his mother's behavior more amenable by psychologically aligning with the Fourth Commandment and fulfilling his father's request. Essentially, the focus was taken from her and placed on him; he did not want to commit a sin nor did he want to displease his father, so he literally followed both commands.

Victor

I was on top of the world. It started to be one of the most exciting nights of my life. I was with Tina, my girlfriend. We were at the park, holding hands, and I was so happy, because I knew she liked me. And I loved her. When I was with her, I felt so safe, like I was in a dream [1]. I wanted to kiss her so bad [2], but I wanted to be gentle, not like my father was with my mother [3]. I wanted to be a different kind of man. A gentle man [4]. We stopped walking and just looked at each other. Then I brushed my lips against her lips, and it was heaven. We clung to each other for what seemed like hours. I didn't want it to stop. I felt like a boy, like a man, like I was okay after all [5]. I walked her home and ran to my home.

   I tried to make it to my bedroom but my father heard me. He called me to the living room and grilled me. I told him I was with Tina. "You, with that bitch. Don't lie to me, Niño. You know you don't want what she got [6]. It's time I put you in your place [7]. You are not my son. You are Daddy's little girl" [8]. He mocked me before but never like this. He was drunk. He had a beer can in one hand and his revolver in the other [9]. I thought about grabbing the gun and using it on him. I hated him, fucking hated the bastard. He told me to sit in his lap. I didn't want to die [10]. "Yeah, yeah, mi mija. That's right, take care of Papi. Show Papi how much you love him" [11]. With that, he told me to strip naked as he played with the revolver. I kept thinking about Tina, about how she would never want me, knowing what I was doing now [12].

CLINICAL NOTES

1. Tina provided a necessary and safe haven for Victor.
2. Victor was reaching a developmental milestone in his life. Unfortunately, the experience of incest was about to obliterate the anticipated natural path of psychosexual and psychoemotional development.
3. Victor was discovering and defining the man he wanted to become by transforming the attributes of his father into their polar opposites.
4. There may have been conflicts with cultural stereotypes and gender-role expectations, particularly in light of the highly demarcated "machismo and marianisma" model of gender expression within the Puerto Rican culture.

5. Victor's feelings of security and gender integrity emanated from within, as a consequence of his mutual and reciprocal interactions with Tina. This was in contrast to Victor's incipient feelings of inferiority that Manuel, his father, as an external source, was seeking to impose.
6. The father was attacking his son's sense of maleness with the intention of cultivating feelings of inadequacy.
7. Victor's father was relieving himself of responsibility by constructing the abuse as a lesson to be learned. In doing so, he was also setting the stage for Victor's invalidation of, reconciliation of, and compensation for the abuse.
8. Manuel was rendering Victor even more vulnerable by manipulating his son's need to feel accepted as a male child.
9. Victor's father was exerting an excessive amount of force in order to assure his son's compliance with the abuse. This is a necessary tactic among perpetrators as it builds a stronghold around their greatest fear—the child's potential disclosure.
10. Victor was perceiving only two options: humiliation or death. Biologically, Victor was in the midst of an acute stress response. Psychologically overwhelmed, he was unable to cognitively appraise the situation in any other way. Sociologically speaking, Victor's subjection to CSA was so incongruent with his perception of gender-role expectations, all but obliterating his current sense of identity.
11. Here, Manuel, the father, was expressing his distorted perception of love to which Victor had to comply in order to maintain a viable bond, however illusory, and to remain alive. Sadly, children view such distortions as emanating from within themselves.
12. Victor began to project shame and humiliation onto his interpersonal relationships and onto his future.

Jake

My parents were killed in a car crash when I was nine and since that time I was staying with some relatives who really didn't want me around [1]. They sent me to this Catholic school, junior high, and I liked it. People there seemed to like me. The headmaster, Father Simon, always picked me to serve mass with him. He told me I was his favorite student, altar boy, and to top it off, his favorite player on the football team. That meant the most to me [2]. I mean, I knew I wasn't the biggest, the fastest or the best, but I tried and he noticed, and that made it worth the world [3].

One day I thought I was the only one left in the gym locker room. I was in no hurry to get home after practice, never really was. Aunt Rita and Uncle Dominic already had five kids and I was a burden [4]. Anyway, I was just taking my time, showering and getting dressed. Then I went to take a pee in one of the stalls. I heard footsteps coming toward me, but didn't think much of it. A janitor, no big deal. When I turned to get out of the stall, I saw Father Simon peering at me through the slats. I was speechless. I thought he thought I must be doing something wrong [5], to be hanging out so late after school. He didn't say a word. He just smiled at me. I was frozen. I thought he was going to be really mad at me. But the smile—I was confused [6]. He tapped the door and it opened. He was a huge man and just stood in the doorway. Then he held his arms out to me, and all I remember thinking was, "What big hands" [7]. I took a step forward, and he put his arms around me. And I began to cry, because for the first time in seven years, I felt like I was someone's son [8].

CLINICAL NOTES

1. Children who have a history of serious losses and who are without viable attachments are often viewed by perpetrators as potential and viable targets of abuse, albeit, under their guise of affection and care. In general, perpetrators evidence a facile capacity toward identifying and selecting vulnerable children—children with unmet emotional needs and, in many instances, prepubescent boys and girls who appear to lack secondary sex characteristics or boys who they believe to have traits commonly perceived as belonging to the other gender. Perpetrating priests, on the other hand, tend to target postpubescent girls and boys, who appear to be older, more developed, and therefore, from the perpetrator's perspective, more inclined to view the sexual interaction as mutual and reciprocal.
2. Unlike Manuel, Victor's father, who attempted to attack Victor's sense of gender identity, Father Simon sought to enhance both Jake's sense of gender identity and mastery. Both, however, were attempting to enforce their own distorted perceptions on the boys.
3. Father Simon seemingly provided support and validation when, in actuality, he emotionally manipulated Jake into a state of dependence and trust. Often, in retrospect, such manipulation is perceived as more hurtful than the actual sexual abuse itself.
4. This sense of being a burden led Jake to seek comfort and safety outside of his foster home.
5. Due to Jake's self-attribution, Father Simon's unexpected presence in the locker room elicited fears of punishment and penance; his biggest fear was that of angering and disappointing Father Simon, and the worst anticipated penance was that of losing Father Simon as a source of safety and comfort.
6. Feelings of perplexity and confusion led Jake to rely more heavily on Father Simon's interpretation of the situation, thereby leaving him more vulnerable to harm.
7. It is common, in states of confusion and shock, to fight the feeling of being overwhelmed by focusing instead on only one aspect of the situation. By

focusing on Father Simon's hands, for example, Jake was also able to block out any other potentially confusing or overwhelming information.

8. Jake was left perplexed by the quick change in his perceptions of the situation. Although Jake feared Father Simon's anger, the headmaster did not appear to be angry or disturbed and, in fact, was offering comfort and acceptance instead. However, Jake did not realize that Father Simon—superficially responding to the boy's significant emotional needs—was actually setting the stage for impending physical, emotional, sexual, and spiritual violations.

Ty

No one knows how hard I tried to be a boy the right way. Nobody [1]. I grew up in a house with seven womens: Grandmama, Mama, Auntie Bess, Auntie Glo and three big sisters, Demarus, Abilene, and Juliet [2]. Gadsden County, Florida, the hot, poor pit of the deep South. When my Auntie Florence and my big cousin Rodney moved to town, I was so happy. I wanted to be just like him [3]. I was ten and he was seventeen. My Mama, my aunts, my sisters, and even my Grandmama tried to push me off on him, but he didn't like that very much. It made him mad, real mad [4].

Once, when he was supposed to be watching me, he took me out to the field. I was happier than a pig in—well, you know. Just to be with him. I thought it was the greatest. I tried to walk like him, talk like him, dress like him. I just wanted to be him [5]. We got to this field where a bunch of his friends were waiting. I was really excited then, because I thought that meant he like me enough to have me tag along. Like I was important, a part of him now [6].

That's not what it was all about, though. Rodney pushed me toward his friends. I just sort of laugh at first, thinking he was playing. But then they circled me and start calling me names. "Queer boy." "Faggot." "Miss Tyler" [7]. I look to Rodney for help, and he just laughed. The circle got smaller and I tried running away but they caught me, threw me down in the mud and took my pants [8]. I was so scared. Two got my arms and two got my legs and they threw me up in the air and I smash the ground. I tried not to cry but I did anyway. They spit on me. Kicked me. Called me "cocksucker" and "fairy." They took their penises out and pissed on me [9]. Then I didn't feel anything. Like a stone, I just lay there. I couldn't even remember my name [10]. And that was only the beginning.

CLINICAL NOTES

1. Ty experienced discord between gender role expectations and gender role efficacy before the subjection activities began, rendering him even more vulnerable. This is important to note in light of Ty's preabuse self-

concept. More specifically, prior to the abuse, Ty perceived himself to be "stupid at bein' a boy. I was my Mama's shame."

2. The lack of male figures in Ty's family left him susceptible as he persistently attempted to comprehend and fulfill the model of masculinity formed in the minds of his female relatives. Such an image, based on social mythology, was an ideal and was both exalted and misconceived and, consequently, unrealistic and unattainable.

3. With Rodney's entrance into the family system, Ty now had a role model rather than a mere role image. For Ty, being "just like Rodney" held the promise of attention, approval, and love from his family.

4. Ty's desperate need to be with Rodney overrode his awareness of the older cousin's negative reactions toward him.

5. With Rodney idealized by the family as the "answer to prayers," the "man of the house," and "Gadsden County stallion," and in light of Ty's preabuse self-concept as his mother's "shame," Ty could not use Rodney as an object of identification. Concerning this, Ty stated: "When you're a skunk, you can't be a cougar. When you're a Ty, you can't be a Rodney." Rather aspire to be like Rodney, Ty wished that he could live within his cousin, or live Rodney's life by proxy so that he, too, could experience the appreciation and respect of others, even at the expense of losing his identity in the process.

6. Ty selectively absorbed information which supported his anxious attachment to Rodney despite environmental signals of disinterest and danger. To maintain his representation of the idealized other, Ty defensively denied, intellectualized, and minimized any indicators that held the potential to uncover the true nature of Rodney's intentions and, accordingly, Ty's authentic responses to them.

7. Here, three dynamics occurred simultaneously. First, Ty was forced to acknowledge that his illusion of Rodney's acceptance was not based in reality. Second, he confronted the fact that Rodney betrayed him and would not protect him from public humiliation. Third, and lastly, he was attacked and degraded where he was most vulnerable—his sense of gender integrity.

8. The other boys were showing Ty that the power and control he so desperately wanted in his life were not his and could be taken from him at any time.

9. Ty was learning a lesson on how peers influence each other's behavior. The group cohesion of the young men, including his cousin, in conjunction with their successful attempts at humiliating, intimidating, and degrading him, served to further isolate Ty from a sense of belonging to his gender.

10. For Ty, the ability to process information was diminishing as his compelling need for acceptance, his fear of losing an attachment to Rodney, his sense of hurt and betrayal, his feelings of vulnerability, and his exposure

to developmentally discordant and premature sexualization became all too overwhelming. He was most likely experiencing psychological and physical immobility, a hypnotic state attributable to an imbalance within the autonomic nervous system. In such a state, rather than the sympathetic and parasympathetic systems working in check, the parasympathetic masks the activity of the sympathetic, rendering a frozen quality within.

SEXUAL ABUSE

Take by assault; lay violent hands on; to use so as to injure or damage; to belittle, denigrate, slur, slander, and defame.

Nicholas

My mama tells me never say "no" to Terry cause he loves me just like a real Daddy [1]. My real Daddy can't love me cause he was bad. Bad people go to jail. But Mama told me Terry is good, not bad like my real Daddy. Mama told me if I'm bad then Terry won't love me anymore and won't love my mama any more and he would leave me just like my real Daddy [2].

All the time Terry tell me he loved me. He make me afraid. I don't like it when he made that bag gush up my bum. I don't like it when he made me play with his snake. I don't like it when he made his snake crawl up my bum [3]. That's what he do to my Mama.

CLINICAL NOTES

1. Terry was in the role of caretaker. However, his "caretaking" activities included: (a) administering enemas for no apparent medical reason; (b) coercing Nicholas into "playing" with his penis; and (c) anally penetrating Nicholas. Thus, "love" became equated with pain and discomfort, and as something expressed against Nicholas's sense of agency and will. Further, Nicholas's formulation of ego defenses was immature and underdeveloped, leaving him ever more vulnerable, exposed, and endangered to the perpetration of pain.
2. Consider the following contextual dynamics: (a) the loss stemming from the absence of his biological father; (b) the mother's unwavering support of Terry; (c) the threats of further loss of love if Nicholas was "bad"; and (d) Nicholas's fear of disclosure. Nicholas's need for attachment, expressed by his loyalty to his mother and Terry, demanded that he disfigure the truth.
3. The most common sexual offense experienced by boys of male perpetrators is coercive receptive rectal intercourse. In this case, such an act was reframed by Terry as a game.

Kip

I was kicking and fighting so hard. I had to be tough. Who do you call on at a time like this? God? He wasn't in my life. I had to depend on me. And for the first time in my life, the first fuckin' time in my life, I wasn't able to do that [1].

I kept thinking, "He's gonna rape me." "No, shitface, he can't rape you. You're a guy" [2]. "Yeah, right, asshole, big fuckin' guy you are, getting yourself in a mess like this."

One look at his eyes and I knew he was gonna kill me if I didn't give in. Do I want to die this way? What if people see my body down here? A raped body? No way, man. I don't want anyone seein' that. So I gave in. I stopped fighting. And I felt the life slip right out of me [3].

You ever have a fuckin' puppet? That's what I felt like, man. A puppet. I was nothin' and he had all the control. Lifeless, man, like a puppet. Even when he cut my clothes off with a knife. Even when he slit my shoulder. Even when he made me suck. Even when he fucked me. I was his puppet [4].

CLINICAL NOTES

1. Fierce independence and autonomy were keystones of Kip's preabused self. Emanating from such characteristics were self-pride and self-efficacy. However, without an awareness of any risk for sexual abuse and, consequently, little or no psychological space in which to contain the abuse, a loss of self began to occur.
2. The experience of sexual abuse was altogether incongruent with Kip's assumptions about gender, sexuality, and victimization. His adherence to the social mythology around the sexual abuse of males inhibited any acknowledgment, let alone the cultivation, of any preventative measures against such an experience.
3. Kip felt like a drowning boy who, when struggling to come up for air, was pulled under again and again. He fought to hold onto something, anything, yet the surrender of his body and of his sense of self was the only option allowing for the possibility of survival at that moment in time. He stated: "Once I saw what he was gonna do, I knew me as a guy and my life as a kid on the streets was never gonna be the same again."
4. The traumatic state associated with sexual abuse is often described as a crashing wave which sweeps away one's identity and one's sense of the world. The shattering of assumptions, about life, about masculinity, about the world coincided with an upsurge of stress-responsive hormones and the fractionation of unity among the senses; what Kip's eyes saw, his ears could not hear, and what his nose smelled, his body could not feel. Kip lay there feeling lost, confused, dazed, and like a puppet—motionless and lifeless. Neurologically, with Kip's dopaminergic system modulating his mood and affect by way of detached calm and his opioid system obstructing the

sensation of pain, diminishing the amplitude of alarm and altering his sense of person, place, and time, it's no wonder why he felt like a puppet. This violent episode of rape also fractionated Kip's continuity of time, demarcating the self into preabuse, abuse, and postabuse compartments.

Palo

All of this was too much for me to take in. We're taught from a very early age to respect our elders. My father and uncles were acting as natural as can be. My cousins, too. Was I the only one who thought this was strange [1]? Or, was I the strange one, the odd man out? And what about my brothers?

I wanted to protect them, to stay by their side, so I set a tent up outside for the three of us to sleep in. That night, my two cousins begged to sleep out with us. There wasn't enough room or sleeping bags, so I said "no." Hearing about this, my father pulled me aside and, well, I had to sleep inside while my two brothers and cousins slept in the tent.

Inside, my uncles and father were drinking, playing cards, and acting crazy. I made my way to the bedroom, desperately trying to fall asleep. I couldn't do it, so pretending to be was the next best alternative [2]. A while later, my uncle came in, drunk, talking incoherently and fell on top of me. I didn't budge. My father and other uncle came in, telling me to wake up. Still, I didn't budge. Then they began tickling me, and I couldn't fake it anymore. They got pretty rough, thrashing their hands all over me. I wanted to scream but didn't want to scare my brothers [3], so I pulled away and got really mad. My father laughed, saying, "If you wanted us to stop so bad, why is there a rise in your pants? How are you going to answer that, son [4]?"

I wanted to die, right then and there. I didn't know how to answer him. My words were saying one thing, my body another. "C'mon, son. You know what you want." What did I want? Why was my body, my cock, hard? Why? I felt like it was giving them permission to do what they did [5]. They took off their clothes and came at me, all at once. I didn't know what hit me. I was thrown off guard. Mouths, hands, bodies, cocks all over me.

I never felt that way before [6]. My head was spinning. I couldn't think. My heart was racing. I could hardly breathe. I couldn't speak. My body felt more and more like a rock. I was dizzy. My vision was blurred. Eventually, all I could do was smell [7]. I knew one was on top of me, one was behind me, and the other was over my face. I smelled whiskey and man scent. I felt like I was going to vomit. I thought I was going to pass out. And I did.

CLINICAL NOTES

1. Palo desperately wanted to receive external validation for his perceptions. However, given the discrepancy between his perceptions and the actions of

those around him, he was unable to do so. The absence of external validation, in the midst of trauma, and opposes the veritable facts by default.

2. Palo learned the importance of pretense—of pretending to see things that
were not there and to feel things that he did not feel. Feigning sleep afforded him a momentary reprieve from exposure to a reality that he was
desperately trying to evade.

3. Protecting his brothers from the abuse, and spending as much time with
them as possible, allowed him to participate in their world—a world where
abuse, at least for that moment, did not exist. Or so he thought.

4. Palo's father was already reconstructing CSA, with an eye toward calling it
anything but incest or childhood sexual abuse. He was also using Palo's
natural physiological response to deflect any responsibility for manipulating and exploiting his son, emotionally, physically, and otherwise.

5. Palo, given his confused and vulnerable state, accepted his father's reconstruction of the abuse as the only viable rationale for his body's response.

6. Palo had no experience in his life to prepare him for CSA. Thus, he could
not associate it with any other memory. Psychobiologically, the amygdala
relies on and functions in accordance with stored information necessary to
assess the gravity of the sensory stimuli it receives. However, Palo's subjection to incest by means of mass perpetration was beyond imagination. Consequently, but understandably, Palo's amygdala had few, if any, internalized
experiences from which to appraise and respond to the incest in an informative manner. This set the stage for his sensations of shock.

7. Given his traumatic state, Palo's sensory channels were constricted to a
point in which only olfaction was in the foreground, while the others re-
cessed to the background. The neuroanatomy of the olfactory tract is unique
among the sensory receptors. Although converted signals of hearing, vision, taste, and touch enter the brainstem and travel to the thalamus, or the
sensory gate, smell, processed as electrochemical data, treks directly to the
amygdala and olfactory cortex.

Matt

Like I said, this didn't happen overnight. Maybe it took the whole summer. It
sped up when she started feeding me alcohol [1]. I was so afraid of my brothers finding out that I stopped sleeping in my bed. I pretended to fall asleep on
the couch every night. Truth is, I hardly ever slept [2].

When she would come into the living room, I always pretended to be
asleep. At first, she would just look at me. Fucking strange. Then she would
touch me. It was the middle of summer and I was sleeping in layers of underwear, sweat suits, you name it [3]. She became brazen, and began putting her
hands in my pants.

Did you ever have the feeling that you were in a movie? That what was happening to you, really wasn't happening, it was just like a movie? Well, that's what it was like for me. Especially this one night, when she managed to take my clothes off. She knew that I wasn't asleep, and she knew that I knew. "It's only a movie. It's only a movie" [4].

She took me by the hand, and led me to her room [5]. I knew what was about to happen. "It's only a movie." She called me by my father's name [6]. She begged me to make love to her. What was I supposed to do? I tried talking my way out. That didn't work. I ran away three times. That didn't work. Couldn't talk to the police. Couldn't talk to a priest [7]. Who the fuck was going to believe me?

She lay there naked. I had never seen a naked woman before. Never touched one. Never kissed one. And here I was, kissing, sucking, on her, in her, making love. And the whole time I held onto the fact that it was only a movie [8].

CLINICAL NOTES

1. Alcohol, for Matt's mother, was a way of increasing his vulnerability and his acceptance of her directives. For Matt, alcohol was a way of escaping from the realities of the situation.
2. Because of his mother's persistence, Matt developed an increased awareness of his surroundings at all times. Hypervigilance, manifested through his lack of sleep, provided for Matt a means of defense against his mother's intrusions.
3. Matt's sense of safety and trust diminished as his mother became more persistent. Although feeling a need to protect himself, Matt also wished to appear as normal as possible in order to keep his brothers from detecting anything strange about life within the home.
4. By defining the experience of CSA as a movie, Matt was shielding himself from the onset of a traumatic state. He was describing derealization, an altered state of consciousness and a core element of the traumatic response. With derealization, Matt experienced a palpable sense of estrangement from the impinging realities of incest. His ego disengaged into a detached observing self and a distant but participating self. The accompanying feelings of unreality maintained a buffer zone around his full-fledged realization of childhood sexual abuse and, consequently, an onslaught of traumatic effects—at least for that moment in time.
5. Unable to escape the situation without alarming his brothers, Matt had to surrender to his mother's directives.
6. In calling Matt by his father's name, the mother not only demonstrated that she "experienced" Matt as his father, and therefore her equal, but also further exacerbated Matt's sense of unreality.
7. Commonly held myths—that sexual abuse does not happen to boys, and if the sexual activities occur with a woman, then the boy is either "lucky" or, if he does not enjoy himself, "queer"—make disclosure of sexual abuse

uncommon among boys. Matt, too, was unable to think of anyone who might have been able to understand his experience of the abuse, much less protect him and his brothers.

8. By holding onto the idea that the incestual encounter was "just a movie," Matt was able to derail his full recognition of the situation and, consequently, its traumatic effects. When watching a movie, one can see and hear the action, but one can not taste, smell, or tactilely experience it. This very willing suspension of disbelief would ultimately interfere with Matt's ability to perceive his mother as a perpetrator and the incest as a form of childhood sexual abuse.

Victor

I knew that my Mom was at work at the bar, but I was still shocked that my father was acting like this in the living room because I thought my brothers and sisters were in the house. When I asked about them, he told me to "shut up," that they were at my grandmother's house staying overnight. This was all set up by him.

My mind was racing: "What am I going to do? What if the guys on the team find out? Can I kill him? Why is my mother always gone? Is he drunk enough to pass out? Does God see [1]?" I had to get to the bathroom. I started out of the room but he threw the can and hit me in the back of the head. I ran to the bathroom and locked the door [2]. He came after me, and I hear this big bang. I thought he stumbled against the door, but he was actually breaking the damn thing down. I opened the door.

He grabbed me by the hair and dragged me into his bedroom and threw me on the bed. I was praying that he left the gun in the living room but soon I felt it against my head. He told me to strip and I did. "Holy Maria, Mother of God, pray for us sinners, now at the hour of our death. Amen" [3].

This was my dad. I was his son [4]. He had a gun. I had nowhere to go, no one to call, no place to hide. My skin was so tight, my heart in my mouth. I wanted to scream but he would have punched me. I wanted to run but he would have caught me. I wanted to fight back but he would have killed me [5].

Holding the gun to my face, he told me to take off his clothes, and like a robot, I did; for now, I felt nothing [6]. It was weird. One second, I'm in a panic; the next, a wave of calm comes over me [7]. I took off his clothes and, like my mother, folded them and placed them in a neat pile on the red chair.

I walk over to the bed, to him, and he takes my clothes off, kissing my body as he does, saying: "bonita, bonita, mi bonita" [8]. I'm so limp, about to fall, and he picks me up and places me on the bed [9]. Everything is so slow. I can't think. I feel nothing except his touch, his body on top of mine. He was trying to put his penis in me, but it wouldn't go. When it did, this fire went through my body. Pain. Excruciating pain. But it wasn't my body any more. I knew it was pain, but it didn't hurt me. It wasn't my body anymore [10].

CLINICAL NOTES

1. Victor, in one sense, was calling on those who could have potentially intervened, but to no avail. Victor believed that God was all-seeing and all-knowing. That being the case, Victor felt even more frightened, as he wanted to shield God from the impending acts of his biological father and he wanted to shield his friends and family from the knowledge of this life-eradicating event.
2. This was a way to "buy time," giving Victor a chance to search for a plan of escape. Decades later, this fact would prove vital to Victor's "rediscovery" that he did not want the abuse to occur and that he, in truth, tried to get away.
3. Victor perceived his behavior as sinful, despite his father's coercive actions. Given his understanding of and perceptions around religion, punishment was sure to follow.
4. The imposition of a new role, especially a gender-discordant and familially antagonistic one, exacerbated the traumatic response.
5. Victor, so overwhelmed by fear, was unable to consider how he did try to prevent the abusive episodes from escalating into other forms of violence, how he complied in order to save his life, or how and why, given the circumstances, "surrendering" was just as industrious as fighting back.
6. Feeling "nothing" is a common manifestation of CSA, perhaps attributable to the psychology of dissociation and defense, the biology of neurohormonal activity, or the psychobiology of both. Whatever the case, feeling "nothing" is often misinterpreted by both subject and observer. In this instance, the father may have viewed Victor's response as signs of permission and desire.
7. Victor was describing the psychic numbing that occurs during and after traumatic incidents which fosters coping and adaptation. Time slows, sensations cease, reality suspends. Such distortions ascend in service of defending the ego against the danger of a full and instantaneous multisensory exposure to reality. Like a healing balm, psychic numbing does not eradicate pain, only one's recognition of it.
9. Victor could not escape from his home without risking his life; with tenacity, he "surrendered" psychically and physically, in order to preserve his will to exist and his dreams of life with Tina.
10. These statements are indicators of dissociation. Dissociation, as a psychobiological operation, disunites the synthetic and integrative network of sensory and communication channels between and among thoughts, feelings, behaviors, knowledge, sensations, and memories. Strategic, protective, and self-preservative, it generates a shift in and modification of consciousness. During Victor's first incestual episode, dissociation gave rise to relief. His ego allocated itself into a detached, observational self and into a detached, experiential self, thereby buffering him from the full

exertosensory and interosensory experience. Additionally, in response to the searing pain of anal penetration, Victor's opioid system rendered a number of palpable effects, including analgesic action, tranquilizing action, a diminished fear response, and a sense of relaxation and weightlessness, as if one is floating through air.

Jake

Nothing else happened that evening. I stopped crying. He hugged me again and wham, the tears came flowing a second time [1]. I had to get out of there.

The next day at school, I could barely look him in the eye. I felt ashamed, flustered, confused [2]. I kept telling myself that I would never be there like that again. But that was a joke, because that afternoon, after football practice, I hung out [3]. After all the guys left, and the coach went home, I made my way to that same stall. I sat there for, I don't know, maybe an hour or so. I got up, peeked out, and the place was dark. It was scary. I wanted to run but didn't want to make any noise. I tiptoed to the exit, and just as I was about to leave, I heard someone call my name. It was Father Simon.

I couldn't see him, because it was so dark, but I heard his footsteps getting closer and closer. My head felt like it was about to burst [4]. He stood before me, felt for my hand, and tugged me, I guess like he wanted me. I did follow him, into the coach's office, still in the dark. He locked the door behind us.

The quiet was so loud. I felt like I was screaming inside, but nothing was coming out. He had a booming voice, but now it was so low, so gentle. "Tell me what you want, Jake. Tell Father what you want. What do you want Father to do?" I couldn't believe what happened next. Please don't ask me why. Please. I said, "Father, Daddy, I want you to love me" [5].

And with that, he held me so close, stroked my hair, kissed my face. When his lips touched mine, I opened my mouth and let him in. Why? Why? I felt his erection and knew that I was Satan's son [6]. Or else why did he lay me on the table? Why did he take my clothes off? Why did he lay on top of me, spread my legs, and press his thing all the way inside of me? And why, when he came inside of me, did he cry? Why? I was Satan's son [7]!

CLINICAL NOTES

1. Jake's fundamental drive was not in search of pleasure but rather in search of a constant object. In addition to his loss of nuclear family and years of feeling unwanted by his foster family, someone was finally showing Jake the emotional care and physical affection that he had been longing for over many years. That he found an expressive object overrode, at least initially, the form and content of what was expressed.
2. The roles and boundaries that characterized their relationship up to this point transformed at the onset of abuse. In other words, (a) sexual abuse

(b) by a priest (c) on the school grounds transgressed the boundaries of their former role sets, that of headmaster and student, priest and altar boy, coach and athlete, thereby creating for Jake a sense of disequilibrium, mystification, and shame.

3. Jake's hunger for nurturance and affection was so strong that it initially overrode his ability to cognitively appraise the situation as dangerous and to viscerally connect with his feelings of discomfort.

4. Given his religious upbringing and his adherence to catechismal dogma, Jake was cognizant of what was right and wrong, good and bad, holy and sinful. Although cognitively he recognized an impending situation that might lead him into "sin," affectively, he was drawn into a situation that allured and mesmerized him.

5. Father Simon capitalized on Jake's need for a father figure and at the same time presented a sexualized invitation. The headmaster construed love as sex, innuendo, and betrayal; Jake yearned for love in the form of parental affection, care, and concern.

6. Even though Father Simon was the one who violated boundaries while preaching on the virtue of chastity, Jake viewed himself as the betrayer, the one who offended against God, morality, and a representative of Christ.

7. Despite overwhelming evidence pointing to Father Simon's manipulative, intrusive, and sexualized behavior, Jake's view of himself as a sinner, and as deserving of supreme punishment, prevailed. Like many priests, and perhaps more so given Jake's context and history, Father Simon was aggrandized to a place of perfection and glorification. In viewing himself as Satan's Son, Jake was able to maintain the idealized object representation of Father Simon while simultaneously the priest's more authentic attributes, such as guilt, betrayal, and sexual aberration, became introjected components of Jake's self representation.

Ty

I was so frightened. Like I was in outer space. It's scary when you can't remember your name [1]. I was just a faggot. My cousin pulled his—can I just say it? My cousin pulled his dick out and I can't believe it. My cousin Rodney was a man. A big man. I guess I wasn't. I knew I wasn't [2]. He sat on my chest and shoved it in my mouth while the other guys took all my clothes off.

I was choking, but he didn't seem to care about me. They were laughing about greasing me up but I couldn't go anywhere, get away. Two of the guys was spreading my legs so far like they was gonna break. Another one of them was kneeled between my legs and just shoved himself right inside my body. I'm not real sure what really happened after that. I felt like I fainted but I really didn't faint. You're gonna think I'm really crazy now but something happened. It was like I was there but like I wasn't really there. Like I was on the dirt, having sex, but then I was up in the tree, looking down at what they was doing to me [3]. I'm crazy, I know.

The part of me that was up in the tree just counted: One. Two. Three. Four. Each one took turns fucking me. Rodney was the last. Five. You ain't going to believe this, what happened next. It was the worst part of all, I think. It's the part that I could never forget, the part that makes me sick to my stomach, the part that makes me wanna cry [4].

After Rodney was finished with me, he signaled for them to go away. One of the guys, I don't even know his name, came back over, pulled his pants down again, and shit on me. He shit on me. That's when the dam broke. One of me was still up in the tree but the me on the ground, I felt it. My heart felt it. You must really think I'm crazy [5].

CLINICAL NOTES

1. Fear, unbridled fear, stimulated surges of cortisol, epinephrine, and norepinephrine, among others, thereby triggering sensations common to stress, but uncommon to Ty. As a boy, Ty was unaware that stress-responsive cortisol could engender feelings of "spaciness." Like many other males with histories of CSA, Ty's inability to remember his own name incited fears of "going crazy," which, in turn, maintained the fear–adrenaline–fear cycle.
2. The very presence of Rodney provoked feelings of emasculation, inferiority, and shame within Ty. Further, Ty did not take into account the impact of puberty and development when comparing the size of Rodney's penis against his own.
3. In an attempt to escape or, at the very least, shield himself from traumatic feelings and sensations, Ty unconsciously fractionated into ego states—one detached but observant and floating above his body, and the other, detached yet participatory, lying on the ground. Decades later, in telling his story, Ty was able to give voice to both ego states, which contributed significantly to the narrativization of his history of CSA.
4. Even though an abuse episode may last for more than an hour, as was the case with Ty, thoughts, feelings, and sensations generated by the experience as a whole may coalesce around one element of the abuse, such as a stated phrase or a particular action. Bearing witness to a man defecating on him—the images, sounds, smells, and sensations—broke though Ty's stimulus barrier and dissociative state, thereby allowing feelings of shame, horror, disgust, humiliation, and despair emerge swiftly to the fore.
5. Statements such as "this sounds really crazy" and "you must think I'm crazy," quite common among males with histories of CSA, indicate sensory mistrust. Social mythology, in tandem with defense strategies required to cope with the abuse, distort reality, leaving Ty and others in a state of quandary as to what is real, what is imagined, what is true, and what is false.

CONCEALMENT

To prevent the disclosure or recognition of; to place out of sight; to mask, disguise, camouflage, retreat, obscure, eclipse.

Nicholas

Mama always told me to tell the truth, so I told her the truth. I told her that Terry made me do things that hurt me. She beat me for saying bad things about Terry [1]. He beat me for saying lies [2].

CLINICAL NOTES

1. Nicholas learned that telling the truth engendered punishment, namely, physical abuse, as well as threats around the loss of love and home. Concurrently, he discovered that upholding illusions brings rewards, such as maintenance of an intact family environment and positive feedback from his caretakers.
2. Nicholas's mother, the nonoffending caretaker, and her boyfriend, the perpetrator, taught Nicholas to mistrust what he sees, hears, smells, touches, and tastes in order to conceal the truth, and to become a master of pretense and deception. Such lessons became, for Nicholas, modes of survival.

Kip

Never, ever, ever in my life did I ever for once think that something like this could happen to me. I heard about it happening to girls all the time [1]. Every day I would see men slapping women, grabbing tits and pinching ass, calling them whores, getting them drunk, slipping them pills and having sex whether the girls or ladies wanted to or not.

So there I am, right? Bleeding from the gash. Naked with my clothes cut off me. Bleeding from my ass. Fuckin' gross. And I'm thinkin', "Fuck the gash, fuck the blood, fuck my clothes. Who the fuck am I really? Have I been fooling myself my whole damn life? Am I really a queer that everyone else can see but me [2]? Am I really some fuckin' misfit, some gender bender?" Never, never, never did I ever have these kinds of thoughts before. "What's this fuckin' world coming to? I don't even know who I am anymore" [3].

He was calling me "pussy boy." Told me if I told he was gonna have me killed. Told me that I wanted it else why did I have a hard-on and shoot? No fuckin' way was I gonna tell [4]. What would people think, that I was a pussy boy, too, 'cause I didn't get away, 'cause I allowed it to happen, and fuck man, 'cause I must have liked it [5]? My cock, man, that did the only talkin' that was necessary. It got hard. It shot. It wanted this whole thing to happen. Yeah. Who was I gonna tell, and who the hell was gonna believe me [6]?

CLINICAL NOTES

1. Kip's environment laid the foundation for risk identification, confrontation, and escape, especially in relation to drugs, alcohol, and gang related activity. However, nobody and nothing prepared him for sexual abuse as a potential life event. Consequently, his brain, when registering the abuse, ignited a vast circuitry of stress responses, given the novelty of and danger inherit in childhood sexual abuse.
2. Unless the abusive experience was fully repressed, cognitive and/or affective seepage was likely to break through the defensive barrier, particularly in the forms of intrusive thoughts and intense feelings, regardless of the defenses employed. In Kip's case, such seepage triggered a sense of exposure as if others were able to see what he was so urgently trying to conceal.
3. Because sexual abuse happened "to girls all the time," but not to boys, Kip had to struggle not only with the traumatic experience, but also with his perceptions of what this experience had turned him into—a "queer" and a misfit—in other words, the polar opposite of how he perceived himself prior to the abuse.
4. Even though the perpetrator enforced concealment in a number of ways, the most salient enforcer of all was Kip's physiological response. All other enforcers were unnecessary and redundant.
5. Kip's beliefs reflected social mythology and therefore were not amenable to the facts that defined or the logic that supported the realities of his authentic experience of CSA.
6. To be sure, the seriousness of the sexual abuse of males is often minimized by adults, with many believing that boys in general, and adolescents in particular, are not psychologically harmed. At this point, it's quite clear that Kip already had internalized social mythology, thereby mistaking myth for truth and, moreover, viewing the self, others, and the world in mythological terms. From his worldview, there were no caring others with whom he could disclose without inciting disbelief and disparaging remarks.

Palo

When I came to, woke up, it was very dark. I had cum on me, in me, my face, my body. I just wanted to get it off of me. I tiptoed to the bathroom because I didn't want to wake anyone up. I was afraid to turn the shower on because it would have been too loud, so I just sat in the bathtub. Every sound, the crickets, the floor creaking, every movement, the curtains from the breeze, made me jump [1]. I couldn't even turn the faucet on. It kept squeaking. Squeaking. It wasn't the faucet. It was me [2]. The tears came on like an avalanche and this sound—I had to muffle my mouth. This sound, big, loud, came out of me and there I was, trying to remain quiet. I couldn't. I just couldn't anymore.

My father came into the bathroom. I was naked, in the tub. I flinched and wrapped my arms around my body. I tried to stop crying, but couldn't. He knelt down at the tub and put his arms around me. I just wanted to die, to disappear, to turn back time [3].

I never saw him like this before. "I love you. You're my first, my son, and I love you." Oh my Spirit. I waited for years to hear my father say he loved me. Not only did he say that, but he called me his son. My Spirit. "I love you, and would never do anything to hurt you." Is this what I have to do to get close to my Dad [4]? Then he began to cry, and I couldn't take that. "Please don't tell anyone, son. Your mother needs me. The family will split up [5]. Please don't tell anyone." That wave was coming over me again, and I wanted it to stop. "Promise me, son. Promise me that you won't tell." "I promise, Dad. I promise." And with that, he hugged me harder, and we both cried. He was—is—my father. How could I disrespect him, be so disloyal and tell? I had to honor him, honor my father. "And I want you to promise me something, Dad. Promise that you won't do this to my brothers. Promise me. Please" [6].

CLINICAL NOTES

1. Palo was in a sensitized state wherein thoughts, feelings, behaviors, and sensations were magnified. From Palo's perspective, this heightened sense of arousal appeared to occur "from nowhere," with little or no sense of its impending emergence. Fear of subsequent abuse and fear of its discovery held constant; as such, they remained unabated, functioning as barriers against the cessation of his state of hyperarousal. Simply, Palo's initial state of hyperarousal, initiated by the occurrence of incest, maintained itself, or habituated, given his incessant fears around the recurrence of abuse and the implications of its disclosure. In essence, Palo's state of hyperarousal developed a pattern of regularity within his central nervous system.

2. As his arousal state habituated, triggers and his emotional reactions to them seemed to grow exponentially, overpowering and numbing his mind. Subjected to this type of chronic stress, the perpetuance and force of the autonomic arousal catapulted Palo, without delay, from trigger to reaction, as if they were one and the same. At the time, he was unable to discern the ways in which his cognitive appraisals of a trigger mediated his biological, psychological, and behavioral responses to it.

3. Palo felt as if he had no sense of an "old self" from which to access inner strength, direction, and alignment between thoughts, feelings, and behaviors. With dissociation and depersonalization, alterations in identity persist for hours and or days and, in some cases, for years after the traumatizing event.

4. Palo was describing depersonalization, a palpable detachment from his self, and derealization, a discernible detachment from the environment, both with feelings of unreality. Even though he longed to hear such words of

love, the context in which they were expressed (e.g., sexual abuse) and the psychobiological depletion resulting from the abuse thwarted his reception of them.

5. The father, as the perpetrator, recruited Palo into a conspiracy of silence by capitalizing on his son's investment in family preservation. This fulfilled the perpetrator's need to conceal the abuse from uninvolved family members and it provided Palo with an opportunity to reconnect with an aspect of his life prior to the abuse

6. In service of protecting his siblings, Palo complied with his father's desperate plea. In essence, his father was asking him not only to conceal the abuse, but to forfeit his birthright to a childhood filled with protection, respect, and unconditional love.

Matt

For a while, I was drunk enough to believe that I was just in a movie, but then it became too real. An erection. Ejaculation. That was real. This was not a movie [1].

I got sick. I tried to pull myself off of her but didn't make it in time. I vomited on her. I was choking on it [2]. She shoved me and slapped me. "What is wrong with you? I just gave you a gift. What in God's name is wrong with you" [3]?

I felt vile. I felt shame. I felt disgusted. Not with her, but with me. My body. My penis. Why? I wanted to know why it did what it did. Thoughts of the way she acted with me always disgusted me before this, but this night my penis got hard [4]. I came inside my mother. I thought my head was going to blow off my shoulders [5]. I wanted the movie back. I thought I was going to lose my mind. It was too much. I couldn't take it in. What was wrong with me? Why was she always telling me how handsome I was? People were always making comments about my body. I was a jock. Big fucking deal. I felt like a magnet for sex, weird perverted sex [6]. My fucking cock betrayed me [7]. Maybe that's all I'm good for. John is the brain. Keith is the wild one. Maybe I was there for sex [8].

"Clean this vomit up and make me a 'Bloody Mary.' Easy on the blood" [9].

CLINICAL NOTES

1. Matt's erection and ejaculation served as verdicts of guilt, ruling out such salient facts as his mother's coercive, intrusive, and manipulative behaviors.

2. Becoming ill or feeling sick after an abusive episode is a common effect. Thoughts of sex or feelings of desire as well as actual sexual experiences can activate the same response. When a boy is actually engaged in abusive sexual activity, a number of manifestations may pervade the defensive wall,

including flashbacks, dissociation, depersonalization, derealization, images of self involved in bizarre sexual scenarios, perceptions of self as a whore, perpetrator, abused boy, sexual deviant, or she-male, exertosensory and interosensory memories of the abuse, feelings of shame, guilt, disgust, and inferiority, sensations of nausea, stomach cramping, and bowel tension, the fear of rejection, and the fear of AIDS.

3. The distorted perceptions of Matt's mother were very compelling for him. Because Matt did not have other ways of finding validation for his reality, he had to rely on the "reality" constructed by his perpetrator.

4. Matt's erection rendered null and void his prior thoughts and feelings about his mother in regards to her invasive, antagonistic, and "unmotherly" behavior. Psychically, he did not identify with the aggressor—he was the aggressor.

5. Primary stress emerged as a result of the sexual abuse and from attempts at enforcing its concealment. Secondary stress manifested whenever Matt felt as if he was on the verge of losing control over the secret. Traumatic effects, for example, panic, palpitations, and paralysis, intensify in response to thoughts such as "Oh my God," "I can't take it," and "I'm going to lose it." Thoughts such as these are analogous to fuel on a fire, for the amygdala will respond to fear, any fear, before the medial prefrontal cortex can acutely analyze the situation at hand and, when possible, constrain the amygdala's conditioned fear response.

6. Matt constructed the experience with his mother as being consensual sex. Given his physiological response, it was difficult, if not impossible, for him to view the experience as incest or sexual abuse.

7. Thus, Matt's sense of betrayal by his body opposed, or perhaps protected him from, his acknowledgment of maternal perpetration and, by definition, maternal disaffection and alienation.

8. Matt's identity was being shaped by environmental feedback that emphasized his physical self. His sense of self-worth, then, was based less on who he was as a person, and more on what his body could do both in terms of enticing and serving others.

Victor

He passed out on top of me. I could hardly breathe. I thought I was going to die. I closed my eyes, held my breath and waited. I couldn't die. I had to take care of my brothers and sisters. I had to keep my family together [1].

I didn't want to make waves. He beat my mother, and she always came back for more. He beat us, and we had nowhere else to go. Divorce was not an option. Puerto Rican women will endure almost anything before getting a divorce. So that was out of the question [2].

He called me "pequeña," and "maridita"—his little wife. Why? He said he would kill me with the gun if told anyone [3]. I was so confused. He was a man, but I didn't want to be like him. Did that make me gay [4]? He was always making comments about women on the street, always looking at porn and wanting to share it with me. I didn't get it. Why didn't it excite me, like it excited him? Did that make me gay? I would hear him in the bedroom with my mother, grunting like a pig. Just the thought of him on top of her made me sick, really sick, vomit and everything [5]. Did that make me gay?

That night, I made a pact with God. If I did everything my father wanted me to do—if I tried to be the best boy I could be—if I tried to be a man, and do all of the things that men are supposed to do—if I did my best at baseball and made my parents proud—if I proved to everyone that I wasn't gay—if I kept this secret from my mother and the rest of the family—would God protect my brothers and sisters from him [6]? If I didn't try something, anything, I knew I would go crazy or die [7].

CLINICAL NOTES

1. The family dynamics around abuse and violence fostered, within Victor, a sense of self-worth based on his ability to discern, and take care of, the needs of others.
2. Victor felt so constrained, helpless, and powerless that only "impossibilities" emerged as possible solutions.
3. The perpetrator, or, in this case, Victor's father, was both the tormentor of Victor's distress as well as his "teacher," modeling for Victor everything that he needed to know in order to keep the reality of the abuse concealed. Further, the father performed another role, that of Victor's self-object, mirroring and confirming for Victor his deviation from gender expectations and the consequences of such, namely, gender shame and humiliation.
4. Victor, like many others, confused sexual orientation with gender identity. This is understandable because sexual abuse typically engenders feelings of emasculation for the boy regardless of perpetrator gender. Emasculation, in turn, incites a fear of homosexuals and, at times, a misidentification of one's homosexuality.
5. Victor was able to accept himself as the receptor of his father's vulgarity. However, his conceptualization of "mother" prohibited him from viewing her in a similar manner.
6. Victor's perception of God was pivotal to the concealment phase. On the one hand, God was punitive—"punishing" him for sexual behavior; on the other hand, Victor was relying on this same God to help him conceal the abuse, prove his manhood, and protect his siblings from their father. Essentially, Victor's internalized representations of the God split vertically into compartmentalized images of infliction, punitiveness, and castigation under one domain and compassion, love, and hope under the other. Even though the mental representations were isolated from one another, they coexisted at the same time.

7. In other words, if Victor discovered that he was gay, if he ever considered himself to be a "failure" as a male, or if he were to find out that his father had abused the younger children, then exacerbation of the traumatic response was likely to follow.

Jake

Satan's son [1]! Is that what you confess to a priest in confession? After you confess you do penance. Kind of like saying, "I'm sorry and it will never happen again" [2]. If I confessed, I would have gotten him in trouble [3]. I couldn't say a word. I didn't want to say a word. I just lay there. On that table. Crying.

I wanted him to come back. I wanted him to hold me. Oh my God, I can't believe I'm telling you this [4]. I was sick. I am sick. I just wanted him to hold me. But I knew I could never let it happen again [5]. I have to make up for it. I felt like I did something so bad, so rotten, that I was so evil that I could make a priest give up his vow of chastity [6].

I'm glad the room was still dark. The school was dark. It was dark outside. I walked home, praying to God to give me the strength to never let me do that again, praying to all the saints to make Father Simon feel okay and still like me, begging Virgin Mary to purify me, and pleading with everyone in heaven to help me keep this secret on earth [7].

I snuck in my house. No one really noticed me anyway. I took a shower and went to my bed in the basement. I was finally glad that no one shared a space with me, because I got down on my knees and prayed again as hard as I could. "Forgive me, God. I'm sorry. I'll never let it happen again. Please make me whole again [8]. Please keep me away from those I can hurt. Please take evil sex out of me."

I finally felt quiet. I felt a little peace. Maybe God would give me another chance. Maybe I can make up for this. I laid so still, not wanting to ruin the little peace. But then I felt the cross on my neck—and it started all over again [9].

CLINICAL NOTES

1. Because God, as Jake knew him, was all-knowing and ever-present, Jake believed that he could not conceal the sexual experience from him. Jake perceived himself as having fallen from God's grace. No longer a child of God, and deserving of "just punishment," Jake assumed an identity fitting of his perceived transgression—Satan's son.
2. From Jake's psychological and sociological space, any type of penance, in and of itself, would have been a mere slap on the wrist. Thus, penance could not have served as punishment for such a mortal sin.
3. The risk of possibly losing his only viable and consistent source of per-

ceived attention and care, particularly in light of a history characterized by loss and neglect, was too threatening.

4. From Jake's view, boundary diffusion, role confusion, physical violation, guilt, and shame were, perhaps, a small price to pay for an affectionate hug.

5. Jake was speaking as if he was the perpetrator, as if he broke a vow of chastity, as if he committed a crime, and as if he was ultimately responsible.

6. Father Simon made no overt attempts toward enforcing concealment. In similar cases, the vow of chastity becomes a safeguard against recognition.

7. Jake felt compelled to conceal the abuse in order to maintain the illusion of love. He called the experience by every name but its own. He was invested in protecting Father Simon because he perceived that his only other option was to lose love and the love object, two calamities of childhood that he did not wish to repeat.

8. For Jake, to feel "whole" again would have required self forgiveness and, ironically so, for sins never committed. Still, he could not refrain from assuming blame and seeking punishment.

9. While memories of the initial episode of abuse triggered fear, for Jake, even nonaligned objects, such as his sacred cross, evoked a similar response simply by association. Essentially, while Jake was processing and adapting to the abuse stimuli, within a day or two, additional stimuli, separate and apart from the abuse experience and environment, ignited the same fear response when coupled with his memories of the abuse.

Ty

Rodney must've hated me. He grabbed me by the throat, banged my head against the ground [1], and told me how much shame I would bring to my family, to my Mama, if I told [2]. Because everyone would really know that I was a faggot. He said people just think it now, but if I told, people would know for sure [3].

My body was crippled kind of—I couldn't move. But I heard every word he said. I wasn't up in the tree anymore. I was just this faggot nigger whore in the dirt with cum and shit all over me [4].

Rodney was right. People would know that if I told. My mother was already ashamed of me. She said, "Miss Tyler, if you don't wise up, if you don't go out there and learn how to be a boy, I'm gonna take your sisters' brassieres, ribbons, and dresses and send you to school that way. Now you ain't a girl, so stop walkin', talkin', eatin', thinkin', feelin', and actin' like one" [5].

I thought, "No, Mama, I ain't gonna tell you. Not gonna tell no one. This is my cross to bear [6]. I'm the mistake. You and no one would believe me anyway. You and everyone would only believe Rodney [7]. He's the real man. I'm the mistake." I didn't want to be rejected anymore. I didn't want to be blamed anymore. Maybe this was my lesson. Maybe, if I tried even harder, keep my mouth shut, and act like Rodney, maybe I could be a man one day [8].

CLINICAL NOTES

1. Ty was threatened, shamed, and physically forced into concealment. There appears to have been no means of escape, and no caring other to whom he could disclose and receive a compassionate response. Rodney, the perpetrator, was aware of, and made use of, these facts.
2. More specifically, Rodney, as perpetrator, aggressively convinced Ty that his silence would ultimately protect his mother, grandmother, sisters, and aunts from knowledge of their boy's evil and behavior. In short time, Rodney was idealized once again, as an icon of hope—hope that the abuse would remain undisclosed and hope that the family would be sheltered from shame.
3. Recognizing that people "thought" he was gay, as opposed to their "knowing," offered a window of opportunity for Ty to try and prove to them that he could "be a better boy."
4. These potent descriptors and sensations, when linked to sexual abuse, can habituate and, with time, generalize into intimate and sexual experiences throughout adolescence and adulthood.
5. The mother used shame, guilt, and other forms of negative reinforcement in order to drive Ty toward fulfilling her expectations of the male gender role.
6. The taunting, derogatory remarks, and the verbally, emotionally, physically, and sexually abusive behavior appear to have been rationalized as "life penalties" for perceived boyhood inferiorities and failings.
7. Rodney was the benchmark against which Ty compared himself and others compared Ty—with Ty ultimately being criticized on all accounts and ostracized by all parties.
8. Survival, in Ty's environment, required not only secrecy but fractionation and concession of his self as well. As a boy, he undoubtedly experienced the apathy, contempt, and maltreatment of others, and in response he learned to experience himself as unworthy, unlovable, and, sadly, as a "mistake."

INVALIDATION

Being without foundation or force in fact, truth, or law; to weaken or destroy the cogency of; to disprove, falsify, dispute, deny, refute, crush.

Nicholas

Mama didn't like me anymore for telling the truth [1]. I don't like it when she don't like me. Said my 'magination's gonna get me in trouble. Make the bad social workers come back. Said my 'magination's gonna get everyone in trouble, make them take me away to jail.

My 'magination. I like it. Big Bird's in my 'magination. God's in my 'magination [2]. When Terry wants to play snake in my bum, Big Bird helps me fly away [3].

CLINICAL NOTES

1. After several attempts at disclosure with physically abusive results, Nicholas discovered that the pursuit of validation led to loss of love.
2. In order to counterbalance the lack of care and corroboration in his external world, Nicholas, with creativity and industry, imbued his intrapsychic world with such qualities in the form of God and Big Bird.
3. For Nicholas, "Big Bird" actually provided what he could only wish for from his environment. Without external protection of any kind, Nicholas resourcefully found an older, wiser, bigger, and protective object to fill that void.

Kip

A nightmare. This was one big fucking nightmare and I kept waiting to wake up [1]. I woke up the next day big time, man, and knew like nothing that this nightmare was more than real.

I skipped school a lot, but that next day, I don't know why, I just went. Got up early and everything. Even tried doing some homework [2]. I kept looking around, seeing if people were looking at me different, or treating me different, and they weren't so I started to chill some. Then wham, bam, man, hit in the head again.

It was health class. Fuckin' teacher, Mrs. Capshaw, she starts asking these questions like: "How many women can expect to get raped?" "How many girls are sexually abused before they reach the age of eighteen?" "One in four, class. The answer is one in four. Most girls are abused by someone they know." And "Why do men sexually harass, assault, rape, and abuse women and girls [3]?" And I'm half-waitin' for her to say something about this stuff happening to boys, but she don't. And I'm half not wanting her to, because I don't know if I could take it. Felt naked [4].

But as she's ramblin' on, I'm thinking she's not talking about what happened to me. She was saying some shit about this group, something like boy man love, or man boy love, or something, about men who want to be with boys and boys who want to be with men, just like it was in ancient history times, and I'm sittin' there thinkin', "You faggot, you. Here's this teacher up there, talking about all of these facts, and the only place you fit in is with that gay stuff. When she's talkin' about that, she's talking about you [5]."

I knew then that the nightmare wasn't gonna be over. I must be gay. I must have wanted it. I must have did something, acted a certain way or something, to make him do what he did and to know he was supposed to do it to me. I'm gonna get AIDS [6].

That night I prayed for the first time in my life. "Dear God, if AIDS can make me die, let me get AIDS [7]."

CLINICAL NOTES

1. Kip's intense focus on the abusive event, coupled with his persistent sensations of shock and fear, advanced a state of agitated introspection which led to feelings of unreality. The conditions that urged Kip's hypervigilance—concealing the abuse, fearing its recurrence, anticipating the actualization of the perpetrator's threats, worrying about accidental disclosure and the reactions of others, not to mention the rape itself—also triggered and restored Kip's psychobiological states of hyperarousal and dissociation.

2. Kip was striving to establish a sense of normalcy by imposing structure and routine. Even though Kip thought he was "going crazy," the imposition of structure and routine afforded him the opportunity to act "as if" nothing out of the ordinary had just occurred. It also gave him a sense of purpose and direction.

3. Kip was distorting reality, shielding himself from overwhelming affect, by means of defense strategies. This was an act of commission. The teacher was distorting reality, exposing the students to inaccurate information, by her adherence to social mythology. However, the teacher was correctly elucidating facts germane to the sexual abuse of female children. This was an act of omission.

4. Because the violent rape, as an event, did not provide a "goodness-of-fit" with Kip's socially constructed gender schema, it could not be readily assimilated into that ready-made cognitive framework. Consequently, he had to accommodate the rape, which required him to change his self-schema, in order to incorporate new data. Still, Kip was on a desperate search for corroboration of his reality, his abuse. The reception of such validation, had it been available, would have required the relaxation of Kip's defenses. Doing so, however, would have given rise to a dreaded feeling of exposure.

5. This is another example of the ways in which adherence to social mythology nullifies the reality of abuse, thus setting the stage for reconciliation and compensation.

6. As a result of the abuse, Kip's masculinity schema and his sense of gender identity were invalidated by the newly accommodated sexually abused male schema. Confusing his sense of gender identity with sexual orientation, Kip's sexually abused male schema was infused with a socially constructed gay male schema. Lastly, this gay male schema included an assumption of AIDS that, from his perspective, was equated with death.

7. Kip was asking God to put an end to the sexual trauma, to silence its effects, and to bring back to life his preabuse sense of self.

Palo

That night marked the first day of the rest of my life [1]. I knew that I could never go back to the way things were before. I never wanted to be like my father, his brothers, or other men that I knew. And here I was, a member of that same tribe [2].

One of the elders in the tribe, of the nation, she taught me how to pray, meditate, clear my mind. I was in the process of learning that when this happened. From the time I stood up in that bathtub, and for months after that, I imagined myself on a circus tightrope [3]. On a tightrope, you must take one step at a time, check your balance and proceed with the next step. If you do that, you won't fall. I did the same thing. I said nothing that would make me lose balance, make me feel vulnerable. I did nothing that would call any attention to myself. I was always looking around, and would only make a move when it felt safe to do so. I labeled everything—people, places, and things [4]. That's danger; stay away. She's safe; proceed. Talking too much is dangerous; be silent. He's coming to get you again; pretend he's not, and come back when it's over [5]. Do whatever you need to do to stay on the rope; when you're still, you feel nothing. When you're still, you won't fall. When you're still, when your mind is clear, you can see whatever you want to see. I kept my eye on the rope, and refused to let go [6].

CLINICAL NOTES

1. This was an indication of how the schematic accommodation process created a new view of self, others, the world and the future for Palo. Thus, like Kip and other cases, Palo could not assimilate the experience of CSA, for it was far too momentous and discordant.
2. The disdain, disgust, and abhorrence that were once directed toward the men of the family were now being directed toward himself.
3. Palo's image of the circus tightrope allowed him to maintain some distance from the effects of his abuse. In terms of positive consequences, the sensory image allowed him to focus on other aspects of his life while maintaining a sense of control against intrusive thoughts or feelings. On the negative side, however, his abuse-related thoughts and feelings became encapsulated in an image that inhibited their direct expression.
4. Given the overwhelming nature of sexual trauma, in addition to a social environment that invalidates such an experience, sexually abused males, like Palo, often reduce people, places, and things down to their lowest common denominators in order to make a chaotic world more manageable and predictable. Thus, all people might be dichotomized as perpetrators or victims, places as good or bad, and things as right or wrong with no shades of gray.
5. Even when Palo would "come back," he was returning to a world of pretense. In other words, during an abusive episode, he had to pretend that it

was not happening, and afterward, he still had to maintain the pretense that it hadn't happened. Thus, Palo was shifting more between layers of pretense and less between pretense and reality.

6. The intrusive repetition of conflictual and overwhelming thoughts, memories, sensations, feelings, and motoric discharges fills Palo's body between sexually abusive episodes. Consequently, defense strategies became essential to his survival, as they helped him to sustain a working level of functionality and normalcy given their ability to buffer the impact of sexual abuse, including his psychic, cognitive, affective, behavioral, physiological, interpersonal, and social responses to it. Here, Palo was indirectly referring to the way in which his defenses were exerted on a permanent basis; they were no longer temporary. For Palo, the defense strategies were necessary, not only to shield him from the full impact of incest, but to conceal it as well. They invalidated his reality so he could survive; they remained faithful to his father's perpetration by suppressing the truth.

Matt

Once it happened the first time, I knew it wasn't about to end. She'd been working up to this for quite some time. I wish I could say that she was retarded, or depressed, or a junkie. I wish I could call her anything but "mother" [1].

Mother and sex. The two weren't supposed to go together. I tried to keep them distinct, in my head, but I couldn't. Every time I thought about mother, I thought about sex. I couldn't stop thinking about what happened. Every time I tried to stop thinking about it, the louder it became. In school. How could I smell it when I wasn't with her?! On the bus. At home. With my friends. In my sleep. Every day, every minute [2].

And it wasn't just the thoughts. It was this awful feeling of shame as well. Shame, like it was the blood in my veins. Shame like, "You mother fucking disgusting bastard. You crazy, sick pervert. You are the lowest of the low. You don't deserve the breath you breathe." I wanted to bang my head against the wall—and I did [3]. I tried drinking more, that didn't work. I tried cocaine, and all that did was make me more tense.

All of this is going on, in my mother's bedroom, inside my head, and I'm still trying to act normal. I felt like I was living in two different worlds—one where no one was supposed to know what was going on and I had to make sure it never came out, and another where the reality of what happened was strangling me from the inside out.

I was like a hammer, a hatchet [4]. I could hold everything in for some time, but then I had to find ways to let it out—to almost pound it out—ways that would still protect the secret. There just seemed to be so much on the inside, and I just had to make it come out without using words [5]. One day when I was in the basement, I saw the sledge hammer sitting in the corner. I grabbed that thing so fast, tore up deep into the woods, and began banging my leg with it. I wanted to break my fucking leg so bad. I was swinging that thing with all my might. "Break, mother-fucker, break [6]!"

CLINICAL NOTES

1. Ironically, there were indicators of pathology, such as depression, drug addiction, and sexual fixation, as well as a number of illegal activities, including procuring and serving alcohol to a minor, abuse, and neglect. However, Matt's schema for mother could neither assimilate nor accommodate such data.
2. Invasive introspection fuels the traumatic response. Triggered internally or externally, Matt's conditioned traumatic fear response emerged by way of visual, auditory, and olfactory flashbacks and memories. Even though Matt's conditioned fear responses germinated during the first incestuous episode, they soon generalized and amplified across time and place.
3. Seemingly, the only way to stop or, at the very least, buffer the incessant psychic conflict was to literally "bang [his] head against the wall." Doing so helped Matt to "explode," rather than implode, by externalizing the anxiety.
4. In many instances like this, the abuse-related content was contained within a sensory image. For Matt, however, the hatchet had no apparent connection to the incest.
5. Words seemed foreign to Matt when he attempted to imbue the abuse with meaning. If his experience of CSA, most likely encoded and consolidated on sensory, affective, and motoric levels, obstructed verbal comprehension, it may have all but impeded his verbal expression. Fractions of his abuse experience, implicitly encoded and stored, defied verbalization until they were explicitly processed years later.
6. With traumatic memories in speechless form, Matt could not access and express his internal pain with words. The sensory image was externalized, bringing forth an association with the abuse in general, and with his mother, the perpetrator, in particular. Unfortunately, the explosive rage was directed toward himself.

Victor

As much as I prayed on it, I couldn't understand. I even stopped praying, maybe for a couple of years, because I thought God was ashamed of me, too [1]. I was so angry with my father for hitting my mother, and the thought of him hurting my brothers and sisters enraged me. But what he did to me—it seemed like I felt nothing about him [2]. How could I? I was the one committing the sin, not he.

First, I was having sex before marriage, and I didn't do everything I could to stop it. So that was one sin. Second, my father was the bugarrōn, the dominant, so no one can say anything about homosexuality. But for me, I was the receptive one, and that's definitely viewed as homosexual. That makes two sins. Also, when something bad happens to you, to respect that God did so much suffering for us, you suffered in silence, did not complain. My mother used to say, "Esto es mi cruz que debo a llevar." This is my cross and it is mine to bear [3].

So, if I told anyone, or even if I admitted it to myself as abuse, then I also had to admit that I was a sinner, a homosexual, a failure as a boy and a son [4]. No fucking way. I knew I was those things, my father knew those things about me, but I didn't want anyone else to know [5]. Just tuck it away. Pretend. Shove it under the rug, just like he shoved me on the bed. And when it's over, board the place up until next time. I got to be pretty good at that [6].

CLINICAL NOTES

1. Victor was attempting to rationalize why, given years of prayers requesting an end to the abuse and violence, his devout petitions were never answered. He concluded that the nonresponsiveness was a form of punishment.
2. Victor invalidated feelings that would have been directed toward his father—rage, disgust, and heartbreak. Because he viewed himself as the sinner, Victor did not feel entitled to feelings of betrayal, disappointment, or horror; rather, he expected such feelings to be directed toward him.
3. Victor saw in Jesus Christ's suffering a correlation (not comparison) with his own—paying a painful price to protect those he loves.
4. Victor's statement was a very cogent indication of his internalization of the social mythology surrounding the sexual abuse of males. Abused boys, regardless of perpetrator gender, struggle incessantly with a sense of failure and gender shame. Victor once asked: "How could I have been my mother's son when I was also my father's 'wife'?"
5. Victor was forced to live in a world of duality. The reality of incest conjured feelings of hopelessness, powerlessness, and shame while the reality around the baseball diamond fostered feelings of mastery, competence, and worth. It was necessary for Victor to compartmentalize these two realities in order to maintain a sense of equilibrium.
6. Prior to the incest, Victor's sense of self-efficacy was fortified through school and athletic activities; after the incest began, his sense of self-efficacy was sustained by his abilities to conceal the abuse and defend against its traumatic impact. Perhaps his ability to vertically spilt representations of self by context helped to prevent the traumatic conditioning of stimuli external to his home environment.

Jake

It was the last day of school. I remember waking up feeling like I wasn't myself, about to jump out of my skin. Pain in my belly. Nervous. I made it to school, but I was really shaking by that point. Almost gagging. The homeroom bell rang. I was at my locker, and it just seemed so loud, louder than ever, like it was piercing my eardrums [1]. I kept saying to myself, "Calm down. Calm down." But the more I said it, the more I became jumpy. I tried making it to my homeroom, but I almost couldn't get my legs up the stairs [2]. There were so many kids around me, like they were screaming, and I just wanted to scream back, "Shut the fuck up!"

I needed to get away [3]. I made it to the bathroom, but there were some kids in there so I just found a stall. I had to sit down, to act like I was really using it. My hands were shaking. My whole body was trembling. Something was wrong with me, really wrong with me. I started to think I was going crazy. I didn't feel like me anymore. I had to look in the mirror. The last person left and I crawled over to the mirror. I couldn't even walk. As I boosted myself up the wall, I saw a reflection in the mirror, and I knew for sure that I was going crazy. When I looked at myself in the mirror, I didn't know who it was [4].

That's when I really began to panic. Someone came in the bathroom, a teacher, Mr. Demos, and I tried to act like everything was normal, but on the inside, I knew that I was losing my mind. I made it out the bathroom, and out of the building, and everything was like I had never seen it before [5]. I knew I was at school, but it was like I was in a different place. I walked up and down that road hundreds of times, but it wasn't the same road anymore. I looked at my body, and I felt like it wasn't mine. I kept saying to myself, "My name is Jake. My name is Jake." And every time I thought that, I didn't know who Jake was anymore. I was scared. I was going crazy. I was gonna die [6].

CLINICAL NOTES

1. Sensory overload was both a precursor to and a condition of acute anxiety in this case. Jake's implicit memories—his conditioned emotional responses, his sensorimotor sensations, and learned unconscious behaviors emanating from the sexually abusive episode—emerged independent of his explicit memory system. In conjunction with his implicit memories, Jake evidenced hyperarousal coupled with dissociation and their concomitant neurological, biological, psychological, and physiological manifestations.
2. The heightened response of the sympathetic, or adrenaline-releasing, nervous system resulting from the fear and stress generated by the abusive episodes appears to have formed an obstruction in Jake's voluntary nervous system, responsible for directing motion and movement.
3. Jake was recoiling from a fear that seemingly had no apparent trigger. Fur-

ther, his response, intense and swift, prompted a need for flight, thereby intensifying the stress response.

4. Jake was in a depersonalized state, with the sensation of being detached from the body and its processes. This triggered for him feelings of unreality, which, in turn, conjured additional fear and exacerbated the stress response.

5. Feelings of derealization were apparent here, as evidenced by Jake's altered perception of a very familiar environment. Depersonalization fostered an internal suspension of identification within himself; derealization engendered a suspicion of his external sense of reality.

6. Jake was describing the two most common fears associated with anxiety and the stress response cycle: insanity and death.

Ty

You might think I'm crazy [1], but Rodney meant everything in the world to me. From way back to when I can remember, I wanted to be just like him. So many times I would be surprised that he would want to be in the same room as me. What Rodney was, I wasn't [2]. Rodney was big and strong and tough and masculine like. Here comes another crazy part. Sometimes, when I was by myself, I would just think about Rodney. I wanted to smell like him, eat like him, talk like him, screw like him, play football like him, and just act like him. It was like a hunger inside of me, so deep, that I wanted to be him. I wanted him to swallow me up, so I would disappear, and I could live inside him [3].

We shared a bedroom. After I got home, after his friends did what they did to me, people there were amazed like, cause I never would get dirty like the other boys, and here I was covered in dirt. Rodney was sitting right there, eating some peach cobbler, when mama asked me where I was. It makes me laugh kinda now, 'cause I told her that I was playing football down by the river and "nothin' really happened, Mama, I just tackled some kid too hard and we both fell in." They liked that [4]. Rodney winked at me, and I knew that everything was gonna be all right. I knew that if I said the right things, people was gonna believe me, and Rodney would like me more [5].

That night, in the bedroom, Rodney said, "You did good, kid." He wrapped his big arms around me, so, so, tight. He kissed me and made love to me [6]. I couldn't be mad at Rodney. He was just everything. I was the mistake. He was just trying to teach me a lesson. He was teaching me how to be a boy, and for that, I would have given him my life [7].

CLINICAL NOTES

1. The experience of sexual abuse taught Ty to mistrust his perceptions. Accordingly, his comments such as "You might think I'm crazy" and "Can you see what I'm saying?" suggest that while he was struggling to make sense of

himself and the abuse, he simultaneously felt invisible, bewildered, and insecure in maintaining a position.

2. This belief was generalized as follows: Rodney is a man; I am not. Rodney is straight; I am gay. Rodney is loved and respected; I am despised and disrespected.

3. Ty's urgent need to feel like he was a respected member of his gender and a valued member of his family could only be actualized in the imagination and through the experience of Rodney.

4. Family members and peers provided Ty with validation for pretense and lies—and invalidation of the truth.

5. Ty was discovering that there were prerequisites to, and for, care—namely, the preservation of the social mythology, the concealment of the sexual abuse, the compartmentalization of thoughts and feelings, and the primacy of helping others think and feel what they wanted to think and feel, regardless of plausibility, reliability, and believability.

6. So desperate for care and validation, Ty would have called any number of people, places, or things "love" if attention of any kind was directed his way.

7. Clinging steadfastly to this illusion of love, Ty had to reconstruct Rodney's manipulations, physical violence, sexual abuse, and general disdain as normal and necessary, a task not easily accomplished and requiring vast amounts of psychic energy.

RECONCILIATION

To settle or resolve differences in accordance with social law; to make consistent or congruent with reality; to be both enemy and ally to oneself.

Nicholas

Preacher Mike likes when we tell the truth. I don't ever want to tell lies, but Mama tells me that my 'magination is all lies—that my 'magination's fixin' to get me taken away. Sometimes I don't not know what is my 'magination and what is my lies [1].

Terry keep sayin' that I'm really a little girl, but I know that was his 'magination cause my private part is a boy's private part. I'm just like Terry [2].

But then my body changed. My body changed into a girl, and I know that ain't my 'magination, cause blood came out my bum, and I know that blood comes out my Mama's bum cause she has to put these plugs in to make the blood stop. I'm a girl, just like Terry told me, and that ain't my 'magination no more [3].

CLINICAL NOTES

1. What is the truth? What is illusion? Nicholas was learning that telling the truth is sinful, and falsifying reality is rewarded.
2. A paradox: On the one hand, Nicholas realized that he is a boy and, in fact, could prove so. On the other hand, he also recognized that the sexual acts perpetrated by Terry were the very acts that Terry employed to convey "love" to his mother.
3. Nicholas constructed a rationale to account for the effects of abuse, without calling anal penetration "abuse," and without making reference to Terry as his perpetrator. In essence, he was assuming responsibility for the ambiguity and the abuse.

Kip

I'm not smart or nothin', but I ain't stupid either. That teacher, she kept calling the girls this happens to, she called them victims. The men, the dudes that do it, they were perpetrators. So what was I supposed to think? What was I supposed to call what happened to me? Sexual abuse happens to girls. Period. Sexual abuse does not happen to dudes. Period. Something happened to me. People who are sexually abused are victims. Sexual abuse only happens to females. Females can be victims, but men can't [1]. So what am I? Am I a perpetrator? What am I supposed to call what happened to me [2]?

The answer was right in front of my fuckin' face, man. Smack, dab, poke my eyes out. I can't be sexually abused, right, 'cause it's not supposed to happen to guys. I can't be a victim, right, 'cause I'm not a woman. I got a hard on when it was happening, right [3]? So what does that tell you? What does that fuckin' tell you?

I'm the blame, man [4]. Something happened to me. I don't care what you call it. It happened and I allowed it to happen. If I was a real guy, I would have been able to get away, run faster, beat the mother fucker up, just get away. But no. I couldn't do any of those things. If I was a real guy, my cock wouldn't have gotten hard. How do you explain that, man? A dick's a dick. If it wants sex, it gets hard. If it's turned off, it stays soft. My cock got hard. What am I supposed to do with that? Just pretend it didn't happen. I hate my fuckin' cock [5]. If I was a real guy, I wouldn't be sittin' here in front of you, talkin' to fuckin' social workers and DSS [Department of Social Services] and all. If I was a real guy, I would have been able to protect myself, like I always have before [6]. So don't go try tellin' me that it's not my fault. I know what I fuckin' did. I know what I failed to do. I know what I am—a cheap white jungle trash faggot whore of a person [7].

CLINICAL NOTES

1. Kip convincingly presents an argument that supports social mythology, validates the teacher's misinformation, absolves the perpetrator of any wrong-doing, and condemns himself. Such information, as presented in his school, leads him further astray.
2. Kip aggressively ask, over and over again, "What am I supposed to call it?" Given the far-reaching implications of the male perpetrator/female victim paradigm, any authentic answer to his call is rendered null and void.
3. Kip's rationalizations, in effect, reduced his erection and ejaculation to a one-factor theory. Taken out of context, and without regard for the ways in which fear, or, for that matter, stimulation in many forms, can provoke such a physiological response, the erection and ejaculation were misinterpreted and ultimately used as weapons against the self.
4. Sadly, Kip cannot see that he is attributing the effect of CSA to the wrong cause. In doing so, he erroneously nullified the perpetrator's guilt and responsibility and, in the act of doing so, vilifies his innocence and credibility.
5. With the perpetrator exonerated, thus leaving no external source on which to direct anger and rage, Kip's penis became the object of aggression.
6. Here, Kip makes reference to the self prior to the abuse, struggling to reconcile the current, abused self, inflicted with mythology, with the remembered self, now idealized in light of the current trauma.
7. Before, during, and after his experience of CSA, Kip received information about himself, based on the perceptions and actions of others. His self-concept, as a "cheap white jungle trash faggot whore," convincingly reflects the information presented by those across his microenvironments.

Palo

The tightrope mind-game worked for me when it came to my father, but failed when it started happening with others. First, it was with my father, but I was learning how to deal with that.

But then my uncle, my Uncle Taron. Oh man, it makes me want to cry just thinking about it. Not my uncle. He was my role model. A warrior, a teacher, so brave, so noble [1]. Uncle Taron—he wanted me, too.

About two months later, John, my cousin—I guess he was about seven or eight years older than me—he starts. We were at this tribal ceremony, camping out in the mountains, learning about the medicine wheel. It was supposed to be this sacred experience, at least that's how I envisioned it. And it was sacred and special, until that last night.

I was mesmerized. I felt so connected to my culture, so enamored and humbled by Morningstar, the medicine woman. Sacred, like I said. But that last night, as I was sleeping in the tent, I woke up to find John inserting himself into me. Once again, just like that first time with my father, I wanted to scream, but nothing came out [2].

How was someone—I—supposed to make sense of all of this [3]? First my father. Then Uncle Taron. John. Then this man in a truckstop bathroom. People just felt like they could have sex with me, when they wanted, how they wanted [4]. One after the other. Pass him around. Bang. Bang. Bang.

I didn't understand. I felt like I was fucking crazy [5]. It didn't seem like a big deal to them. Why was it a big deal to me? What was it about me that was creating all of these experiences in my life? I felt like a sex trap, like bait. I couldn't figure it out. I still can't. What was I conveying to people? "Hey, I want sex, and lots of it, especially if it's incestual, so come on down and get some. Take a number. Stand in line. I'll get to you as soon as I can."

What else was I supposed to think? It wasn't them. They didn't lose sleep. They didn't feel like they were going crazy. They didn't feel out of control. It was me. What is it about me?

CLINICAL NOTES

1. Dichotomous thinking, like the psychodynamic concept of splitting, divides the perception and experience of life phenomena into two distinct categories, typically "all good" and "all bad." For Palo, such maneuvers, in service of adaptation, upheld his idealized image of father and uncle and, as such, exonerated them as well. Unfortunately, in order to maintain this compartmentalization, Palo attributed the "all bad" qualities to himself. Thus, he maintained the illusion that the world is safe, that his family is loving, but that he, somehow, is defective, thereby rationalizing the abuse.

2. Palo could not scream, he could not speak. Although defense strategies serve to protect, they also bring with them a defensive delay, where words, speech, and sound stay embedded within. Palo's memories of CSA persisted with little or no semantic translation. Rather, they remained stealthily organized within his sensory, somatic, emotional, motoric, and behavioral systems, leaving him in a state of wordless alarm.

3. Palo was baffled at the occurrence of subsequent abuse by other perpetrators after his father: his uncle, his cousin, and a man in a truckstop bathroom, among others. In an attempt to makes sense of this, Palo began to view himself as a contaminant—profane, perverted, and befouled.

4. His sense of contamination was so potent as to pervade his self-concept and to become the "thesis" of his rationale for his experience of sexual abuse. For him, it answered the question that haunts so many: "Why?"

5. Feeling crazy and the fear of going crazy permeate the lives of males with histories of CSA. Given the ways in which defenses distort reality, the pressure of concealment, the deceptions of invalidation, and the dilemmas of reconciliation, it's easy to understand why.

Matt

How can you make sense of something like that? I was becoming a basket case. Some days I felt like a big brick wall, like nothing could get in or out [1]. No explosions in my head. I loved those days, or those hours, or even minutes, because sometimes it would change without notice and for no apparent reason. Other times, I felt like the dam would break [2], like I was going to be swept away by those vile thoughts and feelings. Back and forth. Up and down [3]. She's sick. No, I'm sick. This is abuse. No, this is love. It's her fault. No, it's my fault. She's a whore. No, I'm a pervert. Guys are supposed to enjoy sex, just relax. I hated it, so something is wrong with me. Up and down. Back and forth. I was a walking time bomb [4]. I didn't know what to make of this whole situation. My mind changed from one minute to the next [5]. All I know was that I wanted it to stop.

The next time my mother came on to me, I begged her to stop. "Stop what? I don't know what you're talking about." I was shocked to hear her say that. "You know, Mom, the sex." "Matthew, I really don't know what you're talking about. Why would you accuse me of such a thing? Tell the truth, Matthew. Tell the truth. You came into my bedroom. Yes?" "Yes." "You climbed on top of me. Yes?" "Yes." "You were stimulated and you had an orgasm. Yes?" "Yes [6]." "You are no good, Matthew. If I wanted to, I could get on the phone right now, call the police and have you carted away. You are to blame for this, Matthew [7]. You! Something is wrong with you. And don't you ever forget it."

I never did.

CLINICAL NOTES

1. The degree to which Matt felt like a "brick wall" was the degree to which he felt empowered. Behind his brick wall, feelings remained dormant and undifferentiated. So although he was able to feel "nothing" but the fear of feelings breaking through, he was also unable to recognize the authentic truth of his experience.
2. Fear of the abuse recurring paled in comparison to Matt's fear of being overwhelmed to the point of no return. The more he feared and strangulated his feelings, that is, the authentic meaning associated with the facts of his history of sexual abuse, the more haunting and foreboding they grew in his mind.
3. Invalidation strategies and numbing foster an illusion of control; reexperiencing and flooding phenomena engender panic, anxiety, and fear of a return to the original state of helplessness and terror. At any given time, Matt fought to stay with the former and to avoid the latter. Still, his intrusive phenomena sought expression, as they held the facts and meanings of his incestual experience; his numbing phenomena sought expression, too, as

they held his self-preservative intentions to deny, invalidate, and escape the facts and meanings of his sexually abusive experience.

4. Because of Matt's fear of losing control, his hypervigilance over the concealment, invalidation, and recurrence of abuse, and increasingly frequent states of autonomic hyperarousal, there was no time for him to rest his sensitized body, no time to relax his sensitized mind.

5. This refers to the process of sensitization. Given Matt's continual subjection to stress as well as his near-constant state of hypervigilance, he learned to react urgently and immediately to stimuli directly associated with his experience of CSA and to stimuli that threatened his abilities to conceal and invalidate it. Due to the nature of sensitization, triggers extended across his microenvironments and his responses to them progressively intensified. To experience a hyperaroused state, day after day, is exhausting enough. In a constant state of fight—to focus his mind, to control his feelings, to prevent the abuse from recurring, and to create the illusion of "normal"—Matt was unknowingly defeating himself, depleting his psychic and physiologic reservoir ever more.

6. Like many children, Matt had great difficulty in seeing beyond the role and title of "mother." Perpetual questions about what she did or did not do, about what he may or may not have done to cause her to act in such ways, could not be answered truthfully, for such answers were profoundly incompatible with his perceptions of mother. Consequently, his ability to discern and trust his perceptions of reality was overridden by the mother's overbearing and pathologic construction of events.

7. By blaming her son, Matt's mother obstructed his ability to label their interactions as child abuse. If anything, Matt perceived himself as the perpetrator.

Victor

When the place was boarded up, I acted like nothing was happening to me. I was leading a double life [1]. At school, I was totally machismo, and did everything I could to let everyone know it. Fortunately, I was very athletic, a jock, a baseball player. I was always trying to beat something—a school record, a record I already broke. I had easy access to the most popular girls, the cheerleaders, and I flirted with all of them. I was always telling queer jokes in the locker room, and messing with guys that were common targets of the jocks. In the neighborhood, I, like an alpha male animal, kept my territory. At home, when my father wasn't around, I took charge, even with my mom sometimes. She didn't seem to mind.

But in the bedroom, late at night with my father, usually when he would come home drunk, and when my mother was working, I was his mariposita [2], totally submissive, the way he wanted. I didn't question him, didn't struggle anymore or put up a fight. I made an agreement with him to be his puta and he agreed to keep away from my brothers and sisters [3]. He wanted me to grow my hair long, and I did. He wanted me to shave my body, and I did. He dressed me in my mother's nightclothes, and I wore them willingly [4].

It seemed so easy, as long as I was able to keep one world away from the other [5]. Someone in group therapy said it was noble of me to try so hard to protect my brothers and sisters. I got pissed. It shouldn't have been so easy for me to switch back and forth [6]. I want to beat myself sometimes for even thinking this, but I even looked forward to being with my father sometimes [7].

Every birthday, for thirteen years, every Christmas Eve at midnight mass, every time there was an opportunity to make a wish, I wished that my father would say, "I love you." I never dreamed that my wish would come true in the way that it did [8].

CLINICAL NOTES

1. Victor's experience of leading a "double life" personified the internal conflict between his authentic self, now imbued with socially imposed denigrations, and his compensatory self, endowed with socially prescribed behaviors to the extreme.
2. The machismo/marianismo dichotomy represents a socially prescriptive gender role protocol within the Puerto Rican culture. Victor's sense of self-worth was a function of his ability to fulfill the machismo role within and across his microenvironments.
3. As the oldest male child, Victor saw his role as teacher and protector of his younger brother and sister. In negotiating this agreement with his father, Victor was honoring cultural, gender, and familial codes of conduct.
4. Victor's compliance was supported by his understanding of the Fourth Commandment, "Honor thy mother and father," and was perceived to be a guarantee against the violation of his siblings.
5. For Victor, the ease with which he was able to function was due to the vast differences between his two perceived roles, muchacho by day, marianista by night.
6. Victor's sense of self-efficacy was enhanced, not so much by what he achieved in the classroom or on the baseball diamond, but more so by his ability to conceal the abuse and, in his mind, fool others into thinking that he was a respectable male.
7. This produced a great sense of guilt for Victor. At the time, Victor could not see that violent incest was the price he had to pay to hear the words "I love you" and to receive hugs from his father.
8. Victor originally misconstrued this to mean that he prayed for the incest to occur in the first place, and that God was simply granting his deviant wish.

Jake

I was so afraid to let anyone see me [1]. If they did, they would have known that I was going crazy [2]. I made it home. Thank God no one was there. I knew I had to run away, but I didn't know where to go. I just didn't want to stop moving. If I did, I thought I would have become paralyzed, like what was happening to me in the bathroom.

I made it down to the basement, my bedroom, and grabbed my bank and my backpack. That was it. I left the house and never returned there again.

I don't even remember how much money I had with me, but it turned out to be enough to buy a one-way bus ticket to the furthest place I could go that night, and that was San Francisco.

It's so strange to think about this now, because all of this happened so long ago. Either I was a really good actor or people around me, relatives and strangers, didn't give two hecks about me. I mean, this awful thing was going on in my life and no one seemed to notice a thing [3]. How could I be going so crazy in my head [4] and nobody notice? How could I be spending so many late evenings at school and no one question me? How could I have walked through the halls of school, in the bathroom, going half out of my mind, unable to walk, and no one say a word to me? How could Father Simon see me day after day and smile, pat me on the back, do all of the things he did before and act so natural about it? Was this just me? Was I crazy as a loon? Or was I just flighty, nelly, like they say the queers were? Was I a queer? What possessed me to want Father Simon to hold me? Why was I so weak, to start crying in his arms [5]? Maybe all he was doing was feeling sorry for me, trying to comfort me, and I turned it into something blasphemous [6]. I wondered why I was always fascinated with the stories of Mary Magdalene—the way she was stoned, called a whore, cast out by her family. Maybe because I was a whore—a whore for the head-master [7]. And why didn't he stop? He was a priest. He wasn't supposed to have sex. What was it about me that could have made him fall like that? For what I done to him, I was afraid that I would make him burn in hell [8]. Why was I feeling so awful about all of this, and why wasn't anyone acting like something was wrong? I was wrong and I had to bear it on my own [9].

CLINICAL NOTES

1. Like many other males with histories of CSA, Jake felt transparent, as if anyone could see through him, in spite of the defenses shielding him. Additionally, he mistook social mythology for "truth," further burying his authentic self.

2. At the same time, Jake's self-esteem and self-efficacy became hostages to his ability to seemingly convince others that all was well. Perceiving himself

as a good actor, a good deceiver, was necessitated by the fear of recognizing his family's lack of care and concern.

3. Jake was attempting to rationalize the discrepancy between his traumatic response to CSA and the utter lack of response from those around him. Not only did he feel "crazy" as an effect of the trauma, he also felt "crazy" because no one seemed to notice, let alone care about, what was happening in his life.

4. "Going crazy in my head" refers to Jake's experience of depersonalization and derealization. With all that was going on internally and physiologically—distorted perceptions, heightened audition, a palpable sense of estrangement from self, a conspicuous sense of alienation from others and the environment, fear of going crazy, panic attacks, palpitations, and paralysis—Jake could not reconcile the nonresponsiveness of others. Further, his shock and disbelief regarding their lack of reaction heightened and maintained his hyperaroused states.

5. The barrage of questions, so swift in succession, leaving no time for critical thinking of any sort, exacerbated the hyperaroused state.

6. To preserve the illusion of love and care extended by others, on the one hand, and to give some sort of rationale for the sexual abuse, on the other hand, Jake was left with no option but to blame himself.

7. The headmaster and the whore. Jake's use of dichotomous thinking helped him to safeguard his perception of Father Simon as pious, holy, and upstanding, while attributing the guilt, shame, and blame to himself. In dichotomous thinking, if there is a good one, there must be a bad one.

8. Based on the perpetrator's enforcers of concealment, on Jake's desperate need for love, and on the lack of response from those around him, Jake's rationale included self-blame for not being a lovable son, nephew, and student and, in fact, for being so evil a sinner he could bring a priest down from his vows.

9. Reconciling the abuse via self-blame, in turn, justified the need for self-punishment.

Ty

I flip-flop all the time about calling it abuse [1]. I know you said I can call it anything I want to, but I get confused sometimes because other people in the group who had a situation like mine, they call it abuse. There's a part of me, sort of like—please don't laugh—sort of like the "little boy" part of me that wants to believe that Rodney really loved me. And then there's a part of me, sort of like the "man" part, that asks me "what am I even doing here?" And then there's this "friend" part of me, I guess, a friend part that says "I want to be like the guys in the group" (i.e., psychotherapy group) so maybe I should call it abuse [2].

At least once a week for years, Rodney and at least one of his friends would do me rough, beat me up, call me "pussy" and "Miss Tyler" and such. But all during that same time, too, Rodney would hold me tight at night. Do you know what it feels like to know that as a boy, you are such a mistake? I didn't want to be. I just wanted to be loved and accepted like everyone else [3]. But I wasn't right somehow. Even my Mama—I brought her such shame.

One summer, the summer Rodney moved in with us, Rodney signed me up for softball tryouts. He was the coach for the boy's team. He's signing me up, and I'm begging him not to, because it's one thing to be called a "pussy boy" at school and it's another thing to show what a failure you are in front of the family [4]. And my Mama, I knew she and my Grandmama and my sisters and my aunts would be there to watch Rodney.

I was having nightmares and daymares about this the whole week before, just like the sex ones [5]. Rodney and his friends was already gangin' up on me. I knew I didn't know how to hit a ball or catch a ball and Rodney, no matter how much I begged, he wouldn't help me. That afternoon, I pretended to be sick. I ran into the bathroom, pinched myself with tweezers, and went to my Mama, telling her that I think I got the chicken pox [6]. She screamed at me, called me a big sissy and told me to get dressed. All of us, we walked to the park together. I was shaking like a leaf.

When it was my turn to go to the plate, I felt tingly all over [7]. I couldn't even see the ball. I just swung three times and got called out. From the bleachers, I heard the names again: "Three strikes, you're out, pussy boy. Way to go, Miss Tyler." I wanted to crawl into the ground. My Mama grabbed me so hard and pulled me out of the field. She was so mad. She hated me. I brought such shame to the family. When I told her I was sorry, she said, "I was planning on making you an abortion. Now I wish I had."

So I knew I wasn't right. But I had to believe in something. Since I couldn't believe in me, I had to believe in my Mama and Rodney [8]. So you see, if I call it sexual abuse or emotional abuse or just plain old abuse, then that means they really didn't care for me, love me, after all, and I don't know if I can ever be ready to believe that.

CLINICAL NOTES

1. Ty was afraid to label the abuse as "abuse," and his cousin as perpetrator, for fear of the authentic meaning that would eventually emerge.
2. This points to the way in which CSA fractionated Ty's self into shards: this part of him, that part of him, the little boy part, the man part, the friend part, with little or no semblance of an integrated whole.
3. Ty was more than willing to say, do, and/or be anything in order to experience care and affection. Given his overriding fears around the loss of love

or of loved ones, sexual abuse, public humiliation, and familial degradation were small prices to pay if the illusion of love was kept alive.

4. Having experienced taunting and ostracism at school, Ty now anticipated shame and humiliation in front of his family. Ty's developing sense of gender-related self-efficacy was diminishing rapidly.

5. Nightmares, night terrors, and flashbacks are common effects of CSA. For Ty, as well as for many other males with histories of CSA, the manifest content and latent content are vastly similar. Ty's traumatic memories were not only recalled but reexperienced as well, as if aspects of the abusive episodes were recurring again, in the present moment.

6. Ty found a creative way to externalize the pain and, at the same time, found a way to possibly avoid the public humiliation he anticipated.

7. Ty was describing the sensation of "pins and needles," an impression indicating the overstimulation of the autonomic nervous system. In states of high sympathetic nervous system arousal, some brain activity, such as the semantic and episodic encoding of learning and memory, may become inactivated. In response, the central nervous system reverts to sensation-based forms of memory that prevailed during childhood.

8. This is a compelling example of how splitting and dichotomous thinking distort reality. In essence, these strategic maneuvers helped Ty to preserve attachments to an idealized mother, even though she was emotionally abusive and neglectful, and to an idealized male figure, in spite of Rodney's perpetration against Ty.

COMPENSATION

A biological, psychological, and sociological adjustive reaction; correction of an organic inferiority; make reparation; atone and pay for the penalty.

Nicholas

Mama said that Terry touched me in my 'magination. That the blood was my 'magination, too [1]. So when the social workers came and I said it happened in my 'magination, they went away. Mama hugged me, and Terry took us to Pizza Hut [2].

CLINICAL NOTES

1. Nicholas compensated by revising the reality of abuse in service of gender integrity and family cohesion.

2. Nicholas's efforts toward concealment, invalidation, reconciliation, and compensation were reinforced by those most important to him.

Kip

I couldn't stop my head from thinkin'. Faggot. Whore. Victim. Perpetrator. Just sex, sex, sex, all the time, sex. I couldn't make it stop. And if I saw it, that was even worse. Like when my moms would have her boyfriend come over, and I would see the two of them walk up the stairs to her bedroom, I would get sick, real sick, like heaving and vomiting and stuff [1].

I couldn't jack off anymore, cause every time I did, I thought about what happened and it made me nuts [2]. I stopped going out with girls, 'cause every time I tried to kiss them, or even just talk to them, I thought they could see right through me [3]. I stopped hangin' outside with my friends, 'cause I was afraid that I would bump into that man again and that he would tell everyone. So I stayed in my room. Only went out when I had to. Only went to school enough so I wouldn't be flunked or held back. I was always lookin' for excuses for gym class [4].

One day, the gym class was swimming, and I had to sit in the locker room. There was this fat guy, Tony, and I saw that fat made your dick look small, almost make it disappear [5]. So that's when the eating started.

I ate and ate, everything in sight that I could. It took a while, but then the fat started to grow. I wasn't running around anymore, playing sports or anything, just eating and eating. I started wearing really big clothes to make me look fatter [6]. I didn't want anyone to see my body, or to look at me and think about sex. I hated my body. My body meant sex, and I didn't want anything to do with that [7].

And I found things that would make my head stop pounding. Like the food. I would get so stuffed that I wouldn't be able to think or feel, just felt like a dead piece of wood [8]. Just kept getting fatter and fatter. Some kids even called me "fatso" but I didn't care. I wanted to be so fat that I couldn't see my dick when I looked down.

But after a year of this, after sixty pounds, I could still see my dick. And I still hated it just as much [9].

CLINICAL NOTES

1. For many males with histories of CSA, the experience of sex and, for some, simply the thought of sex can trigger nausea, heaving, vomiting, and the sensation of an uncontrollable bowel movement. The immediacy of Kip's stimulus/response cycle further aggravated his feelings of sexual shame and gender inferiority, as he felt so out of control.
2. Kip's inability to masturbate points to the relevancy of primary process thinking. For him, the thought of masturbation was akin to the behavioral action of masturbation, whereby both thought and action equally incited feelings of shame, guilt, and self-degradation. Thus, Kip punished himself for crimes uncommitted.

3. Kip felt transparent. To see "through" him was to expose oneself to contamination. Kip believed that he had to protect not only himself from his sexual feelings, but others as well.

4. Gym class often evokes a feeling of terror for males with histories of CSA. The fear of exposure, devaluation, and mockery is too much to bear. Further, given the perceived uncontrollability of his penis, Kip was afraid that he might possibly get an erection in the shower or locker room, thereby proving, beyond a shadow of a doubt, his deviance and culpability, and thereby inciting further public humiliation and shame.

5. Kip felt unworthy of being male. He did not feel banished by his gender; no, he believed he deserved to be banished from his gender. Compulsive eating was the first step on his mission to minimize the presence and function of his penis.

6. Feeling intensely emasculated by the abuse, as if he lost all rights and roles associated with his gender, Kip attempted to find some semblance of comfort in a quasi-androgynous presentation. In one particular session, he stated: "I don't got a right to this hair growin' on my legs, the fuzz on my face. I'm not a real man and I never will be."

7. Kip began to associate sex with abuse, violation, power, and control. Whenever thoughts, feelings, or desires associated with sex emerged, he simultaneously felt like both the abused and the abuser.

8. Both the anticipation and act of compulsive eating, including the hoarding and hiding of food, engendered an altered state of consciousness, wherein Kip felt a sense of nothingness, a sensation of floating in spite of his being full. Because obesity was his superficial goal, the bloatedness from overeating and the tightness from clothes too small were viewed not as discomfort but as indicators of success.

9. Kip's penis became for him the external evidence of his failure to protect himself from abuse, and of his deviance for experiencing an erection and ejaculation. His only means of anticipating relief from the constancy of hyperarousal, intrusive thinking, guilt, and shame was to somehow render it senseless.

Palo

I sound like a broken record, right? Well, I was one back then. Father. Uncle. John. Truckstop. Father. Uncle. John. Truckstop. Neighbor. The list grew. And that's exactly how it was in my head. Incessant. Nonstop. I wanted to know why. Why me? Why so much sex? Why? Why? Why [1]?

I had to come up with an answer, or go crazy. One or the other. That was it. I didn't want to go crazy, even though it seemed appealing at times. I prayed to everyone and everything I knew to pray to—the earth, the moon, the spirits, the totem. Nothing. No answers. So I thought some more, and figured it out.

There's a native teaching about the earth, and how it has no spare parts. Everyone, everything has a purpose to fulfill. Well, what was my purpose? I thought my purpose was to be a teacher for my people [2].

"Wrong, Palo. What is your purpose? Let's see here. What are your unique gifts? What can you do like no other? What can you contribute that will bring joy and pleasure to you and others? Hmmm. You're a failure as a male, given your recent foray into darkness. You're a failure as a son, for disrespecting your father. You're a failure as a brother, for failing to protect your siblings. You're a failure as a student this year, going from 'A's' to 'D's' in one fell swoop. What does that leave, Palo? Oh yes. Sex. That is your unique gift. You certainly have a way about you, Palo, a way like no other. The way you walk, the way you talk. That way about you that lets people know what you're really good for. And what is that? Blow jobs and taking it up the ass are contributions that bring joy and pleasure to those around you. You're a faggot, Palo. A whore. Trash. Garbage. A hole. Shit. Scum. Crud [3]."

So that's the answer I came up with. And it seemed to work. It matched with what people were doing to me [4]. How else could I explain my father, my uncle, my cousin, the trucker, and the teacher? They told me what I was good for, so I built my life on that [5].

CLINICAL NOTES

1. The succession of perpetrators in Palo's life was bewildering to him. The self-knowledge he gleaned from such rampant sexual abuse—that he was a whore, a faggot, a failure, all things that males are not supposed to be—was so incongruent with his previous sense of self, cognitive dissonance was sure to emerge and infiltrate his mind, and incessantly so. No doubt, he was bound and determined to answer the question, "Why is this happening to me?"

2. Palo was striving to find his niche in life with a view to fulfill his stated purpose of becoming a teacher for his tribe and Nation. The occurrence of sexual abuse in his life, along with abuse effects, and the meaning both held for him, could not be assimilated and integrated into a comprehensible life story. Where he came from, and what he planned to do, was one thing; what happened, and where he could go as a result, was another.

3. Given Palo's sacred views around the roles of son, brother, nephew, friend, and tribe member, and the ways in which he honored blood relations, it was far too unlike him, and far too risky, to express feelings of rage, betrayal, and shame toward his perpetrators. Because these feelings could not be directed outward, they found expression within. In doing so, Palo was protecting himself from the repercussions such direct expression could elicit, and, at the same time, he was protecting the perpetrators who had provoked these emotions. Sadly, in order to protect others, he had to turn against himself.

4. Understandably, Palo sought and found people and experiences that confirmed his "sexually abused male" self-schema. The validation and corroboration of a negative self-schema are as compelling as affirmation of a positive one. Further, such experiences helped Palo to make sense of his world, because the external was not matching the internal. Palo found success in failure.

5. Internalizing the messages received from his history of sexual abuse, Palo began to build life goals congruent with them.

Matt

When she confronted me about the truth, this strange feeling came over me. I don't know if I can explain it. It was like a steamroller came over me, crushed me, and I knew that I would never be the same again. Matt was gone—the Matt that I knew myself to be. From that moment on, I felt like a square peg in a round hole. Nothing seemed to fit anymore, to make sense or be real anymore [1]. I didn't know what the truth was anymore.

How could I call it sexual abuse or incest when my body responded the way it did? By the time it got to the point of sex, I stopped fighting her, running away from her. I guess I wanted her to have sex with me. She was my mother. I thought she was sick, depressed, crazy, or an alcoholic. I was her son. I was supposed to take care of her [2]. I should have stopped her, understood her better. But I didn't. I let it happen.

What does that say about me? And how could I really blame her? She was sick. Something was really wrong with her. Whether it was the alcohol or some mental thing, I don't know, but something was very wrong and she couldn't help it. So how could I call that sexual abuse? And that's my mother we're talking about. A mother. Not a dirty old man who hides in alleys and preys on vulnerable children. My mother. So how can I call it abuse [3]?

Everything I ever came up with was a reason not to call it abuse. And I didn't want to be a square peg in a round hole anymore. I wanted to feel like myself again [4]. I wanted to feel like a real person. So I just stopped looking at the whole thing like it was crazy and just accepted it. Accepted the facts.

I had sex with my mother. I wanted it. I got a hard-on. I was good at it. People liked looking at me. People didn't praise me for intelligence like my older brother. People didn't blow me off, like I was worthless, like they did my younger brother. People, not just my mother, but friends, parents and sisters of friends, girls at school, people on the street, men and women, they liked what I had, and so I started giving it away, to anyone who wanted it [5].

CLINICAL NOTES

1. The perpetrator and social mythology teach children to mistrust their perceptions, suppress their feelings, deny the truth, and blame themselves.

Attempting to discern the difference between fact and myth, with little or no validation for the truth, leads to confusion; confusion, in the midst of chaos, obliterates one's view of self, others, and the world, as was the case with Matt.

2. Matt believed his duty as a son was to respect, honor, and care for his mother. What remained the unexpressed part of the equation was, "And she was supposed to care for and nurture me."

3. This statement highlights the cognitive dissonance experienced by Matt. His mother's impositional statements, namely, "You are to blame, Matthew," and "Something is wrong with you," diametrically opposed and disputed the authenticity of his self-concept, that of being a good son and brother with inherent value.

4. Matt wanted to feel like himself again, in other words, like his authentic self. Unfortunately, his authentic self was embedded beneath his abused self, his invalidated self, his reconciled self, and his compensatory self.

5. As a result of his incestual experience, Matt was learning that self-worth was a function of his ability to entice and please others, while simultaneously concealing, invalidating, reconciling, and compensating for his authentic perceptions and feelings.

Victor

I was fine as long as no one knew what was really going down [1]. I knew I was a fraud from the get-go, but I couldn't let anyone else find out. It was like building a great wall around me and the only person who could get inside was my father. He was the only one who could see what I truly was—a freak and failure as a boy [2]. Whenever he came for me, and whenever he was finished, I made him promise that all would be well with my brothers and sister. For that reason alone, I let him do what he did to me.

On the outside, people saw the other Victor, the one I made sure they would see. I was everything a boy, a young man, and man was supposed to be, only to the extreme [3]. If a friend ran five miles, I ran ten. If a guy from the other team hit a home run, I made sure I hit two. When my cousin drank six beers, I drank ten. I pumped my body. I wanted to be the biggest. I wanted all of the girls to want me, and I did everything I could with them, everything they would allow. I teased and beat up the boys that were called queers. I joined the marines, because they only wanted a few good men, and I wanted to be their best. Went to college on a baseball scholarship and tried to break every existing record when it came to pitching. I was team captain, fraternity chaplain, and student government president. I made it to the college world series and got drafted by the pros. I got married and started a family. It was always about being bigger, better, and the best [4].

I kept trying and trying to make my way to the top, but it always seemed out of reach [5]. I was trying too hard to keep the secret, to make up for it, that

I was killing myself in the process. But that didn't stop me. Nothing did, until the worst call of my life came through.

It was Provi, my sister. She was calling from a hospital in Miami. I could hardly understand her through the tears. Bernardo, my youngest brother, killed himself. The note said he couldn't take it anymore—the sex, the lies, my Dad. Provi said she understood. She had been there, too. I wanted to die. I wanted to die for Bernardo, to bring him back. I wanted to die for Provi, for failing to protect her [6]. But Bernardo's death said, "No, but you will die, if you don't learn to live."

So that's why I'm here. It's time to live. Or at least learn how with some peace.

CLINICAL NOTES

1. Victor was suggesting that his feeling fine was a function of his ability to compartmentalize his life, conveying a different set of facts, a different series of personas, depending on the situation at hand. In every instance, every circumstance and situation, there were truths to be shielded and lies to be told. With each altered state of consciousness come its own congruent memories, thoughts, feelings, intentions, states, traits, and behaviors.
2. In other words, Victor was letting down his guard and exposing a socially imposed self-concept. He did not realize that the impositions inflicted by his father and enforced compliance were necessary to initiate and maintain the incestuous relationship and necessary in terms of concealing, invalidating, and reconciling it.
3. Unbeknownst to Victor, his source of motivation was not only the internalized impositions and consequently how he came to view himself, but the fear that others would perceive him in a like manner.
4. Bravado and machismo were compensatory measures enlisted by Victor to vindicate himself in the public arena while suffering the horrors of family violence and incest in private.
5. Yet no matter how far Victor reached or how much he attained, he could not, at that time, acquire what he needed most and wanted so desperately: for the abuse to stop.
6. Victor's guilt for "failing" to protect himself paled in comparison to his sense of guilt for "failing" to protect his brother and sister.

Jake

So there I was, fifteen years old, in San Francisco, and scared as hell. My first night there, I was picked up by the police for loitering at the bus station. They called my family back in Ohio. I got shipped back that same night, but when I got back, I got placed in foster care, this group home, until I was eighteen.

At the group home, all the faces were new. When one of the other residents asked me my name, I said "Jake." That's the first thing that came out of my mouth. My real name was Andrew, but now it was Jake. I liked that new name. Jake. It was strong. I got to be a new me [1]. Whenever anyone asked me a question about my past, I just made something up. After a couple of weeks, the story of Jake was finally coming together.

I told people that I was sent to the group home since I was too much trouble for my family, fighting, stealing, doing drugs. I kept it simple. They bought it. I acted like a demon, a terror, just to keep people in their place [2]. When I left the group home at eighteen and went to work, I kept the name, Jake, and kept the story.

It wasn't as easy as it may sound. Yeah, it was fun, being someone else, but I also couldn't let anyone get too close, and I couldn't forget about Andrew [3]. Sometimes, it felt like the truth was going to bust out of me, especially when I was around Lena, my wife. She wasn't my wife then. We met at work. I really tried to keep her at arm's length, at least, but she found her way into my heart. I don't know how. She just did. She was always asking questions about my family, and after I told her the story I had, she wanted more. I couldn't give that to her.

I tried every way to get rid of her, to break up with her, but she just wouldn't go away. I would be sitting with her, on a date, and I felt like two people, Jake and Andrew, instead of one [4]. I started drinking, every day, and that helped a lot. I was able to keep Andrew down [5].

CLINICAL NOTES

1. Andrew, as a name, represented who he was, where he came from, what he experienced and the losses in his life; Jake, on the other hand, compensated for all he perceived himself not to be.
2. To be perceived as the compensatory self, as inauthentic as it may be, is thrilling and exhilarating. For Jake, hope of a brighter future was built on illusion, which was created to mask the imposed shame. Unbeknownst to many, Jake's compensatory self overlaid his authentic truth.
3. To forget about Andrew was to forget about the abuse. Jake could not do that. Nightmares, night terrors, and flashbacks hindered him from doing so. Invalidation, reconciliation, and compensation remained constant for years. Additionally, limbic-system abnormalities, resulting from protracted stress, may have obstructed the explicitly encoded facts and implicitly encoded meanings of his sexually abusive experience from transforming into words and, consequently, from integrating into a cohesive narrative.
4. Compensating for the abuse, by definition and action, kept the abuse memories and aftereffects alive. Jake would continue to feel like two people until both were integrated into a united whole.
5. Drinking, and often excessively, served at least two purposes for Jake: It helped convey his desired image of a tough street kid, and it helped repress the embedded memories of the past straining to surface.

Ty

I knew from jump street that I wasn't gonna be the best boy in the world, but for a while I tried hard to find the place for me [1]. I knew it wasn't sports, or fixin' cars, or playin' roughhouse, but I prayed to God, every morning and every night, to help me be a boy that could make my Mama proud. Grandmama used to say that if God wasn't answering your prayers, you just wasn't praying hard enough or right enough. So I tried praying in every way I could—on my knees, standing up, eyes open, eyes closed, in every room, up in trees, at different times during the day and night. All kinds of ways, but I don't think He ever heard me [2].

When Rodney moved to town, I guess my hopes and prayers about being a decent boy was shot to hell. And I mean hell for real, cause Grandmama would sometimes say that Rodney had the devil in him, and that the devil was gonna get me, too, if I didn't watch my step.

I wanted so much to be a boy—the right way. I would talk to God and I would say, "God, I know that you are all-loving and all-caring and such, but why God, why did you give me a penis when Rodney and my Mama and so many of the folks in town call me a girl? What am I supposed to do with this thing, God [3]? What do you want me to be?"

I didn't know where to turn for an answer. I just wanted people to love me, that's all. My Mama was ashamed. My sisters had their own lives. Rodney moved back to Chicago. People in town were always calling me names, beating me up, trying to get sex, throwing stones, shoving me in dog and horse and pig shit.

How much more was I supposed to take? I felt like I didn't deserve my—can I say it—penis. I hated my penis [4]. The more it grew, the more I hated it. I knew that I would never grow into a real man, the way one is supposed to be. So I said, "God, if I can't be good at being a boy, maybe I can be good at being a girl [5]."

One morning, Grandmama was downstairs, cooking breakfast, screaming up at me to get up, get ready for school. But I was already up for hours, in my room. I took a long bath. The night before I bought a dollar dress from the Salvation Army. I snuck a bra and panties from the five and ten. I made falsies from old nylons in the basement, and found an okay pair for me. I took an ace bandage from the bathroom to bind me. I borrowed makeup from my sisters' purses. And I got an old afro wig from the hair lady next door, sayin' it was for my sick aunt with cancer.

By now, Grandmama, Mama and my sisters was screaming for me to come down and go to school. I took one last look at myself in the mirror. Now, God, now I was the girl everyone wanted me to be [6]. I knew that once I walked downstairs like this, I would never return. And that's what I did. Down the stairs. Grandmama fainted. Mama threw a lamp at me. The sisters laughed. And I cried all the way to Atlanta [7].

CLINICAL NOTES

1. Ty was striving to discover that special psychological and sociological space in which he could function most effectively. In other words, he was trying to find microenvironments and relationships congruent with his need for acceptance and validation, yet compatible with his self-concept and his understanding of the world and others.

2. No matter how hard he tried, Ty felt like failure, as a boy and as a son, believing he transgressed against and violated social and familial expectations. Further, he felt deserving of punishment for bringing disgrace and dishonor to his family and gender. In his mind, such "failures" rightfully merited and earned abusive treatment.

3. Ty equated a penis with power and potency, masculinity, and aggression. His view of self was the very antithesis of these qualities. For Ty, his penis was a constant reminder of all he was not and all he desperately wanted to be.

4. A delay in the development of Ty's secondary sex characteristics, namely, the growth of facial and body hair, muscular development, and the deepening of the vocal register, contributed to his negative self-concept. Moreover, with Rodney as the benchmark for all things male, including penis size, large stature, athleticism, and popularity among both genders, Ty felt unworthy as a male and thereby undeserving of his penis.

5. In pursuing this line of thinking, Ty was using his history as a foundational base from which to create a present niche as well as a future. This was not a sign of an organic gender identity disorder or transsexualism. Ty did not intend to psychologically align himself with attributes socially allocated to females; however, the information he received from others regarding his failure as a boy, as a son, as a brother, as a cousin, as a peer, and as a male certainly paved the way for this idea.

6. Ty was simply searching for a way to feel validated and to be accepted. This compensatory sense of self was based on the following data: (a) how Ty was looked on by others; (b) how Ty was treated by others; and (c) Ty's perceptions, based on the significance he placed on the information received from others, as to his inherent value and worth. The development of this compensatory self was also based on feelings of inferiority as a male and a desperate need to find his place in the world.

7. With all that had gone on, this was Ty's first reference to tears. He stated: "Before that, there was no tears inside me, only hope to make everything better. When you cry, you know hope is gone."

THE CYCLE CONTINUES

Double-minded, half-hearted, having many faces; to oscillate, pendulate, fluctuate; legacy, birthright, something received from the past.

Nicholas

God will punish me if I lie [1]. Mama will punish me if I tell the truth [2]. Sometimes I feel like a ping-pong ball [3].

CLINICAL NOTES

1. Nicholas lived in great fear of offending God, for he believed God, along with Big Bird, helped him "fly away" during episodes of sexual abuse. His ego functions and defenses were his greatest resources.
2. At the same time, Nicholas lived in great fear of offending his mother, for without her, he would be alone in the world.
3. His feeling like a ping-pong ball points to the oscillations between the authentic truth and the perpetrator-imposed "truth." Over time, Nicholas grew unable to discern one from the other. Sadly, the latter prevailed.

Kip

I hate my dick. I hate my ass. I hate my whole fuckin' body. I hate goin' to the bathroom [1]. Rather be constipated for weeks and take that pain than have to go to the fuckin' bathroom. Makes me sick when I do. For real sick. Vomit sick—when I go to the bathroom. And I have to be around a shower else I won't even go [2].

You're probably gonna cart me away when I tell you this—. You know, I don't even care right now. Just don't care. I hate my dick so much that I try to hurt it [3]. With pencils. With hangers. With anything I can get. I know it's sick. I know something's really wrong with me. But I just can't help it. I gotta do something to make the pain go away [4]. Was the only thing I knew to make me chill, get me to go to sleep. But it just gets worse and worse—the pain— and I gotta keep using something bigger and bigger to make it go away [5]. Last week, when I got mad and shoved a rusty nail inside, that's when I really hurt myself, couldn't make the bleeding stop. So there I was in the emergency room. Couldn't talk. Couldn't feel a thing. That's when the doctor called DSS.

I hope that was enough to make me stop. How many doctors will it take to make me stop? How many times to the emergency room with a spike in my dick will it take to make me stop [6]? I'm afraid I might die next time [7].

CLINICAL NOTES

1. Kip's anus and rectum were penetrated by the perpetrator's penis and fingers. During the sexual assault, some fecal matter was expelled. Rather than feeling violated by the perpetrator, Kip felt as if he had contaminated him. Ever since then, Kip equated bowel movements with filth, contamination, and shame.
2. If and when Kip was able to empty his bowels, certain conditions had to be met. First, he had to be alone. Privacy was nonnegotiable. Second, he had to have access to a sink or a bucket of water in order to wash himself while wiping. Third, he had to have access to a shower to bathe his entire body afterward. Similar protocols and conditions are relatively common among males with histories of CSA.
3. Kip believed that he could express his pain to no one without some form of humiliation, taunting, or insensitive response. From his vantage point, the only way to express his rage and, at the same time, conceal his secret was to abuse his penis.
4. Pain was the price Kip had to pay in order to engender the endogenous opioid effects of analgesia, euphoria, and diminished feelings of inadequacy. Stress-induced analgesia, according to Kip, helped him to survive. It prevented him from registering and experiencing pain, physical and emotional, as he defended against the traumatic effects of his violent rape. Initially, the self-injurious behavior gave rise to a detached state of consciousness and, at times, feelings of euphoria.
5. However, in order to achieve such an anticipated state, Kip had to progressively increase the "dose," as one would have to do with exogenous opiates. Thus, Kip had to progressively use bigger and more dangerous implements until finally he had breached his penile urethra beyond full repair. A common progression begins with safety pins, moves to plastic straws and pencils, and on to metal objects such as screwdrivers and drill bits.
6. So desperate for feeling states of detachment and calm, and relying solely on this progressive method, Kip was unaware, and could not conceive of, other ways in which to produce the a desired state. At the same time, he was cognizant of the negative consequences, but could not stop.
7. Kip's fear indicated an unactualized sense of hope beneath the distress and desolation propagated by the sexual abuse.

Palo

I couldn't wait until I was eighteen [1]. I didn't want to be another Native American child in the foster care system. I wanted to fight that system. I wanted to go to college and become a lawyer. I also wanted to get married to a wonderful woman and make babies and raise a healthy family. You see, I did have a dream [2]. Used to, anyway.

I went away to college on a scholarship. I felt like a captive bird set free. I was fine for a week or two, going to classes, meeting new people. But then those thoughts came back: "Palo, you're a freak. Palo, you're fucked up. Palo, you're a queer. Palo, you're a mistake. Everyone knows, Palo. They can see right through you [3]."

I couldn't listen to the professor and I couldn't take notes. I tried using a tape recorder but couldn't concentrate enough to listen when I got back to the dorm. I wanted to run away but didn't know where to go.

At the cafeteria one day, I met this beautiful girl. Autumn. Autumn Dawn. We started talking and for this brief moment, I forgot about Palo [4]. I just was so happy to be with Autumn.

We started dating, and after a week of that, she knew something was up. I was hot and cold [5]. When I was away from her, all I could do was think of her. When I was with her, I felt like I was going to explode from all the stuff inside me that I was trying so hard to hide. I didn't want her to think that I was like all the other men in this world, but if I didn't act like all the other men, she would think something was wrong with me and get suspicious [6]. I felt like I was a pony's tail—wag here, wag there, wag up, wag down. I would break up with her and then beg her to come back to me. To be with her, I had to drink. When the drinking wore off, I had to run.

I couldn't make my mind up about anything, kept forgetting things [7]. One semester I wanted to be a psych major, the next one a history major. Sophomore year I was back into law, but later that year I switched to biology. I wanted to be with Autumn and then I was afraid to be with Autumn. One day I would tell her I loved her and the next day I acted like she meant nothing to me. Sometimes I thought I was gay and sometimes I thought I was straight [8]. But all the time I knew I was fucked up. I can't believe that Autumn was putting up with all of this.

Right before graduation, I asked her to marry me and she said "yes." I couldn't believe it. I was so happy. I ran across the campus, after seeing her that night, jumping up and down like a kid. I stopped by the library, to return an overdue book, and for some reason, went into the men's room on the second floor. I didn't need to be there.

I'm sitting there thinking, "Palo, what's up? What are you doing, Palo? Why are you ruining what you have with Autumn, Palo? Get out of here, Palo." A hand came from under the partition, from the next stall. It touched my leg. I wanted to run. I wanted to stay. He slipped me a note written on toilet paper. "Palo, it's me, Josh." I felt like I was struck by lightening [9]. I tore out of there and ran like the wind back to my dorm.

I sat on my bed, trying to catch my breath. Instead of calming down, I started to feel like I was going crazy. I was sweating. My heart was pounding so loud I could hear it. I looked down at myself and felt like I wasn't Palo anymore. I looked at my hands, my feet, my arms, my legs, my face in the mirror, and felt like I was looking at someone else's body, someone else's face, anybody but Palo's. I felt myself slipping away [10].

I crawled into bed but couldn't sleep. At graduation the next day, I pretended to have laryngitis so I wouldn't have to speak. I thought I was on my way to crazy, and that it was just a matter of time. I didn't know what to do, where to go or who to ask for help. I thought if I did, they would put me away.

I knew I had to do something, because I was scheduled to start law school in the fall. I never thought I would make it till then. On graduation night, my family didn't show. I was trying to hide from Autumn. She found me drunk, in the corner of the pub. As soon as I saw her, I began to cry.

So I told her everything. I thought I was going to make her sick. I thought she was going to think I was crazy. I thought she would never want to see me again. But she didn't. She just hugged me, and cried, too.

CLINICAL NOTES

1. Palo coped with a childhood rife with incest, sexual abuse, family alcoholism, and family violence by means of fantasizing about what life would be like once he turned eighteen: Incredible, free of abuse, free from its effects, happy, peaceful, blissful, with all of his dreams coming true. Although such coping strategies served him as a boy, instilling a sense of hope and promise, as an adult, they engender a sense of defeat.
2. Palo lost his dream along the way. It became apparent, once again, when he had the opportunity to identify and give meaningful expression to the losses and gains associated with his history of CSA.
3. Palo anticipated that moving away from his family would stop the abuse memories and effects from shadowing him.
4. On his continuing search for anyone or anything to help him "forget," Palo unknowingly invalidated the truths of his childhood and reinforced his need for environmental distractions and external loci of control.
5. Palo's fantasy of life being better than what was occurring in the present moment, in addition to his perpetual impulse to escape the present moment, which often included oscillations between intrusion and numbing, contributed significantly to his sense of being a "pony's tail," in other words, at the whim of his feelings and fantasies.
6. Palo had little sense of how he could possibly personify "masculinity," separate and apart from his father, uncle, and other perpetrators, because to do so otherwise, from his perspective, would surely reveal all that he was so desperately trying to hide, namely, the truth.
7. Palo experienced years of hyperarousal. With such extensive and prolonged sensitization comes psychic, sensory, cognitive, emotional, and physiological depletion. Further, abnormalities in hippocampal functioning, resulting from protracted stress, mutate the formation of and interrela-

tionships within the brain, leaving as a consequence potential impediments to explicit memory and narrative recall. Palo's conditioned fear response exemplified the disengagement of the amygdaloid–hippocampal relationship and, consequently, the implicit–explicit systems of memory and, most concretely, the CSA facts from their meanings. Unfortunately, Palo was unaware of such repercussions, and attributed his inability to make up his mind to personal inferiority and failure.

8. A cardinal effect for males with histories of CSA, regardless of perpetrator gender, is confusion around gender identity and sexual orientation. Palo's fluctuations between "I think I'm gay" and "I think I'm straight" were founded on the following gross rationalizations: "I was abused because deep down inside they know I'm gay" and, alternatively, "I am going to turn gay because I was abused."

9. That Palo was recognized in the bathroom by Josh, another student, was too much to tolerate. Palo felt exposed, as if all the layers of concealment and invalidation were demolished, leaving only his greatest fear, that of being perceived as a deviant and gay.

10. Palo was acutely and succinctly describing depersonalization in the midst of panic.

Matt

I was asked to leave a sex addicts' therapy group because I admitted that I was actively acting out [1]. Yes, we, the group members, agreed to refrain from acting out and no one at that point talked about the truth in the group, even though most of us saw each other at SLAA (Sex and Love Addicts Anonymous) meetings and heard each other talking about what was really going on. We were acting out, but we didn't talk about that in the group, because if we did, we would be kicked out, and that's what happened to me.

I was shocked. I was shamed. I couldn't believe it. I was trying to get help. I wanted someone to help me stop acting out.

It's like a shadow, always following you [2]. You may not always be able to see it, but you know it's there. And sometimes it seems so much bigger than you are. If I tell the truth, I have to say that I was pretty much always in a state of acting out. I was always flirting, always trying to, I guess, get someone to want me [3].

You see, it's really not a sexual thing, in that I'm not acting out to have sex. It sounds crazy, but the relief is not in having sex. I'm a pretty physical person. I work in construction. I run five miles a day. I'm always on the move. However, no matter what I do, when the shadow is bigger than me, I can't work it out physically. That's my danger zone, when I can't seem to shake the shadow.

I can't sit still. It's a tension, a tension inside me that won't dissipate no matter what I do. I call my sponsor, I talk to friends, I try to distract myself, but nothing works. It's like I'm setting myself up to act out and, at the same time, I'm doing whatever I know how to do to keep myself from acting out [4]. I know I'm not going to beat it, no matter how hard I try.

I'm just feeling real shamed right now. Doing it and talking about it are worlds apart. But I want to do this. I need to talk about this. It's just very difficult. I'm an exhibitionist. That's my way of acting out.

It's one thing to do it at a nude beach. Everyone around you is in some state of exposure. For me, that's fine for a while, but when I can't control the shadow, I act out in places where I can be arrested [5]. Libraries. Clothing stores. Parks.

It's quite simple. God, that sounds so strange, but it is. This is so—shaming [6]. God, I just find a place and act as if I'm supposed to be there. For instance, if I'm at a library, I act as if I'm there to read a book. If I'm at a department store, I act as if I'm there to try on new clothes. I find someone, usually a woman, usually someone who looks innocent and meek and I begin to expose myself. If I'm at the library, I might just lean my chair back far enough for her to see. If I'm in a dressing booth, I will leave the door ajar enough for her to see. When she seems to be unfazed or accustomed or whatever, I'll lean my chair back further, or I'll step out of the dressing room, more exposed.

I don't want her to call the management. I don't want her to call the police. I don't want her to run away disgusted. I want her to—just to like me.

Afterwards, that's the worst part. During the acting out, and even for a little while after, I'm detached [7] and that's just fine with me because I know that in a short while, the shame is going to come crashing like a wave [8]. It's like I'm drowning in it and can't escape it. It would be so easy for me to stay in bed for three days after each acting out episode, and sometimes I do. Sometimes, though, I can't. I have to go to work. I have to get myself to a meeting. And it takes every ounce of strength I have to get out of bed, to get out of the house. I can't look at anyone. I don't want to see anyone. I just want that feeling to go away. Maybe not bad enough, though, because I haven't been able to stop.

CLINICAL NOTES

1. Many agencies and therapists hold the policy that any form of compulsive or addictive behavior (e.g., drugging, drinking, sexual acting out, bingeing, purging, etc.) must be fully cessated for a certain period prior to admittance into treatment. Matt was reaching out, asking for help. His termination from the treatment program in some ways affirmed his long-standing belief that falsifying the truth was necessary to maintain ties and attachments.
2. Matt was describing his compulsion to act out, as ever-present, always menacing, and invariably damaging. Still, it was compelling, harboring the offer that the next time will be the best time.

3. Matt's history of mother-perpetrated incest taught him that self-worth was a product of his ability to fulfill the needs of his others and to nullify his own.

4. For Matt, the positive consequences of acting out, namely, a sense of validation, euphoria, and self-worth, were more compelling than the negative consequences, such as the possibility of discovery, the possibility of legal sanctions, and the possibility of public humiliation; the positive consequences were predictable and immediate whereas the negative consequences tended to be unpredictable and delayed.

5. This points to the progressive nature of invalidating, numbing, and compulsive strategies. Risk factors become necessary additions to the process of achieving the desired and anticipated outcomes.

6. Shame is a pervasive feeling, not limited to a particular behavior or a specific context. Cognitively, shame is supported by the core belief: "Something is wrong with me."

7. As with many others, Matt's typical acting-out cycle included a desperation for love and acceptance prior to his acting out, a sense of detachment during it, and feelings of despair soon after it. Ironically, the anticipated outcomes of euphoria were illusory, for they leased very little space and time in this process.

8. Matt was describing how shame broke through the increasingly ephemeral numbing effects, lasting, at times, for days. Even though the positive consequences dissipated quickly, if generated at all, and the negative consequences intensified and multiplied over time, the former remained more compelling than the latter.

Victor

I knew I didn't want to live the lies anymore. I just wanted to be me. Everything seemed to be a lie to me [1]—my career in baseball, my career as a sports anchor, my marriage—everything except my being a father to Bobby and Eva [2].

I didn't want to lie anymore, at home, on the job, anywhere. I knew my marriage was a lie, but I didn't know why. The hardest thing I ever did was telling my wife that it was over. And getting the divorce [3]. I couldn't even give her a reason. I just knew I had to go. She was stunned, and understandably so. I knew I loved her, but I wasn't in love with her. And I wanted the feeling of being in love—for her, with someone special, and for me, too.

I remember the first time I told Kevin that I loved him. Here I was, a man, a dad. My marriage didn't work out but I didn't make a connection. This man comes along. Kevin. I thought he was just my friend, my buddy. I started to feel these things, things like I never had with Teresa [4]. I kept shoving them away. I kept thinking, "I'm a man. I'm not supposed to have these thoughts about another man. That's a sin." But the feelings kept growing. The more they grew, the more I shoved them away [5]. I shoved Kevin away. One night we went to a baseball game. I drank a little too much. In the parking lot I picked a fight with him. I criticized him up and down, told him that I didn't want to be his friend anymore and that I wished I had never met him. I just kept shoving him [6]. Finally he swung back and I wrestled him down. He got loose and ran. I thought he was going to get killed, running across the main drag. I ran after him, down to the river. He told me to get the fuck out of his life until I was ready to tell the real truth. He just walked away. I thought I might never see him again. And I said it. "I love you, Kevin [7]." Then bang. Anxiety. From nowhere [8].

CLINICAL NOTES

1. Victor's perception that "everything seemed to be a lie" points to the layers of imposed truth, that is, the invalidated truth (e.g., nothing bad really happened), the reconciled truth (e.g., it was my fault anyway), and the compensatory truth (e.g., I can't let you see how bad I am on the inside), all concealing the authentic truth (i.e., the facts and meaning of CSA).
2. This was one major facet of Victor's life uncontaminated by the effects of CSA. Essentially, his father represented what not to do, how not to be. Victor, in parenting his children, inverted his father's attitudes, beliefs, and behaviors into their polar opposites. Although this strategy afforded him the opportunity to define and convey love and nurturance in a constructive way, he was constrained by it as well, given the dynamics of dichotomous thinking and psychic splitting.
3. Victor's fantasy of an ideal family, necessary, in his mind, to make reparations from the past, was predicated on a heterosexual orientation. Just as gender dichotomizes human behavior into socially sanctioned male and female categories, the machismo construct dichotomizes males into superior/acceptable and inferior/deviant categories. Victor associated heterosexuality with the former and homosexuality with the latter, thus inhibiting the emergence, identification, and ultimate acceptance of his authentic orientation. Further, as a male who happened to be gay and as a male who happened to be a father, Victor experienced great difficulty in reconciling the two. To accept his authentic orientation was to dissolve the dream.
4. Victor was taken aback on two counts. First, he was surprised that he experienced feelings at all, given his superior and long-standing defenses against them. Second, Victor was astonished, not only at the presence of such feelings for Kevin and the absence of such feelings for Teresa, but at the momentary bliss that accompanied these new feelings.
5. The more his feelings intensified, the more they contradicted his schemata for masculinity, marriage, and fatherhood.
6. Defended against his authentic orientation and his romantic and sexual feelings toward Kevin, Victor viewed Kevin as the enemy, when in reality he was an ally.

7. This was a catalytic moment for Victor; it precipitated change in his desire for, and his ability to express, the authentic, rather than the compensatory, truth.

8. Still, Victor was perplexed as to why he experienced an intense anxiety response upon revealing his true feelings to Kevin. At the time, he did not realize that anxiety was in response to a number of conflicting yet converging beliefs: who he wanted (i.e., Kevin) and who he should have wanted (i.e., Teresa); his authentic orientation (i.e., homosexuality) and his preferred orientation (i.e., heterosexuality); and ultimately, who he was and who he thought he should be.

Jake

Lena and I got married, had three kids, but a lot of it's a blur to me, since I was drinking so much [1]. Lena seemed fine for the most part. Her dream was to be a mother and that kept her busy till the kids grew up and moved out of the house.

Then it was just her and me. Me and Lena. And I couldn't stand it [2]. There was nothing to distract her anymore. She was wanting from me what she had been getting from the kids. The closer she came, the further I moved away. The alcohol was all I cared about. I couldn't stop. I was always on the verge of losing my job. I always tried to stay one step ahead of the alcohol, to cover its tracks, but not more than that, because it became the love of my life [3].

Lena started accusing me of having an affair. I was in a way, wasn't I? Not with a woman. Lena and me—we hadn't been—didn't have—you know what I mean? We didn't have relations—you know—for about fifteen years. Our anniversary was coming up. I could never forget the date, but never wanted to remember [4], or have anyone make a big deal about it. Just another day was fine with me.

Lena said she wanted it to be different this year, special. On the anniversary day, I came home from work and she fixed this special dinner. All through it I knew what she was up to, what she had planned. I pretended to fall asleep [5] after dinner, but she kept nudging me, dressed in this slinky, you know, whatchamacallit. She was saying how much she wanted me, how much she loved me, how much she has missed being with me over the years. I couldn't pretend to be asleep anymore. I had to do what she wanted.

We went up to the bedroom, and the moment we started kissing, I started sweating, choking, heaving. I started crying. I thought I was going off the deep end. I wanted a drink so bad. I wanted to be out of that bedroom so bad. I just kept looking at her, knowing that she deserved to be with a man, not with me. I calmed down some, trying to pass this off as stress from work or something. She started kissing me again, this time on top of me. And then it happened [6]. I—I—please don't think that I'm—I lost my—I lost control of my—bowels—

and please don't—all over the bed [7]. I wanted to die. I went to the bathroom in a daze [8]. Cleaned up and left the house. And didn't come back for three days. I was on a binge.

When I stumbled back in that Sunday morning, I guess she couldn't take it anymore and arranged an intervention that afternoon without my knowing it. My wife, my son, my daughter, their families, my boss, two neighbors—wanted to send me to a rehab. I was yelling. I was denying I had a problem. I said it was all in her imagination. And she said, "No, Andrew, it's your imagination that got you here in the first place [9]."

She knew of Andrew all along, but never told me. I knew of Andrew all along, but just couldn't put him into words [10].

CLINICAL NOTES

1. Jake experienced blackouts for decades. Blackouts are akin to partial amnesia, with alterations in, but without loss of, consciousness.

2. As it can be for more than a few males with histories of CSA, Jake felt exposed around the person with whom he felt close, for she, from his vantage point, and due to such closeness, held more than enough ammunition to penetrate his walls of defense.

3. Jake was not after the "high" one can get from alcohol; he was on a mission to forget, not only his history but his present life as well, because it is through the present that memories of the past emerge. Although for some, blackouts are viewed as signs of hitting rock bottom, for Jake, such experiences were the irresistible, given that drinking to such a state elicited, for him, an "I don't care" attitude about the past as well as a lapse in memory about the present.

4. Jake was "forgetful" in many areas of his life. He viewed memory like an intricate structure of dominos: Release one, and they all come tumbling down.

5. Jake was so accustomed to concealing and invalidating the truth that playing possum in this context seemed to be the most natural thing to do. From situation to situation, day to day, he was invariably on the lookout for an exit. Interestingly, his life work involved the design and manufacturing of doors.

6. Prior to this moment, when Jake thought about sex, he often had olfactory flashbacks, which commonly led to choking and other autonomic and physiological reactions. In this moment, Jake's psychic, sensory, and nervous system circuitry overwhelmed itself.

7. In efforts to avoid defecation and his negative associations of it, Jake would intentionally constipate himself, regularly, for two weeks or more. His olfactory sensation of feces upon thinking of sex, coupled with his fear of losing control of his bowels, accomplished just that.

8. Jake was mortified, felt humiliated, dirty, and disgusting, the very things he experienced during his first episode of incest.
9. Astonishingly, Lena knew all along, not the details, but the disguise.
10. With protracted stress, the amygdala tends to overact, the hippocampus tends to overload, and Broca's area does not let a word escape. For this reason, Jake understood more than he could say. Splitting, dissociation, depersonalization, and derealization as well as other factors contributed to this process as well.

Ty

Some old lady in church said, "Be careful what you wish for, God's gonna give it to you." I been wishin' my whole life for love and all I got to show is just lots of memories of sex [1]. I always wanted to be a nurse or such. Somebody that does something good for somebody else [2]. But I ain't made that happen yet [3].

I don't know what to say about what my life has been like since I was a kid. I would like to tell you that I am happy. That I live in a little stone house with a swing on the porch and a dog in the yard. That I have a partner who loves me for me. And that I am trying to help people who got lost in life some way.

That's what I would like to tell you. But you would know that was a lie, right?

CLINICAL NOTES

1. Ty believed that sex was the gateway to love. He felt inferior across the domains of race, gender, and class; as an African American male with a sporadic history of employment, in addition to his being a male with a history of CSA, Ty viewed himself as second-rate on all accounts. When searching for partners, he was most attracted to men who were "rugged, wealthy, and White," all that he wanted to be, and, in his mind, all that he was not.
2. One of Ty's greatest desires was to give to others what he did not receive in his own life. However, a depleted sense of self-efficacy in the domains of education and work, in tandem with negative personal hypotheses about his life purpose, impeded the actualization of his dream.
3. For Ty, wishes and dreams were escape valves from his reality, not initiatives toward goal attainment. He lived according to the proposition: When someone loves me, then I will be happy, then I can go back to school, then I can get a good job, then I can have a home, then, then, then all will be well.

4. Ty was revealing goals and aspirations, all within the realm of possibility. However, from his perspective, such outcomes were disproportionately greater than his sense of self-worth.
5. Perhaps for the first time in his life, Ty was ready to explore the truth of his experience, unencumbered by his prolonged need to protect his mother and perpetrator. A moment such as this can initiate the validation of his horrific history of sexual abuse, violence, and neglect.

This chapter presented the authentic truths of seven males with histories of CSA. Application of the SAM model of dynamics and effects underscored their experiences by way of intrapsychic, interpersonal, familial, social, and cultural concepts, patterns, and themes. Now the SAM model can be translated into a philosophy of practice, treatment objectives, practice principles, practice analogy, and interventions.

PART TWO

CHAPTER SIX

THE SAM MODEL
OF PHILOSOPHY OF PRACTICE

A PHILOSOPHY OF PRACTICE is fundamental to the provision of conscious, viable, and purposeful services. It holds an overall vision of the sexual abuse of males and a view of its treatment. Although human behavior theories, practice models, and intervention strategies are central elements of biopsychosocial therapy, a philosophy of practice is perhaps even more critical, because it provides the lens through which all knowledge, values, principles, and skills filtrate. Finally, it specifies an integrated network of perspectives from which to conceptualize and execute practice that is systemically reasoned, culturally sensitive, gender specific, and developmentally congruent. This chapter presents the SAM model philosophy of practice.

THE SAM MODEL PHILOSOPHY OF PRACTICE

The philosophical perspectives that undergird the SAM model of practice are as follows: (1) the ecosystems perspective; (2) the multisystemic, multitemporal determinism perspective; (3) the parallel processes perspective; (4) the theoretical perspective; (5) the conceptual perspective; (6) the developmental perspective; (7) the relational perspective; (8) the dynamics and effects perspective; (9) the fact and meaning perspective; (10) the boy's perspective; (11) the self-determinative perspective; and (12) the strengths perspective. All perspectives recognize that childhood sexual abuse (CSA) is both a biopsychosocial phenomenon and, for many, a personal life event generating a myriad of effects, initial and long term, and conscious and unconscious. These effects, viewed in context, are conceptualized as purposeful and resourceful responses toward coping with, adapting to, and mastering the experience of CSA (Courtois, 1999; Herman, 1992; Lew, 1990).

The Ecosystems Perspective

To view a person such as SAM independent of impinging systems, and to view a biopsychosocial problem, such as CSA, independent of the person–environment context is to promote a vacuous understanding and, potentially, clinical negligence. Individuals, families, and groups, as well as intrapersonal, interpersonal, and social problems, must be viewed in a life context—that is, with respect to the biological, psychological, and sociological systems through which they occur and wherein they are experienced. Such an undertaking requires an ecosystems perspective (Bronfenbrenner, 1977, 1979; Garbarino, 1977, 1986; Germain & Gitterman, 1996), from which past and present, moment-to-moment, reciprocal interactions between and among individuals, families, groups, and environmental systems can be addressed within a multitemporal and multivariate framework.

A false dichotomy of biology, psychology, and sociology prevents a therapist from holistically understanding the dynamics and treating the effects of childhood sexual abuse. Human beings are endowed with chemically encoded information at the cellular level that makes each a member of the human species and each a unique individual. The human being, as an adaptive system, relies on its biology and psychology to discriminate, act on, and respond to the social environment. Transactions within social environment hold the capacity to promote or prevent biological or psychological well-being.

Working knowledge of biological factors is critical for understanding the ways in which SAM's brain, central nervous system, metabolic system, and immune system, among others, respond to CSA as well as initiate and maintain its effects. Knowledge of psychology is fundamental to appreciating the vast array of systems, constructs, and strategies that arise from or may be germane to SAM's subjection to CSA—cognitive appraisal, object relations, hyperarousal, dissociation, splitting, self-concept, cognitive dissonance, sensitization, habituation and generalization, and compulsive behaviors, to mention a few. Likewise, a conceptual and applied understanding of SAM's greater social context is imperative, including, but not limited to, his relationships with parents, caretakers, siblings, relatives, neighbors, teachers, and ministers, as well as relations with gender, sexual orientation, and racial, ethnic, socioeconomic, religious, and cultural reference groups. Such an understanding would also encompass institutional practices, policies, and procedures as they relate to the prevention, detection, and treatment of childhood sexual abuse. Further, knowledge of the social environment in which SAM, his perpetrator, and his family live is essential as it holds the socially constructed attitudes and beliefs that foster the existence of sexual abuse in the first place. For example, the myths around masculinity, femininity, sexuality, and abuse emanate from the macrosystem, an "invisible" yet uncompromising domain. To be sure, the macrosystem enforces concealment of CSA, requiring SAM to invalidate, reconcile, compensate for, and finally disown his history of childhood sexual abuse.

For example, when subjected to CSA as a sociological event, the experience is filtered through SAM's sensory receptors (Perry, 2001). The reception of sensory data successively commences a cascade of cellular and molecular processes that modify neuronal neurochemistry and cytoarchitechture, which, progressively, alters the structure and function of SAM's brain. Upon the boy's recognition that something violent is about to happen, fear registers in his amygdala (LeDoux, 1992). Unable to anatomically and psychologically accomodate the penetration of his father's penis, for example, he dissociates (Gartner, 1999). While dissociated, immune-boosting chemicals traverse to his internal organs to fight and ameliorate potential infection or injury (McEwen, 2000a). While dissociated, SAM vertically splits the internal representation of his father into the caring provider and the raging abuser (Grotstein, 1985). The next day at his soccer game, SAM, while dissociated, looks to his proud father in the stands after scoring a goal. In the shower room, SAM overhears other boys yelling about a teacher: "Mr. Adams, what a fag! He must like to get butt-fucked!" That night, as his father penetrates him once again, and unaware of the impact of social mythology, SAM reframes the abuse as homosexual activity, noting that such event would not be occurring if something wasn't intrinsically wrong with him. Given the protracted nature of CSA and his ceaseless and untold fears around a recurring episode, SAM's brain may be intermittently and vigorously steeped in chemicals, resulting in the suppression of hippocampal functioning (Bremner, 2002), thereupon producing memories, conscious or unconscious, absent of localization in space and time (van der Kolk, Burbridge, & Suzuki, 1997). Unless dissociated, he continuities to cognitively appraise the incest as an indication of his failure as a boy. Time and again, the action and efficacy of ego defense mechanisms may promote partial or full amnesia upon SAM's exposure to subsequent episodes of CSA (Terr, 1994). People seldom notice; SAM rarely discloses. Over the years, SAM's guilt for experiencing pleasure, his shame for failing to prevent the abuse from occurring, the dissociation between his implicit and explicit systems of memory, his fear of rejection by family, peers, and "society," his fear of losing an attachment, and the social bias toward the masculinization of perpetration and the feminization of victimization calculate prominently in this biological, psychological, and sociological concealment process (see, e.g., Carballo-Dieguez & Dolezal, 1995; Kellogg & Hoffman, 1997; LeDoux, 1992; Lew, 1990; Gordon, 1990; Sebold, 1987; Siegel, 1995; Sorenson & Snow, 1991; Spiegel, 1997; Woods & Dean, 1985).

Given his brain's lack of spatial or temporal context, his mind's inability to integrate the facts and meanings and his social environment's lack of support and validation, SAM's memories cannot become autobiographical (Siegel, 1999); rather, they remain wordless, free-floating, and with the capacity to materialize sensorially without apparent reason (Herman, 1992). Thus, biology, psychology, and sociology form a unitary system, or a person–environment gestalt, in which these tripartite systems mutually and reciprocally influence each other.

From the ecosystems perspective, therapists can interview, study, conceptualize, intervene, and evaluate by way of the intrapersonal domains, such as the cognitive, affective, behavioral, biological, historical, and spiritual, as well as the interpersonal domains, involving micro-, meso-, and exo-level relationships, and the social domain, highlighting macro-level blueprints. In this way, assessment, treatment, and evaluation, as parallel processes, are steadfastly biopsychosocial in nature, encompassing both internal and external systems, and highlighting the mutual, reciprocal, and interactive processes that elucidate the ecosystems perspective. More specifically, the ecosystems perspective directs therapists to take into account the SAM–environment interface, each with their own histories, developmental courses, and dynamics and effects, with each impinging on the other.

Multisystemic, Multitemporal Determinism

Across helping professions, academicians, therapists, theoreticians, and researchers engage in points/counterpoints as to the presence or absence of the unconscious, the utility or futility of social constructions, and the disuse, misuse, or overuse of posttraumatic stress disorder as a diagnostic category; CSA and SAM, however, are not so amenable. To the extent that a model of practice concerns itself with only one or a few seemingly relevant causal sources, its applicability, practicality, and reliability are greatly diminished. Sexual abuse effects are not circumscribed in a way that yields to linear causality; in fact, activating (e.g., developmental triggers such as SAM's first date, first sexual experience of choice, and birth of child), mediating (e.g., prior history of coping with trauma, early disclosure coupled with familial and judicial validation), and consequential (e.g., secondary elaborations of effects, therapeutic amelioration of effects) factors are often varied and numerous.

In light of the realities of the sexual abuse of males, as experienced in houses across the country, as disclosed in clinical settings, and as indicated by an evolving knowledge base, a complex of reciprocal determinism is both congruent and necessary. Although it may be easy to bring one CSA dynamic and one CSA effect to the foreground, to identify such a linkage as cause and effect is imprecise and inappropriate. Without question, a multivariate understanding of SAM is indispensable.

The philosophical inquiry into, the study of, and treatment directed toward the sexual abuse of males must recognize the intricate and permeating relationships between and among the intrapsychic, cognitive–affective–behavioral, and biophysical systems across the life span and within a transacting and interdependent multidimensional environment. That being so, the SAM model philosophy of practice holds the following assumptions about human behavior in the social environment:

1. For every action, there is an equal and opposite reaction. Thus, change in one part of a system impacts all parts of that system, including itself (Bertalanffy, 1968).
2. Interaction between the self-system and the environment is bidirectional; that is, it actualizes a process manifesting reciprocity (i.e., to give and take alternately; action/reaction) and/or mutuality (i.e., having the same reaction, one for the other) (Garbarino, 1977).
3. A system, be it individual, family, or group, strives for a goodness of fit between itself and the environment (Bronfenbrenner, 1977).
4. Biopsychosocial problems are viewed as outcomes of the transactions between and among many complex variables (Hollis & Woods, 1981).
5. All psychic events hold influential meanings and causes (A. Freud, 1936; Strupp, 1992).
6. All psychic events are influenced by the psychic events that precede them (Brenner, 1986).
7. Thoughts influence feelings; feelings influence behaviors; behaviors influence subsequent thoughts and feelings (Bandura, 1986; Mahoney, 1974).
8. Individuals, families, and groups search for and strive toward meaningful goals (Brower & Nurius, 1993; May & Yalom, 1995).
9. Individuals, families, and groups construct their own versions of reality through what they have experienced and, in turn, through what they have learned and, in turn, through what they perceive (Brower & Nurius, 1993).
10. Adaptation is a function of the perceptions of self, others, the world, and the future (Beck, 1993; Janoff-Bulman, 1992).
11. The greater social environment and, in particular, the macro level of the ecosystems perspective provide the context for understanding CSA as a social phenomenon and as a personal life event (Garbarino, 1977, 1986).

The Parallel Processes Perspective

Assessment, intervention, and evaluation are parallel processes, mutual and reciprocal in nature, guiding and informing one another throughout the duration of treatment. As data are solicited through the assessment process, interventions are formulated and executed, thereby generating more data, which can be assessed, analyzed, and utilized to create clinical hypotheses, treatment goals, and interventions with and for SAM. Furthermore, treatment success is dependent on the efficacy and the continuity of the assessment process. This is irrespective of such factors as short term/long term, psychodynamic/cognitive behavioral, or individual or group treatment. Assessment must be excellent notwithstanding the choice of treatment modality.

The sexual abuse of males knowledge base and the biopsychosocial practice knowledge base, in tandem, form the foundation from which treatment goals and objectives are operationalized into interventions. Interventions supported by a rationale promote purposive and deliberate practice. A rationale is comprised of the following: (1) a definition of the intervention; (2) a systematic description of its execution; and (3) its anticipated outcomes (see chapter 9). Developing interventions in this manner provides a cogent link between theory and practice, and between treatment goals and outcome, thereby enhancing practice congruency and efficacy.

For any type of evaluation, it is important to have definable, observable, and measurable treatment goals (Bloom, Fischer, & Orme, 1995). These outcomes can be either short term or long term. However, if the assessment is vague or incomplete, then the outcomes will be insufficient in their scope, failing to reflect either the actual target change areas or SAM's biopsychosocial context.

Case facts exist in a vacuum if therapists don't go beyond their occurrence and existence, if they don't reach for client meaning—in other words, the substance of the data, its signification and how it is conceptualized, rationalized, and operationalized by SAM. Facts alone (e.g., sexual abuse from ages 3 through 7, mother as perpetrator, father institutionalized) remain benign, and open to clinical imposition, until they are anchored in client meaning. Intervention exists in a vacuum if therapists do not elicit from SAM, let alone understand, his particular dynamics and effects, and the manifestations of each, both historic and current. Evaluation exists in a vacuum if the assessment goals are not operationalized into objectives, if objectives are not operationalized into treatment strategies, and if such strategies are not founded on anticipated outcomes, which, when definable, observable, and measurable, can be evaluated for efficacy.

Theoretical Perspective

The exclusive use of any one theoretical lens inevitably results in a type of "tunnel vision" that prohibits the identification of aspects of CSA external to that theory or, at the very least, greatly diminishes their importance. In other words, if the therapist's understanding of sexual abuse is limited to theories that only address abuse effects, or focus entirely on one major effect, such as posttraumatic stress disorder, then there is a risk of imposing specific sequelae onto individuals who may or may not, in the real world, experience those reactions. In other instances, a therapist may want to acknowledge and work with dissociation as an effect of CSA. Yet, depending on the school of thought, dissociation can be conceptualized as an unconscious intrapsychic phenomenon (Vaillant, 1992), a deliberate and avoidant behavior (Deblinger & Heflin, 1996), or, in some cases, a nonentity in the realm of human behavior (e.g., Ellis, 1995; Wolpe, 1990).

The limitations in expression and understanding, resulting from the utilization of only abuse-related theory, can be moderated by familiarity with other, non-abuse-related theories. Often these theories, such as systems, cognitive-behavioral, and psychodynamic, can provide a broader perspective through which the therapist can comprehend and conceptualize the complexity of material presented by SAM. Although symptoms such as flashbacks, repressed memories, and numbing or flooding are generally applicable only to those who have undergone a great deal of stress, anxiety, or trauma in their lives (and within that population, only a circumscribed subset), concepts such as assimilation, accommodation, schemata, and defenses are universal and hold relevance for all human beings—including, but not limited to, those with histories of CSA.

For example, by using a broader perspective to understand that SAM utilized defenses in no way restricts him to, say, the use of denial or repression. Not only does this understanding allow for a greater range of expression from SAM—one that can more accurately reflect his authentic and idiosyncratic responses—but it also allows his reactions to be viewed in context just as they are engendered and experienced in context. This broader knowledge base further serves the therapist and the client in understanding the normalcy and the congruency of patterns over SAM's life span.

Unless the abuse is seen in its context of actualization, intrapersonally, interpersonally, and socially, all abuse dynamics and effects are inevitably consigned to the individual, pathologizing SAM and denying the significant impact of the social environment. This further reinforces the perpetrator's perceptions and validates the social mythology surrounding sexual abuse rather than encouraging SAM's true expression of his unique experiences and reactions.

Conceptual Perspective

The therapist's biopsychosocial conceptualization of SAM is far-reaching, in that it suggests the terminology to be employed when assessing, intervening on behalf of, and evaluating the progress of males with histories of CSA. The therapist's words, as tools, convey an understanding of his or her perspective around sexual abuse as a personal matter as well as a biopsychosocial problem; these perceptions transmit to colleagues and clients alike.

One of the most common terms, historically and currently, permeating the sexual abuse literature is *victim*. This term is compelling, in that it properly places blame for CSA on the perpetrator, and with those who did not intervene, rather than on the child. Unfortunately, it holds negative connotations as well.

First, to address or describe SAM as a "victim" is to do so with regard to his abusive experiences but without regard to the growth and development that continue to emerge in response to, in spite of, and irrelevant to his history of CSA. Next, it serves to keep SAM fixated on the abuse, constraining him not only by time, but also within the psychological and sociological space of its occurrence. Consequently, events that took place before, during, and after the abuse receive only secondary or cursory attention. Further, the male perpetrator/female victim paradigm, by definition and design, allocates the "victim" role to females. A term like this one serves to disavow SAM, while simultaneously validating the social mythology concealing and invalidating, and thereby exacerbating SAM's experience of CSA.

Another term that has gained popularity in the literature is "survivor." Unlike "victim," the term "survivor" connotes images of resourcefulness and perseverance. However, like the term "victim," it remains bound to the time, place, and space of the abuse. Further, it does not necessarily place credit for having survived on SAM. He could alternatively have survived due to luck or to the "mercy" of the perpetrator. Moreover, to simply survive is, in and of itself, limiting and invalidating. "Survival," as treatment terminology, simply implies that SAM hung on, held out, and pulled through. It does not connote the learning, creativity, or growth—the breadth and depth of living—and the way SAM has turned, or can turn, tragedy into triumph.

"In recovery" is another common phrase utilized in treatment circles. Although, like the others, it holds positive connotations—to retrieve, to regain, and to restore—it unfortunately carries with it a disease implication in our society. Such terminology, then, becomes tainted with the idea that there was, or is, something "wrong" with SAM and that he is in the process of recovery, of being "cured." It is also a term that has become increasingly popular in the drug and alcohol field—an area that may, or may not, have any personal relevance to someone with a history of sexual abuse. Lastly, it is, again, a term bound to, and limited by, the abuse.

Although the ease of having a single term to distinguish a male with a history of sexual abuse is alluring, it is also misleading. In fact, anytime that one chooses a particular label to describe SAM, such as "victim" or "survivor," the label will necessarily limit, and therefore inevitably fail to capture, his true essence. In respect to the sexual abuse of males, the selection of only one specific term reinforces the separation of those aspects that have already been fractionated within and from the self, thus further inhibiting the integration of the abuse into individual and collective histories.

A Developmental Perspective

Although many people view sexual abuse as a discreet episode that occurred in the past, given the profound nature of this biopsychosocial problem, it is highly unlikely not to affect one's functioning in the present, or even in the future. In order to truly grasp the full range of SAM's being, it is necessary to view his history as evolutionary in nature—rather than fixated or "stuck" at the point of trauma. By keeping a pattern of awareness that combines intrapersonal, interpersonal, and social dynamics with preabuse, abuse, postabuse, and current perspectives, both the therapist and SAM can work toward a true integration of his experiences. Further, by integrating the past and the present, the abuse can, eventually, be seen as a part of the SAM's history much the same way that going to school was a part of his history—important, significant, and life changing, but not necessarily overwhelming, dictatorial, or shame-based.

Therapy, as a process toward integration, will eventually afford SAM an understanding of the connections between the past and the present, of the present to the future, and in doing so, help him regain a sense of feeling "whole" (Meiselman, 1990; Siegel, 1999). Cyclically then, this new awareness can help the client to gain an even greater understanding of events, both abusive and nonabusive, in the past—thus helping to increase his understanding of the present, and so forth. Through this process, which is both cyclical and dynamic in nature, SAM is afforded the opportunity not just to recover memories and to reclaim what was lost, but also to build on what already exists.

Relational Perspective

CSA and its treatment both occur within a relational context. Some theories promote this notion by viewing the relationship as a curative factor (e.g., psychodynamic, object relations, person-centered), whereas other theories demote this notion, regarding the interventions as curative (e.g., behavioral, cognitive-behavioral). To separate intervention from interventionist is to perceive the treatment process vacuously. The clinical relationship is a modus operandi (Courtois, 1988, 1999; Wilson & Lindy, 1994). Therefore, it is crucial that therapists be knowledgeable about human behavior and problems in a social context, facile in translating such knowledge into efficacious interventions and competent in evaluating treatment and progress, as well as masterful in initiating, developing, maintaining, and terminating relationships.

Across theories, the therapist is alternately conceptualized as a teacher, a trainer or an expert, often leading, directing, or determining the course of treatment. Given the context of sexual abuse, wherein SAM's authentic responses have been repeatedly contradicted, the therapist cannot act simply as the director of the therapeutic process without running the risk of replicating the same abusive dynamics. It is always appropriate and helpful for the therapist to provide opportunities for SAM to give direction to the course and depth of his therapy. No matter what the context—private practice, foster care, community mental health center, prison, psychiatric unit, or seminar—SAM is entitled to choice and has the right to self-determination. By presenting options, reaching for client feedback, and mutually deciding on directions for treatment, the therapist presents SAM with another occasion to build on his evolving sense of self-determination and self-worth.

When SAM is able and willing to focus on sexual abuse as a central issue, the therapist must make a decision as to whether to continue with him or to refer him to another treatment resource. If therapy is to progress, the therapist must be ready and willing to accept SAM's perceptions of his abuse, be able to conceptualize sexual abuse as happening within a greater social context, and view SAM's coping and adaptational strategies, present and past, as both beneficial and natural, even when they might be considered maladaptive in his current context. This acceptance not only lends validation to SAM's thoughts, feelings, and experiences, but also helps to increase his objectivity and sense of trust in terms of what he perceives, senses, and knows to be true.

Throughout the treatment process, the therapist is alternately a guide, a witness, and an ally (Herman, 1992) to SAM and must be able to transition from one role to the other in response to both SAM's wants and needs at any given time, as well as in accord with particular phases of, or interventions during, treatment. For example, as SAM tells his story, the therapist simultaneously acts as a guide in order to help provide structure, as a witness to events once kept concealed, and as an ally to provide support for SAM.

During the early phases of treatment, it is important that the therapist not dispute SAM's self-attributions, his misattributions, or any other perceptions around the abuse. Doing so diminishes the environment in which SAM can express his authentic feelings. Further, it is evidence that the therapist is not taking the time necessary to understand the rationale behind SAM's perceptions. This will inevitably convey to SAM that the therapist does not comprehend, and cannot relate to, his biopsychosocial reality.

However, with patience and acceptance, the therapist has the ability to place CSA in context, both micro and macro, without being perceived as attacking or as threatening. From intake to termination, CSA can be explored in a broader social context. This presents SAM with numerous and necessary opportunities to see, hear, and experience not only the therapist believing in the reality of sexual abuse, but also understanding the contemptible and often irrepressible intrapersonal, interpersonal, and social dynamics and effects. As a result, two vital consequences arise—validation and affirmation. Such interactions and outcomes, for SAM, are invaluable.

This contextual analysis also offers SAM the chance to realize that the therapist views his reactions as a natural response to an unnatural event. For example, since SAM often presents stating that he feels as if he's "going crazy," the therapist, without arguing directly with him, can gently dispute this reaction in a way that promotes an empathic understanding. The therapist, with the insight that there are many lies inherent in sexual abuse—lies about love, lies about trust—could say to SAM: "For years now, you've had to pretend that something that has happened, has not, and you had to pretend that something that does hurt, does not. From where I sit, it's easy to understand why you might feel as if you are 'going crazy.'"

It is also important for both the therapist and SAM to realize that the clinical relationship is mutual but is not meant to be reciprocal. Boundaries exist to maintain the intention and integrity of the treatment process and to protect both parties from exploitation or misuse. Despite these boundaries, however, it is a relationship in which there is a give and take (i.e., mutuality), only the giving and the taking are not of the same things (i.e., reciprocity).

Whereas the client is "giving" of himself, disclosing and telling the truth, the therapist is "giving" support, guidance, hope, knowledge, and skills. It is the client's, not the therapist's, wants and needs that are the focus, and the client's expressed feelings and points of view that are encouraged and sought by the therapist. The focus must remain on SAM because the personal wants and needs of the therapist are rarely stepping-stones to the eventual goal of integrating his history of abuse within his life story.

However, as many other microrelationships in the SAM's life are expected to be both mutual and reciprocal, it is natural for him to impose a social model on the therapeutic relationship. This may be because a social model feels more comfortable and familiar, or because the client believes that when his needs override the wants or needs of another, he is, consequently, acting like a perpetrator.

Yet SAM's sense of self-worth is externalized, that is, a function of his ability to tend to the needs and demands of others. This is a consequence of the abusive relationship, wherein he was required to take care of, respond to, and protect the perpetrator from others who might find out about the abuse. Thus, if the boundaries are blurred within the therapist/client relationship, SAM may respond by repeating this role of caregiver to the therapist rather than focusing on his own needs.

It is vital that SAM have the opportunity to perceive and experience the therapist as someone who is receptive, interested, sincere, and giving, but not as someone who needs to be taken care of or protected. Given his overarching tendency to care about others, this frees SAM to explore, identify, and learn how to meet his own needs without simultaneously attempting to balance the wants and need of another person. Such an opportunity is unique to the therapeutic relationship and is also of great worth to SAM.

The fact remains that, since sexual abuse meanings and effects originated within a relationship, constructive change must take place in a relational context, too. While the abusive relationship yields exploitation, betrayal, and mistrust, the clinical relationship provides SAM with the opportunity to have an emotionally corrective experience infused with trust, integrity, care, and respect, both for self and for others. More to the point, within the clinical relationship, this developing knowledge can be translated into viable skills that can eventually generalize across any number of settings and circumstances.

Dynamics and Effects Perspective

Dynamics refer to intrapersonal, interpersonal, and/or social forces that initiate and maintain the sexually abusive relationship; the ways in which the boy was subjected, the sexual activities involved, and the ways in which secrecy was enforced. The effects of sexual abuse are conceptualized as the consequences engendered by the dynamics, such as invalidation, reconciliation, and compensation.

Dynamics are located across all systems, from micro to macro. The individual dynamics (e.g., the resistance to accepting signs of disclosure from the child), the dynamics of the perpetrator (e.g., manipulation used to enforce consent), and the social dynamics (e.g., social service messages and interventions aimed almost exclusively toward females) are all interactive and of equal importance to understanding the full context of the sexual abuse of males.

Initial effects are those that are manifested during and between abusive episodes. Aftereffects develop shortly after termination of the abuse and may persevere for months, years, or decades (Finkelhor, 1986). Effects are also experienced and/or defended across systems (in the living room, on the playground, and at church) and across the life span, including developmental milestones such as the first date, high school graduation, first consensual sexual experience, marriage and partnership, and parenthood, to mention a few. SAM is continually involved in a cycle of concealment, invalidation, and reconciliation. At any given moment, he is concealing the abuse while trying to believe that it did not happen; simultaneously, he is assuming responsibility for its occurrence while compensating for its effects.

Finally, to view effects independent of dynamics is to pathologize the client by locating the problem as lying solely within the self-system. Conversely, to view dynamics independent of effects is to "politicize" the society by locating the problem as lying solely within the greater social context. In the former, all attention is given to the individual with little effort being made to effect social change; in the latter, there is much discussion concerning the magnitude of the problem, but little effort made to provide treatment services that could tangibly help SAM. Thus, treatment must take into account the nature of the interaction between dynamics and effects, which is both fluid and dynamic.

Facts and Meaning Perspective

While the treatment of sexual abuse may seem like, and often is, a fact-finding mission, it is imperative that facts be infused with client meaning. A fact, such as "Nicholas was sexually abused by his mother's boyfriend," in and of itself, lacks contextual meaning. Consider, now, that fact, coupled with the client's points of view: "I wanted it to stop, 'cause it hurt me bad . . . but I didn't want it to stop, 'cause Terry wouldn't love me no more and he would leave my Mama." The fact and meaning, in tandem, place the sexual abuse in context, reflect and affirm SAM's authentic experience, point to conflict within and between intrapersonal, micro, and meso systems, and suggest windows of opportunity for intervention. However, a fact independent of contextual meaning opens the door to assumptive thinking, projection, and, quite conceivably, false logic and misinterpretation.

Thus, it is important that SAM delineate not only the facts of his story, but the cognitive and affective meaning imbuing the facts, for they hold and reveal the story behind the facts, the story behind the story. To explore, identify, and experience the facts and meanings is to establish, tell, and reclaim the truth as SAM knows it to be.

At the same time, it is critical that SAM be "in charge" of the facts of his story. Memory is viewed as a state-dependent process (Perry et al., 1995; van der Kolk & Fisler, 1995; van der Kolk, 1997), mediated by biological factors, such as SAM's stress response, hippocampal functioning, and efficiency of Broca's area (Bremner et al., 1999; Chu, 1998; Rauch et al., 1996), psychological factors, including depth and degree of dissociation, the cognitive accommodation of abuse-related schemata, and the presence or absence of splitting (Davies & Frawley, 1994; Janoff-Bulman, 1992; Pearlman & Saakvitne, 1995), and sociological factors, for example, lack of opportunity to verbalize the experience to others, fear of rejection by others, and an infiltrating sense of gender shame (Bauer et al., 1998; Fivush & Schwarzmueller, 1995; Lisak, 1995); all of these serve to impede the process of transposing implicit memory into explicit memory and, ultimately, translating the abuse experience into a cohesive autobiographical narrative (Schore, 1996; Siegel, 1995, 1999).

With maximal respect for SAM's memories of CSA and the factors that mediate their retrieval, it is critical that he be perceived as the one in command over the facts of his story, when they emerge, under what conditions, and what meaning they hold. The therapist is not the retriever of SAM's memories, but the receiver. Memory retrieval is neither a tactic nor a goal (Courtois, 1999). As SAM spontaneously conveys his memories by way of uncontrived and noninvasive means, he and the therapist rely on content and process interventions applicable to any form of legitimate psychotherapy. "The aim is not to develop deeper and deeper memories of more and more abuse; rather, the patient must gradually face and accommodate the occurrence and meaning of any abuse as it is known and resolve associated feelings" (p. 154). That is SAM's charge, if he chooses to accept it.

The Boy's Perspective

The reconstruction and reintegration (Briere, 1996a; Herman, 1992; van der Hart, Steele, Boon, & Brown, 1993) of the abusive experience must be founded on the boy's perspective, regardless of SAM's chronological age. The boy's perspective holds the facts of the abuse and the cognitive and affective meaning associated with them. More often than not, the perspectives of adults with histories of abuse, as well as their perpetrators, family members, and significant others, are mediated by mythology around the abuse or, at the very least, adult sensibilities. The former includes notions such as "If you got an erection, then it wasn't abuse" and "You must have wanted it to happen"; the latter is often expressed as "Well, that happened such a long time ago. It shouldn't have any impact now." The story told from these perspectives is vastly different from what SAM experienced as a boy.

Thus, it is important that SAM tell his story, from his boyhood perspective, in his own way. Typically, SAM will disclose his history in a piecemeal fashion—moving from the general to the specific, from dissociated to emotionally laden content, from seemingly neutral to shame-based disclosures, and from adult sensibilities to boyhood authenticity. Authentic fact and meaning will only come when the therapist presents consistent indicators of receptivity and comfortability with SAM's topic and terminology and is capable of actively and empathically listening to and understanding his life story.

Self-Determinative Perspective

Self-determination promotes SAM's right to exercise choice, which, in turn, helps him to reestablish a sense of agency. Therapists need to remember that, even when they disagree with SAM, he is making the best possible decisions with the information available to him at any given moment. Moreover, excepting times whereby SAM may be dangerous to himself or to others, he has the uncircumscribed right to decide how to conduct his own life. The client is also entitled to change his opinions and/or behaviors at any time. It is important to realize, however, that self-determination is moot unless SAM has the knowledge and ability to take advantage of potential options presented to him. For example, if SAM is not familiar with certain needed resources available in the community, then he will not be able to make an informed decision.

One of the tasks of the therapist is to validate SAM's self-worth and honor his dignity by providing options and support, enabling him to maximize his quality of life. For instance, SAM might express an interest in therapy around CSA but be unsure of how to proceed. The therapist can present various options to him (i.e., individual therapy, group therapy, a support group, or the option to do nothing at this time); in turn, both can explore the positive and negative, and short-term and long-term, consequences of each option. The way in which these options are introduced and explored must be in a manner that is both supportive of and encouraging to him, as well as validating of his fears, concerns, expectations, anticipations, and ambivalence.

While presenting different options to SAM, the therapist encourages him to make his own choices, as SAM is the locus of control of the therapeutic process (Chu, 1998). It is the therapist's task to offer guidance, but SAM must arrive at his own decision as to how he wishes to proceed. In this way, the therapeutic relationship can provide an environment that enhances and fosters the self-determination of the client. By allowing SAM to devise his own plan of action, the therapist is affirming, and building on, his decision-making abilities. Although the therapist generally acts as the guide for the therapeutic process, it is important, given the context of sexual abuse, that the client be offered every opportunity to take a leadership role, or at least an egalitarian role, so as to not, in any manner, replicate his previous experiences with imposing relationships that have overridden or discounted his will in the past (Briere, 1996a; Herman, 1992; Sgroi, 1989).

Strengths Perspective

An exploration and identification of both SAM's strengths and challenges is an integral part of the treatment process. If strengths remain unacknowledged, SAM is denied access to inherent or cultivated resources. An exclusive focus on strengths and potentialities, or, conversely, on dysfunctions and pathologies, however, amplifies the illusion of mutual exclusivity; if "this" exists then "that" does not. Furthermore, it intimates that a person with psychopathology is inherently weak and that a person without dysfunctional behavior is inherently strong. Given the context of CSA, however, this logic is insensitive and, moreover, inaccurate.

If psychopathology is present, it can be framed as a natural and spontaneous response to an unnatural and premeditated event (Courtois, 1988). Its existence need not diminish the therapist's appreciation of the creativity, endurance, and potentialities of SAM. If the therapist is unable to perceive and articulate SAM's strengths, then given his skewed view of self, he may walk away from the therapeutic process simply having his belief in the social mythology enforced and having his authentic self disregarded yet again.

Strengths can be conceptualized as positive characteristics, traits, intentions, competencies, capabilities, capacities, attitudes, attributes, resources, talents, and aspirations within self-systems and across microsystems (Saleeby, 1992). It may be easy to identify surface strengths, that is, strengths that are easily recognizable, at first or second glance—a sense of humor, perseverance, or comfort in expressing emotions. In contrast, embedded strengths, embryonic, yet with potential, are often overlooked and untapped. For example, the intention to laugh at one's foibles, the ability to express emotions freely, and the resource of historic perseverance frequently lie dormant beneath beliefs such as "I'm a failure as a male" and "I don't deserve to have a good life," as well as feelings of shame and inferiority. Still, they are strengths, with the potential to arise from obscurity.

Whether surface or embedded, strengths help therapists to understand how SAM has developed and achieved in defiance of CSA and its effects. Not only that, strengths warrant a name, for, like any other aspect of life, it is only through acknowledgment and identification that inherent or ascribed meaning can come to light. Without a name, a potential strength remains idle or latent, with little or no value.

SUMMARY

This chapter presented 12 philosophical principles germane to developing and executing a treatment protocol for the effects of childhood sexual abuse. The SAM model philosophy of practice is in accordance with the ethical codes of several professional organizations, including the American Psychiatric Association, the National Association of Social Workers, and the American Psychological Association. A practice philosophy is key, for it imbues the therapeutic endeavor with guideposts, values, and meaning. In essence, these 12 philosophical principles comprise an applicable standard of practice in the treatment of males with histories of CSA.

CHAPTER SEVEN

PREPARATORY EMPATHY

THE NOTION OF *EMPATHY* derives from the Germanic concept of *einfuhlung*; the "ein" prefix implies something from outside moving into something else; "fuhlung" is the noun version of the state of feeling; thus, "einfuhlung" literally translated denotes one person feeling into another. Empathy, as a psychotherapeutic skill, encompasses two primary actions: (1) the act of impartially perceiving, reflecting on, and conceptualizing the client's person/environment configuration of dynamics and effects (Bowlby, 1988; Winnicott, 1960), and (2) the act of accurately communicating such an understanding to the client (Strupp & Binder, 1984; Kohut, 1959) with objectivity and tolerance. Thus, empathy is personified as and evidenced by (1) the therapist's proficiency in entering and beholding, psychologically, cognitively, affectively, and physiologically, a client's inner world, for example, his or her conscious, preconscious, and unconscious mental activity; (2) entering and beholding the client's external being, within and across microenvironments; and (3) entering and beholding his or her phenomenological points of view, both historically and currently (Wilson & Lindy, 1994), as well as (4) the therapist's adeptness in synthesizing and making sense of the incoming data (Lichtenberg, Bornstein, & Silver, 1984) and (5) the therapist's dexterity in expressing, verbally and nonverbally, the client's surface and underlying experience (Kohut, 1959). Metaphorically, the therapist functions like a pendulum, beginning with an invitational stance, decentering into subjective and active participation in order to identify with SAM's history of CSA within the greater context of his life story, then moving back into objective detachment, wherein the therapist contemplates SAM's dynamics and effects with a sense of neutrality and centering once again to accurately and sensitively reflect SAM's multidimensional experience.

PREPARATORY EMPATHY

Empathy is a cardinal component of therapy; not only can empathy be sustained through the therapeutic process (Pearlman & Saakvitne, 1995), it can also be employed as a preparatory measure in working with SAM. This chapter focuses on the ways in which a beginning therapist or a therapist new to the field of childhood sexual abuse can attune to the established dynamics and effects within the sexual abuse of males knowledge base and to the potential motivic forces and impacts of therapy before treatment begins. With a view toward the cultivation of preparatory empathy, topics in this chapter include the sexual abuse of males knowledge base, the therapeutic alliance, the role of the therapist, SAM's presentation in therapy, their egalitarian relationship, safety and trust, transference and countertransference, and policies and procedures that support and advance the therapeutic process.

The SAM Knowledge Base

Without question, the sexual abuse of males knowledge base is an indispensable resource. Although commonly viewed as "embryonic" or in its early stages of evolution (Gartner, 1999; Mendel, 1995), it holds a number of instructive documents, including reviews of the literature (e.g., Holmes & Slap, 1998; Watkins & Bentovim, 1992), empirical studies (e.g., Bagley et al., 1994; Paul et al., 2001; Spencer & Tan, 1999), clinical reports (e.g., Morrell, Mendel, & Fischer, 2001) and books (e.g., Gartner, 1999; Hunter, 1990a, 1990b; Lew, 1990). There are a number of other excellent references within the general CSA knowledge base. Please refer to the references for authors and titles.

Childhood sexual abuse can be conceptualized by way of its dynamics and effects, within the context of biological, psychological, and sociological theory and research. In terms of the sexual abuse of males empirical base, it is imperative that the therapist have a working knowledge of the dynamics and effects most commonly associated with SAM. For example, prevalent dynamics include perpetrators' selection criteria, their subjection strategies, the rationales they construct and uphold to initiate and maintain the sexually abusive relationship, the ways in which they expose a boy to drugs, alcohol, pornography, and enemas, their use of physical violence, threats, and bribes, familial and social responses to a boy's abuse, and the dynamics of social mythology, to mention a few (see, e.g., Kelly et al., 2002; Lamb & Edgar-Smith, 1994; Lisak, 1995; Melchert & Parker, 1997; Mendel, 1995; Spencer & Tan, 1999).

Initial effects, that is, outcomes manifesting within 2 years of the abusive episodes (Finkelhor, 1986) encompass a divergent array of symptoms and coping strategies, including the acquisition of sexually explicit knowledge, penile and perianal erythema, concentration difficulties, enuresis, encopresis, invalidation tactics, dissociation, splitting, self-blame, dichotomous thinking, nightmares and night terrors, sexually transmitted diseases, and trauma symptomology (see, e.g., Fontenella et al., 2000; Gully et al., 2000; Kinard, 2001; McLeer et al., 1998; Wells et al., 1997). Aftereffects, or symptoms and coping strategies experienced by boys and adolescent and adult males with histories of CSA 2 or more years after the first abusive episode, vary in terms of their chronology and chronicity. They include, but are not limited to, habituated and generalized fear responses, autonomic dysregulation, prolonged use of defense strategies, overreliance on compensatory procedures, confusion around gender identity and sexual orientation, compensatory maneuvers, repetitive relational patterns, workplace difficulties, compulsions and addictions, anxiety, depression, and posttraumatic stress symptomology (see, e.g., Dilorio et al., 2002; Fondacaro et al., 1999; Gill & Tutty, 1999; Olson, 1990; Lisak & Luster, 1994; Teicher et al., 1997).

In essence, the knowledge base holds lists of dynamics and effects in a one-dimensional format—the word. An effective method of conceptualizing a biopsychosocial problem, and elucidating its dynamics and effects, is the What–How–Why formula. In general, *What* is the first level of conceptualization, the acknowledgment of the existence of a dynamic or effect and its definition. *How* is necessary because it illuminates the processes by which something emerges or the mechanics by which something works. Such processes and mechanics may concern, for example, how the use of force is differentially employed by male and female perpetrators or how an abused boy's confusion between sexual orientation and gender identity reflects corresponding social constructions, and so on. *Why*, too, holds significance, as it provides a rationale, a reason why a dynamic is universal, why a constellation of effects emerges disproportionately among males or why a certain effect generates secondary elaborations. *What*, alone, merely identifies and defines; *How* and *Why* bring both the phenomena and, consequently, the conceptualization to a more concrete level.

As a case in point, when considering encopresis as an initial effect highlighted in the sexual abuse of males knowledge base, the *What* might be defined as the involuntary or, in some cases, intentional impaction or discharge of fecal matter (Morrow et al., 1997). As for the *How*, withholding, purposefully or otherwise, promotes the formation of large stool in the rectum. Such an obstruction, over time, may induce the bowel to malfunction. And the *Why* of encopresis may result from a number of interrelated factors correlated with CSA, including a loose anal sphincter and poor anal tone (Bowen & Aldous, 1999; Gully et al., 2000), discomfort in the bathroom (Kolko et al., 1988), shame associated with the genital and anal area (Spiegel, 1997b), and the misuse of enemas for nonmedical reasons (Spiegel, 1998). If the encopresis is involuntary, it may be due to the physical effects of the abuse in the anus and rectum. A number of biological, psychological, and social factors impinge on SAM's ability to discern if and when a bowel movement is necessary: (1) the physical pain engendered by the penetrating penis; (2) discomfort from the effects of penetration, such as anal fissures, irritation, spasms, and pain; (3) SAM's sense of abuse-generated gender shame linked to his genital and rectal regions; (4) his fear and avoidance of public and private bathrooms; and (5) the intermittent cycling of impaction and loss of control. Consequently, constipation occurs and, in due course, liquid stool leaks around the impaction. Although the impaction may not be intentional, SAM, in dreading another episode of sexual abuse, may purposefully expel fecal matter in order to repel the perpetrator. In either case, the CSA effect of encopresis gives rise to its own biopsychosocial aftermath, including, within the microdomain, the frustration and confusion of parents, taunting and rejection from peers, and anger and aggression from the perpetrator. For SAM, or the self-system, biopsychosocial effects of encopresis include potential bowel malfunction, the risk for toxicity, an increase in shame and humiliation, a decrease in self-esteem and self-efficacy, and the need to isolate from others. Thus, the rippling consequences of CSA dynamics and effects are not confined to the sexually abusive relationship. Rather, they eventually encroach upon and across SAM's microenvironments—the neighborhood, his school, his church, and the ballpark.

Working in this way, especially for therapists new to the CSA field, bridges the conceptual with the applied, minimizes the tendency to reify concepts—that is, treating concepts as if they are human entities, rather than expressions of human behavior—and bridges the theoretical with the empirical or the abstract with the concrete. Further, addressing the *What, How,* and *Why* of phenomena enhances the explanatory power of the therapist's conceptualizations, adds depth and dimension to his or her analyses, and anchors such phenomena in SAM's biopsychosocial context. Additionally, the therapist's knowledge-driven and ecosystemic formulation contributes to the standard of care necessary to inquire into, understand, reflect, and validate SAM's experience within the confines of the therapeutic relationship.

The Therapeutic Relationship

The relationship forged by SAM and therapist is, perhaps, the most critical and efficacious of all the foundational elements of the therapeutic process (Courtois, 1988; Herman, 1992). It can be conceptualized along the lines of Bowlby's (1988) and Winnicott's (1960, 1962) holding environment, a place for safekeeping and a relationship that encompasses a repository for the client's pain along with a reservoir of therapeutic empathy, hope, and healing. From intake to termination, a holding environment can be operationalized by the regularity of sessions in terms of time and space, the consistency of opening and closing rituals, the steadfastness of the therapist's relational stance, adherence to the integral boundaries and limitations of the therapeutic relationship, and the empathic and supportive constancy provided by both the therapist and the therapeutic process (Winnicott, 1965).

The therapeutic relationship is unique in comparison to other interpersonal relationships and fundamental to the majority of therapeutic approaches. More specifically, the ethically sound, theory-driven therapeutic alliance can be transformative for SAM (Gartner, 1999; Meiselman, 1990; Pearce & Pezzot-Pearce, 1997). As he begins to talk about and eventually reexperience, in the safety of the therapeutic space, his emotionally laden, intrapsychically defended, and interpersonally concealed abuse dynamics and effects—for example, the betrayal, the shame, the dread of being perceived as deviant, the fear of going crazy—change begins to occur. And when both the therapist and the therapeutic process generate for and with SAM intrapersonal points of view and interpersonal processes unlike those he experienced as a boy and contrary to those he anticipates and fears, then constructive change deepens.

The therapeutic process offers the structure and the therapeutic alliance generates the security that facilitates the unfolding nature of the treatment wherein trust builds, defenses relax, bona fide meaning emerges, myths recede, and the author of an embedded abuse story finds his voice. The process advances slowly; the alliance develops gradually (Davies & Frawley, 1994); and all along the way, empathy deepens. The explicit and implicit limits and boundaries inherent in the therapeutic process function to initiate and sustain a viable and nonexploitive therapist/client working atmosphere, protect SAM's right to and privilege of privacy, and foster the actualization of his goals and aspirations. Further, such a special and unique relationship can only begin, exist, and terminate within the treatment setting. Dual relationships solely serve to exacerbate a client's sense of boundary diffusion and role confusion. Accordingly, the therapist can occupy only one position and hold only one purpose in SAM's life (Courtois, 1988).

THE THERAPIST

The therapist's interpersonal stance (Herman, 1992; Pearlman & Saakvitne, 1995), specifically, his or her relational availability, emotional responsivity, and session-to-session consistency, contribute to the formation and safekeeping of the holding environment (Bowlby, 1988; Winnicott, 1962). Held in this way, SAM can begin to experience a sense of safety more acutely, delve into his subjective world more deeply, remember the abuse dynamics and effects more fully, and explore, identify, and express the meaning emanating from his history of CSA more authentically.

Central to the therapeutic alliance and the sustainment of empathy is the therapist's ability to be both participant in and observer of the therapeutic process (Davies & Frawley, 1994; Herman, 1992). This dual function is not dichotomous in nature—that is to say, if one participates then one cannot observe—but rather complementary in form. As a participant, the therapist enters into the subjective world of SAM in order to understand his experience; as an observer, she or he examines and notes phenomena as they occur in SAM's life with particular regard for the conscious and unconscious, the internal and external, his biology, psychology, and sociology. As a participant, the therapist joins SAM in articulating the dynamics and effects of his history of CSA; as an observer, he or she empathizes with SAM and validates his experience, giving credence to his history of CSA, both verbally and nonverbally, with the understanding that traumatic remnants and shards impacted him then, influence him now, and shape the experience of the therapeutic relationship.

As SAM's cocreator of the therapeutic alliance (Gartner, 1999), the therapist engages in a number of different but reciprocal roles: that of guide, ally, witness, and caretaker surrogate (Courtois, 1988; Herman, 1992). As ally, the therapist holds with the utmost regard SAM's request for help and harbors an unflappable commitment to the integrity of the therapeutic process. Grounded in theory, guided by clinical wisdom, and informed by the sexual abuse of males knowledge base, the therapist as ally normalizes and contextualizes SAM's abuse effects, respects the creation of and the purpose undergirding his defensive strategies, appreciates and works through the transferential and countertransferential elements of the therapeutic relationship, and from beginning to end, strives to cultivate SAM's sense of agency, humor, and hope (see, e.g., Chu, 1999; Friedrich, 1996; Gil & Johnson, 1993).

As guide and educator, the therapist (1) imparts valuable information about the therapeutic process, (2) provides data regarding the dynamics and effects of CSA that demystify SAM's experience, (3) develops and modifies interventions so they are gender specific, ethically and racially sensitive, and developmentally congruent, (4) operates within a frame that accommodates both the therapeutic necessity of in-depth uncovering work and SAM's readiness and emotional state at any given time, and (5) helps SAM discover and cultivate empathy for the disowned aspects of the self, all in service of reintegration (see, e.g., Crowder, 1995; Meiselman, 1990; Salter, 1995). And, as witness, the therapist upholds a persevering and stabilizing presence as SAM reconstructs his history of abuse, listens actively to his authentic recollections, holds his pain, shame, and loathing, honors his resistance, understands his ambivalence, and empathizes with the boy he was and the man he wants to be.

THE CLIENT

When SAM embarks on the therapeutic process, he brings with him not only a history of childhood sexual abuse, but also a compelling legacy of CSA, explicitly, a history of intrapersonal, relational, and systemic invalidation. From the moment he was first subjected to CSA and perhaps until the moment he enters the clinical room, SAM's perception, experience, and understanding of his harrowing past have been contravened and disavowed, certainly by the perpetrator, most likely by himself, and without question by the social environment in which he was born to prosper and grow.

Pervasive and unimpeded personal and social invalidation engenders its own enduring effects. In the midst of nullified childhood horror, his experience rendered void by others, SAM is left uncertain as to the facts of his story and of the genuine (albeit camouflaged) meaning infiltrating the facts. Without a doubt (but for his own and those who don't believe him), what he saw, what he heard, what he smelled, what he tasted, what was touched, and what he thought or felt were invalidated in service of the perpetrator's pathology and social mythology.

Invalidation, to be sure, is far-reaching. To cite a particular example, SAM's language, as a matter of course, is notably filled with pronouncements such as "I think I'm making a big deal out of nothing" and "It sounds like I'm exaggerating or trying to be dramatic" and phrases such as "it was sort of like," "kind of like," "um, like, you know," and pervasive questions, including "Do you see what I'm saying?" and "Am I crazy or what?" (Lew, 1990). SAM not only learns to mistrust his perceptions of the abuse (Briere, 1996a), but as mistrust generalizes across microsystems, he also learns to mistrust himself, others, and the world in which he lives (Janoff-Bulman, 1989; Klein & Janoff-Bulman, 1996). Rarely certain that his perceptions are accurate or, for that matter, in the ballpark and scarcely sure that anyone perceives or experiences life as he does, SAM perpetually throws doubt on his sense of normalcy and sanity. Additionally, in order to compensate for his palpable sense of confusion and perplexing sense of transparency, SAM tends to communicate with the pedantic tone of an academician—cautiously metered, grammatically exact—and at the expense of authentic meaning and spontaneity. By the same token, SAM may have refined a seemingly indifferent style of communication, allowing him to maintain a gender-directed illusion of emotional control and to act "as if" all is well (Lew, 1990).

How challenging it is for SAM, after weeks, months, and years of systemic invalidation, to perforate his authentic self, to discern his thoughts and feelings about what happened then and what is occurring now, to recognize his inherent worth and to ascertain his purpose in life. Even if he could reach inside his silences, find his thoughts and feelings and put them into words, he fears that others simply could not understand, let alone respect, what he has to say and what he would like to do. But he can and will unearth the particular words and discover the only voice that can author and narrate his story of childhood sexual abuse.

Indeed, SAM is the primary locus of control in this therapeutic endeavor (Briere, 1996b; Faller, 1988). Therefore, it is critical that the therapist be cognizant of and sensitive to the power dynamics of the relationship (Courtois, 1988, 1999), even if he or she does not view and/or experience himself or herself as "powerful." The fact remains that the role of therapist is imbued with notions of authority, scholarship, expertise, and specialization. Still, she or he must strive to create and sustain an egalitarian relationship and, in doing so, help SAM to reclaim from brutality and unmistakably experience his rights to agency, dignity, and equality.

AN EGALITARIAN RELATIONSHIP

Just as there are dynamics that initiate and maintain the sexually abusive relationship, there are dynamics that undergird the therapeutic alliance. On that ground, SAM and the therapist, their relationship, and the therapeutic process hold the potential to "replicate" his abuse dynamics. Simply on the face of it, the therapist is often perceived as an expert, a role model, and an authority figure. SAM, once again, is in a vulnerable position, fearful of yet dependent on the therapist. SAM, alone but for the therapist, plays with a sand tray, lies on a couch, or sits in a chair; what they say and do remains behind closed doors where confidentiality is key. Therapy harbors social stigma; SAM often feels a sense of shame and inferiority around "having to go to therapy," just as he does for having been sexually abused. In therapy, money is exchanged for professional services; in sexual abuse, currency, perhaps money, special privileges, gifts, and the like, are exchanged for sex. Moreover, if SAM is subjected to the needs of the therapist—for example, to his or her discomfort with sexually explicit language, emotionally volatile expression, or avoidance due to unanticipated countertransferential reactions—SAM will likely and spontaneously revert to the role of caretaker and consequently abdicate his own truth, just as he did with the perpetrator. To be precise, the therapeutic relationship—like any other relationship—holds the potential to both harm and to heal.

To buffer against harm and in light of SAM's history of betrayal and injustice, the therapeutic relationship is most equitable and efficacious when coconstructed by SAM and the therapist (Gartner, 1999). In concert, they build an egalitarian alliance (Bolton, Morris, & MacEachron, 1989; Briere, 1996a; Courtois, 1999; Crowder, 1995; Herman, 1992; Meiselmen, 1990; Salter, 1995) that sets the context for change, with SAM as the change agent and the therapist as an agent of empathy, guidance, and support. SAM is the expert when it comes to his history of abuse (Crowder, 1995); the therapist has expertise in the art and science of sexual abuse therapy; the therapist facilitates the therapeutic process and SAM holds responsibility for his own amelioration. Together, they cocreate the transference and countertransference dynamics and effects throughout the course of treatment (Gartner, 1999), just as they mutually consider treatment plans, intervention strategies, and indicators of goal attainment. In this relationship, SAM has the freedom to agree and disagree without consequence, to negotiate issues around the timing, pacing, and context of uncovering work, to take a break, to leave and return, all without judgment, simply with understanding (Courtois, 1988). As cocreators, though, SAM and the therapist must keep the pathways of communication as open and frank as possible.

As for the therapist, he or she must not only believe in an egalitarian approach, must not only explain this type of relationship to SAM, but more importantly must cocreate a relationship wherein SAM has the experience of equality, validity, and worth. It is one thing for a therapist to speak of self-determination; it is another for the therapist to personify and model self-determination, to see and access such characteristics within SAM, and, moreover, to employ interventive strategies that can potentially create the experience and outcome of self-determination. It's one matter to talk of safety and trust, as many therapists do; it's fully another when the therapist operationalizes trust into concrete actions, for example, starting on time, finishing on time, scheduling sessions at the same time every week, utilizing the same opening and closing rituals, keeping one's word, remembering facts of SAM's story, retaining the content of last week's session, and so on. Working in this way subtly yet persuasively conveys reliability, congruency, and consistency over time. In due course, trust, for SAM, transforms from an abstract notion to a cognitive, affective, behavioral, relational, and kinesthetic experience.

Safety and Trust

Gender directives, emanating from the macrosystem, are dichotomous and intractable. In the face of CSA, not only do they incite harm around SAM's personal sense of security and adequacy, they also obstruct him from accessing the self-generated capacities necessary for bettering the effects of CSA (Lisak, 1994a, 1995). CSA, personified by the perpetrator, breaches SAM's sense of security and trust (Crowder, 1995). Entrapped by social mythology and stripped of any sense of positive identity that may have been evolving, SAM brings to therapy diminished self-care capacities, a ruptured ability to trust, and an acute or obtuse fear of impending danger.

The therapist cannot provide for SAM a privileged immunity from harm within and across his microrelationships and environments; that not withstanding, the therapist can certainly create and sustain a context in which SAM can learn about safety and trust. Here, though, words are not enough. The therapist must not merely rely on assurances of safety, assertions of trust. He or she must furnish for SAM the experience of safety and trust. As SAM apprehends with his senses the therapist's reliability, dependability, security, and congruency over time, trust begins to build. As the therapist provides multiple opportunities for SAM to explore and express his firsthand impressions—what he knows, what he thought, what he sees, what he felt, what he believes to be true—and steadfastly responds with empathy and validation, trust begins to take hold. And as the therapist not only assures SAM that he will not be rejected or demoralized but also consistently communicates acceptance and respect, trust emerges more palpably.

The therapeutic milieu deserves special consideration when working with SAM. Central to providing a sustaining and generative environment is the understanding that SAM's discernment of safety is subjective, that the therapist can not "make" SAM "feel" secure, but SAM can come to perceive, sense, and ultimately experience "safety" vis-à-vis the therapeutic relationship and process. Thus, it is important that the therapist routinely assess SAM's level of comfort and reach for his feedback (Bolton et al., 1989). More often than not, preferences remain unstated until they are gently elicited (Briere, 1996a; Crowder, 1995). In group therapy, Matt felt extremely uncomfortable sharing a sofa with another group member, as is the case for many males with histories of CSA. Jake, on the other hand, preferred the sofa; because he spent much of his life avoiding other males, this gave him an opportunity to gain comfort within their proximity. Palo, among many others, felt more comfortable in a chair that faced the door, thereby maintaining his vantage point on the exit and promising him the shortest route of escape, if necessary. When feasible, it's important to provide within the therapeutic room as many options as possible so that SAM can choose on any particular day what is most comfortable and safe for him.

SAM is likely to feel more comfortable if the office is clean, open, and free of noise. Clocks are important, too, as they serve as subtle cues as to the preciousness of time in therapy. If the space is large enough, a circumscribed play area, perhaps with a sand tray, puppets, finger paints, and other art supplies, subtly serves as a noninvasive reminder of childhood for adult males with histories of CSA and provides a therapeutic work area for younger males. For males of any age, the room might contain a specified area or closet that contains "memory boxes" or designated folders to safeguard intervention-generated materials, such as portraits of self before, during, and after the abuse, a sexual abuse autobiography as well as a future autobiography, significations of fears, dreams, night terrors, and life goals, and any other therapeutic productions related to abuse history and abuse amelioration. Discernible rituals around the retrieval of the memory box and returning it to a safe place promote constancy and dependability (Karp, Butler, & Bergstrom, 1998; Pearce & Pezzot-Pearce, 1997). For older males, an analogy might suffice, rendering the same outcomes. To illustrate, in place of a memory box, Ty imagined an "everything bag." At the beginning of each session, he "opened" the bag, retrieving whatever contents were necessary at the time—memories, surplus from the prior appointment, the facts and meanings of his story, and so on. Toward the end of every session, he "closed" the bag, leaving it with the therapist. Between sessions, this inhibited the major interference of abuse-related content, because Ty learned to forestall such contemplation until the bag was retrieved and "opened" once again during the next session. He stated: "Keeping my story at the office is like keeping my cash at the bank. I always know where it is, I take it out when I need it and I can keep putting more into it. I just wish I had as much money as I got memories."

The therapist can employ any number of interventive strategies to promote safety and stability. At the onset of therapy, such preparatory strategies might include the following: (1) maintaining an open and inviting stance; (2) acquainting SAM with the therapeutic process, perhaps through metaphor, but definitely with emphasis on experiential aspects; (3) informing him that therapy tends to be long-term, that therapy on a short-term contractual basis is available, and that symptoms, at times, appear to be getting worse instead of better; (4) reframing the emergence of overwhelming memories and intrusive effects as a sign of readiness to work through them rather than as an indication of "losing control"; (5) teaching SAM ways to manage stress, contain intrusive memories, thoughts, and feelings, and the skills to control and ultimately ameliorate compulsive and interfering effects; (6) enhancing his self-soothing skills; (7) fortifying SAM's skill base around affect tolerance and regulation; and (8) providing psychopharmacological treatment or referrals if necessary (see, e.g., Bolton et al., 1989; Briere, 1996a, 1996b; Courtois, 1999; Draucker, 1992; Friedrich, 1996; Gonsiorek, Bera, & LeTourneau, 1994; Herman, 1992).

Additional interventive strategies include: (1) using the same language as SAM, especially when it comes to his abuse-related perceptions, sensations, impressions, beliefs, emotions, behaviors, and the like; (2) sustaining empathy; (3) acknowledging and normalizing ambivalence; (4) reflecting the meanings embedded in SAM's verbal and nonverbal content; (5) focusing more, at least initially, on content (e.g., presenting problem, abuse-related material, personal goals and aspirations) than on process (e.g., relational patterns, transference themes); (6) emphasizing cognition over affect, especially at the onset of therapy, as the former tends to be experienced as less threatening than the latter; (7) helping SAM put feelings into words as a way of familiarizing, demystifying, and normalizing affect; (8) working from the surface to the embedded, for example, from behavioral manifestation, to defensive strategy, onto underlying conflict or anxiety; and (9) reaching for SAM's feedback, always (see, e.g., Chu, 1998; Crowder, 1995; Davies & Frawley, 1994; Gartner, 1999; Meiselman, 1990; Salter, 1995; Whitfield, 1995).

The preparatory phase is also a time in which SAM has the opportunity to assess his current life situation. Before embarking on the first abuse-focused treatment objective, it's advisable that SAM achieve a sense of order and predictability across microrelationships and microenvironments. Since the exploration of CSA and its effects is often distressing and unsettling, it is beneficial if other disruptive factors can be kept to a minimum for the duration of treatment. For example, any treatment of sexual abuse-related concerns is best postponed until major life changes, such as those regarding work or relationships, have been accomplished, or have been contracted to remain at their current status. To illustrate, Jake and his wife initially agreed to postpone a marital separation until his individual therapy was well underway. In the meantime, they entered couples counseling and, after working through a number of significant issues, decided that a separation wasn't necessary after all. Similarly, in terms of Matt's treatment plan, in-depth work central to his abuse history was delayed due to a pending court case. In the meantime, he and the therapist focused on stress management and symptom abatement.

Further, there may be certain behaviors that SAM acquired along the way in order to distance himself from the abuse, including the misuse of or addiction to drugs and alcohol, or compulsions around sexual behavior, gambling, and work, among others. Self-injurious behaviors such as self-mutilation, suicidal gestures, food or sleep deprivation, social isolation, or passive participation in volatile relationships, all jeopardous to his health and well-being, may also be notable factors in SAM's life (Chu, 1998; Hunter, 1995; van der Kolk, McFarlane, & Weisaeth, 1996). Such self-destructive and self-injurious behaviors serve multiple functions. First, many anesthetize SAM in one way or another, offering repose from acknowledging and accepting CSA as a fact of his life and from enduring its effects (Herman, 1992). For instance, Matt's compulsion to reenact abuse-related dynamics was, in part, driven by the endogenous opioid discharge he experienced during the incest and, years later, while sexually acting out. Second, when actualized, compulsive and self-destructive behaviors confirm SAM's sense of shame, deviancy, or pathology, thereby creating congruency, as the external behaviors generate beliefs and emotions that match the internal perceptions of the self (Hunter, 1995). To illustrate, Matt's internalized albeit socially imposed beliefs, including "I am worthless unless I please others sexually" and "Any son who has sex with his mother is an insane pervert," emerged to the fore, evoking feelings of guilt, shame, and despair upon cessation of the morphine-like effects of stress-induced analgesia (SIA). Third, the repetitive nature of self-destructive behaviors detours SAM from cultivating more self-soothing strategies, reinforcing his reliance on invalidatory measures to prevent or cope with the emergence of the fractionated shards of his abuse experience (van der Kolk et al., 1997). Continuing with Matt, the tangible effects of SIA compelled him more persuasively than his abstract notion of self-care. SIA held hope and promise; self-care remained enigmatic until Matt contracted to learn and rehearse self-soothing skills and ultimately employed them as a means of interrupting his cycles of sexual compulsivity. Fourth, in many instances, self-destructive behaviors represent symbolic or literal reenactments of SAM's abuse dynamics and effects. The intention is mastery; the outcome is often degradation and despair (Davies & Frawley, 1994). Dynamically, Matt's compulsive reenactments typically involved older women with a penchant for sadomasochistic domination. In this way, the reenactment paralleled the incestual relationship with his mother. The historic episodes incited hyperarousal, uncontrollable retching, and feelings of powerlessness and emasculation, whereas the contemporaneous episodes represented attempts toward prevailing over such effects.

SAM's risky behaviors and destructive activities are purposeful; as such, they are not freely suspended or promptly transformed (Courtois, 1999). Compulsions, addictions, and other invalidation strategies present a potential therapeutic impasse, if not paradox: On the one hand, if SAM continues to employ the invalidation strategy, he will not be able to work through abuse dynamics and effects fully and effectively; on the other hand, if he relinquishes the invalidation strategy, without self-care, self-soothing, alternative coping, and social support procedures in place, he will likely encounter an overflow of intrusive phenomena, most certainly a high-risk situation for relapse. Thus, before engaging in the treatment of sexual abuse effects, SAM and the therapist must acknowledge the behavior in question and decide if it can potentially be a major impediment. If so, these concerns must be assessed and addressed and/or suitable referrals must be made to alternative treatment facilities. Further, if external or collateral medical or psychiatric care is not indicated, then SAM and the therapist can formulate a contract, not necessarily to stop the behavior, which would only serve to increase its compelling nature, but to learn about the behavior—its dynamics and effects—and how to make alternative choices regarding the behavior.

Often this includes a contract holding that SAM will call before engaging in any of these activities and simply state "I am consciously going to (binge) (purge) (act out sexually) (get drunk)." Although this is not a foolproof measure in terms of behavior cessation, it does increase SAM's awareness of his intentions and actions, reframing them in terms of conscious choice. Additionally, in calling the therapist's voice mail, the behavior is no longer a secret. When an intention is verbalized, it receives more forethought and recognition than when simply acted out in silence. Ironically, because the behavior in question frequently remains unactualized, its dynamics can be explored and alternative options can be considered. SAM now has the chance to survey more constructive choices with a view toward achieving similar outcomes minus compulsivity and self-destruction—for example, the feeling of control from purging but now from yoga or the sensation of cordiality from alcohol but now from volunteering at a food bank. Furthermore, by acknowledging the behavior, verbalizing it, and discussing alternatives, SAM begins to develop his own rationale for the new behavior. With the therapist providing the framework for making a decision, SAM is given the opportunity to explore and identify both positive and negative and short-term and long-term consequences of his actions. (Refer to the "Change Chart" intervention highlighted in chapter 10.)

To illustrate, Kip, on a number of occasions, called the voice mail, stating, "I'm consciously going to binge on junk food and I don't care how fat I get," just as Palo, from time to time, phoned to say, "I know what I'm doing. I'm going to the truck stop or biker bar to act out sexually." These externally different but dynamically similar behaviors were compelling for both Kip and Palo and both led to the same end—a sometimes palpable and at other times illusory sense of benumbment. Kip called it "being in the zone of zero"; Palo referred to the outcome as "feeling alive although it's never been as good as the first time." More often than not, the act of verbalizing a destructive intention and the shock of recognition associated with such a verbalization, in fact, prevented the behavior from occurring, thereby offering opportunities to examine the impetus behind the intention as well as more constructive alternatives without the interference of guilt and shame that so often follow such enactments. In exploring dissimilar methods that yield similar outcomes, Kip discovered that participating in an intramural cross-country running squad—starting slow but soon amassing significant mileage—diminished his level of stress and produced a sense of calm. As an unanticipated by-product, Kip developed friendships unlike any he experienced beforehand. In a like way, Palo, after experimenting with several activities, found that actualizing a long-dormant passion for woodcarving gave rise to conspicuous and sustaining feelings of enthusiasm, accomplishment, and well-being.

In working through these preparatory tasks and issues, SAM begins to establish a pattern of congruity, safety, and self care (Briere, 1996a; Chu, 1998; Herman, 1992). Such care can extend to his micro environments and relationships as well. For example, SAM can cultivate or make use of his social support system, including friends, family members, his physician, church, self-help groups, and Internet support groups for individuals with similar histories, among others. He can create a sanctum in his home, a special place for retreat and relaxation. If SAM is a boy or adolescent, the therapist can work with SAM's caretakers in a number of ways, such as (1) providing psychoeducational materials regarding the dynamics and effects of CSA and the processes and outcomes of therapy; (2) providing simple skill-building around listening to and talking with SAM about his abuse experience with particular emphasis on understanding, empathizing with, and managing invasive effects, coping strategies, and problematic behaviors; and (3) providing referrals to agency and community resources (e.g., medical, forensic, legal, and therapeutic). Securing the cooperation and cultivating the support of caretakers advances and fortifies the abuse amelioration process for everyone involved, especially for SAM (Deblinger & Hefflin, 1996; Faller, 1988; Friedrich, 1996; Pearce & Pezzot-Pearce, 1997).

In spite of such preparatory measures, and even if he eliminates self-destructive behaviors from his coping repertoire, the fact remains that SAM is likely to experience the notions of safety and trust as foreign. However, by listening actively and responding empathically, by extending SAM's genuine sense of hope and confidence in the therapeutic process, by intervening on purpose, in creating one opportunity after another for SAM to practice self-determination, and by holding the horror, pain, and triumph that infuse his sexual abuse history, SAM can experience security, dependability and stability, three vital components that operationalize safety and trust. And, as SAM begins to exclude self-destructive behaviors and replace them with growth-promoting actions, a sense of self-worth and value begins to burgeon. In a potentially convincing way, the ground is fertile for SAM to transform personal hypotheses into facts about a deserving self, a caring and responsive other, and a world that, although not immune from danger, continues to offer opportunities for joy, contentment, and living on purpose. Once again, the therapeutic relationship is key.

Transference and Countertransference

Depending on the therapist's or agency's theoretical orientation, as well as constraints around time, session allocations, and resources, transference and countertransference may be addressed centrally, peripherally, or not acknowledged at all. In simple terms, transference is an unconscious process involving the reexperiencing of perceptions, attitudes, expectations, feelings, impulses, and reactions; these phenomena were typically transacted within a significant relationship in a historical context but are now displaced onto another in a current context (Davis & Frawley, 1994; Kohut, 1977). Such thoughts, feelings, and behaviors were congruent with the historic relational configuration in which they first occurred; however, they appear seemingly out of sync with the current attendant conditions of the relationship. Regarding SAM, transference manifests when he personifies from his past emotionally laden wishes, fantasies, conflicts, relational patterns, and traumatic dynamics and effects and reexperiences them in the present by way of projecting them onto the therapist.

Countertransference, of course, is a potential element of any therapeutic relationship—in fact, of every relationship in life, whether it is recognized as such or not (Chu, 1998). Simply put, countertransference encompasses the therapist's cognitive, affective, behavioral, and physiological reactions to SAM as a person, for example, his race, gender, age, sexual orientation, and social class, as well as to the material he presents (Wilson & Lindy, 1994). This includes SAM's verbal presentation (e.g., the facts and meanings of his story and the ways in which he communicates them), relational dynamics (e.g., his interpersonal style, his transferential material), and nonverbal communication (e.g., emotionality, body language). Countertransference also comprises the therapist's conscious and unconscious reactions to and defenses against such data and, like SAM, the displacement of cognitive, affective, behavioral, and physiological reactions arising from the therapist's past (Pearlman & Saakvitne, 1995).

TRAUMATIC TRANSFERENCE

Common transferential material among males with histories of CSA includes the phenomenon of traumatic transference (Gartner, 1999). The emotionality and relationality around people in positions of authority have been malformed by the experience of terror and the experience of helplessness (Herman, 1992). Authority is not limited to the workplace or the therapeutic room; in relationships, SAM unknowingly for the most part delegates sole dominion of himself to others in his life, be they boss, colleague, therapist, partner, or spouse. So under the influence of others, so easily impelled by a furled glance, so quickly persuaded by a contradictory opinion, he sways direction, changes points of view, revises his perceptions and feelings, as if his very being is under the jurisdiction of another. To do otherwise is to diminish his sense of self-efficacy and worth, both functions of his ability to perceive clearly with his senses the wants and needs of others and to oblige them expeditiously.

In traumatic transference, SAM unconsciously anticipates that at any moment in time, the therapist will take advantage of him in some form or fashion, just as the perpetrator did weeks, months, or years ago (Spiegel, 1986). Within, between, and across therapy sessions, SAM transitions from one relational stance to another, posthaste. Sometimes SAM thinks, feels, acts, and relates as he would if his perpetrator were present (Davies & Frawley, 1994; Lister, 1982) and as if social mythology suddenly infiltrated the therapeutic working space. In quick succession, SAM, in response to authentically conveying a fact and meaning of his history, feels guilty for breaking the concealment injunction. Fearing an onslaught of repercussions, SAM tenaciously clings to the hope and promise personified by the therapist. However, the therapist, relegated to the role of rescuer, does not have the ransom to free SAM from his usurping belief that action such an as telling his truth is cause for punishment. And punish he does.

Within any given session, there are many passages, just like the example above: from truth to terror, from terror to dependency, from dependency to helplessness, and from helplessness to assailing the self. Returning to therapy after another 3-week absence, Victor emphatically stated: "Look, you say how important it is to tell the truth, and when I do, you can't help me! You can't make these feelings go away! I'm vile. Why would you want to help me anyway? Just say it! I know you're thinking it! I'm a 'good-for-nothing but shit' Puerto Rican whore of a cocksucking faggot and I don't deserve to live! I can't take it anymore! Every time I want to leave you don't force me to stay and every time I come back you are still here acting like I actually mean something. Why are you here every time I come back? What do you want from me? Just fuck me and get it over with. [Silence] Oh, God, I feel detached. Really detached. [Silence] I'm so sorry. Can you forgive me? I'll leave if you want me to." [Victor folds and begins to cry.]

Detecting, comprehending, and conceptualizing transference of any kind is, in part, a function of the therapist's ability to identify and empathize with SAM's verbal and physical expression of unconscious dynamics, conflicts, defensive constellations, and internalized relational paradigms with self-objects (Gartner, 1999; Wilson & Lindy, 1994). Victor's expressly stated declarations convey a number of traumatic transference dynamics: (1) the shifting view of therapist from collaborator to omnipotent protector to perpetrator-by-proxy to parent surrogate; (2) Victor's shifting stance from collaborator to abandoned boy to vicious attacker (of therapist and self) and to discardable client; (3) Victor's displacement of wrath from perpetrator to the therapist; (4) Victor's introjective identification with the perpetrator; (5) his explicit expectation of abuse from the therapist; and (6) the summoning of dissociation and depersonalization as a neutralizing yet disconcerting balm, effaced enough for the self-state of "Victor as sexually abused boy" to emerge with authentic feeling. In this brief moment, the balance began to shift from a once unwavering and deep-rooted identification with the aggressor to the nascent exposure of the traumatized self. Beyond conjecture, traumatic transference holds the potential to elicit traumatic countertransference.

TRAUMATIC COUNTERTRANSFERENCE

As caretaker of the therapeutic environment in which SAM, at age 5, 15, or 55, tells his story of childhood sexual abuse, as guide of the process that leads

SAM from socially imposed mythology to undisguised authenticity, and as witness to the heinousness his little body, his developing mind, and his burgeoning spirit endured, the therapist may find himself or herself inundated with intense emotions such as horror, rage, fear, and disbelief, overcome with intrusive reactions, such as vivid imagery, nightmares, and hypervigilance, or deluged with numbing responses such as avoidance, detachment, and depersonalization (Courtois, 1988; Wilson & Lindy, 1994). In essence, the therapist, empathically attuned to SAM's revulsion, his confusion and fury, his sense of inferiority, shame, and dishonorment, secondarily experiences the effects of CSA, that is, traumatic transference (Herman, 1992), a natural and anticipated derivative of working with CSA that harbors the potential to impact the therapist both internally and externally, thereby forestalling empathy (McCann & Pearlman, 1990).

Empathy, a critical skill necessary to work clients of any background, can potentially foster therapeutic inoperativeness when working with SAM (Gartner, 1999). As the therapist actively listens to and empathizes with the horrific details of SAM's history, as the therapist absorbs SAM's experience of being subjected to intentional cruelty, and as the therapist and SAM, together, work through traumatic reenactments, such exposure can render its own aftermath (Gil & Johnson, 1993). The shattering of basic assumptions of self, others, and the world (Janoff-Bulman, 1989) and the threatening of identity, worldview, and spirituality schemas (Pearlman & Saakvitne, 1995), common effects endured by individuals, families, and groups with histories of trauma, can, in the therapeutic setting, serve to sever the empathic linkage (Sullivan, 1953), as the therapist experiences traumatic countertransference (Herman, 1992; Ochberg, 1988), sometimes referenced as secondary traumatization (Figley, 1995). Thus, the therapist's capacity for and expression of empathy, a primary source of both success and failure in the therapeutic enterprise (A. Freud, 1936; Fromm-Reichmann, 1950; Kohut, 1959), carries with it benefits as well as costs. Among the benefits, empathic inquiry and responsivity, balanced with self-care in both personal and professional domains (Gartner, 1999), often increase relational strength, content, and value and fortify the therapist in containing SAM's traumatic material. Sustained empathic inquiry can deepen the therapist's ability to understand and validate, thereby inciting in SAM a willingness to disclose more fully. In maintaining a balanced, tolerable, and viable empathic stance, the therapist may, as a by-product, experience an evolving sense of confidence, self-efficacy, and mastery.

Regarding the potential costs of sustained empathic inquiry and responsivity, if the therapist's stance reaches a point of strain, that is, if the therapist becomes overwhelmed by traumatic transference, or fears its occurrence so much so that the therapist unknowingly or intentionally employs avoidance measures, the focus can shift from SAM to the therapist, as the therapist experiences lapses in attention, avoidance reactions, a sense of helplessness and inferiority, irritability, and psychic overload, among other countertransferential responses. A number of these negative effects coincide with the characteristics of "burnout" (Courtois, 1988). If taken too far, or not addressed by self-contemplation, supervision, therapy, and/or peer consultation, unacknowledged and traumatic countertransference runs the risk of diminishing the therapist's ability to intervene effectively and the risk of rupturing the therapeutic alliance, thereby disrupting SAM's progress in treatment and possibly his sense of hope regarding the value of therapy.

Traumatic countertransference reactions can typically be categorized under two main headings: avoidance, and overidentification (Davis & Frawley, 1994; Gartner, 1999; Pearlman & Saakvitne, 1995; Wilson & Lindy, 1994). Following are a few examples under each category, beginning with avoidance. In grappling with the facts and meanings emanating from SAM's history of abuse, the therapist may convey a sense of discomfort, thereupon signaling to SAM a need to curtail his language, buffer his facts, conceal their meanings. Experiencing a sense of embarrassment in response to contextual language, for example, "fucking," "blow jobs," "cock," and "pussy," the therapist may unwittingly mute SAM's communication by imposing a more comfortable vocabulary, such as "intercourse," "fellatio," "penis," "vagina," or "private part." In doing so, the therapist invalidates SAM's abuse history and experience to such a degree that he feels as if he is telling the story of another. And he is.

While struggling with the savage yet unfeigned details of SAM's history—impregnation of his mother, enforced prostitution by his father, ritualistic abuse by a priest—the therapist, defending against the horror of it all, may unintentionally divulge a sense of disgust and disbelief whereupon the holding environment begins to enclose, losing the breadth and depth necessary to invite, accommodate, and honor SAM experience as SAM lived it, as he knows it to be. Nicholas, during his first session, stated: "I got so much inside my head, so many truths and so many lies. Only a giant can hear me." Similarly, Palo, within seconds of his first phone call, said: "I've been to three of you [therapists] already and now I'm looking for another one. I don't want someone to get angry for me. I don't want someone getting disgusted by me. I want someone who is big enough and strong enough and willing enough just to listen, just to be there. Am I asking for too much?"

In creating an environment wherein stories of childhood sexual abuse, with their inherent barbarity and inhumanity, come to life, therapists endeavor to protect their own immunity from exposure to molestation effects. Some find themselves in an existential void, wondering how a society permits and even condones such cruelty against innocent children; many question their ability to help, given the pervasiveness and devastation of CSA. Some suspect the intentions of others. Others question the very world they live in. More than a few remember a world they once knew, safe and benevolent; many (at one time or another) momentarily wonder what they're really trying to do. In striving toward excellence but feeling incompetent and overwhelmed, the therapist may consign to oblivion his or her professional and personal wellsprings, such as the knowledge base, an acquired skill base, clinical wisdom, and a sense of purpose and self-efficacy, and, that being so, may intervene randomly or unknowingly find ways to avoid sessions or terminate the therapeutic relationship (Herman, 1992).

Philosophically arguing in favor the male perpetrator/female victim paradigm, and resisting an attack made on this frame of reference, the therapist may forgo interventions and therapeutic processes that would bring forth, work through, and ultimately validate SAM's history of CSA. This personifies the social mythology that, on the one hand, initiates and maintains the sexual abuse of males and, on the other hand, simultaneously conceals and invalidates it. In such a case, the therapist may decline to conduct an in-depth assessment of SAM's history, impede his intention and need to tell his story, or, because SAM is male and by default only "congruent" with one role of the paradigm, perceive SAM as if, and consequently respond to him as if, he is a perpetrator. Conversely, the therapist, needing to subscribe to the male perpetrator/female victim paradigm yet wanting to work with SAM, may unintentionally emasculate him by attributing socially constructed and culturally allocated traits imbuing the role of victim. In any case, diametrically conceived theoretical frameworks emanating from the iconic feminization of victimization and the masculinization of perpetration exclude the stark reality that adults of both genders hold the capacity to abuse and children of both genders bear a risk for abuse.

Countertransference can also be exacerbated by overidentification. Impervious to the emergence of survivor guilt, often expressed in the question "Why him and not me?" or, for that matter, overidentifying with SAM, wishing to care for him in ways that SAM was not treated as a child exposed to CSA, therapists may overextend the customary limits and boundaries of their work. Indicators may include prolonged sessions, "emergency" sessions, late-night phone calls, home visits, preferential treatment around fees, requesting favors from SAM, or thinking about or fantasizing about SAM, outside of work, and all to the point of interference with or negligence regarding other responsibilities and activities. "Interventions" like these run the risk of crossing the very boundaries established to uphold professional integrity and to protect SAM. Similarly, the therapist, unconsciously yearning to rescue SAM from the realities of his history and from the therapeutic processes necessary to reintegrate the fractionated effects of CSA, may, in fact, collude with his protective tendencies—those employed to depersonalize his authentic memories, dissociate from the pain of recognition, and invalidate the devastating consequences in spite of his perpetual plight with them. The degree to which the therapist views SAM as helpless is the degree to which the therapist preserves the traumatic transference, sustains the traumatic countertransference, and undermines the amending potential of the therapeutic relationship (Briere, 1996a; Herman, 1992).

In another direction, the therapist may capitalize on SAM's history of abuse, voyeuristically delving into the sexual details of his experience to the exclusion of other dynamics, focusing on the sexual compulsions or sexual problems with little regard for the array of divergent effects, or overemphasizing SAM's experience of CSA to the point of dismissing the myriad of other experiences that comprise his biopsychosocial history. SAM, in essence, becomes an object of the therapist's curiosity (Courtois, 1988); at times, his therapy becomes the subject of discussion, particularly when the therapist endeavors to impress colleagues, family, friends, and SAM with war stories and the glory of therapeutic success. In doing so, the therapist derails the therapeutic process, as SAM is no longer the agent of change but a sideshow exhibition.

Finally, that the therapist may have a history of CSA is, in and of itself, neither asset nor liability. The meanings, however, enveloping and generating from such an experience, both conscious and unconscious and both authentic and socially imposed, can impact the therapeutic process (Chu, 1998; Gartner, 1999; Meiselman, 1990; Pearlman & Saakvitne, 1995). In general, males with histories of CSA fear that on disclosure they will be perceived as "gay," "sexually deviant," and as a potential perpetrator (Spiegel, 1997b). Similarly, females with histories of CSA have apprehensions of being viewed as "damaged goods," "whorish," and blameful (Courtois, 1988). Therapists with histories of CSA are not immune from such effects, nor are they immune from social mythology.

Unfortunately, the allied therapy professions—social work, clinical psychology, psychiatry, marriage and family therapy, and counseling psychology, for example—convey the message that to be perceived or recognized as a therapist with a history of CSA is akin to being viewed as incompetent and impaired (Pearlman & Saakvitne, 1995). Thus, when the therapist is identified as a "survivor" of CSA by self-disclosure or the presumption of others, his or her value as a service provider depreciates at once. A shadow remains, silent but invisible. Such professional mythology then, like its social counterpart, eclipses the therapist's record and potential for work, enforces concealment, generates shame, and fails to recognize the great dispersion among the ways in which therapists with histories of CSA cope with sexual trauma and work with SAM.

On the one hand, a therapist with an integrated abuse history may use the experience of childhood trauma to his or her advantage, and for the betterment of SAM. With a history of CSA as a resource, therapists often have an uncanny ability to empathize and understand SAM in a way that fosters the therapeutic alliance (Courtois, 1988). On the other hand, a therapist with an undetected or unintegrated history of CSA may find that his or her traumatic background impedes the therapeutic process, as evidenced by avoidant and invasive countertransferential reactions to SAM and the material he presents (Pearlman & Saakvitne, 1995).

A therapist compensating for abuse aftereffects and with an unconscious mission to defend against their emergence may experience or engage in any of the following, among others. To begin, a therapist may, in attempting to neutralize his or her potent sense of powerlessness, cultivate SAM's unreserved dependence (Courtois, 1988), unmindfully suspending favorable opportunities in the direction of SAM's self-actualization.. She or he may show great partiality to SAM if his facts and meanings are "less traumatic" and little acceptance if his facts and meanings are "more traumatic" than the therapist's, given his or her need to feel special. A therapist contesting a pervasive sense of shame and inferiority may find himself or herself abdicating the roles of witness, ally, and guide, finding comfort in their turnabout, whereby SAM becomes the caretaker and the therapist becomes the attendee.

When it comes to boundaries, a therapist with an activated and unresolved history of CSA may find it particularly difficult to work with both process and content parameters. Process parameters include guidelines around length of sessions, contact between sessions, fee agreements, and intervention strategies; content parameters concern the boundaries around client material and therapist observations, interpretations, and reactions. The fear of being viewed as a "perpetrator" often leads a therapist to hold overly permeable or permissive boundaries, indulging SAM's every request, impetuously acquiescing to his body language before he has a chance to express an opinion, and tacitly condoning behaviors that would be unacceptable with other clients. Alternatively, the fear of being viewed as a "victim" is equally potent, and defensive and compensatory measures may include the enforcement of overly inflexible boundaries—canceling sessions if SAM arrives late, terminating the case if SAM accrues a balance, deterring phone calls between sessions—with little or no regard for SAM's particular circumstances at a given time.

In a similar way, a therapist with an abuse history may harbor a debilitating sense of gender shame. Because American culture tends to uphold the male perpetrator/female victim paradigm, males with histories of CSA are viewed as feminine, flawed, and/or gay (Crowder, 1995). Some male therapists unconsciously endeavor to project themselves as a man unlike all other men. In sheltering his image as a nurturing male, such as a therapist may seek refuge in containment interventions. From his perspective, ventilation strategies run the risk of overwhelming SAM and, consequently, run the risk of shattering his intended image. Even though the benefits of emotional ventilation include, in the short term, relief and tension reduction and, in the long term, an increasing familiarity and comfortability with authentic emotional expression, the cost of being perceived, by SAM or by the therapist himself, as manipulative, overbearing, and without regard (traits often attributed to the perpetrator) is far too great. Comparably, a female therapist with an operative sense of gender shame may avoid altogether the strategies necessary for in-depth and iterative exploration and description, given the probability that such interventions would elicit graphic details of sexually abusive acts. Unable to appreciate the underlying therapeutic utility or to willfully accommodate the explicit facts and corresponding meanings for fear of being perceived as a voyeur, whore, or perpetrator, the therapist involuntarily overshadows healthful strides toward the therapeutic goal of abuse integration.

Finally, SAM often asks the therapist if he or she has a history of CSA. While there are no hard and fast rules around this matter, the therapist must always contemplate such self-disclosure within the realm of therapeutic, as opposed to personal, gain (Crowder, 1995). Before the therapist discloses an abuse history, he or she should explore the driving impulsion behind such an intervention. Is he doing so out of countertransferential necessity, that is, with an unconscious hope of receiving a particular response from SAM, such as respect, support, or consolation? Is she doing so in order to dodge a therapeutic impasse, countertransferential revelations, or SAM's uncovering work (Pearlman & Saakvitne, 1995)? And is the therapist disclosing a history of CSA with SAM's personal and clinical needs in mind?

Just as significant others often perceive SAM, upon disclosure of CSA, as deviant, guilty, inadequate, inferior, and a failure as a male (Burges et al., 1984; Davies, 1995; Ray & English, 1995; Weihe, 1990), comparable to the way he perceives himself (Gill & Tutty, 1999; Ray, 1996; Wells et al., 1997), SAM, upon abuse disclosure by the therapist, may, in fact, attribute such qualities to the therapist. Even though SAM states that he is okay with this new knowledge, and even though he appears to be so, he may, more through action than words, take on the role of caretaker. Like a shot, he feels guilty about burdening the therapist with his "problems." Perhaps he will come to use the therapist's apparent success in overcoming the effects of CSA as a weapon against himself for failing to achieve such a status. Although a therapist may self-disclose with the intention of serving as a beacon of hope, the therapist may ultimately discover that he or she is viewed by SAM as a distress signal.

In light of the evocative nature of countertransference and the benefits and costs of empathic bonding, not to mention the roles and responsibilities of the therapist and the intricacies and dilemmas inherent in the therapeutic process, a therapist's personal experience as a patient is essential to his or her personal growth and professional development, and, ultimately, to SAM's experience in and outcome of therapy (Davies & Frawley, 1994; Gartner, 1999; Pearlman & Saakvitne, 1995). Additionally, it is critical that therapists buttress their professional endeavors with clinical supervision and peer consultation, extend their professional activities to include research, writing, and presentations, and fortify and counterbalance their professional duties with viable self-care strategies. Excellent references in the areas of transference and countertransference with regard to CSA include *Therapy for Adults Molested as Children* (Briere, 1996s), *Rebuilding Shattered Lives* (Chu, 1998), *Healing the Incest Wound* (Courtois, 1988), *Treating the Adult Survivor of Childhood Sexual Abuse* (Davies & Frawley, 1994), *Betrayed as Boys* (Gartner, 1999), *Trauma and Recovery* (Herman, 1992), and *Trauma and the Therapist* (Pearlman & Saakvitne, 1995).

The Therapeutic Window

The two most common errors generated within the therapeutic relationship are the therapist's failure to explore, identify, and, consequently validate (let alone work through) a client's history of CSA, and the therapist's untimely or vehement use of uncovering strategies (Lebowitz, Harvey, & Herman, 1993). In terms of the former, the therapist may rely solely on sustainment techniques or, in fact, be so nondirective that the therapist altogether circumvents SAM's history of abuse (Briere, 1996a). In doing so, the therapist, regardless of intent and by default, condones the perpetrator's actions and ultimately reinforces SAM's invalidating, reconciliatory, and compensatory strategies.

As for the latter, the therapist's agenda as well as certain interventions may hold precedence over SAM's particular wants and needs of the moment, leaving him overwrought. Ill-seasoned and frequently executed with fervor, such strategies may include: (1) the use of invasive uncovering techniques, for example, hypnosis, age regression, and drug induction; (2) the premature and untimely introduction of evocative interventions, such as psychodramatic role play, family sculpting, guided imagery, and systematic desensitization; (3) pushing for defended content with little or no recognition as to "how" or "why" the ego defense strategy is there in the first place; (4) imposing on SAM suggestive or evocative hypotheses and interpretations before he has been presented with opportunities to arrive at them at his own pace; (5) the overzealous working through of client material in order to be compliant with his insurance allocations, in terms of both number of sessions and financial compensation; and (6) generally controlling the focus, direction, and intensity of the therapeutic process. Both types of therapeutic errors—failure to work through and overzealous intervening—yield the right of way to more risks than benefits (Briere, 1996a; Courtois, 1999; Herman, 1992).

If reintegration of the sexually abusive experience is the ultimate goal (Chu, 1998; Meiselman, 1990), then therapy must draw forth the dynamics and effects of SAM's history of abuse, including his memories, myths, beliefs, emotions, injunctions, ego defense strategies, and conscious coping maneuvers. Together, the therapist and SAM strive to increase his awareness of them, relieve symptomology, differentiate his authentic meaning from social impositions, recontextualize the meaning of the abuse, and promote resourcefulness and mastery in the cultivation and actualization of life goals and aspirations (see, e.g., Crowder, 1995; Gartner, 1999; Meiselman, 1990; Rieker & Carmen, 1986). The therapeutic window (Briere, 1996a; Cole & Barney, 1987), as an interventive analogy and strategy, is one of many tools that can be utilized throughout the therapeutic process in service of such treatment outcomes.

Building on the work of Briere (1996a) and Cole and Barney (1987), the therapeutic window in this context is conceptualized as an opening to admit a particular aspect of SAM's history of CSA, offering him a psychological space and vantage point from which to explore, identify, contemplate, understand, empathize with, and ultimately work through the dynamics and effects. As a preventive measure against unduly overwhelming SAM, thereby inciting his use of well-armed defense strategies, the therapeutic window can be regulated by a window frame. In framing the window, SAM and the therapist cooperatively and coactively adjust to and account for the selection of content, the timing and pacing of exploration, and the intensity of SAM's responses. Working within the circumscribed window frame allows for an in-depth focus of one aspect of SAM's history, and it helps both the therapist and SAM strike a balance between containment and ventilation without excessive stress. Nicholas stated: "I like the window. I like it cause you can always see out it and the sun always shines in it so you don't have to hide."

More concretely, in working with the therapeutic window, SAM is afforded the opportunity, moment by moment, session by session, to present, gain comfort in, and contemplate the dynamics and effects of his sexual abuse history in a progressive manner. The therapist, as partner and guide, continually counterbalances sustainment and advancement interventions in response to SAM's working within the parameters of the therapeutic window—in other words, above the frame of avoidance but below the frame of overstimulation (Cole & Barney, 1987). As the therapeutic process evolves in a stepwise manner, the therapist assesses SAM's capacity to work within the defined window frame; if he feels relatively safe and comfortable, the therapist can help SAM delve more deeply. If the therapist or SAM overshoots or exceeds the therapeutic window frame, wherein the timing, pacing, intensity, and content eclipse SAM's cognitive and affective regulatory capacities, he is likely to employ defensive strategies to buffer the experience and to regain a sense of equilibrium (Briere, 1996a). At this juncture, the therapist must first help SAM to ameliorate his distress, and then expand his skill base to more effectively work through the emerging material (Gartner, 1999). Alternatively, if SAM or the therapist continually undershoots or falls short of the therapeutic window, denial, dissociation, and social mythology are reinforced and SAM incurs the loss, that of advancing toward the therapeutic goal of reintegration (Briere, 1996a). Palo said: "The idea of a window helped me to focus. Before I learned about the window, I felt anxious and all over the place. After I learned about the window, I was able to hone in on one subject or concern at a time. I needed that."

In addition to the window frame, the therapeutic window has an adjustable sash, holding any number of windowpanes from which to view a phenomenon dimensionally. For example, a sash separating two windowpanes can highlight the divergent perspectives of SAM and his perpetrator, track the intentions of the authentic self versus the compensatory self, and simultaneously show SAM's authentic meaning in contrast to socially imposed meaning. In a like manner, a sash holding three window panes can differentiate problem-solving alternatives and the positive and negative consequences of each. Kip stated: "I kept thinking too much about what other people kept thinking of me. Sometimes when I got confused about what I thought and what they thought, I would make their part of the window real dirty and my part real clean so I could only see what I was thinking. I didn't need to deal with their dirty thoughts of me."

The therapist must be continually mindful, however, to work within this adjustable and regulatory frame. As therapy progresses, the window frame expands accordingly, encompassing the breadth and depth of SAM's experience; at any given moment, the window frame contracts if the field of vision is too stressful or overwhelming. Or, for that matter, SAM can shut the window at the end of a session, sealing off the admission of material that may interfere with his work and home life, and open the window once again during the next therapy session. Jake stated: "I install windows and doors for a living so the idea of a window was very comfortable for me. It just made a lot of sense to me seeing my past and seeing my present and my future that way, sometimes through tinted glass, sometimes through a crack in the window and sometimes I just had to replace the whole damn thing to really see the truth."

Expectancies

Preparatory empathy can be employed by the therapist as a means of anticipating SAM's biopsychosocial context and potential frame of reference upon engaging in therapy. If SAM is a minor, his entry into therapy is most likely prompted by a court mandate in close proximity to disclosure. Given the efficacious nature of ego defense strategies and the persuasive properties of social mythology, he is predisposed to minimize the initial effects, some because of dormancy or intrapsychic detachment, others due to guilt, shame, and fear of repercussions. That being said, the knowledge base reveals that the vast majority of boys and adolescent males with histories of CSA rarely disclose (Gries et al., 1996; Keary & Fitzpatrick, 1994; Lamb & Edgar-Smith, 1994) or receive clinical services (Brown & Anderson, 1991; Gold et al., 1997; Jacobson & Richardson, 1987). If SAM is an adult, secondary elaborations of the abuse— for example, sexual dysfunctions, relational problems, anxiety, depersonalization, and process and consumptive addictions—rather than the abuse experience itself, hasten his entrance into therapy.

For many boys, effects have yet to germinate into symptomatology, although memories are recent and clear; for men, symptoms often coexist with voiceless memories, although a conscious connection between the two remains severed. Regardless of age, SAM will likely enter therapy with preconceived ideas about treatment based on images from the media. These can include negative conceptions suggesting that therapy requires the use of hypnotic techniques, "memory" drugs, or electrodes, that the therapist has total control and can read SAM's mind, or that a full-throttle purging of emotions will be required by a therapist who is a complete stranger to SAM. It can also include positive, but equally inaccurate, images, such as the therapist as a "miracle worker," rescuer, and protector, or the idea that telling the story once will "cure" him.

Accordingly, SAM may have questions about the validity of treatment based on these images. For example, although the media often depict therapy as a place to dredge up repressed memories, SAM has often suppressed the meanings, rather than repressed the facts of his history of CSA. He may wonder then, since he already has substantial recall of the abusive events, why he should bother. Jake stated: "I already know what happened to me. I just don't know what it's all supposed to mean." Where SAM may not fully understand the connection between past events and current thoughts, feelings, and behaviors, he often doubts the therapist's ability to provide anything he cannot furnish for himself as it pertains to the abuse experience.

He may fear that the therapist will repeatedly ask, "SAM, what are you feeling?"—a question to which SAM often answers, "I have no idea." This impasse, and SAM's fear of not being able to meet the therapist's expectations, is further compounded by a service delivery system that allocates a set number of sessions to SAM for his complete "recovery." The pressure of these demands often triggers, within SAM, feelings of apprehension about, and skepticism about, the treatment process. Contemplation of therapy gives rise to other concerns as well. He wonders if the therapist has a history of CSA. He wonders about the therapist's sexual orientation. He wonders if the therapist is a mother or father. He wonders how long therapy will take to complete. Such questions are quite common, and SAM, particularly as a late adolescent or an adult, inquires into these matters.

For the first three, the therapist's history of CSA, sexual orientation, and parental status, there is no standing order. Some suggest giving simple and honest answers to such questions (Crowder, 1995); others recommend erring on the side of caution, because the outcomes of such disclosures cannot be determined and may, in fact, impede the therapeutic process (Spiegel, 1998). Regarding the length of treatment, it's important that SAM be informed that therapy tends to be more long term than short term and that symptoms seem to get worse before they get better (Courtois, 1988). However, it is equally important that SAM be presented with options. For example, he and the therapist can contract to work in 12-week intervals. Within each interval, the work is circumscribed and task oriented, thereby fostering the likelihood of more tangible goal attainment. After one or two intervals and depending on SAM's resources, he and the therapist can negotiate a contract that includes long-term interventions or they may continue working within circumscribed periods.

Lastly, there is often a distrust of the clinician's motivation for wanting to work with SAM. Often unable to imagine why anyone would want to become a therapist, and why anyone would want to listen to his story, let alone believe him, SAM fears there must be something deviant and perverted about the therapist. It may also be helpful from the onset of treatment for the therapist to clearly explain to SAM that the therapist appreciates constructive skepticism, and that SAM has no reason to blindly trust either the therapist as an individual or therapy as a process. Trust evolves, and is a function of congruency and consistency over time. Doubt and mistrust, when presented as normal and fair reactions to a new situation, validate SAM's authentic responses, helping him to deactivate and relinquish his learned compensatory reaction of pretending that he feels safe and trusting. It also begins to teach him how to assess situations and to build trust. As a starting point, the therapist can encourage SAM to adopt a stance of neutrality, with allowances for caution and reservation. As their relationship progresses, the therapist teaches by example and SAM learns through experience. SAM's experience of the therapist—of the therapis's sensitivity, genuineness, humor, acceptance—evolves slowly, moment by moment.

Exploration and validation of SAM's anticipatory concerns gradually establishes confidence and reliance in the fact that he has a point of view and that he can begin to trust it and give it a voice. The therapist's empathic presence and communication help SAM begin to perceive the therapist not only as a human being who has a genuine interest in him, but as someone who can also believe in his authentic self and, at the same time, understand the compelling nature of his compensatory self. In time, SAM will experience the therapist as someone who realizes that fear and comfort, love and hate, and attraction and repulsion, for example, can coexist in the same time and space. Finally, the therapist is someone who knows for certain that SAM's sense of agency and sense of self-determination are paramount priorities.

SAM is likely to hold expectations around the therapeutic process as well. Thus, the preparatory phase of sexual abuse therapy must include exploration of and explanation for what treatment realistically can and cannot provide. For example, therapy cannot produce instant cures for SAM's problems, it cannot offer friendship or a sexual relationship, and it is not a panacea for pain. Similarly, neither can therapy eliminate the past nor make him forget, provide a concrete response to the unanswerable and existential question "why did this happen to me?," replace what was lost in childhood, or provide a therapist who does a "search and rescue," that is, does the work for SAM.

Treatment can, however, cultivate an unique relationship in which SAM can learn or relearn about care, trust, affection and intimacy in a nonexploitive context. It offers a safe environment for SAM to explore and identify his authentic meaning around the abuse, wherein conflictual or defended thoughts and feelings can emerge in noninvasive ways. Therapy offers opportunities both to mourn losses and to acknowledge gains resulting from having been subjected to an abusive experience. Over time, SAM learns to place the abuse in context and integrate it with all other aspects of his life so that it is no longer dictatorial, overwhelming, or all consuming. Therapy, too, helps SAM transform knowledge into practical and self-affirming skills. Through the action of therapy, SAM gradually reclaims and actualizes his authentic self as well as his dreams of and goals toward a fulfilling life. By proactively placing realistic expectations on and around the therapeutic relationship, the therapist helps create a safe, predictable, and sustaining environment for SAM.

POLICIES

In order to further cultivate realistic expectations about the treatment process, and in order to provide SAM with a pragmatic framework as to what he can rightfully expect from the therapist and what the therapist expects from him, information on issues such as length of sessions, contact between sessions, extra sessions, and payment policies is best conveyed when grounded in forethought and discussed prior to or during the first session. More specific issues, such as working with collaterals (e.g., husbands, wives, partners, children, perpetrators, etc.), appropriate touching, attendance under the influence of drugs or alcohol, and contact with the client during a therapist's absence or vacation, can be addressed during the preparatory phase or as they present as issues within the therapeutic process. Regardless of when they are discussed, it is important that the therapist formulates a rationale for these policies in advance so as to foster clarity for, and to maintain consistency with, SAM. It is also important for the therapist to present these policies in writing as well. As is especially common at the beginning of the therapeutic process, SAM may be dissociated or feel overwhelmed at the time of discussion. Built-in opportunities for him to reference back to session content, polices, procedures, and ground rules at a later time can augment his comprehension and decrease the possibility of misinterpretation.

Adherence to policies that are definable, observable, and, if possible, measurable contributes significantly to the creation of an environment where expectations are realistic, boundaries are defined, communication is clear, the therapeutic relationship is open, and the therapeutic process is therefore sound and reliable. As a by-product, policy adherence provides a countercharge to SAM's long-standing experience of ways in which explanations, namely, those of his perpetrator, contradict actions.

Given the betrayal, exploitation, boundary diffusion, and role confusion in SAM's past, the therapist can talk about boundaries and consistency with little or no impact on his expectations. The most binding and compelling communication about these issues—in fact, the only way in which SAM is going to be able to see, hear, feel, and experience the difference between the therapeutic alliance and the relationships of his past—is to be faithful to and abide by the boundaries, parameters, and policies of the clinical practice. In this way, SAM learns that the relationship is not about exploitation, violation, or intimidation. He might experience such reactions within the relationship, but the policies and parameters, when maintained consistently over time, act as safeguards against the very things SAM fears.

Further, by working with the therapist to understand the need and rationale for these policies, a mutual understanding is developed—that the policies are not random and that the boundaries are really there to protect SAM and to maintain the integrity and intention of the relationship. This communication also enhances SAM's sense of self-determination and control within his environment. Thus, when the therapist has a well-established sense of his or her boundaries and expectations, then SAM can learn about consistency, trust, and respect for the clinician's intentions, for himself, and for remembering, reexperiencing, reintegrating, and change.

SUMMARY

This chapter presented a number of treatment components that are integral to the treatment process involving SAM. Preparatory empathy helps the therapist to anticipate not only the dynamics and effects associated with SAM's history of childhood sexual abuse, but how such dynamics and effects may be experienced across SAM's microenvironments and reenacted within the clinical relationship. Preparatory empathy can be contemplated with regard to SAM's potential transferential reactions as well as what the therapist may anticipate in terms of countertransference. The therapeutic window, as an interventive analogy and strategy, contributes to the therapist a systematic way of executing the working-through process and offers SAM a means of focusing on content, regulating generated affect and building upon his internal resources. Anticipating SAM's frame of reference helps the therapist attune to the potential expectancies, questions, and dilemmas SAM may bring and that, unacknowledged or unadvised, could create a therapeutic impasse from the start. And practice polices, grounded in forethought, help demystify the extraordinary process of therapy.

CHAPTER EIGHT

THE SAM MODEL
OF TREATMENT AND OBJECTIVES

A PERSONAL MODEL OF PRACTICE can and will develop over time (Crowder, 1995). The capacity to translate science into art, theory into practice, philosophy into practice principles, and knowledge into interventions is infinite. Throughout this evolutionary process, however, practice must remain purposeful, reliable, and replicable. Practice without a conceptual framework, independent of the knowledge base, and short of interventive rationales, is accidental and arbitrary.

The conscious use of theory, the intentional/teleological development of interventions and corresponding rationales, and the decisive execution of interventions, as well as the mindful development and implementation of evaluative procedures and analytic strategies, systematize practice and promote treatment efficacy. Practice founded upon the mission of biopsychosocial justice, freedom, and equality, and guided and informed by state-of-the-art knowledge and intervention, advances professional autonomy, the expert delivery of services, and, hopefully, consumer growth and satisfaction.

In simple terms, it is imperative that therapists conceptualize and articulate childhood sexual abuse (CSA) and its effects and conceptualize and articulate the treatment of CSA. Only in doing so can therapists create, modify, select, and/or borrow interventions that can actualize constructive change. This chapter presents the SAM model of treatment and treatment objectives.

THE SAM MODEL OF TREATMENT OBJECTIVES

The SAM model of treatment, like several of its counterparts, is conceptualized as a stage-by-stage process (see, e.g., Chu, 1998; Courtois, 1999; Deblinger & Helflin, 1996; Lebowitz, Harvey, & Herman, 1993; van der Hart et al., 1993). Therapy is progressive and circuitous: progressive, in that each phase emerges from, and is influenced by, preceding phases; and circuitous, in that each phase and every objective iterates, in cycles. Thus, the therapeutic course recognizes that the exploration, identification, and working through of adverse effects and the acquisition, practice, and integration of constructive coping strategies, beliefs, and behaviors are recursive in nature (Courtois, 1999; Crowder, 1995; Sgroi, 1989).

Therapy, however, is not viewed as repetitive since each "repetition" is grounded in previous and progressive learning, insight, and knowledge. With CSA, newly constructed thoughts, feelings, and behaviors typically evolve through many iterations before the old, imposed ways are transformed into and succeeded by authentic thoughts, feelings, desires, dreams, actions, coping, and behaviors. Therefore, treatment does not cessate at the acquisition of insight or knowledge.

The Foundation

The SAM model of treatment objectives, like the SAM model of dynamics and effects, is founded on the ecosystems perspective (e.g., Bronfenbrenner, 1979; Garbarino, 1977; Garbarino & Eckenrode, 1997) of childhood sexual abuse (e.g., Harvey, 1996; Wurtele & Miller-Perrin, 1992), derives from a developmental understanding of CSA (e.g., Finkelhor, 1995; Putnam & Trickett, 1993; Pynoos, Steinberg, & Wraith, 1995), and employs a multivariate conceptualization of CSA (e.g., De Bellis, 2001; Finkelhor & Browne, 1985; Wurtele & Miller-Perrin, 1992) and the change process (e.g., Herman, 1992; Spiegel, 1998). Further, it integrates philosophical principles, concepts, and interventive strategies from ego psychology (e.g., A. Freud, 1965; Hartmann, 1964), object relations theory (e.g., Kernberg, 1976; Winnicott, 1965), self-psychology (e.g., Kohut, 1977, 1984), self-developmental theory (e.g., Erikson, 1963), interpersonal psychology (e.g., Bowlby, 1973, 1980; Sullivan, 1953), social-cognitve theory (e.g., Brower & Nurius, 1993; Janoff-Bulman, 1989), cognitive-behavioral theory (e.g., Bandura, 1986; Beck, 1976), trauma theory (e.g., Figley, 1985; van der Kolk, 1987), systems theory (e.g., Germain & Gitterman, 1986; Meyer, 1983), and social psychology. The SAM model of treatment objectives presented here is conceptualized as an initial phase of therapy on a long-term treatment continuum. It is congruent with the sexual abuse of males knowledge base, compatible with the major theoretical orientations that predominate the helping professions, and amenable to both individual and group treatment modalities.

It must be noted, however, that the SAM model of treatment objectives is simply one way to approach the beginning phase of long-term treatment. Therapists are encouraged to accommodate SAM's particular wants and needs, to adapt philosophical principles and modify intervention strategies in accordance with SAM's age and developmental capacities, and to be sensitive to his biopsychosocial context, as no one model holds a "one size fits all" guarantee.

Therapeutic Goal and Treatment Objectives

SAM, as a whole person, fractionates into shards—shards of sensations, knowledge, feelings, images, visual memories, auditory memories, olfactory memories, gustatory memories, and kinesthetic memories, thereby creating an array of altered states of consciousness and sensations of heightened reality (Herman, 1992; Krystal, 1988). SAM's traumatic memories appear lifeless, with no words to speak, no voice to speak them. CSA fractionates unity among the senses; what the eyes saw, the ears could not hear, and what the nose smelled, the body could not feel. CSA fractionates thought from feeling, fact from meaning, meaning from experience, and experience from context. CSA fractionates the continuity of time, demarcating SAM into preabuse, abuse, and postabuse selves. The whole, once greater than the sum of its parts, splinters into shards.

The essence of therapy, then, is to help SAM explore, identify, and express the dynamics and effects of his experience of CSA and to bring back to its original and authentic state the meaning emanating from the abuse (Rieker & Carmen, 1986). The primary treatment goal is as follows: SAM will author and narrate his story of childhood sexual abuse, from a developmental and experiential perspective, in order to reclaim his history and integrate the past with the present.

Goals, typically global, conceptual, and general, are operationalized by treatment objective. The following treatment objectives comprise one of many therapeutic paths. In following this format, SAM will:

1. Acknowledge a history of CSA in order to begin the change process (Briere, 1996a).
2. Explore social, cultural, familial, interpersonal, psychological, and biological dynamics and effects of CSA in order to identify facts relevant to his history (education) (Spiegel, 1998).
3. Infuse the evolving facts with contextual meaning in order to bring his cognitive and affective points of view associated with them into the foreground (Meiselman, 1990).
4. Analyze the various points of view in order to differentiate authentic meaning from socially imposed meaning (Rieker & Carmen, 1986).
5. Recount his story of CSA, from the perspective of first person, present tense, in order to affirm and validate his history as experienced (Herman, 1992).
6. Specify and describe losses and gains generated by his experience of CSA in order to grieve the former and claim the latter (Courtois, 1988).
7. Formulate and execute a goal-based project, based on a CSA effect or constellation of effects, in order to build upon and generalize his progressive skill base (Crowder, 1995).

Goals operationalize into objectives; objectives actualize by way of interventions. Even though the SAM objectives are introduced in a step-by-step manner, just as treatment unfolds in a stepwise manner, they do not comprise an exact prescription. Thus, some males with histories of CSA will not, upon embarking on the therapeutic process, follow the progression as stated; some will work on particular objectives much longer than others; others will bypass certain objectives for any number of reasons, perhaps returning to them at a more conducive time.

THE TREATMENT OBJECTIVES

Objective 1

> SAM will acknowledge a history of childhood sexual abuse in order to begin the change process.

ACKNOWLEDGING THE ABUSE

Before utilizing a practice model for the treatment of sexual abuse, it is important that SAM be willing and capable of acknowledging its current or historic existence. This includes the admission of sexual abuse as a personal event as well as the identification of the perpetrator(s). However, the ways in which the abuse is communicated are not as important as SAM's ability to acknowledge its occurrence in the first place. SAM may use different language than the therapist, may disclose the abuse from a dissociated state, or may use a combination of verbal and nonverbal expression with which to communicate the event(s).

Regardless of form, this acknowledgment is momentous for both the therapist and SAM. First, it helps to define where SAM is and where he wants to begin and it supports the therapist in formulating, with SAM, the client-based goals of treatment. Additionally, without this acknowledgment, the therapist merely assumes, and perhaps incorrectly, the source of SAM's expressed effects.

Second, this acknowledgment benefits SAM because it signals his readiness to give expression to experiences previously concealed. Simply, yet persuasively, the act of acknowledging the abuse begins to erode the compensatory self originally erected to both hide and, ironically, to make sense of the abuse. It is a conscious step toward countering the schemata and defenses established to conceal, invalidate, reconcile, and compensate for the abuse. Step by step, SAM moves toward creating an integrated identity whereby authentic thoughts, feelings, and behaviors can be identified, expressed, and validated, and from which connections between the past and the present, and between the authentic and the compensatory selves, can be realized.

And, step by step, SAM begins to accept his experience of CSA and its history of effects. Although initial acknowledgment is a momentary event, as the therapeutic process unfolds, there is more to acknowledge, more and more to accept. Thus, acknowledgment and acceptance are incremental in nature. Acknowledgment requires SAM to consider as true the occurrence of abuse, the intentions and actions of the perpetrator, and the historic and current manifestation of sexual abuse effects. Acceptance calls for SAM to give credence to the facts and meanings of his story as he remembers them to be, the industrious coping strategies he employed to brave and bear up against the abuse, and the numerous losses and gains generated by the experience (Bolton et al., 1989; Courtois, 1988). The degree to which SAM is able to referee and reduce the severity of concealment injunctions, invalidation strategies, reconciliation measures, and compensatory efforts is the degree to which he will be able to progressively advance into the depths of acknowledgment and acceptance. SAM's sensory receptors and memory are key. The more he is able to remember—that is, to see, hear, think, touch, taste, and feel by way of the mind, body, and being of the boy he once was—the closer he is to the defenseless and undisguised truth. However, as noted throughout this chapter, intervention strategies that manipulate SAM's states of consciousness, attempt to break through his defensive barrier by way of invasive means, or strive to retrieve memory independent of SAM's will or readiness are contraindicated given their risk-benefit ratio, their capacity to induce autonomic hyperarousal, emotional dysregulation, and psychic decompensation, and the controversy surrounding them in clinical and nonclinical circles.

ORIENTATION

At this point, SAM and the therapist enter into an orientation phase. The orientation phase encompasses four main lines of work: (1) familiarization with the therapeutic process; (2) normalization of the traumatic response; (3) stabilization of symptoms and effects; and (4) acquisition of self-care strategies. Based on the therapist's comprehensive state-of-the-art assessment and SAM's readiness for in-depth work, this phase of treatment may be relatively brief or, in some cases, require substantial time, attention, and effort on both their parts.

In terms of orientation to the therapeutic process, the therapist guides SAM in learning about and developing an appreciation for the role of the therapist, the role of the patient, their mutual commitment to cocreating and sustaining the therapeutic relationship, and policies and procedures such as attendance, fee schedule, notification of absences, latenesses and vacations, phone calls between sessions, requests for extra or emergency sessions, and the like (Courtois, 1999). The presentation of this material tends to be straightforward; however, it is critical that the therapist reach for client feedback in all of these areas so as to ensure a mutual understanding. It is around these very policies and processes that SAM's transference and the therapist's countertransference are likely to emerge and where resistance is likely to surface. Thus, a clear understanding regarding "what" these therapeutic processes mean, "how" they operate, and "why" they are vital to SAM's experience of and outcome in treatment is essential.

Concerning orientation to the traumatic experience, the therapist takes an active role in helping SAM develop a framework of understanding his traumatic past vis-à-vis the therapeutic process. First and foremost, the therapist must normalize his sexual abuse effects (Courtois, 1999; Gartner, 1999). Far too frequently, SAM's guilt and shame preclude a cognitive appraisal that engenders understanding, compassion, and empathy. The therapist conceptualizes sexual abuse effects as reasonable and creative biological, psychological, interpersonal, social, and spiritual responses to an atrocious event, whereas SAM, on the other hand, conceives sexual abuse effects as verdicts of his emasculation, deviancy, and craziness. Core beliefs like these, even when embedded underneath layers of defenses, form a slippery slope.

Critical points include the following:

1. Symptoms are likely to get worse instead of better. Jake stated: "I'm glad I knew this from the start. From watching a program on PBS, I thought that with sexual abuse therapy, you spend a weekend in a room with a bunch of people like you, holding teddy bears or something, talking, telling your story, crying, and hugging, writing a letter to your perpetrater, and then leaving like everything is okay now. That is not what therapy was like for me."
2. The points of view of SAM as the boy who was subjected to CSA may be very different from the points of view of SAM, as the adolescent, young man, or adult who coped with such a history.
3. Just like therapy, sexual abuse and its effects are not reductionistic phenomena. That SAM may feel both love and hate toward his perpetrator, that he may, on the one hand, desire change but, on the other hand, find that he detests it as well, or that he may mistrust yet respect the therapist simply signify the coexistence of two contrasting points of view or two divergent states of affect.

Management of abuse-generated effects or symptoms comprises the third aim of the orientation phase (Briere, 1996a; Chu, 1998; Davies & Frawley, 1994). Prior to engaging in in-depth exploratory and ameliatory work, it is critical that SAM evidence the following (when applicable and/or obtrusive): (1) reduction in his hyperarousal response; (2) reduction in the use of invalidation strategies including compulsions around food, work, sleep, sex, drugs, and alcohol; (3) reduction in the use of dissociative, avoiding, and/or numbing invalidation strategies; (4) reduction in hyperreactivity to abuse-related stimuli; (5) reduction in intrusive reexperiencing symptomology; (6) regulation of the fear–adrenaline–fear cycle; (7) reduction in anxiety and mood-based symptoms as well as other comorbid symptomatology such as obsessive–compulsive behaviors and sleep disturbances; and (8) and reduction in and regulation of self-injurious behaviors, such as cutting, biting, head banging, and the like.

A number of cognitive and cognitive-behavioral interventions show promise in the amelioration of these effects. Strategies such as stress management, relaxation, grounding, self-monitoring, the chaining of thoughts–feelings–behaviors, self-talk, and self-soothing, among others, are quite amenable to the orientation phase in that they tend to offer systematic directions and render definable, observable, and measurable outcomes. Moreover, interventions like these create parameters around a defined behavior or symptom, making the process of amelioration more manageable in the eyes of SAM. Additionally, they do not require in-depth exploration, which is indicated only when SAM acquires the ego resources, the regulation of symptoms, and the stabilization of activities within and across microenvironments.

Orientation to self-care, as the fourth aim, is evidenced by the stabilization of activities within and across microenvironments. Unfortunately but understandably, self-care may appear to be a foreign concept to SAM. During this orientation phase, SAM may have to consider ways in which to correct potential obstructions to the therapeutic process, including workplace conflicts, school-based problems, relational difficulties, and financial complications, all of which may divert his time and attention away from therapy, tax an already fragile psychic economy, and usurp whatever internal and external resources that may be accessible at the time.

Further, it is vital that SAM create as much consistency as possible in and around his activities of daily living, such as eating, sleeping, hygiene, and exercise. In terms of eating, Ty stated: "I was always going to fast food places—McDonald's, KFC, Taco Bell—when I did eat, which wasn't every day. My therapist asked me if I would make myself a home-cooked dinner, 'nutritiousness,' he said, 'not like the fast food but good food' and I just laughed cause I did not do that in years. But I did. And when I took the fork to my lips and began to chew, these tears just gushed out of me. I was taking care of me. Now he wants me to cook every day." In terms of sleeping, Kip revealed: "I gotta be at school at 8 but I don't sometimes fall asleep till 3 or 4. When I go to sleep I keep waking up and going to the frigidare to eat. Sometimes I keep food snuck under my bed. My moms never cleaned the room so it don't matter none. I'm trying to be on a different routine now—doing boot camp exercising after school and deep breathing when I want to fall asleep. That helps me to stay sleeping better. The food though, I ain't wanting to give that up yet."

As for hygiene, Matt disclosed: "This one summer, I stopped brushing my teeth and showering. I didn't plan it that way, it just seemed to happen. But after a week or so, people didn't want to be around me. They avoided me. And I was fine with that. I didn't want people looking to me for sex, and I didn't want to be around people, because the only thing I seemed to know how to do with them was to have sex. Neglecting my body seemed to work. At least for that summer. At least until I couldn't stand to be around myself." And, regarding exercise, Nicholas stated: "I am afraid to run and play. When I run and play my heart beats loud. When my heart beats loud I get afraid. When I get afraid I think of Terry [his perpetrator]. When I think of Terry I have to go with Big Bird again."

SAM'S DECISION TO PROCEED

A primary intention at the onset of therapy is to help SAM render an informed decision about a process where therapist-based and process-based surprises or unknowns are kept at a minimum. In order to do this, the therapist and the client need to form a mutual understanding regarding their roles and activities in relation to the treatment process.

It is quite natural for SAM to be ambivalent about his goals around treatment. On the one hand, he may want to be in therapy with the aim of ameliorating the abuse effects; he may simultaneously, on the other hand, fear the process of change and not want to talk about his experiences of abuse to anyone, particularly a stranger. Nicholas stated: "If I told you the real truth, then all of bad things Terry's said will happen, they will really happen. So I don't want you to ask me any stuff about the truth." Expressing a similar sentiment, Kip commented: "If I talk about this, the dam'll break and I'll be flooded like Johnstown was and lose control." And, Ty relayed: "Please don't take me for rude, but I don't know if I really want this [therapy]. Nothing against you, but if I call it 'abuse' like the books do and the TV does, then I'll stop being who I am and don't know who I will be after that. And, most of all, I want to believe that Rodney deep down really loved me. I just gotta."

SAM may also fear that change will be so extensive that his only identity—the one fabricated to conceal, invalidate, reconcile and compensate for the abuse, and the one still standing—will disappear, and that he will be left adrift, not knowing who he is. This fear is particularly potent for SAM if he has experienced depersonalization, a terrifying and intimidating sense of estrangement from the self. Or he may also fear that, if and when he tells his story, the therapist will agree with his negative self-images imposed by the abuse. Palo revealed: "What scares me most about you and about therapy is that, sooner or later, you're going to see that I am a fraud, that underneath I am my father's whore and a failure as a brother." In a like way, Jake stated: "Every time I tell another part of my story, I'm just waiting for you to say, 'See, you are Satan's son. You are evil. You deserve to be punished.'"

It is important at this point that the therapist normalize these fears, self-concepts, and reactions and acknowledge that, simply by presenting for treatment, SAM is making a significant step toward change. Both his desires and his apprehensions need to be addressed—to be given equal time and validation—for they are both equivalent and component aspects of SAM's presentation. Overlooking or underrating either side reinforces his sense of ambivalence, that of both wanting and fearing change.

Treatment at this stage can be conceptualized, then, not as a battle in which one side will eventually conquer the other, but as a process through which both aspects of his ambivalence can merge together. Here, one aspect of self, which wants to tell the truth and acknowledge the past, can utilize the strengths and perseverance of another aspect of the self, one that helped SAM to survive and to develop despite the traumatic childhood he so boldly surmounted.

ASSESSING HIS CURRENT LIFE SITUATION

A discussion of a multimodal assessment protocol is beyond the scope of this book. Excellent resources include the following: for children, *Child Sexual Abuse* (Faller, 1989); and for adults, *Males at Risk* (Bolton et al., 1989), *Healing the Incest Wound* (Courtois, 1988), and *Recollections of Sexual Abuse* (Courtois, 1999). In addition to conducting a comprehensive biopsychosocial assessment, the therapist can utilize the Trauma Symptom Inventory (Briere, 1995; Brier, Elliott, Harris, & Cotman, 1995), a compact self-report checklist comprising the following categories: Dissociation, Anxiety, Depression, Sleep Disturbances, and Post Sexual Abuse Trauma. This instrument yields a number of anticipated outcomes for both SAM and the therapist, including (1) a tangible understanding of SAM's sexual abuse effects across divergent domains, and (2) a conceptual understanding of the potential linkages between his abuse dynamics and expressed or dormant effects. In general, a thorough assessment provides a vantage point from which to view SAM's initial effects and coping strategies as contextually creative, normative, and adaptive. However, as they habituate across time and generalize across microenvironments, SAM and the therapist may come to discover that such abuse-generated effects and coping strategies, unnecessary, impedimental are and/or destructive (Briere, 1995; Briere & Runtz, 1988). If interested, please refer to a knowledge base resource that centers on the assessment process.

SAM'S RATIONALE

Before further therapy can pragmatically begin, it is essential that SAM clearly define his own rationale for entering treatment. Not only does this afford him a sense of self determination and freedom, but it also establishes that he is capable of at least entertaining the possibility that his world can change. This "leap of faith" may be a transitory state at this point, but it introduces a sense of purpose and lays the foundation for all further work. It also begins to cultivate a sense of hope. Please refer to the "Change Chart" intervention, discussed and illustrated in chapter 10.

It is critical that SAM negotiate and modify his goals throughout the treatment process. He may enter therapy with the goal of symptom management but soon discover that he also wants to work through his traumatic past. Alternatively, he may at the start wish to work through his history of CSA only to discover such an undertaking is contraindicated for any number of reasons, including the presence of coexisting conditions or circumstances related to psychopathology, health status, family obligations, time constraints, and debilitating fear, for example (Chu, 1998; Courtois, 1999).

The first transition from Objective 1 to Objective 2 should evidence the following: (1) SAM's acknowledgment of an abuse history; (2) SAM's identification of his perpetrator; and SAM's evolving but viable capacity to (3) recognize the traits of affective states; (4) differentiate thoughts from feelings; (5) employ self-soothing skills; (6) tolerate the emergence of abuse-related content; and (7) maintain stability across his microenvironments, particularly in the areas of school, work, social support, and significant relationships.

Objective 2

SAM will explore dynamics and effects of childhood sexual abuse in order to identify facts relevant to his history.

In this phase of treatment, the emphasis is on SAM's working with the facts of his history of CSA while beginning to place the realities of the abuse in their rightful biopsychosocial contexts. For this, psychoeducation is key. Psychoeducation is intended to elucidate the realities of sexual abuse by creating a context from which SAM acquires an understanding that sexual abuse exists not only as a personal event, but also as a social phenomenon generating its own set of powerful dynamics and effects. Context-specific analyses build an awareness of the person/environment interplay; without it, SAM may find it difficult, if not unrealizable, to differentiate his authentic story from the one socially imposed on him. Although analyses of the social dynamics that initiate and maintain the sexually abusive relationship are not typically part of a therapeutic protocol, it is virtually unfeasible to explore, understand, and validate SAM's history of CSA and its effects absent of social context (Crowder, 1995). Furthermore, it is illusory to disregard the fact that both SAM and his therapist are members of a culture that not only subjects boys to CSA but conceals and invalidates it as well. Thus, psychoeducation around this objective and throughout the treatment process provides for SAM a cognitive framework (Herman, 1992) that (1) normalizes the effects of CSA; (2) demystifies the treatment process; (3) functionally maintains a sense of distance from overwhelming affect until a more stable therapeutic alliance emerges; and (4) offers a structure to therapy, in general, and an orientation to the sexual abuse of males knowledge base, in particular, until SAM's internal resources can serve him in acknowledging, experiencing, and containing his authentic story of CSA. This treatment protocol, however, does not advocate the canvassing of memories or the employment of invasive memory retrieval strategies, nor does it require random and excessive reliving or undue abreaction that in many instances results in retraumatization, disintegration, and premature termination for SAM (Courtois, 1999).

Thus, the therapist relies on tried-and-true techniques to elicit SAM's history of abuse—his memories, thoughts, feelings, assumptions, conclusions, and the like. With respect for SAM's comprised sense of agency, his defense constellations, the psychobiologies of hyperarousal and dissociation, his implicit and explicit systems of memory, and, perhaps most importantly, SAM's right to discover his authentic truth, the therapist allows the clinical process to take root. As SAM becomes acclimated to the therapeutic process and environment, as he actively engages in the working alliance, as he begins to trust the therapist's intentions, and as his defenses begin to relax, SAM's story unfolds without the assistance of specialized retrieval strategies. SAM will speak when he is ready, and when he knows the therapist will be able to accommodate his horror. Matt stated: "I never told anyone about my incest. When I came into therapy, I wasn't about to divulge everything during the first few sessions. I heard too many stories about therapists in it for the money or therapists who had sex with their patients. I needed time to discover what was going to happen or likely to happen before I could share such a deep and painful secret." Victor revealed: "I was desperate for help and knew I had to get it, but when I came to the first session, I realized that I was talking to a complete stranger and there I was supposed to talk about incest—about penises and fathers and boys and blood—and I couldn't do it. I remember sitting there wondering what was going on. I felt so numb inside, almost as if I was imagining that I was abused as a kid, that it was all in my head." Still, Palo stated: "I was ready to go from the beginning. The therapist encouraged me to wait until I felt comfortable but I wanted to tell as much as I could during the first meeting. And I did."

When exploring the realities of abuse, there must be an inclusion of both the factual and the mythical elements of the abuse experience(s). Unbeknownst to SAM, he has likely put under quarantine the mythology around the sexual abuse of males, isolating it from the social and cultural context that sustains it, internalizing its prejudicial meanings and integrating it into his perceptions of self, thereby making it his own and, therefore, seemingly authentic. Common myths include the following: (1) Erection and ejaculation equal consent; (2) boys are less defenseless than girls and therefore less affected by CSA than girls; and (3) if a boy is sexually abused, it is only a matter of time before he perpetrates against young children (Gonsiorek, 1994).

When it comes to mythology and authenticity, it is important to keep in mind that, in SAM's psychological and sociological space, what is real to the therapist is often mythical to him and vice versa. As a counterbalance to social mythology, psychoeducation provides a context for SAM to eventually identify and evaluate the social myths and "facts" that he has learned along the way and to dispute the relevance and the validity, as appropriate, of both the content and the source of what he "knows."

To begin, SAM must convey some facts. Initially, Kip listed the following as fact: (1) "I let someone fuck me." (2) "I must be gay." (3) "I'm a failure as a boy." In light of the tendency to reveal myths as facts, it is critical that SAM be presented with information that fosters the development of an alternative knowledge base. Disseminated information can include, for example, the actual incidence or prevalence rates of the sexual abuse of males, highlighting the fact that approximately one of every six boys will be sexually abused before the age of 18 (Leverich et al., 2002; Melchert & Parker, 1997; Neisen & Sandall, 1990; Paul et al., 2001; Ratner et al., in press). This new frame of reference, as a substantiated fact, dramatically contradicts the social myth that sexual abuse doesn't happen to boys. During this type of process, SAM's authentic experience of CSA, heretofore oppressed by social mythology and invalidated by his defenses as well as the responses of others, emerges and emends slowly—improbably at first and, without exception, inconducive to speed or force.

Psychoeducation can also include the dynamics and effects of sexual abuse. During this interventive phase, Kip's subsequent but still evolving list of "facts" were delineated as follows: (1) "I was physically taken down by a man." (2) "He was older than me." (3) "He was one foot taller and more than 100 pounds bigger than me." (4) "He was high on crank." (5) "He threatened to kill me." (6) "He slashed my clothes and underwear off with a knife." (7) "He raped me." (8) "I got a hard-on." (9) "I thought I was gonna die." (10). "My ass bled." (11) "I prayed for the first time in my life." (12) "I felt all dead inside. . . ."

In a key way, an alternative knowledge base generated by empirical data begins to challenge mythology. To illustrate, the physical responses of a boy during abuse can be addressed and reframed. One myth asserts that if SAM was physically aroused during the abuse, then he must have wanted it to happen. The reframing of this "belief" necessarily includes psychoeducation around basic anatomical principles. The reality is that a boy's penis is sensitive to both emotional and physical stimulation irrespective of context and intent. Knowledge like this provides SAM with an alternative basis for understanding his own physiologic reactions and, by design, credibly disputes his socially imposed interpretations of such reactions. (Eventually, this alternative basis for understanding CSA will help SAM discover an alternative placement of responsibility and blame for the abuse, that is, on the perpetrator.) This is not to suggest, however, that one discussion of a particular issue or, for that matter, of any point of concern will modify SAM's point of view immediately. Defenses, rationalizations, compulsive behaviors, and socially imposed views of self, others, and the world mutate slowly, like deep wounds, over time, and by degree. It does suggest, however, that SAM has the liberty to explore and reclaim his authentic truth.

Ironically, adaptation to CSA plays a very significant role in aiding and abetting SAM's adherence to social mythology. To begin, SAM's defenses serve as a buffer between him and the realities of his abusive experiences. By way of subjection, sexual abuse, concealment, and invalidation, SAM inherited, and often excels in, an ability to dissociate from, depersonalize, and deform his authentic realities of CSA. Naive, traumatized, and simply trying to live through one horrific moment after another and with little reprieve from anticipating the next, SAM's boyhood body and mind offer refuge to the fractionated shards of his abuse encounter. Further, the greater social environment conceals and invalidates his reality by supporting social mythology. Consequently, SAM must learn how to disentangle fact from myth, authentic meaning from imposed meaning, his voice from the cacophony of others (including that of the perpetrator), and ultimately, his reality from the socially constructed reality surrounding the sexual abuse of males.

Up to this point, given the greater social context, SAM had little choice but to conceal, invalidate, reconcile, and compensate for the abuse. Psychoeducation gives him the opportunity to recognize that there are forces greater than himself, greater than the relationship in which the abuse occurred, and, in fact, that no one, and no organization, is exempt from the influence of these mythologies. Still, the void of disparity between authenticity and mythology is vast and, for many, linked only by a bridge of ambivalence. As SAM enters into the process of addressing abuse related issues, he inevitably encounters some feelings of ambivalence about the treatment process as well. This manifests both inside and outside the treatment room. Ambivalence is often expressed by way of polar shifts in SAM's thoughts, feelings, and behaviors, including transitions from striving to accept as true his perceptions of the past, to perjuring himself for stating anything of the kind; from feeling hopeful, to disheartened; from disclosing fully, to emphatic recantation; from attending regularly, to abstaining without notice; from empathic concern, to caustic indifference; from seeking authenticity, to concealing it; from countermanding his truth, to endorsing the perpetrator's lies, and so on.

On the one hand, as SAM learns about the realities of childhood sexual abuse and takes another step toward understanding the lies inherent in it, he experiences a sense of relief, as if a burden has been lifted. By way of psychoeducation and the knowledge base, he slowly, in a piecemeal fashion, comes to understand his battle with social mythology, gradually recognizing the united front between his perpetrator and the myths. He feels validated in knowing that many others share his experience, that he was, and is, not alone, and he begins to view his coping strategies in a new light. On the other hand, SAM may feel threatened. Quite often, he wonders if his abuse identity, fortified with such mythology, is really a false self. Victor asked and answered in this way: "Who will I be if I give this up? I already lost myself once; I don't want to lose myself again. I have a handle on who I am now even if I think it's my fault and that I was asking for it and that I'm pretty much a failure as a guy. I'm afraid to change. Who will I be then?"

Around the time of his abuse, in order to make it from the perpetrator's grasp to the school yard and back home again, SAM had to alter his authentic perceptions of reality to align with the perpetrator's view and with the social view. By doing so, he had to certify the myths as reality. For example, Ty labeled the incest, not as abuse but as "coming out early." Nicholas believed that he was a freak of nature, a "she-boy," taking his perpetrator's and mother's words as gospel truth. Matt saw himself as the perpetrator, his mother as victim. The only opportunity to cry out against such hypocrisy was in his sleep, with consciousness closed, eyes shut, and defenses at ease. Now, he is being asked to alter his reality again. At this moment, and many more to come, SAM stands before the steep face of a new vista—at the precipice of accepting the truth as truth—a mountainous task, indeed. Just as SAM vacillated between truth and lies at the time of the abuse, he will do the same in therapy.

This ambivalence, or simultaneously conflicting thoughts and feelings, is a common dynamic of the treatment process and represents a positive sign that new information and ideas are under consideration. Ambivalence is not to be mistaken for disinterest, nor does it indicate that SAM isn't working hard enough. He is not suggesting that a view to a "new reality" is impossible; perhaps he's simply wondering whether or not it is possible for him. By examining, disputing, and challenging myth and authenticity, SAM is developing an ability to discern his thoughts and feelings, perceptions and reactions, and goals and aspirations from those around him. Simultaneously conflicting thoughts, feelings, intentions, and actions, however, often generate anxiety.

Anxiety can be conceptualized as conflict that emerges between two discrepant perspectives. For example, when SAM experiences discrepancies between "who I am and who I think I should be," "what I think or feel and what I should think or feel," "what I'm doing or what I think I should be doing," the conflict between the two discordant points of view ignites with anxiety. In treatment the belief, "I should keep this to myself" is highly incongruous with the action of telling the story to the therapist (or to the group). The assumption "Sexually abused boys become perpetrators" and the personal hypothesis "Because I caused someone to abuse me, I deserve to be punished" collide with the wish to develop a loving and intimate relationship based on trust and equality. To be sure, SAM confronts discordancy from merely contemplating an incongruous perspective. Acting on one could be paralyzing. As a result of these intrapsychic and, in some cases, existential conflicts, it is not uncommon for SAM to have feelings of unreality as well as intense guilt or shame, often coinciding with panic attacks or fear of repercussions. If well defended during the day, anxiety may manifest in nightmares and night terrors during sleep.

For example, cognitive flashbacks, sudden visual images associated with an abusive episode, affective flashbacks, that is, shuddering surges of negative affect bypassing the defensive wall, somatic flashbacks, or the sensation of pain or discomfort in a part of the body subjected to the abuse, and kinesthetic flashbacks, a multisensory reexperiencing of the abuse, are commonly roused by environmental triggers and are even much more likely to occur when SAM is feeling vulnerable from anxiety. In a state of unrest, the defensive barrier may fall short of the threshold necessary to fully shield SAM from affect, thereby allowing abuse-related content in the form of a flashback to emerge. Paradoxically, when extremely focused on work, for instance, or when experiencing a sense of comfort, the defensive barrier may wane, allowing abuse-related content to seep through. The triggers, however, are similar in either case. For Nicholas, such triggers included hearing about or seeing a snake. For Jake, sexual overtures from his wife as well as lovemaking scenes on television or in movies often instigated flashbacks to the abuse. And whenever possible, Palo dodged small groups of men as a means of defending against the emergence of anxiety. Abuse-related nightmares and night terrors operate by a similar dynamic.

These reactions are natural responses to both childhood sexual abuse and to telling the story. What disconcerts SAM, time and time again, is that the triggers strike in the present whereas the content of the flashbacks and night terrors ricochets from the past (Chu, 1998; Crowder, 1995). Given the difficulty of discerning the trigger's connection to the response it elicits, not to mention the sensation of reliving the historic abuse in the present moment, it's no wonder that SAM feels "crazy" and out of control. Furthermore, because these fear-laden responses, conditioned by the amygdala, seem to be random, out of context, and with minimal, if any, connection to the present, SAM would like to—and will try to—make them disappear. Quite commonly, SAM endeavors to invalidate the traumatic symptomology by way of drinking, drugging, overworking, and acting out sexually, among many other avoidant and screening strategies. However, doing so only serves to reinforce the potency of the abuse-related content or aftereffects and to make them more compelling (somewhat akin to the "Don't think about pink elephants" syndrome.) Panic-filled thoughts such as "Oh my God I can't believe this is happening," "I'm going crazy," and so on further contribute to the intensity, just as gas induces an inferno from a flame.

Initially, SAM often feels out of control when these intrusive memories occur, but he can learn to regulate his reactions when they emerge (Briere, 1996a). Rather than fight or flee, the therapist can help SAM to confront the anxiety, accept that it's surfacing, and stay with it—as if riding a wave that builds in intensity but soon crests and wanes. Gentle reminders about who he is, where he is, and how he is, such as "I'm SAM, I'm in the office, I'm okay," help to ground him in the here and now—diminishing the urgency of the current trigger, the potency of the historic material, and the acuity of the stress response. Also, diaphragmatic breathing from the first sensation of anxiety can often fully inhibit, or at least diffuse, the interrelated biological, psychological, emotional, and physiological reactions. Until integration can occur between and among the shards of SAM's abuse history, wherein the past remains fractionated from the present, thoughts disconnected from feelings, and facts from their meanings, it is essential that the therapist ground SAM in the here and now, by providing a place where he can find support, options, validation, and connection. The therapist personifies an anchor, and this sense of boundary and security allows for further exploration.

Even without these particular flooding responses, focusing on sexual abuse issues can be extremely disquieting for and upsetting to SAM. In favor of minimizing anxiety responses and maximizing the potential for safety and progressive learning, the therapist employs a gradual and systematic treatment approach (Briere, 1996a; Courtois, 1999). This affords SAM the time to develop a greater capacity for emotional regulation before and while working through more defended, threatening, conflicted, and disrupting material.

To achieve this end, the therapist must be willing to move back and forth and between SAM's preabuse, abuse, postabuse, and current perspectives. This process enables SAM to utilize his own distancing abilities in order to protect himself while still maintaining focus on his history of abuse and currency of effects. Furthermore, the strategy of weaving forward and back again creates threads of meaning through SAM's experiences and permits both SAM and the therapist to uncover and appreciate the seed, the roots, and the trees of his current thoughts, feelings, and behaviors.

Understandably, SAM is often unable to differentiate between his authentic self and his compensatory self, between what is reality and what is fiction, and so forth. His abuse experience, from its recognition onward, was inundated by sensory overload, shielded by ego defense strategies, burdened by the perpetrator's injunctions, and overridden by socially constructed schemas and mythology. The very same may be happening today, months, years, or decades from the last sexually abusive episode. Thus, his bona fide truth remains encumbered by planks of personal, relational, social, and cultural impositions. Essentially, as concealment of his abuse and the invalidation of its occurrence and effects have happened not once but many times and in many contexts, it follows that SAM's authentic facts and his uncorrupted meanings associated with his abuse experience must be similarly imbedded under layers of social mythology, denial, self-blame, and compensatory rationales and behaviors. For example, Palo stated: "When I told my aunt, a medicine woman, about the abuse and my anxiety, she told me that I was like four corners of a room, but the room had no walls. The first corner, that's who I was before the abuse. The second, me during the abuse. The third, who I was after the abuse. And the fourth, who I am now. My medicine, she said, was to build the wall, to connect the four corners, and to live in that room for it was my life. What she didn't tell me was how frightening it would be."

By mirroring SAM's natural oscillation tendencies in the therapy process, alternating between preabuse, abuse, postabuse, and current perspectives, SAM is enabled to unearth these layers in the multicontextual manner in which they evolved. There is additional comfort for SAM in that he will not be required to stay in any one area too long, thereby minimizing the risk of becoming "stuck" or overwhelmed. By taking advantage of SAM's natural tendency to alternate between attention and dissociation, this therapeutic process can simultaneously uncover more information and enhance SAM's sense of comfort and control. Throughout, the therapist continually assesses SAM's current state as well as his willingness and readiness to proceed. At any given moment, the therapist must be prepared with a variety of interventive strategies that serve to pace, modulate, advance, stabilize, support, and sustain SAM on his trek toward abuse resolution.

When this objective is completed, SAM will have identified as many facts as possible that elucidate his experience of CSA. Additionally, he will have a developing capacity to normalize and contextualize his abuse-generated responses. Further, he will have gained additional experience in modulating the affect generated by his gradual exposure to abuse-related content. Slowly but surely, SAM rediscovers his history.

Objective 3

> SAM will infuse facts with contextual meaning in order to bring cognitive and affective points of view into the foreground with the facts.

As is often the case, SAM remains incognizant of the padlock between his experience of CSA and its generated effects. Neither the perpetrator nor social mythology inform SAM that he is blameless or that shame springs from social forces promoting abuse and from the perpetrator, not himself. They do not inform him about the horror and terror of it all, nor do they tell him about guilt, flashbacks, dissociation, emasculation, inferiority, panic, and the night terrors he comes to know so intimately along the way. They in fact help SAM believe that he was abused because he deserved to be abused. They in fact teach SAM to conceal and invalidate his authentic truth, to dissociate from what is real and to personify what is false. For these reasons and many more, SAM spends his childhood and adulthood in a wayward excursion to find normal.

Here, the therapeutic window comes into play (Briere, 1996a; Cole & Barney, 1987). As the window frame expands to include fact and meaning, the gradual augmentation of biophysiological attunement, cognitive comprehension, and emotional expressiveness becomes a function of SAM's ability to increasingly acknowledge and experience abuse-related content while decreasingly relying upon invalidation and defense strategies. This type of systematic, regulated, and graduated exposure operationalizes the third treatment objective by helping SAM "to evoke traumatic material but to process it in a sufficiently different way that it loses its potency and spontaneous and uncontrolled emergence" (Courtois, 1999, p. 210).

Therapy provides a context for SAM to understand the links between CSA and its effects, between his past and his present. The therapist can help SAM to reconstruct his past, to discover, understand, and integrate the fractionated shards of his abuse experience into a cohesive and evolving whole (Courtois, 1999; Crowder, 1995; Meiselman, 1990; van der Kolk, McFarlane, & van der Hart, 1996). The reconstruction and reintegration of SAM's abusive history unfold along three dimensions. It is important to keep in mind, however, that psychoeducation does not stop here, but rather continues to play a crucial role throughout the therapeutic process.

The three dimensions through which SAM is encouraged to relate his experiences are the facts, his cognitive points of view, that is, his beliefs and attitudes about the facts and his emotional points of view, or his affective responses to the facts (see "Facts and Meanings" intervention in chapter 10). In each of these dimensions, SAM reviews his abuse experiences in a slightly different manner. This repetition allows SAM to follow a natural progression of revelation leading to more facts, more meanings. And, because he most likely experienced numerous episodes of abuse, and in some cases subsequent abuse by another perpetrator, the fact that SAM was abused (even if he calls it by another name) can rarely be shielded from consciousness, but the significance such an event holds, embedded in the meanings, tends to be fractionated off. In no way will the facts of SAM's history change. Yes, he will strive to do so and, in fact, will often use therapy as a resource to accomplish this seemingly feasible but utterly impossible outcome. However, at intervals and by degrees, SAM gradually realizes the constancy of facts and the malleability of meaning. Understanding that meanings can change becomes his harbor of hope.

More specifically, by simply presenting the facts of his abuse, SAM maintains his defenses that serve to invalidate and deny the significance of the abuse thus preventing him from becoming overwhelmed. Next, while SAM begins to attach a point of view to the factual realities of his abuse, he is still able to preserve some distance while exploring the discrepancies between what he was taught and his authentic responses. And finally, SAM is encouraged to make a connection between the facts, the differing points of view, and his emotional reactions. For example, Jake stated the following fact: "I was abused by a Catholic priest." His cognitive point of view revealed: "Sex with a priest and sex before marriage and sex with another guy are sins so I must be punished." On the third iteration, Jake's affective point of view was voiced in this way: "I feel evil, like Satan, worse than a whore. That makes me undeserving of any real love." The first statement represents a fact of his story; the cognitve and affective points of view comprise the meanings imbuing the fact. By constructing and repeating the story in this way, SAM can explore his history in a progressive, multilayered context similar to the way in which his understanding of the abuse was first created. This process, guided by the therapist's moment-by-moment assessment and informed by the CSA knowledge base, naturally and noninvasively affords SAM the opportunity to gradually decrease his reliance on invalidation strategies—avoidance, stress-induced opioid discharge, addictions, and compulsions—and to simultaneously increase his exposure to traumatic material—implicit memories, explicit learning, dissociated affect, and negative schemata—in tractable increments (Cornell & Olio, 1991; Pearlman & Saakvitne, 1995). Further, by working in a gradual and cumulative manner, one fact at a time and from the less intimidating facts to their more threatening affective meanings, the therapist and SAM are more likely to create an experience of mastery rather than a symbolic reenactment of his abuse history (Lebowitz et al., 1993). In this way, deconditioning and desensitization of the traumatic material begins to occur (Briere, 1996a; Rachman, 1980; Siegel, 1995).

Quite commonly, CSA dynamics, such as the perpetrator's threats and social injunctions warning against concealment, and CSA effects, including the initial traumatic response, habituated autonomic arousal, and generalized fear patterns, interrupt the flow and continuity of narrative processing at some point in time (van der Hart et al., 1993; van der Kolk, Burbridge, & Suzuki, 1991). However, verbal expression is not the only way that the facts and the cognitive and affective points of view might be presented. Often the abuse-related intrapsychic, cognitive, affective, and physiologic content is encapsulated in some variant of a sensory symbol. For example, Kip contained abuse elements in a visualization of a hand reaching inside and crushing his heart. Alternatively, Palo encapsulated the abuse kinesthetically through the sensation of being weighted down, as if carrying a yoke across his back.

Facts and meanings, encapsulated in this manner, may inhibit SAM's ability to verbalize the realities of his abuse. First of all, the symbol was actually created in a traumatic state, recording the event without words, and second, the sensory phenomenon summarizes so much information that simple speech may, at first, fail to adequately convey the true meaning behind the symbol (Hartman & Burgess, 1993). "A picture is worth a thousand words," but for SAM, this "picture" could be olfactory, auditory, kinesthetic, gustatory, visual, or any combination among the sensory receptors. Furthermore, the chosen symbol may, on the surface, appear to have minimal, if any, association or relevance to the actual abusive experience that it contains.

In order for SAM to identify the content within the symbol and to verbalize his experiences, the implicit symbols first have to be acknowledged. If the abuse-related content cannot be verbalized, then the sensory image can be externalized. The initial mode of communication, in many instances, can parallel the mode of encapsulation. For example, if the symbol is visual, then the communication could be conveyed through painting or drawing. If encapsulated kinesthetically, then the symbolic expression could be through movement or position. Once the symbol is externalized, then both the image itself and the particular mode of its containment can be examined to understand and verbalize the meaning it holds. Due to the very act of externalizing these images in a safe, controlled environment, SAM is also able to connect all of his sensory modalities and, eventually, to integrate both the symbol and the meaning that it embodies into his greater story. Essentially, this strategy, like many others, helps SAM to noninvasively transform his implicit memories into an explicit mode, thereby contributing to the clarity, assimilation, and resolution of his traumatic past (Siegel, 1995).

For SAM, the longer the abuse is concealed, the more defenses are necessary to invalidate its meaning. Consequently, as with the exploration, identification, and interpretation of symbols, the process of reconstructing the abuse is, by necessity, incremental in nature as well. As the gleaning of some facts exposes others, SAM discovers an increasingly broader range of his abuse history. The cyclical nature of this progressive technique also gives SAM time, between each go-round, to assimilate the emerging facts and meanings. And the gradual, controlled, and stepwise exposure to the facts and meanings—from memory to cognitive recognition onto affective expression or from the symbolic to the somatic onto the verbal—in tandem with the support of the therapist and the structure of the therapeutic process, produces the recontextualization of meaning and the reintegration of the fractionated self (Meiselman, 1990; Rieker & Carmen, 1986).

JUST THE FACTS

By focusing simply on the presentation of facts, SAM slowly immerses into his past without becoming overwhelmed by the totality of the abusive experience(s). On the one hand, SAM often presents with the expectation that an early, emotionally cathartic experience will act as an elixir, ensuring brief treatment and "curing" him of CSA's devastating and enduring effects. On the other hand, SAM may fear that an emotionally cathartic experience will overwhelm him: that he will go crazy, that he will somehow lose himself, with no chance of returning from it. For others, whose authentic meanings are consistently mediated by dissociation, denial, and suppression and/or regulated by perpetrator, familial, gender, and social prohibitions against acknowledgment and disclosure, the very notion of having a cognitive or affective point of view remains foreign.

Because much time and attention has been devoted to establishing a therapeutic alliance, the security provided by this relationship allows SAM to deliberately and purposefully delve into the past and yet return to the comfort and safety of the bond evolving with the therapist in the present. For SAM, by focusing solely on the facts, he will learn about pacing himself, uncovering the realities of the past with determination and preparedness, and sealing them off when necessary or appropriate. For the therapist, focusing on the facts, and just the facts, is not intended to prohibit SAM's affect, but merely to decrease its dictatorial role. Further, by means of stepwise exposure, the therapist is afforded numerous opportunities to assess the impact of both the content and the consequences of the social mythology, schemata, and defenses on SAM.

ESTABLISHING A POINT OF VIEW

During this iterating segment, SAM again has the chance to communicate the facts of his abuse. This time, though, he does so with the intention of discovering the multiple points of view attached to each fact. At this juncture, then, SAM explores the facts one by one. During one session, Kip conveyed the following fact: "When I finally told my Moms about the attack, she threw the phone book at me and called me a 'faggot.'" Through exploration of the situational factors involved in that scenario, including the role of motherhood, Kip's disclosure and his mother's response to that disclosure, a point of view emerged. During this process, Kip stated: "My mother must be right. Something really is wrong with me. I am screwed up." Shortly thereafter, he contested with the following: "Maybe she was saying that to hurt me. I don't feel gay."

Establishing a point of view serves as a bridge for SAM between the recitation of the facts of his abuse and the connection of affect to them. In other words, it creates a basis from which SAM will incrementally discover how his feelings relate to his abusive experiences. Although SAM is still able to maintain some distance exploring his points of view, it nonetheless brings him one step closer to unearthing the authentic meaning fractionated within his story of abuse.

EMOTIONAL CONNECTION

By this time, SAM has recited the facts several times. As a matter of course, the shock of recognition upon hearing himself voice the realities of abuse is diminishing. In fact, there is a developing sense of familiarity with the facts. Now SAM can explore the facts and their points of view, one by one, and begin to discover his feelings which lie underneath. The focus here is not on reliving the abusive experience, but rather on identifying corresponding affect. This process still allows SAM to maintain some distance, however, because the abuse continues to be discussed retrospectively, in the past tense, regardless of whether it happened 2 weeks or 20 years ago. (Refer to the intervention entitled "Facts and Meaning" in chapter 10 for a systematic and graphic presentation of this process.)

Connecting an affective point of view to the facts and cognitive points of view is often very challenging for SAM. Exposure to childhood sexual abuse forces children to cope and adapt by means of denial, dissociation, and other ego defense strategies operating to buffer the cognitive and affective significance of such trauma. Before, during, and after CSA, gender-role socialization processes direct males to detach emotionally and act rationally. To be sure, CSA conjures potent emotions, such as fear, helplessness, panic, powerlessness, and sadness, all socially allocated to the female gender and, by default, disallowed as valid and appropriate for the male gender. Thus, both CSA and gender-role socialization, in tandem, inhibit SAM's range of accessible affect, one reinforcing the other, leaving his emotions tightly caulked.

As a boy, SAM, while simultaneously coping with the facts of CSA, must also not forget to act fearlessly, hide the pain, and force back the tears even though his authentic feelings are fear, devastation, and sadness (Bolton et al., 1989). Taking this emotional methodology into manhood, SAM, consciously or otherwise, recognizes that the two most accepted forms of expression are anger and neutrality—the former, for its sensations of power and control, and the latter, for its apparent freedom from any affect at all. This does not imply that SAM is devoid of feelings such as guilt, shame, terror, or joy. However, emotions like these are generally experienced involuntarily and are perceived as overwhelming, thereby indicating, from SAM's perspective, a lack of control.

SAM might even understand his emotions cognitively, while kinesthetically or experientially they remain foreign to him. Therefore, SAM must go through a relearning process. Although he disconnected from his body during the abuse, in one way or by multiple means, he now needs his body in order to appreciate the depth and range of human emotions. One way for him to accomplish this is to reconnect with his physical being. Given the physiological manifestation of and responses to emotions, SAM can build on his affective range by tuning into and understanding his body's experience of affective stimuli. To begin, the therapist works with SAM to explore, identify, and describe his internal experience—the physiological manifestations, for example, clenched jaw, respiratory rate, feeling flushed, heart rate, and sensations in the stomach; the cognitive precursors and maintainers, for example, predispositional thoughts (e.g., "I don't like talking about this") and emotively exacerbating thoughts (e.g., "I'm going to lose control if we keep this up"); behavioral indicators like laughing out of sync or pounding a fist; and material sensations, such as awareness of his body's contact with the chair or the posturing of his hands. This type of exploration and description serves to familiarize SAM with different feeling states while at the same time helping to ground him in the here and now. These two anticipated outcomes contribute to the desensitization of the adrenaline based fear–affect–fear cycle (Briere, 1996a). As his body begins to work as an antenna for a greater range of affective responses, it then becomes more than simply a harbor for the abuse effects.

Kip began to explore the feelings associated with the fact and cognitive points of view regarding his abuse disclosure. Questions such as "How do you feel about that?" or "What did that feel like?" tend to yield little. However, when exploring and describing the accordant feeling state triggered by his mother's derogatory remark, Kip was able to deduce the corresponding emotional point of view in the following way: "It was like, like um, getting punched, in the chest, hard to breathe. I wanted to scream back at her but my mouth almost couldn't open, freaky, like it was crazy glued. She just walked away after throwing the phone book at me. I thought I was losing it. My breath, I couldn't catch my breath. But then I remembered what you said about breathing deep. Then what you said about just opening your mouth to let words come. So when I went to my room, I opened my mouth and there was a sound like a tortured cat. And then I cried. I guess you call that being hurt and sad. Really sad."

As SAM achieves this objective, he will indicate an ability to differentiate thought from feeling and fact from meaning. Additionally, he will have gained a sense of comfort with his emotionality, a sense of congruency between and among thought, feeling, and behavior, and a burgeoning sense of autobiographical continuity.

Objective 4

SAM will analyze the various points of view in order to differentiate the authentic from the socially imposed.

By this stage in the treatment process, SAM has highlighted a number of facts and their corresponding cognitive and affective points of view. Now it is imperative that he have the opportunity to discern and appraise the sources of his abuse-generated thoughts and feelings. In keeping with the SAM model treatment philosophy, the focus is less on the facts and more on the points of view. Thus, the intended outcome of this process is the differentiation between SAM's point of view and that of others.

When clients come into treatment, their goal, more often than not, is to change the facts of the story—the facts of their history. The facts of Ty's story, such as "I was beaten up and abused by my cousin Rodney and his gang. They fucked me. I bled. One shit on me. I tried to tell my Grandmama. I couldn't get the words out," are all too common and, unfortunately, unamenable to change. Only the meanings associated with CSA can change, not the facts (Crowder, 1995). Such meanings are, as a matter of course, socially imposed; therefore, SAM's truth cannot be told, nor can it be validated, without a thorough examination of the social context in which boys are sexually abused, and the very social context in which they internalize its mythology. SAM cannot identify and reclaim what is authentic until social impositions have been explored, identified, unveiled, disputed, and relinquished. This objective initiates that process.

Following are some common beliefs held by SAM, as well as corresponding sources.

BELIEFS IMPOSED BY SOCIAL MYTHOLOGY

1. Sexual abuse only happens to girls.
2. Sexual abuse does not happen to boys.

3. Males are perpetrators; females are victims.
4. Males cannot be "victims" and "victims" cannot be males.
5. If sexual abuse does happen, you must have wanted it.
6. If you were "abused" by a male, you must be gay.
7. If you were "abused" by a male and didn't stop it, you really wanted it.
8. If you were "abused" by a female, then it's really not abuse.
9. If you were "abused" by a female and did not like it, then something is wrong with you.
10. If you have a history of abuse, you will become a perpetrator.

BELIEFS IMPOSED BY THE PERPETRATOR

1. "I love you. That's why I'm doing this to you."
2. "You better learn now: Love hurts!"
3. "Mothers don't hurt their children. Mothers love their children. You just don't know how to love."
4. "If you didn't want it, you would have stopped me."
5. "I was just trying to be affectionate with you, son. Now your erection proves to me that you are a sexual pervert. You can't blame this on me."
6. "If you tell anyone, they will think you wanted this to happen."
7. "If you tell anyone, you will ruin my life."
8. "You're a fag, a queer, a mistake, a she-boy. I'm only giving what you deserve."
9. "I'm only trying to teach you. Don't be an ingrate."
10. "All boys do this. Billy and his Daddy across the street do this. It's a secret code. This is how boys become men."

BELIEFS GENERATED BY OVERUSE OF DEFENSES

1. You can see whatever you want to see.
2. It's normal to feel nothing.
3. Don't let your guard down, or the dam will break and drown you.
4. Don't worry if you can't remember. It must not be important.
5. It's only a movie—except this time you're the actor and the audience.
6. If you really cared, you would be feeling something.
7. So, you don't feel like yourself. Fake it!
8. If you don't like a certain thought or a certain feeling, just nuke it.
9. It only looks real, but it's really not.
10. Pretend! Pretend! Pretend!

COMMON BELIEFS HELD BY SAM BUT IMPOSED BY CSA

1. "It really wasn't abuse."
2. "It was my fault."

3. "I am a mistake. Something is really wrong with me."
4. "I wanted it to happen."
5. "I should have wanted it to happen."
6. "My erection and ejaculation prove that."
7. "I really must be gay."
8. "I am a whore. I'm going to turn into a perpetrator."
9. "Maybe God made a mistake. I should be a girl."
10. "I deserve to be punished."

Abuse-generated schemata are widely spattered, impacting views about the self, the perpetrator, love, sexuality, relationships, the social environment, and the future, which, in turn, incite core states of emasculation, shame, powerlessness, inferiority, self-blame, humiliation, hopelessness, fear, and despair, among so many others. Given the robust and bewildering nature of abuse-generated cognition and affect, it is important that SAM learn about the ways in which certain statements provoke and intensify overwhelming feeling states. In keeping with the construct of reciprocal determinism, or the ways in which thoughts influence feelings, feelings impact behaviors, behaviors prompt new thoughts, and so on (Beck, 1993; Ellis, 1995), the therapist can work with SAM to become mindful of cognitive antecedents to deluging affect and cognitions that tend to exacerbate affect once it has emerged. Examples of antecedent cognitions include "It's my fault," "Something is wrong with me," and "I deserve to be punished"; "This is gonna make me go crazy," "I'm out of control," and "I want to jump out of my skin" are examples of exacerbating cognitions. As SAM learns to trace backward from affect to cognition, and develops an awareness of his particular antecedent and exacerbating thoughts and beliefs, he can also acquire skill in anticipating and averting problematic cognitions by means of thought stopping, positive self-talk, thought disputation, reframing the thought sequences as "old tapes," and grounding techniques (Briere, 1996a; Deblinger & Helflin, 1996). This will help SAM build a stronger base from which to discover, reexperience and reintegrate the multivariate aspects of his abuse history.

Sexual abuse beliefs can be viewed as authentic to the self, or internalizations of social impositions, "as if" they belong to the self. If the source truly is oneself, and the beliefs are viewed as authentic, SAM, in many cases, might want to retain them. Why? There's strength and power in that stance. For example, if SAM, in referencing the abuse, believes "it is my fault," he can also strive to do something about it, thereby cultivating a sense of empowerment in a situation rife with powerlessness. Moreover, powerlessness is antithetical to male gender mythology and socialization, making such a stance all the more compelling.

However, if SAM believes that he is a "whore," and, at the same time can see that he has not always believed that about himself, change can occur. If SAM can recognize that, in fact, the perpetrator and perhaps others in his microenvironments conveyed similar messages to him, that is, imposed those beliefs on him, then he has an opportunity to claim or disown them. To do so, SAM must question the source.

Questions such as "Where did that view come from?" or "Who's voice is that?" enable SAM to identify the author of these perspectives. This provides him with another opportunity to explore the validity of various viewpoints with the intent of determining if the derived meaning is authentically his or was inflicted. For instance, in the Kip example, the label "faggot" was socially imposed by his mother, causing him to doubt the legitimacy of his hetero-sexual orientation. Once he identified his mother as the source of this point of view and disowned it as his, he began to relinquish the confusion around his sexual orientation. Thus, over time, by placing the abuse in context, SAM will come to understand that his disparaging beliefs and his slanderous feelings as well a myriad of other CSA effects make sense and, in fact, he will come to realize that some of the symptoms were imaginative and resourceful responses to childhood deception, violation, and indignity (Courtois, 1988).

As SAM meets this objective, he will evidence an ability to analyze a behavioral chain, from trigger to thoughts to feelings to action and on to the consequences of such. He will have developed the capacity to discern the sources of internalized beliefs as well as an evolving skill base from which he can manage, modify, dispute, or validate them. Additionally, he will have gained experience in relaxing defensive reactions in service of discovering his truth.

Objective 5

SAM will recount his story of abuse, from the perspective of the first person, present tense, in order to confirm and validate his history as experienced.

In the process of identifying the facts of his sexual abuse, attaching cognitive points of view and connecting emotional responses to them, SAM, in authoring his story, continues to maintain a retrospective stance, that of looking back upon his abusive experiences. Now SAM will narrate his autobiography (Crowder, 1995), but this time from the perspective of first-person present tense, as he would have told it while in the throes of CSA (Herman, 1992). Utilization of the first-person present tense vis-à-vis this treatment objective is intended to support SAM in integrating his preabuse, abuse, and postabuse experiences and reactions within his evolving sense of self.

Often, however, it is far more comfortable for SAM to continue speaking about the abuse in the past tense and in very general terms. Although this is understandable, given that SAM's weeks, months, or years of exposure to so-cial mythologies and overuse of defensive strategies have yielded so-called "sensibilities," it is important that SAM utilize the first-person present tense in the telling of his story in order to circumvent these distancing maneuvers. Such sensibilities are highlighted in the following examples.

Nicholas stated: "I'm a big boy now, and you a big, big boy, so I don't want you to cry." Kip expressed: "If I were stronger then I wouldn't have to be here. I wouldn't be having these problems. And besides, you'll probably feel sorry for me and that's the last thing I want." Palo revealed: "Telling my story will only shock and disgust you, therefore I shouldn't do it." Matt disclosed: "I need to protect you from the vileness. I don't want to ruin our relationship or make you terminate my case." Victor asked: "If I tell you what really happened to me, you might think that I will become perpetrator, or that something is really wrong with me. If I tell my story then you might come to believe that I really am a whore and a faggot and that I really wanted it, so what's the point?" Jake inquired: "It was so long ago. Why am I making such a big deal about it now?" And Ty whispered: "It really wasn't bad. He loved me. I think he loved me. That's the only way he knew how to love me."

"It." They call sexual abuse "it." This, as well as other sensibilities, may be expressed directly or indirectly, prior to or during the telling of the story. Because they serve as barriers to disclosure, it is important for the therapist to help SAM identify their existence, explore their source(s), consider the degree to which they are authentic or imposed, and determine whether they serve or disserve SAM's intention to tell the truth.

Actually, it is important that SAM identify and eradicate as many barriers as possible before he tells his story in the first-person present tense. Despite lengthy bouts of dissociation, and as much as SAM might want to deny the reality of his experiences, his history of abuse cannot be changed and therefore still plays a major role in his present life and future ambitions. Dissociation, depersonalization, and suppression, among other defense strategies, have served to segregate and compartmentalize these abuse experiences from his identity. The perception "This isn't happening to me," once a momentary reaction at the onset of CSA, over time transforms into the core belief, "This didn't happen to me. What I see I don't see; what I know I don't know; what I think and feel isn't really real" (Rieker & Carmen, 1986). Like a missile led astray, this core belief remains operative until silence is broken. Narrativization, in the form of first-person present tense, allows SAM to intentionally and noninvasively integrate the abuse-generated and contextual data generated thus far, including his memories of the abuse, its dynamics and effects, his points of view regarding the abuse, and his emotional reactions to the abuse.

In contrast with the fact that social mythology renders SAM's abuse experience seemingly unreal, the first-person present tense authenticates CSA by framing it as a factual occurrence in his life with a designated place in his history. The language of first-person present tense heightens the connection between the author and his story, the present and his past, and the importance of being truthful and the cogency of his truth. The language of third-person past tense, by its very nature, promotes distance from the subject and the detachment of fact from meaning. In this case, a third-person passive voice is akin to invalidating the abuse by supporting the notion, "this didn't really happen to me." However, the first person, as expressed through "I," "me," and "mine," and the present tense, as expressed via the "here and now," supports and advances SAM in becoming the proprietor of his past.

Ultimately, it is from the first-person present-tense perspective that abuse-related desensitization occurs. SAM's mere exposure to the facts of his story, regardless of person and tense, may connect him to the traumatic event but continue to distance him from the dissociated aspects of his abuse story, thereby doing little to ameliorate the abuse effects (Briere, 1996a; Rachman, 1980; van der Kolk et al., 1996). By way of the first-person present-tense perspective, SAM is likely to remember more fully, reexperience more sensorially and relay more authoritatively his abuse experience as it occurred, thereby assisting in the progress of emotional discharge and relief. Operationally, this process serves to decondition SAM's traumatic memories and effects (Briere, 1996a).

In pursuit of the rectification of CSA effects and reintegration of CSA into an evolving life history, SAM does not simply "relive" a sexually abusive episode but, in fact, begins to decondition CSA memories and effects (Siegel, 1995, 2001). Deconditioning requires a number of facilitating elements (van der Kolk et al., 1996). First, as highlighted in Objective 2, the therapist must facilitate SAM's graduated exposure to the content of his abuse history. Second, as per Objective 3, SAM progressively integrates fact with cognition and affect in a stepwise manner (Briere, 1996a). Third, therapy must introduce an element absent from and at variance with the sexually abusive episode (Foa, Steketee, & Rothbaum, 1989). In this case, the therapist as ally, witness, and guide, the therapeutic relationship as an anchorage of trust, and the therapeutic environment as a refuge of safety together comprise the new element. Fourth, therapy must introduce an element capable of setting in motion a memory network of CSA-related sensorial memories. In this context, telling the story from the perspective of the first-person present tense noninvasively rekindles traumatic memories but this time in the presence of a caring other.

SAM does not narrativize his sexual abuse history simply for the sake of reconjuring the past. Over time, the iterative experiencing and expulsion of abuse-related content neutralizes the cognitive, sensory, affective, semantic, motoric, and behavioral memories. This iterative deconditioning process helps SAM to desensitize the amygdala and transform implicit memories into an explicit narrative. Explicit processing of the sexually abusive experience— when it happened, who abused him, where it occurred, what he saw, how he felt, who knew, who did nothing, where he hid his bloody underwear, the perpetrator's threats, the prayers for it to stop—promotes the establishment of hippocampal and cortical circuits which, in turn, facilitate the storage of a progressively metabolized and neutralized form of memory (Siegel, 1995). The therapist's steadfast presence and empathic responsivity—her facial expressions, his tone of voice, an understanding and acceptance that SAM has so desperately desired—not only maintain attunement with SAM but contribute to his synaptic growth, brain plasticity, and development of a new internalized relational model (Schore, 1996).

In fact, SAM's actions throughout the therapeutic process thus far—that of acknowledging the facts, attaching a point of view, forming an emotional connection, and telling the story in the first-person present tense—represent a fundamental leap toward attaining command (by effort) over abuse-generated imagery, invasions, compulsions, and other effects, over their unbridled emergence, and over his intense and unnerving responses to them. Furthermore, by breaking the silence and reclaiming the personal significance of the abuse, SAM moves forward, gradually and steadily, toward liberation from his past— a past that does not dictate the present, and a present that can now be utilized to create a future of his choice.

In the telling of his story, SAM is restrained only by the requirement that it be in the first-person present tense—from SAM's perspective as a boy— regardless of his current chronological age. In all other respects, SAM has as much latitude as he wishes. Sometimes, he might wish to write his story out beforehand and to then read it aloud to the therapist, or to the group, if applicable. More often than not, SAM comes to the session prepared to read verbatim from his notes but once the story begins, the notes are often placed to the side.

To further signify storytelling, SAM might also wish to utilize boyhood momentos, photographs, as well as other items that help him convey his authentic truth. For example, Zach, who had been a child prodigy on the piano, was sexually abused by his concert master during preparation for a debut performance. Feeling shocked and shamed, and not knowing how to stop the abuse or who to tell, he purposefully began to make mistakes. When that strategy failed, he simply withdrew from his work on the piano. Consequently, Zach was replaced and since the age of 11, he never returned to or completed the piece that he had been working on so diligently. Twenty-seven years later, participating in a group for adult males with histories of CSA, Zach told his story. Before speaking, he sat at a piano. After flipping through a number of sheets, he began at the very bar where he had left off years ago, now completing the unfinished concerto.

There are other options for SAM as well. He can decide where to sit, where others, including the therapist, sit, whether he wants people to ask questions or offer comments before or after the telling of his story, whether or not to bring a friend or significant other, whether he would like his story tape recorded, among many other options. Of course, in a group setting, the use of recording equipment and the presence of collaterals must be agreed on in advance, by the group as a whole. The purpose of these options is to create as much comfort and safety as possible for SAM so that the story can be told with as much authenticity as possible.

The therapist's role, of course, is key throughout the abuse resolution process but particularly so as SAM relays his story. This phase of treatment presents another opportunity for the creation of moments of meaning, that is, moments of transaction within the therapeutic dyad that personify the establishment of a new and ameliorating set of implicit memories for SAM (Stern, 1998). This points to the notion of brain laterilzation and specialization. The left cerebral hemisphere specializes in analytical, logical, and sequential processing; it is linear and time sensitive. The right cerebral hemisphere specializes in intuitive, schematic, emotional, and holistic processing; it is more amenable to sensory perception than abstract thought (Schore, 1994). SAM's story, generated in a graduated manner, from fact to meaning, helps elevate the abuse-generated content to a cortical level whereby it can be processed explicitly or consciously (Siegel, 1995, 1999). Akin to the interactions between caretaker and child, nonverbal transactions within the therapeutic dyad—SAM's tears, the therapist's expressive empathy, their attunement and attachment, the therapist's acceptance, SAM's security—are recorded implicitly (Schore, 1996). The therapist's attention to both the explicit and the implicit aspects of SAM's story as well as attention to the cultivation and sustainment of an egalitarian relationship, characterized by unconditional positive regard, mutual respect, and empathy, create change for SAM at the cellular level (Liggan & Kay, 1999). As the relationship progresses, as he bravely tells his story and as he receives empathic responses, SAM implicitly senses, stores, and encodes a new relational model (Siegel, 1995).

Further, SAM does not merely convey a linear fact; he integrates it with contextual meaning. Nor does he simply reexperience an abuse-generated memory; rather, he and the therapist cognitively process the facts and meaning. Their right-brain to right-brain communication (Schore, 1996) and their left-brain to left-brain reflection and analyses (Siegel, 1999) combine to create a narrative that represents the evolving integration of his explicit and implicit systems of memory, the evolving synthesis of history and currency and, perhaps, the evolving integration of his preabuse, abuse, and postabuse selves. Little by little, conditioned fear responses, defensive constellations, feelings of emasculation, perpetrator injunctions, negative schemata, and socially imposed meanings, once processed, understood, and no longer necessary, give way to SAM's authentic truth. Thus, psychotherapy, as art and science, impacts SAM biologically, psychologically, and sociologically.

PROCESSING OF THE STORY

Initially, SAM may have many responses to telling his story. He is exhausted. He is elated. He is surprised. Even though the content of his story is disturbing, he often experiences, cognitively and/or affectively, a sense of accomplishment. In fact, storytelling in this context is customarily perceived as a life-changing event, shattering the secrecy and letting others glimpse the authentic self behind the compensatory self. SAM realizes, on some level and to some degree, that he is migrating from secrecy to disclosure, from mythology to authenticity, from fear to action, from dissociation to integration, and from one who has invalidated his history to one who is claiming it.

Through the process of telling the story, with as much authentic meaning as possible, SAM has the opportunity to reexamine attribution. He begins to see that he was violated and overpowered, and his submitting to the abuse was actually wise, the only viable strategy available to ensure survival both psychically and physically. By narrating, listening to, and experiencing his story in the first-person present tense, SAM can also appreciate that it was natural for him to want to survive, just as it was natural for him to comply with an elder, to get an erection in the face of danger or stimulation, and to conceal the abuse when confronted with threats and manipulations. Although SAM most likely accommodated the abuse at the time of its occurrence, unable to integrate the facts and meanings into preexisting schemas, he now begins to assimilate his history of CSA by way of authentically understanding what happened in childhood and attaching new meaning to the experience and its biological, psychological, and sociological importations (Courtois, 1999). Indeed, SAM is in the process of creating new memories, reclaiming his sense of self and overriding social mythology. Victor stated: "When it was happening, I, of course, couldn't call it incest. If I disrespected my father I disrespected God's commandments. In my culture, the man who dominates, you know, penetrates—he still maintains his machismo. He's still a man. In my mind, when he was doing this to me, I had to pretend that I wasn't his son, just his puta. When he did this to me, I couldn't be Victor any more. But now I see that I was always Victor. My father was a sick man. I don't like to say this, but he was a criminal. He stole my childhood. He betrayed my mother, his wedding vows. He stopped being my father. I never stopped being his son. I lost Victor once, but never again." So while SAM's sense of agency at the time of the abuse was unlawfully seized by his perpetrator, he is now in the process of repossessing it by stating the facts, infusing them with contextual meaning, and placing responsibility for the abuse on the perpetrator.

Ironically, such a catalytic event, which may have been weeks, months, or years in the making, often engenders a loss of equilibrium. Furthermore, SAM may fear that the perpetrator's threats will come true (even if the perpetrator is dead). Or he may fear that he is a traitor, breaking faith with others invested in concealing his abuse. After the initial sense of elation and accomplishment dissipates, SAM may feel exposed and vulnerable, thus arousing a need to retreat and, possibly, to recant. Additionally, SAM, overwhelmed by this perceived sense of exposure, may vacillate between emotional connection and detachment and/or experience an increase in anxiety and depressive symptomology.

As the unconscious becomes conscious, as defenses relax and feelings emerge, and as SAM strives to "do different to create different," he enters uncharted territory endowed with beliefs once embedded, feelings once foreign

and actions in service of his well-being. All of this can be disconcerting for
SAM, as historically familiar yet life-diminishing coping strategies give way to
adaptive measures that, in their newness, seem unwieldy, clumsy, and without
proof, only promise. For more than a few, CSA effects and coping responses
appear to be getting worse instead of better (Courtois, 1999).

It is important to normalize all of these reactions given the biological,
intrapsychic, cognitive, affective, and behavioral transitions required to tell the
story in this manner. Reactions to telling the story, such as guilt, shame, anxiety, conditioned fear responses, the emergence of additional explicit memories, depression, and hyperarousal, among others, are natural and expected
and SAM needs to be reassured that they will, in fact, diminish with time. His
joy and excitement, disbelief and triumph, may intermit as well. But nothing
need diminish his sense of pride, accomplishment, and his memory of this
momentous occasion. It should further be acknowledged that the telling of
SAM's story is in bold opposition to social mythology, to his defenses and to
the lies he had to believe in order to maintain concealment. Telling the truth,
not an easy task for SAM since much of his current identity, in substantial
measure, functions to invalidate and compensate for the abuse, as it is built on
distortion, imposition, and myth, all but nearly entombing his plain yet sober-
ing truth.

Through the social forces that mandate SAM's concealment of his abuse as
well as the invalidation strategies that allow him to maintain this myth/truth
duality, SAM has effectively compartmentalized perception from recognition,
the real from the imaginary, and the authentic self from the compensatory self.
Telling the truth threatens this compartmentalization by fostering a budding
sense of cohesion and wholeness for SAM. Even though the voice of illusion
may currently be stronger than SAM's authentic voice, the telling of the truth,
its subsequent validation, and the recognition of an empathic and understanding other are very compelling experiences for SAM.

Further, as SAM's authentic self emerges, replete with schemas congruent
with the reality of CSA, not its mythology, self-incrimination begins to cease—
for accusing himself, for being unable to prevent the abuse, for enjoying aspects of it, for despising himself, and so on. In time, as his thoughts, feelings,
and behaviors align with his newly augmented understanding of the contexts
of his abuse (both in the past and in the present), he takes another step toward
unshackling the guilt and shame that have burdened him since subjection.
And, as perpetrator culpability overshadows self-blame, a new realization cautiously surfaces into view—that the abuse was not a reflection of his self-worth
but rather the perpetrator's pathology (Crowder, 1995). This, like many other
recontexualized beliefs about the abuse, transforms slowly and emerges gradually, a little at a time.

Throughout this process, and in noninvasive ways, self-care and self-soothing skills evolve, thoughts link with feelings, facts merge with meanings, significant memory lapses narrow, and traumatic contents begin to metabolize.

SAM now has a narrative of his abuse experience—accessible and valid; coherent and cohesive—that can be integrated within his evolving life story (Brown et al., 1998; Herman, 1992). Yet, in spite of these positive albeit abstract consequences, SAM may, after the telling of his story, also feel apprehensive or uncertain. He may also continue to feel vulnerable, to oscillate between attachment and disassociation and to experience feelings of derealization or depersonalization. In addition, SAM may also fear that, because he does not feel completely different, that all of his work thus far has been ineffectual in "changing" him. This primarily stems from the misperception that the story is the endpoint. SAM may not realize that love, self-respect, healing, and, in fact, all growth processes are infinite. Jake stated: "When I came into therapy, I wanted to tell the story and leave. I thought the story would be a dead-end. Where do you go from there? I didn't realize what a turning point it would be. I always thought that if you talked about something painful, you made it worse. I'm learning that the opposite is true." Palo revealed: "Being here [in therapy] reminds me of my Lakota teachings. The gift that you get in therapy and the gift that you get in life is that learning is eternal. Telling my story showed me how far I had come. At that point, I began to forgive myself, almost to love myself. And I know that until I take my last breath, I can learn to forgive myself for fully and to love myself more deeply. That's the gift."

At this point, SAM has the capacity to transform emotionally conditioned implicit memory into an explicit narrative and the ability to cognitively analyze the experience. In this way, he unites the past with the present, synthesizes the implicit with the explicit, and integrates thoughts, feelings, and behaviors into a cohesive narrative. He will likely evidence a developing sense of agency, cognitive flexibility, and emotional comfort, as well as a consolidating sense of identity as the lines of demarcation around the abuse experience slowly give way to autobiographical continuity.

Objective 6

SAM will identify losses and gains in order to grieve the former and claim the latter.

After telling his story once, and many times thereafter, SAM is often left wondering why he does not feel remarkably different. He may also find himself wondering what to do next. This sense of confusion may stem from the fact that, given the emotional connectedness he experienced when telling his story, SAM, perhaps for the first time, also glimpsed the impact of the many losses associated with sexual abuse. Existential anguish ensues (Courtois, 1999). Matt asked: "Why did this happen to me?" Jake wondered: "Who could I have been if I didn't have to spend most of my life running from the abuse, from him and from my mind?" Kip stated: "I can't tell if I'm a loser or if I just lost who I was supposed to be. I want to be the boy I was before but, fuck man, I don't know if I'm ever gonna be him again." Even though SAM may strive to avoid grief and mourning, and understandably so, the therapist and therapeutic protocol cannot.

There are a multitude of losses associated with CSA, both tangible and intangible. While tangible losses, such as the physical loss of his virginity, or the loss of relationship with his perpetrator (and possibly with others as well), are of great importance to SAM, the significance of intangible losses should not be underestimated, even though they are not explicit, observable, or necessarily palpable. Some, but by no means all, of these intangible losses include the following: a sense of belonging to one's gender, of belonging to one's family, of belonging to one's peer group, of feeling safe, of feeling "normal," of innocence, of living life without the shadow of sexual abuse effects and the fear of its recurrence, of the freedom to experience life without secrecy and shame, of an integrated self, of familial continuity (if either SAM or the perpetrator were removed from the nuclear or extended family system), of the ability to trust oneself, others, and the world, of the belief that others may provide unconditional protection and care, of knowing that one is valuable because life is valuable and not because of what one can provide to others, of the ability to experience sexual development along an average and expected developmental continuum, of control over one's body, of a sense of body integrity, of being able to choose one's first sexual experience, of parenting without the fear of perpetrating or of being perceived as a perpetrator by others, and of the ability to experience love without the fear of betrayal.

Even though intangible losses customarily remain unidentified by SAM, their corresponding affect, nonetheless, intermittently permeates his conscious awareness by filtration. Without identifying these losses, the affect remains insulated from meaning, leading to confusion and disequilibrium. The losses generated by the experience of CSA and its effects are likely to give impetus to some of the most evocative and intense therapeutic tasks (Courtois, 1988). As SAM not only identifies but also reflects on the depth and breadth of loss, a period of grief and mourning are sure to follow (Herman, 1992). As painful as this may be, if SAM does not honor and grieve the losses, he may continue to engage in a compelling but futile search for his childhood, regardless of age (Briere, 1996a).

However, as SAM mourns the losses, he begins to realize that he cannot repossess them nor, in fact, claim them for the first time, by reason of their occurrence in childhood. But he can and will work through them. As SAM identifies and expresses these losses, he establishes a sense of congruency between cognition, affect, and behavior, as well as between past, present, and future. Over time, this will, in turn, help him maintain a sense of integration and cohesion.

Additionally, the identification and exploration of these losses is essential to the treatment process, given the dynamics of childhood sexual abuse. For example, if SAM, the perpetrator, or his family (even the therapist for that matter) invalidates sexual abuse, they, by definition, invalidate the losses emanating from it. Therefore, in order to validate the reality of the sexual abuse, SAM and the therapist must also bear witness to the losses. Only when these losses are given a name can the authentic meaning associated with each one be acknowledged, expressed, and released. SAM begins to realize that he was not responsible for the abuse in any form or fashion and that in truth, it was the perpetrator who unlawfully robbed his innocence and intercepted, at least temporarily, a number of life-affirming possibilities. Additionally, SAM begins to recognize that he cannot alter his history, but he can certainly affect and direct his future toward life goals emanating from passion and purpose.

Toward that end, it is equally important for SAM to recognize and respect the gains acquired as a result of his abusive experience(s). However, due to the dynamics of the sexually abusive relationship, many of SAM's strengths and resources have been overshadowed by guilt, shame, and secrecy. Yet as a result of the sexually abusive relationship and coping with its aftermath, SAM has indeed gained many skills. As SAM and the therapist explore, identify, and name his strengths, including the survival skills he blindly and instantaneously acquired upon subjection to CSA, they too honor his will, ingenuity, and spirit. Regardless of how instrumental his survival skills were then or how ineffective they may be now, they, and SAM, command respect (Courtois, 1988).

SAM's strengths may include, but are not limited to, an increased compassion for vulnerable others, an awareness that he is able to persevere in the face of extraordinarily adverse circumstances, a vast amount of mental energy that can now be channeled in directions of his choice, a highly developed sensitivity to environmental cues, a proficiency at viewing life from multiple perspectives (given the necessary survival strategy that often required him to reconcile mutually exclusive information on a daily basis), and an aptitude for discovering and employing resources within (due to the scarcity of resources without); even characteristics that were once seen as liabilities, such as dissociation and detachment, can now be utilized in constructive and productive ways.

Although the losses were imposed by others, the gains were not. No one helped SAM to persevere—the perpetrator certainly did not—and the abuse was most likely concealed from others who could have potentially intervened. In order to survive, SAM was forced to turn inward for courage and tenacity. Accordingly, the gains are inherently of SAM's creation, and therefore are his for the taking. A show of appreciation for these gains, in conjunction with the realization and acceptance of his losses, begins to bring a sense of closure to the abusive experiences, contributes to the wholeness of self, and liberates SAM to forge ahead in his life, with burdens diminishing, with dreams flourishing.

At this stage, SAM is able to explore and, more importantly, give a name to various aspects of his life experience, including losses and strengths. As he authentically appraises and apprehends the sense of loss, the notion of gains, he begins to reclaim his sense of power. He also has a newly identified resource from which to draw strength.

Objective 7

SAM will formulate and execute a goal-based project in order to build on and generalize his skill base.

SELF-MASTERY PROJECT

Although therapy is quite often a formidable task for SAM, the vast majority of challenges and dilemmas materialize not in the therapeutic setting but outside of it (Crowder, 1995). Thus, the therapeutic process not only includes skill-building but also the generalization of skills from the clinical setting across SAM's microenvironments and within his microrelationships. Skill-building and skill generalization require a great deal of time and effort, as well as patience, encouragement, rehearsal, and reinforcement (Courtois, 1988). Up to this point, treatment has focused on the abuse as it relates to the past and present. SAM will continue to reconstruct his story, and objectives 2 through 6 can be repeated as new information is discovered and reclaimed. Now, however, treatment will incorporate a more global approach, focusing on SAM's present and future as well as on his overall lifestyle. The self-mastery project is designed to help SAM identify personal goals, to explore their meaning, to set steps for their attainment, and to provide recognition for their accomplishment.

In selecting goals, SAM often states, "I don't know what goal to pick" or "Why don't you pick one for me?" Such sentiments can lead to a process characterized by resistance, frustration, and deprivation. Asking "What do I want to accomplish or learn?" is more likely to yield a process delineated by interest, resilience, and gratification. As SAM develops his self-mastery project, the therapist's role is to help him identify his target areas of change, to describe them accurately, and to set realistic goals, expectations, and outcomes. The therapist also helps SAM to monitor his progress, acts as a witness to his perseverance and growth, and assists him in accurately ascribing attributions for the achievement of the goals.

Target areas for change might be selected from any of the losses that he would like to ameliorate, any of the gains that he would like to build on, or any of the coping mechanisms (e.g., eating, anger, drinking) that he would like to change, reduce, or refocus. For example, some common aftereffects associated with the sexual abuse of males include compulsions around food, sex, alcohol, and work, among others. Compensatory behaviors like these provide SAM with positive consequences that, in the short-term, are more commanding than the negative consequences. Answering the following questions can produce viable projects and subgoals: (1) What positive and negative consequences is the compulsive behavior providing me? (2) How might I achieve these or similar positive consequences in a more constructive way?

With the therapist, SAM can develop a client-driven project that is definable, observable, measurable, and realistic. The most important aspect of the goal, however, is the current and potential meaning it holds for SAM. The focus continues to be on the development of his authentic self, and as SAM selects and explores his target for change, his sense of self-determination can also be reinforced. Just as aftereffects, like compulsive caretaking and a sense of inferiority, have generalized from the abusive experience across many domains of SAM's life, so too can the new skills acquired during treatment generalize as well, from the clinical room to any number of microrelationships and environments. As SAM develops new skills in the clinical setting, and starts to apply them to other areas of his life, his sense of mastery will naturally evolve. This sense of self-mastery helps SAM to counterbalance present and future stressors with the evolving intrapersonal and environmental resources now available to him for adaptation and growth.

However, before setting out to accomplish his goals, SAM must explore, identify, and assess potential barriers to their attainment. Answering the question "What would my life feel like, look like, be like, or how would people react to me if this goal is achieved?" can clarify his thoughts, attitudes, beliefs, feelings, and fears, all with the capacity to reinforce or undermine this process. Most importantly, SAM must decide if his chosen goal will actually affect the changes he wants to establish and experience in his life. As a case in point, SAM may suggest, at least initially, a goal around weight reduction or physique enhancement. While exploring this goal, he may confront an embedded fear: "If I lose weight, people might start looking at my body and expect me to be sexual. The thought of it makes me want to run." He may discover that his actual goal—to feel comfortable with and in his body—is, to a large extent, quite different than the one he had originally chosen.

Once SAM identifies and selects a specific goal, his self-motivation can heighten if the goal is partialized into a series of smaller steps or subgoals. For each subgoal, then, an action plan can be developed that includes a concrete definition of the subgoal, the strategies necessary to achieve it, potential problem areas and contingencies, and the cognitive, affective, and behavioral indicators of goal attainment. For example, a goal toward anger regulation could be partialized in the following manner: (1) define anger; (2) identify its cognitive, affective, behavioral, and physiological indicators; (3) monitor for indicators; (4) once identified, place indicators in context of person, place, and circumstance; (5) explore and identify triggers associated with anger; (6) explore and identify corresponding thoughts; (7) explore and identify corresponding feelings; (8) explore and identify corresponding behaviors; (9) explore and identify body reactions; (10) trace the chain from trigger to anger; (11) focus on thoughts influencing the anger response; (12) dispute, challenge, and/or affirm the validity of such thoughts; (13) explore and identify feelings underlying anger, such as disappointment, sadness, and fear; (14) analyze sources of anger; (15) experiment with ways to avoid venting anger against self or others; and (16) cultivate skills to express anger truthfully, directly and nondefensively.

By identifying the component parts, partialization establishes both a systematic way for SAM to achieve his goal and a way in which he can assess his progress and address any barriers. Goal partialization contributes to the project's manageability; moreover, given the series of subgoals, it offers one turn after another for SAM to feel a sense of accomplishment. Thus, SAM doesn't have to wait to the very end to experience a sense of achievement. These accomplishments, both large and small, afford SAM additional opportunities to further cultivate his sense of self-determination and self-mastery, which will, over time, become self-fulfilling.

Once an action plan is established, SAM can execute it. Several techniques can aide him in this process. For example, journaling can provide a process record for SAM that he can also use as a guide for accomplishing future goals. Additionally (or alternatively), self-talk can be beneficial. It can help SAM reinforce the importance of his goals, be used as a calming technique, or be an avenue of self-praise. These techniques are also advantageous—as SAM addresses his fears, his expectancies, and his accomplishments—in helping SAM to develop ways of self monitoring when the therapist is not present.

Self-monitoring strategies are helpful throughout but particularly so as SAM gets closer to achieving his goal, as he is more likely to palpably apprehend the fears associated with goal actualization. As an illustration, when SAM selects and works toward a goal related to weight reduction, body building, or joining a singles association, fears underlying intimacy and sexuality may emerge to the foreground as he begins to receive feedback from others in response to the actualization of his goal. Further, depending on the context, fears of failure and success and the fear of losing or changing his identity can mount as well. It is therefore important for the therapist to individualize SAM's self-mastery project by addressing his particular fears and vulnerabilities and expressing an appreciation for his strengths, determination, and problem-solving capacities.

At this time, as well as throughout the entire therapeutic process, evaluation must be viewed as a critical component. Evaluation of the goals, the processes, and the outcomes is all essential in building SAM's knowledge of self, skill base, sense of self-determination, and self-mastery. For example, as each partialization goal is actualized, the therapist and SAM can assess the efficacy of employed strategies, refine the upcoming action plan in light of current progress, and outline skills necessary to achieve the next subgoal. Additionally, it will prove beneficial if they define and differentiate the impact of intervening variables, such as the type, frequency, and cogency of reinforcement strategies, SAM's cognitve appraisal of the change process, positive and negative expectancies concerning goal attainment, and the presence, absence, and quality of his social support system, to mention a few. The more concrete the goal, the more systematic the strategies and the more tangible the reinforcement and evaluation procedures, the better SAM will be able to replicate similar projects outside of the clinical room and generalize the acquired skills across his microenvironments.

It is important that both the therapist and SAM recognize that the outcome of the self-mastery project is less important than the actual process—the application of new skills, the development of new ideas, and so on. The process is key, and the accomplishment of SAM's subgoals will buttress his a sense of self-efficacy despite the eventual outcome. Furthermore, both must accept that there will continue to be fits and starts. Although the goals might change, or one of the partialized steps might become the actual goal, what SAM learns from this experience will be of far more value than the attainment of any particular end. New goals can be established at any time.

As SAM completes this phase of treatment, he will likely evidence an increased capacity to: (1) accept his abuse history as a life fact; (2) attribute responsibility for the abuse to the perpetrator; (3) distinguish his authentic truth from perpetrator injunction and social imposition; (4) identify emotional triggers; (5) differentiate internal cues from external cues; (6) cognitively appraise events from various perspectives, including his own; (7) regulate emotional responsivity; (8) maintain stimulation far from the extremes of hyperarousal and dissociation; (9) neutralize abuse-generated memories; (10) differentiate remembering from reexperiencing; (11) identify sensory and somatic states and transform them into words; (12) cognitively reappraise schemas related to self, others, sexuality, and abuse; (13) intercept escalating stress by means of active problem solving; (14) synthesize his preabuse, abuse, and postabuse selves; (15) integrate his abuse experience into an evolving life history; and (16) anticipate the future vis-à-vis love and work independent of abuse-generated effects and implications (see, e.g., Cornell & Olio, 1991; Friedrich, 1990a; Marmar, Foy, Kagan, & Pynoos, 1994; Meiselman, 1990; Siegel, 1995; Spiegel, 1998b).

The Next Step

At this point, SAM and the therapist may contract to work through new material that has emerged, rework some of the previous objectives, ameliorate particular effects such as compulsive behaviors, relational difficulties, and mood disorders, explore, identify, and actuate a life mission independent of the abuse, or terminate. Termination, of course, can be evocative, particularly for SAM. Ty stated: "I was afraid to leave therapy, especially the group. In the last session, I kept my crying on the inside until I saw that everyone had tears on their cheeks. I was afraid that it would be like when I left home and never talked to anyone again." Nicholas stated: "I was scared to not go to therapy. I was scared that I would not [be] protected anymore. The therapist helped me to meet Wanda, my advate [advocate], and my foster Momma and foster Daddy take me to therapy parties [reunions] where I get to see all the other boys that are my friends." It's important that the therapist clearly state to SAM that he is welcome to return to therapy at anytime, with any therapist, and that doing so is not a sign of regression but, in fact, a sign of self-care.

While it is necessary and critical that SAM and the therapist allot ample time to address potential feelings of fear, sadness, and abandonment, it is equally important that they explore, identify, and make meaningful the therapeutic milestones as well as any stumbling along the way. SAM has transformed himself. With courage, blind faith, and some trepidation, too, he found his way to the truth.

Costs and Benefits

As with any therapeutic endeavor, it remains critical that the therapist and SAM recognize that although sexual abuse therapy is invaluably beneficial in many ways, it also holds a number of risks. For example, if the therapist is unfamiliar with the sexual abuse of males knowledge base, including its biological, psychological, and sociological components, the therapist may unintentionally fail to understand, assess, and validate SAM's authentic experience of CSA. Rather than promote constructive change, the therapist ultimately colludes with SAM's hearty system of invalidation and with the social mythology surrounding the sexual abuse of males. If the therapist lacks the capacity to titrate SAM's exposure to traumatic material and/or if SAM does not have the ability to tolerate and regulate states of hyperarousal and dissociation, additional stress may ensue. If therapists employ controversial memory retrieval techniques, utilize interventive strategies of any kind without the proper training and supervision, and/or override SAM's legitimate wants and needs in service of their own, then they place SAM at risk for decompensation, dysregulation, or premature termination.

Therapists would not and could not dedicate their professional careers to the amelioration of CSA effects if they did not believe in the efficacy of the therapeutic process. In acknowledging a history of CSA, identifying, processing, and disclosing its implicit and explicit facts and meanings, desensitizing its traumatic effects, honoring the losses and gains, and building a future, all within a rational, systematic, and stepwise fashion, SAM experiences a number of benefits. SAM is likely to evidence: (1) significant improvements in health status and immune function (Harber & Pennebaker, 1992; Pennebaker, 1993; Pennebaker, Kiecolt-Glaser, & Glaser, 1988); (2) an evolving base of adaptive skills, including self-reflection, regulation of affect, and emotional expression (Briere, 1996a; Courtois, 1999); (3) a germinating sense of identity consolidation and autobiographical continuity (Siegel, 1995); (4) a memory system that is progressively coming under his control (Herman, 1992); and (5) a sense of hope and promise about the future independent of his abuse history (Spiegel, 1998).

Therapists can substantially decrease the risk and promote the benefits of this SAM's therapeutic experience by: (1) conceptualizing and executing theoretically sound and/or empirically grounded treatment in such a way that advances SAM toward his goal of resolution without placing him at risk for retraumatization in any form or fashion; (2) welcoming him into the clinical space; (3) maintaining distinct and consistent boundaries that promote safety and security; (4) inquiring into SAM's history with courage and competence; (5) modulating the interventions so that he can work well within the poles of dissociation and hyperarousal; (5) noninvasively helping him to transform implicit and explicit memories into a cohesive narrative; (6) bearing witness to his first-person experience of childhood sexual abuse; (7) empathically responding throughout; (8) validating his losses and gains; and (9) supporting him as he discovers dreams, goals, and aspirations (see, e.g., Chu, 1998; Crowder, 1995; Davies & Frawley, 1994; Pearce & Pezzot-Pearce, 1997).

TREATMENT OUTCOME STUDIES

Treatment outcome studies employing males with histories of childhood sexual abuse and utilizing structured treatment protocols have yielded a number of statistically significant and clinically significant improvements among boys (e.g., Berliner & Saunders, 1996; Cohen & Mannarino, 1993, 1996, 1997a, 1997b, 2000; Friedrich, Luecke, Beilke, & Place, 1992; Gothard & Heinrich, 1999; Hack, Osachuk, & De Luca, 1994; Hoier & Inderbitzenn-Pisaruk, 1987; Hall-Marley & Damon, 1993; Lanktree & Briere, 1995; Larzelere, Collins, & Collins, 1993; Stauffer & Deblinger, 1996; Sullivan, Scanlon, Brookhouser, & Schulte, 1992) and men (e.g., Chard, Weaver, & Resick, 1997; Paivio & Bahr, 1998; Smith, Pearce, Pringle, & Caplan, 1995), particularly in the areas of anxiety, depression, internalizing behaviors, externalizing behaviors, trauma symptomatology, distorted thinking, attribution of blame, guilt, shame, self-control, self-mastery, and interpersonal relations.

Data across studies support the systematic development, piloting, and refinement of both individual and group modalities of psychotherapy. The effect sizes rendered by the execution of individual and group treatment models tend to be similar (Reeker, Ensing, Elliott, 1997; Weisz, Weiss, Han, Granger, & Martin, 1995). However, aggregate studies of treatment outcomes for CSA indicate that, in general, effect sizes tend to be larger for females when compared to males, larger for adolescents when compared to children, and larger for samples recruited for research when compared to samples generated within a clinical setting or by a treatment agency (Weisz, Weiss, et al., 1995).

In terms of theory-driven models, behavioral, psychodynamic, experiential, and cognitive-behavioral have all been shown to render statistically significant effect sizes as well as numerous indicators of clinically significant outcomes (Price, Hilsenroth, Petretic-Jackson, & Bonge, 2001). Still, the vast majority of treatment outcomes studies have assessed the efficacy of practice models that employ cognitive-behavioral interventions such as thought-stopping social skills training and knowledge acquisition.

In light of the dispersion of dynamics highlighted in the literature, such as age of onset, perpetrator gender, abuse duration and frequency, sexual acts and responses to disclosure, in conjunction with the myriad of effects, for example, substance abuse, sexual compulsivity, dysregulated brain chemistry, fear of the emergence of secondary sex characteristics, among numerous others, the question—What works for whom and under what circumstances?—must remain a cornerstone of intervention development, execution, and evaluation. CSA's dynamics and effects are multitudinous and variant; accordingly, effective treatment cannot be consolidated into an invariable protocol (Spiegel, 2000).

Without question, it is imperative that service protocols, treatment models, and helping professionals ensure a goodness-of-fit with client interest and need. Within and across treatment rooms, multiple modalities of service (e.g., individual, dyadic, family, group), multiple (and integrated) models of practice (e.g., psychodynamic, systems, social-cognitive, cognitive-behavioral), multiple levels of service (e.g., inpatient, partial day, outpatient, home visits) may be necessary for different clients or for the same client at different times (American Academy of Child and Adolescent Psychiatry, 1998; Courtois, 1999; Finkelhor & Berliner, 1995; Saywitz, Mannarino, Berliner, & Cohen, 2000). As always, treatment content and execution must be gender-appropriate, racially, ethnically, and culturally sensitive, and developmentally congruent (Spiegel, 1998b). Whatever the case, modality or context, the standards of care remain constant (Courtois, 1999).

SUMMARY

This chapter presented the SAM model of treatment objectives. As safety is established, trust builds; as trust escalates, defense and avoidant strategies relax; and as defenses abate, fractionated shards of the abuse, such as repetition compulsions, behavioral reenactments, and intrusive symptomatology, transform into memories. Memories coalesce into an evolving abuse narrative, the narrative incorporates abuse-related cognition and affect and all elements of SAM's abuse experience. Cognition and affect are the pathways by which socially imposed meaning defers to authentic meaning. And, over time, authentic meaning around the abuse experience integrates into the personal history of the self.

CHAPTER NINE

THE SAM PRACTICE MODEL: AN ANALOGY

THE EXPERIENCE of childhood sexual abuse (CSA) fractionates SAM, as a boy, and SAM's life, as he knows it, into shards—facts short of meanings, truncated feelings, fragments of knowledge, splintered senses, demarcated time, and a boy divided against himself. On that ground, SAM's story of CSA, his truth, remains shattered, embedded, and incomplete. This chapter presents a treatment analogy. It has been employed primarily with adolescent males. Ironically, adult males as well as therapists have found it to be useful as well, particularly in terms of conceptualizing and demystifying the treatment process. Kip stated: "When DSS made me come to therapy, I told them I didn't want to do that touchy-feely kind of hug and cry and talk about feelings for an hour every damn week. They showed me this piece of paper from the therapist that talked about a kid named SAM and him being on an excavation. We were learning about that in science class. I thought to my self, 'If therapy is gonna be like that, I want to go.'" Jake commented: "All I knew about therapy was what I saw on TV. It either looks dangerous, or seductive or too emotional or what not. Thinking about therapy in terms of an excavation—I could get into that. It helped me to understand what I was trying to do without all the psychobabble. I got the point of it all."

SAM AND HIS ARCHEOLOGICAL DIG

Archeology is the scientific study of history, of heritage. The exploration, un-covering, collection, synthesis, and analyses of remnants from SAM's past cul-tivate an authentic truth and understanding about his life . . . before, and including, today.

SAM will uncover the facts and meanings of history—his story of child-hood sexual abuse—with the intention of reconstructing his past as authenti-cally and fully as possible. Archeology fosters the preservation and validation of such a history.

Archeologists work in groups; SAM and the therapist comprise an excavation team. SAM and the therapist will investigate the terrain of his life. Together, they will uncover, layer by layer, the shards, relics, and artifacts of his history—the memories, surface and embedded, the facts, chronological and contextual, and the meanings, natural and man-made.

The initial phase of an archeologic investigation is reconnaissance. At this juncture, SAM and the therapist, as the archeological team, conduct a preliminary survey to acknowledge the need and desire for such an expedition, define the boundaries of this venture, collect pertinent data, and advance a rationale for doing so.

The site for excavation is SAM's biopsychosocial experience of CSA. The initial task is acknowledgment of sexual abuse as an aspect of one's history. It is a conscious and contemplative action in service of deconstructing the schemas and defenses established to conceal, invalidate, reconcile, and compensate for the abuse.

The excavation team will canvass the treatment terrain. Exploration and articulation of the bounds and borders, including policies and procedures, ground rules and contracts, and roles and functions of the participants, are critical to SAM's making an informed decision. Further, by working with the therapist to understand the need and rationale for these policies, a mutual understanding is developed—that the policies are not random and that the boundaries are there to protect SAM and to maintain the integrity and the intention of the excavation site, finds, and team. Clear and direct communication enhances the relationship and the endeavors of the team.

Excavation calls for tenacity and tolerance. The team can expect to encounter variable conditions, some unpleasantly rough, others pleasantly surprising. Thus, preparation, with great attention to detail, is necessary. That being said, SAM makes a commitment to self, agreeing to initiate and/or maintain stability and consistency in biopsychosocial functioning—that is, care about eating, sleeping, and body functioning, and stability and consistency in housing, resources, education, employment, daily activities, and social support.

At this point, SAM also commits to the excavation endeavor, the treatment process, exploring, identifying, and analyzing the positive and negative, and near and distant, consequences of such a decision. Yet before such a venture can truly begin, it is essential that SAM be able to clearly define and articulate his own rationale for embarking on this endeavor. Not only does this foster a sense of self-determination and freedom of choice, it also establishes that he is capable of at least entertaining the possibility that he and life as he experiences it can change.

At the end of this phase, the topography, including detailed descriptions of SAM's life before, during, and after the abuse, as well as graphic delineations of the excavation enterprise, will be generated, mapping the course to follow.

The next phase of an archeological expedition focuses on the contour of the landscape. Here, the archeology team explores and renders, in detail, the topography of his experience prior to the unearthing of his past. The topographic detailing includes the presentation of data and in-depth discussion around the dynamics and effects of CSA, as well as the social context in which it occurs.

Psychoeducation is intended to promote the realities of sexual abuse by creating a context from which SAM can begin to develop an awareness that sexual abuse exists not only as a personal event, but also as a social phenomenon that can, and does, generate its own set of powerful dynamics and effects.

Recording takes place throughout the excavation process. Field notes, journals, mapping, goal-setting, drawing, photographs, and forms of many kinds chronicle this venture.

Next is the excavation phase. At this stage, the emphasis is on SAM working with the finds of his sexual abuse experience while beginning to place the realities of the abuse in their proper biopsychosocial contexts. Excavation brings to light the site—SAM's history of CSA—as it was authentically experienced: subjection strategies, the dynamics of sexual abuse, the initial effects, the enforcers of concealment, the ways and means of invalidation, his reconciliatory rationale, compensatory measures, and aftereffects. Excavation also uncovers the continuity of effects and alterations within a site and the relationships between and among what occurred before, during, and after.

Excavation and recording occur in phases, layer by layer. The excavation team unearths layer upon layer, truth upon truth. Through to the bedrock, that is, truth in its natural state, each layer of SAM's history of CSA conveys facts and meanings—one thing or another about intimidation and terror, erections and ejaculations, intrusion and numbing, blaming, and undoing.

Depending on conditions and time, SAM may dig deeply into one circumscribed area or may simply work with the surface of another demarcated area. Exploration and negotiation are primary processes here, helping SAM to choose if, how, where, when, and why he wants to make his way. Otherwise, digging hastily, randomly, and aggressively can destroy the finds before they are fully unearthed and brought to light. No false moves, then. No unnecessary machinery.

The clinical room becomes the screening area. No find, no shard, no fact, no meaning, no memory, no sensation, past or present, will be recorded as insignificant; nothing is above or beyond initial analysis. The intentional uprooting of a shard, with little or no regard for its cultural context, just like the detaching of CSA facts and meaning from their biopsychosocial context, renders the shard, renders the fact and meaning, incomprehensible, and maximizes the risk of socially biased misinterpretation.

The facts that embody SAM's history of CSA are indelible; they will never change. Meaning, however—the beliefs, attitudes, feelings, and values that bring the facts to life—can and must change! Meaning must change so that the experience of CSA relinquishes its iron-handed hold on SAM and is relegated to a position wherein it is viewed as a notable yet uncontaminated aspect of his life story.

The three dimensions through which SAM excavates his history are: (1) facts of CSA; (2) cognitive meaning; and (3) affective meaning. By repeating the story in this way, SAM can explore his history in a progressive, multilayered manner, similar to the way in which his understanding of the abuse was created in the first place. This progressive and circuitous process builds an awareness of the person/environment interplay, which is the only way SAM can differentiate his authentic finds from what was socially imposed on him.

In order to do this, the therapist must be willing to constantly oscillate between SAM's preabuse, abuse, postabuse, and current perspectives. This process allows SAM to utilize his own distancing abilities in order to protect himself while still maintaining a focus on his abusive experiences. Too much distancing can erode the finds; a balance between approach and avoidance contributes to their emergence and preservation.

As SAM excavates the abusive experience within the psychological and sociological contexts through which and in which it occurred, he becomes aware of how the abuse itself, his perceptions of it, the meaning he ascribed to it, and the initial and long-term effects rendered by it were infused and, in some ways, imposed by social mythology. With every dig, SAM's authentic responses advance toward the foreground.

The reconstruction phase follows. In chronicling his history, SAM describes and classifies the finds, thereby placing them in the actual contexts from which they first arose. In other words, telling the story reveals the ways in which SAM authentically experienced CSA, the sociocultural beliefs surrounding CSA, and the ways in which SAM adapted to and coped with CSA given his sociocultural context.

More specifically, SAM will again tell his story, but this time from the first-person present tense as he would have told it while the abuse was actually occurring. The utilization of the first-person present tense during this phase of the expedition is intended to serve SAM in integrating history with this day and age and building a future on this new foundation.

SAM now turns to processing the finds. In this phase, excavated finds uncover and tell the human story of the sexual abuse of males. CSA violates nature; it obstructs development; it desecrates dreams of what could have been. Thus, losses; thus, gains.

It is vital, then, that SAM have the opportunity to explore, identify, and grieve the losses born of his history of sexual abuse. CSA also requires children to survive seemingly beyond their reach. Gains, both surface and embedded, exist as well, but they, too, must be identified and given a name, for only then will they hold value. The acknowledgment of these finds, in conjunction with the realization and acceptance of remnants lost, begins to bring closure to the abusive experiences and liberates SAM to forge ahead in his life.

Last, but certainly not least, is the survey phase. It addresses the question: Where do we go from here?

The excavation project, up to this point, has focused on the abuse as it relates to the past and present. SAM will continue to reconstruct his story; excavation and analyses will recur as new information is discovered and reclaimed. Now, however, the team will incorporate a more global approach, focusing on the present and future as well as on SAM's overall lifestyle.

The self mastery project is designed to help SAM identify his goals, explore their meaning, formulate steps for their attainment, take action, and provide recognition for their accomplishment. Simultaneously, SAM must be presented with opportunities to transfer what he is learning as a member of the excavation team, and as a result of this expedition, to other aspects of his life. Once again, this points to the premise of translating knowledge and insight into constructive action, but now across contexts.

The excavation of SAM's history, and his liberation from CSA effects, bring to light a present day and future age imbued with hope and promise.

SUMMARY

This brief chapter presented a practice analogy. It is based on the SAM model. During the orientation phase of treatment, it may be helpful to certain males who hold disdain for psychotherapy, who have a number of misconceptions, or who simply could benefit from a little story that appears to have little to do with therapy. This analogy can also be employed during the termination phase, as it may serve as a springboard for highlighting the tasks, achievements, and outcomes encountered along the way.

CHAPTER TEN

INTERVENTIONS FOR SAM

THIS CHAPTER PRESENTS a number of interventions developed or modified for males with histories of childhood sexual abuse (CSA). They can be adapted to fit the particular needs and attributes of SAM. Each intervention is presented in the following format: (1) definition of the intervention; (2) a systematic description of its execution; and (3) its anticipated consequences. Graphs or charts of selected interventions are included throughout.

THE CHANGE CHART

Definition

Given the ways in which childhood sexual abuse creates a line of demarcation between the authentic self and the abused self, and considering the ways in which shame and secrecy promote the development of the compensatory self, decision making can be particularly challenging for SAM. A frequent and recurrent effect of CSA is a diminished ability to differentiate between authentic perceptions, beliefs, and desires and those biopsychosocially imposed via the sexually abusive relationship. The sense of self is often subjected to and overridden by the perceptions of others: fag, girlie-boy, sissy, deviant, sick, whore. The question "What do I want, what do I need?" is often outweighed by the following queries: What do others want from me? What is expected of me? How would a "real" boy act in this situation? What will be discovered about me if I do this or do that? How will this decision influence the secret?

With so much occurring intrapsychically, just in terms of survival, important decisions may be overlooked, circumvented, or overdrawn until it's too late, or made impulsively, without much forethought. The "Change Chart," based on decision theory, provides direction and focuses SAM's attention on factors that need to be identified and examined prior to making a decision.

Description

The "Change Chart" can be diagrammed by SAM, or therapists can present blank charts to clients in a 2 × 2 × 2 matrix format. Structurally, this intervention encompasses the following elements: (1) decisional options (e.g., to enter a group vs. to refrain from joining a group; to prevent further episodes of sexually compulsive activities vs. to continue to act in sexually compulsive ways); (2) the anticipated consequences of each option, both immediate and delayed; and (3) the anticipated positive and negative consequences within each time frame. In other words, clients will generate and explore positive and negative consequences for each option, as they are expected to occur immediately after the decision is enacted, and as they are expected to occur in the long term. Following consideration of consequences individually, they are assessed globally. After weighing both sides, an informed decision can be made.

Additionally, particular attention can be directed toward goals and intentions embedded in the consequences, impediments and conduits to such goals, and indicators of points of view regarding self, the decision under consideration, others, the world, and the future. Thus, the data generated via this intervention go well beyond the decisional options; the data also render a rich person-in-situation configuration.

To summarize, the therapist can guide and inform SAM through the following:

1. Identify a decision to be made.
2. Determine decisional options.
3. Consider the immediate and delayed consequences for each option.
4. Explicate positive and negative consequences for each option within current and future timeframes.
5. Assess each consequence and articulate its meaning.
6. Look for indicators, patterns, and themes that may support or hinder goal attainment.
7. Assess the overall viability of each option.
8. Decide, knowing that a new decision is only a moment away.

Anticipated Outcomes

The "Change Chart" presents SAM with an opportunity to diagram the options available in a given situation, fosters the projection of anticipated or possible consequences that may lead to differing outcomes, and illustrates the costs and benefits of each option. Thus, the anticipated outcomes include: (1) identification of problems or concerns that can be addressed in treatment; (2) identification of client-based goals; (3) identification of motivation toward client-based and treatment goals; (4) identification of barriers to client-based and treatment goals; (5) indicators of self-concept; and (6) development and/or betterment of self-directed decision-making strategies.

Matt

CHANGE CHART

Date:	Immediate Consequences		Delayed Consequences	
/ /	**Positive**	**Negative**	**Positive**	**Negative**
TO CHANGE:	• Know that I'm finally dealing with the abuse in a positive way • Be with others who are like me, who understand me and accept me	• Have to deal with feelings • No more denial • Frustration • Anger • No more sexual acting out • Lose friends who are sex addicts	• Learn how to love • Learn how to have sex • Learn to accept my history • Learn how to like myself • Put the sexual abuse behind me	• What if I find out that it was really my fault or that I really wanted it • Getting more memories • Getting more feelings
TO STAY THE SAME:	• Keep acting out sexually • Stay numb	• Guilt for not doing something to change my life • Feel shame and disgust all the time • Keep hating my body	• Just stay numb from all of the sexual acting out • Say "Fuck you" to everyone by showing them that I really am a no good whore after all	• AIDS • Death • Shame • Suicide

FIGURE 10.1. The Change Chart

Finally, whenever the change process becomes too overwhelming, challenging, or difficult, and when SAM contemplates termination, he can review the initial change chart to remind himself of the anticipated positive and negative consequences, and ultimately of why he decided to change in the first place. Throughout the treatment process, the "Change Chart" can be used toward making any number of decisions. Up-to-date versions of any change chart can be generated, taking into account progress made and goals achieved.

Clinical Example

Matt's "Change Chart" is presented in Figure 10.1. He and the therapist worked on it together. Matt's completed form reveals a number of useful data. First, his immediate consequences were concrete whereas his delayed consequences were abstract. For example, his anticipated loss of friends and acting out were tangible and palpable; his wanting to learn to like himself and put the sexual abuse behind him were not. He stated: "When I hear people talking about self-love or caring for themselves, I feel like I'm listening to a foreign language. It just doesn't compute in my brain." Thus, from his perspective, the anticipated losses were far more compelling than the potential gains. Moreover, the sense of loss generated by his anticipated immediate and negative consequences overrode the inaccessible sense of danger associated with delayed negative consequences, particularly his anticipation of AIDS, death, and suicide. Further, Matt's episodes of sexual acting out evoked a commanding discharge of endogenous opiods. The positive consequences of sexual compulsivity, namely a sense of euphoria at times, numbness at others, was his "self-prescribed medicine." At the onset of therapy, he had no other interests or activities that could elicit an equivalent sense of calm.

Second, Matt exposed his self-concept, that of a "no-good whore." Initially, he did not realize that he had internalized his perpetrator's derogatory remarks. Nonetheless, such a self-concept was viewed as a robust impediment to the actualization of his stated goals. Unfortunately, his self-concept at the time was congruent with his acts of genital mutilation (i.e., "keep hating my body") and his pervasive feelings of guilt, shame, and disgust yet incompatible with his anticipated positive consequences, such as learning how to engage in sex in a more constructive way and advancing beyond the effects of his abuse history. Third, Matt's delayed negative consequences regarding the generation of additional memories, corresponding feelings, and his fear in realizing that he was responsible for the incest induced intense fear. He stated: "If I give up the sexual acting out and deal with the incest, and in that process get more memories and feelings, I won't be able to numb them out. I'm not sure if I am ready to do this. But I'm willing to give it a try." Matt's "Change Chart" was used not only as an assessment tool but also as a springboard to concretizing his delayed positive consequences, providing them with more clarity, meaning, and definable steps toward their actualization.

ACTION CONNECTION WITH SODAS

Anxiety, panic attacks, posttraumatic stress, night terrors, sleepwalking, and the like are common effects of CSA. Through experience, SAM has learned to remain ever vigilant to any thoughts, feelings, and behaviors, or to any person, place, or thing, that has the possibility of exposing his secret of CSA. Notwithstanding such vigilance, many of CSA's anxiety-related effects appear to come from nowhere, and with little or no warning.

Impacted by the original stressor of CSA, and now coping with its effects, SAM may not have the wherewithal to systematically analyze his intrapsychic and behavioral actions in order to cope more purposefully and to regain a sense of control. He may not have the time, energy, or capacity to appreciate the differences between intentions and outcomes, between thoughts and feelings, between historic triggers and present-day stimuli; all seem one and the same. The "Action Connection" is a viable resource toward gaining self-knowledge, and translating it into constructive and purposeful action. It was initially developed and piloted at Columbia University under the direction of Robert F. Schilling, PhD.

Definition

The "Action Connection" is based on cyclical determinism (i.e., thoughts create feelings; feelings generate behaviors; behaviors incite thoughts, thereby perpetuating the cycle), operant conditioning (where actions are preceded by antecedents or triggers, whereas emerging from such actions are consequences, both positive and negative), and problem solving (where options and their consequences are employed to guide and inform the generation and actualization of solutions).

Description

Learning about and developing a behavioral analysis and problem-solving approach to stressful situations in general and to coping with CSA effects in particular presents SAM with a flexible and adaptable skill that can be developed in one context, but over time generalized across many contexts. With that in mind, the therapist will help SAM achieve the following:

1. Identify and describe a trigger, or antecedent event.
2. Define, in concrete terms, thoughts associated with this event.
3. Define, in concrete terms, feelings associated with this event.
4. Recognize the importance of stopping this process before an undesired, random, and/or destructive behavior occurs.
5. Define the problem/circumstance in concrete terms
6. Generate at least three options or possible solutions to the problem.
7. Specify positive and negative consequences for each option.
8. Evaluate each option in terms of intention, time, and resources.
9. Select an option.
10. Execute the selected option.
11. Evaluate the problem-solving process.
12. Acknowledge oneself for completing this process, whether or not the desired outcome was achieved.

Anticipated Outcomes

The outcomes associated with this intervention are numerous and can vary across clients. First, the "Action Connection" provides SAM with an opportunity to view his behavior in context. More specifically, he will learn that thoughts, feelings, and behaviors are interconnected, as in a chain. This chain is preceded by a "trigger"; it ends with consequences. Thus, SAM has an opportunity to analyze his actions, in a systematic way, in context, in light of intrapersonal and/or environmental stimuli, and with respect to effects, both positive and negative, generated by such actions.

Second, rather than respond mechanically, randomly, or with the feeling of having no voice or choice, the "Action Connection" prompts SAM to generate possible solutions to a new problem, as well as cognitive, affective, and/or behavioral alternatives to an ongoing problem. Doing so fosters a sense of purpose and personal power.

Third, through contemplating anticipated consequences across the options, SAM learns to link his intentions with congruent outcomes, thereby approaching life goals, dreams, and desires provocatively. Fourth, by analyzing the options, consequences, and themes and patterns among them, clients not only come to understand "what" they are doing, but also the reasons "why." Thus, SAM reflects not only on the facts of his current life situation, but on the meaning infused in his actions as well. Fifth, clients cultivate a more logical way of perceiving, analyzing, understanding, and solving problems, and learn there usually are a number of ways to achieve the same outcome.

Finally, the "Action Connection" highlights SAM's expectancies and sense of self-efficacy. It helps him generate a number of options he perceives as viable, and it brings his beliefs, such as about his ability to execute such options, into the foreground.

Clinical Example

Palo's "Action Connection" is presented in Figure 10.2. In terms of backstory, Palo, then 18, was playing basketball with Jimmy, his best friend, and Mr. Carter, Jimmy's father. Palo stated: "Everything was fine. I was having a great day. One of the first in a very long time. My father and uncles were at a week long sun ceremony, so I decided to take a break from college work for the weekend and visit my family. That Saturday morning, as I was playing basketball and laughing and just feeling a glimpse of my old self, I began to notice Mr. Carter's hands. I got really self-conscious, thought they could tell what I was thinking—I mean, I didn't even know what I was thinking but I had to get out of there. I felt like I was going to jump out of my skin again."

By this point in the therapeutic process, Palo had learned how to use the "Action Connection" when attempting to solve a problem or dilemma. He listed three possible options: (1) calling his therapist; (2) visiting Autumn, his girlfriend; and (3) going to the P.O. He used the initials P.O. rather than state, "Going to the post office to get picked up for sex," which he later disclosed. His options and consequences exhibited a number of significant items. First, the majority of his anticipated negative consequences across the first two options were indicators of his self-concept, projected onto the therapist and girlfriend. Evidently, he felt transparent at the time, unable to prevent anxiety-provoking and derogatory beliefs about the self from spilling over his defensive and compensatory veneer. Second, he characterized the therapist and girlfriend as "safe," which was palpably different from his anticipation of "feeling safe" from an anonymous encounter at the post office. As per his state of consciousness at the time as well as corresponding perceptions and affect,

Palo

Action Connection

Trigger	Thoughts	Feelings
Playing basketball with Jimmy and his Dad — Mr. Carter's hands	I don't want to think about his hands — I want to get out of here	Weird Confused Sad Jumpy

STOP!
OPTIONS!

1. Call Joe

Positive Consequences	Negative Consequences
Calm Down.	He'll think I'm weird.
He'll understand.	He'll think I'm queer.
He is safe.	He'll think I'm a perv.

2. Go to Autumn's Place

Positive Consequences	Negative Consequences
Have fun.	She'll think I'm bogus.
Feel safe.	Feel like I'm a failure as a guy.
See her mom.	Get emotional if she says I love you.

3. P.O.

Positive Consequences	Negative Consequences
Get Held.	Sick feeling
Feel safe.	Punished by God
Be liked.	Make Joe mad

DECIDE!   (OPTION 1)   OPTION 2   (OPTION 3)   OTHER

ACTION!

~~#3 Go to P.O.~~

#1 Call Joe

SELF-PRAISE!

Nothing's written in cement

FIGURE 10.2. Action Connection

the first option would have provided understanding, the second would have offered a sense of fun, but the third, and most compelling option, would have engendered feelings of safety, the sense of being valued, and the opportunity for affection. The affection that could have been offered with option 2 also held the potential to incite negative feelings about the self; such was not the case for option 3. After the incident, Palo stated: "I did what you told me to do. I filled out the form. I looked at my options and I picked number three."

Palo went to the post office. In this particular city, as with many others, the post office was put to use as a nighttime way station for adults interested in sex with young people. Palo continued: "I got there. I felt all numb inside. It was during the day, Saturday but closed, but people could still see me standing there, yet I still went there to—I'm not sure why I was going there but I did. After a while, a few cars circled around. I saw this one guy with an old Pontiac. There were toys in the back seat. I went with him. After we got to his house, I saw pictures of his children. He had really big hands, too. I was just standing there and he told me he wanted to have intercourse with me. He came over to me and started kissing me and pulling at my clothes. I told him I wanted a hug. He laughed and told me to get naked. I told him I had to run to the bathroom first. I got in there and knew I wanted to leave. I felt like some sense had just knocked its way into my brain. I looked around the bathroom and saw a window. I opened it, climbed out, jumped about six feet and ran as fast as I could to a payphone." Palo contacted his therapist. During their conversation, Palo briefly reported what had happened, namely, that he had decided to take action with option 3 but then changed his mind and selected option 1.

Palo's "Action Connection" presents a number of important details, including Mr. Carter's hands. Palo was sexually abused by his father. On several occasions, while being penetrated, Palo, on his stomach, could see nothing but the father's hands clasped around his chest. During such times he heard his father say "I love you." This intervention helped Palo to see that he did not want to engage in a sexual encounter after all. He in fact wanted to be loved; however, his only way of actualizing "love" at the time was through sexual means, an illusion at best. Similar to many other males with histories of CSA, significant aspects of Palo's story were encapsulated in sensory images. This interventive strategy fostered another opportunity to translate implicit memory into an explicit narrative and to outline more effective and direct strategies that could lead to care and support.

FACTS AND MEANING

The facts of childhood sexual abuse—the fact that it occurs, the fact that it has occurred in many of our clients' lives—are etched in history. The power of healing, the potency of change, is not a function of the facts around CSA, but of the meaning emanating from such histories. Historic facts cannot and will not change. Meaning can and will!

It is SAM's cognitive and affective points of view that create meaning around the facts. For many sexually abused boys, the facts, in and of themselves, appear to be benign because the points of view have been suppressed or otherwise detached, denied, or depersonalized along the way.

Definition

"Facts and Meaning" is a stepwise intervention, providing SAM with an opportunity to identify facts that describe his sexually abusive history, to infuse each fact with a corresponding belief and to align each fact and belief with a relevant feeling. This intervention is founded on the construct of cyclical determinism (i.e., thoughts influence/create feelings; feelings influence/create actions; actions trigger thoughts, and so on) and on the construct of ego defenses (i.e., strategies intended to protect, often by disengaging fact from meaning). It is cyclical in nature.

Description

The facts come first. The therapist can begin by eliciting client-driven facts, one by one, without much processing of any kind. Client disclosure and subtle validation on the part of the therapist are the main elements at this point. Trying to verbally validate moment by moment, overextending empathy, and the like tend to draw too much attention to what SAM is attempting here, with self-consciousness and shame as common impeding consequences.

SAM is typically amenable to such a restrained beginning. By focusing first on historic facts, he recognizes that it won't be necessary to ponder his point of view about the facts, or to delve into any feelings associated with them. Just the facts!

At this stage, given the structure of "Facts and Meaning," and SAM's detached presentation, it's important that the therapist match the seemingly neutral nature of his disclosure. Because the facts are often experienced as benign, at least superficially, it's critical that the therapist empathize, at this phase of treatment and in this stage of the intervention, in a congruent manner.

Once SAM has begun listing his facts, the therapist can inquire as to the experience of having relayed such data. From the client's perspective, it's one thing to have thought of these facts for weeks, months, and years; it's another thing to say them aloud and to hear them in the presence of one who cares without judgment. During this stepwise process, a shock of recognition occurs—the shock of spoken words once held silent, the recognition of the self as subject.

At this point, the client can begin going over the facts again, one by one, this time with the therapist inquiring as to his points of view. What are his thoughts about these facts? What does that fact mean to him? And one by one, SAM will go through and relate a belief with each fact. Throughout the span of the intervention, more facts might emerge. And during this process, more than one belief per fact may surface as well.

After SAM has had an opportunity to state the facts, and to state the cognitive meaning associated with such facts, and has had an opportunity to talk about them, he is often beyond the shock of recognition, and now can begin to look at his emotional points of view. So once again, beginning with each fact and corresponding cognitive point of view, SAM will begin connecting emotional points of view to the facts and beliefs.

To be sure, more facts might emerge, and more thoughts and beliefs about the facts might emerge. Also, we now have the feelings associated with the facts emerging, too. Given the cyclical and spiral nature of this intervention, SAM can begin and end, with many opportunities to begin again.

In sum, the therapist helps SAM to do the following:

1. Acknowledge a history of CSA.
2. Reflect on his history in a systematic manner.
3. Identify facts that illuminate the experience of CSA.
4. Distinguish facts from beliefs, beliefs from feelings, and facts from feelings.
5. Correlate beliefs with each fact.
6. Relate feelings to each corresponding fact and belief.
7. Repeat steps 3–6 as necessary overtime.

Anticipated Outcomes

Although it may seem as if SAM is merely reciting facts, his newfound voice is much more than that. The very act of disclosing is pushing through the secrecy—a barrier that has created so much of the trauma associated with CSA. Not only is SAM revealing and releasing facts emanating from his experience of CSA, but he is also confronting potential beliefs regarding threats about disclosure. He's bravely facing the fact that his perpetrator may have threatened to kill him, may have threatened to hurt someone close to him, may have said that "if you tell anyone, everyone will think you're gay," or "if you tell anyone, God is going to punish you for making something like this happen."

The identification and communication of fact and meaning is a cyclical process—and a building process, too. One fact leads to another, one belief leads to a set of surface feelings, and surface feelings lead to those embedded and protected. This intervention minimizes anxiety by beginning with facts and working toward meaning, by beginning with the cognitive and working toward the affective, by beginning with the surface and working toward the defended. It gently engages thoughts and feelings, the past and the present, and eventually, the preabused or authentic self with the abused and compensatory selves.

SAM is building his story, on his way to telling his truth, in a manner that is noninvasive. SAM is building his story—a story waiting to be told, so healing can be his to keep. This is the most compelling anticipated outcome of all.

Clinical Example

Figure 10.3 presents Kip's "Facts and Meanings Chart." Less than a year after Kip's rape, he was also sexually abused by the boyfriend of his mother. Kip's chart shows a number of clinically relevant points. Structurally, it reveals terse facts, vivid beliefs, or cognitive points of view, and figurative feelings, or emotional points of view. In terms of feelings, Kip communicated in similes—"I felt: (1) like I was scum; (2) like I was nothing but a hole; (3) like I wasn't fifteen anymore; and (4) like fucking Heaven." His direct access to affective states was limited to feelings of anger and hate. In such states, with excitatory neurotransmitters discharging abundantly, he was able to physiologically and psychologically experience a sense of power and potency. Other feelings, however, especially ones tinged with vulnerability, remained dormant behind his defensive shield. For example, Kip stated "I don't know" in response to how he felt when his aunt intervened. Authentically, he felt astonished, relieved, elated, and grateful. As can be seen, he was significantly more verbose in the cognitve realm, as indicated by the detailing and specificity of his more cerebral points of view. It wasn't until Kip told his story in the first-person present tense that long-dormant feelings from both sexually abusive experiences emerged and were fully expressed.

Finally, it's readily apparent that Kip's self-image as a "whore" was socially imposed by the perpetrator and ultimately validated by his mother. It was not authentic to Kip, although he thought and felt it to be so. When he completed his "Facts and Meanings Chart," about 20 pages in length, and traced his experience, page by page, column by column, Kip discovered the source of his negative self-concept. He stated: "All of you [clinical team] been trying to tell me that I'm not a whore but I didn't believe you. I couldn't believe you, no matter how hard you were trying to make me. I needed it in black-and-white. And I got it! I got it right here."

WHOSE VOICE?

By this stage in the treatment process, SAM has highlighted a number of facts and their corresponding cognitive and affective points of view. Now it is imperative that he have the opportunity to discern and appraise the sources of meanings. In keeping with the SAM model treatment philosophy, the focus is less on the facts, and more on the points of view.

When clients come into treatment, their goal, more often than not, is to change the facts of the story—the facts of their history. Facts, such as "I was

FACTS AND MEANING

Kip

Facts	Beliefs	Feelings
1. I was abused by my mother's boyfriend.	He was drunken bastard.	I felt like I was scum.
2. He raped me, shoved his penis inside me.	He was like a fucking animal, so smelly, a wicked fucker – like just the thought of it makes me want to throw up. It makes me sick.	I felt like I was nothing but a hole. For him to fuck.
3. He keep calling me a "pussy-boy whore."	He was right, right? For why would I get a hard-on, right? Just like the first time. Why would from him doing this thing to me make me cum?	I feel so guilty. Like how could I be so rotten to make that drug dealer and my mother's boyfriend do that to me?
4. He kept me locked and tied in the house for two days.	He tricked me, lied to me, locked all the doors, told me to take medicine when my stomach hurt, and he drugged me, the motherfucker. Just kept me in the fucking smelly bedroom. I couldn't even go to the bathroom without him.	I felt like I wasn't 15 anymore. Like I was five or six and couldn't take care of myself and couldn't say the words of what he was doing to me.
5. On the third day, he went out for a while, and I ran out the house and told my aunt.	I was fucking tired and getting raped. I was praying to God and St. Jude that she would believe me, and she did. Didn't ask why or how or anything. Just took care of me. Took me to the hospital.	Fucking heaven. I started crying and losing my breath, then nothing came out of mouth. I didn't feel like me anymore. I didn't know my name.
6. My aunt called DSS.	She was brave. She knew my mother and her boyfriend, and knew that they wouldn't help me. She knew better. Knew that if she left it up to my mother, it would be all pretend.	I don't know.
7. My mother didn't believe me.	That woman is amazing. I don't know why I was so surprised. She put me in foster care for eight years after I was born. She would do just about anything to keep her man – one of her many men – even if it meant giving up her kids. She did.	I hated her for that. She said I was a "whore," just like he said, and that I was gonna be punished by God and burn all up in hell.

FIGURE 10.3. Facts and Meanings Chart

sexually abused by a priest when I was in third grade. I was penetrated. I bled. I tried to tell my parents. They told me I was going to hell" are all too common and, unfortunately, unamenable to change. All that can change are the meanings associated with sexual abuse. Because such meanings are, as a matter of course, socially imposed, SAM's truth cannot be told, nor can it be validated, without a thorough examination of the social context in which boys are sexually abused, and the very social context in which they internalize its mythology. SAM cannot identify and reclaim what is authentic until what's been socially imposed has been explored, identified, unveiled, disputed, and relinquished. This intervention initiates that process.

Definition

"Whose Voice?" is a treatment strategy that offers SAM an opportunity to examine the source of his beliefs and the source of his feelings, and to differentiate authentic meaning around the abuse from meaning that was socially imposed by the perpetrator, family members, peers, social workers, and social constructs, among others sources.

Description

SAM examines each belief, one by one. Some common beliefs include: (1) I am a faggot; (2) I am a whore; (3) I did nothing to stop it from happening; (4) I wanted the perpetrator to love me; (5) it was my fault; (6) my erection/ejaculation proves it; (7) something is really wrong with me; (8) if I tell, everyone will know I am a sinner; and (9) if I tell, then the perpetrator's threats will come true. These types of beliefs may be authentic to the client, or they may have been socially imposed.

Sexual abuse beliefs can be viewed as authentic to oneself, or socially imposed and internalized "as if" they belong to the self. If the source truly is oneself and the beliefs are viewed as authentic, the client, in many cases, might want to retain them. There's strength and power in that stance. For example, if SAM believes "it is my fault," he can also assert himself to do something about it, thereby cultivating a sense of empowerment in a situation rife with powerlessness. Moreover, powerlessness is antithetical to male gender mythology and socialization, making such a stance all the more compelling.

However, if SAM believes that he is a "whore" and at the same time can see that he has not always believed that about himself, change can occur. If SAM can recognize that, in fact, the perpetrator and perhaps others in his social context conveyed such messages to him, that is, imposed those beliefs on him, then he has an opportunity to claim or disown them. To do so, SAM must question the source.

Thus, the therapist will help SAM accomplish the following:

1. Examine each belief.
2. Distinguish the source by asking: Who does this sound like? Where did this come from? When did I hear this? How did I react when I heard this? Did I always believe this to be true?
3. Identify the source of the belief.
4. Discern if the belief is authentic or socially imposed. Ask: Did I come to this experience with this belief? Do I believe it to be true? Would I believe it to be true if I heard it coming from another male in a similar situation? A female? Did someone want me to believe this in order to conceal the abuse? Does this belief invalidate my experience? Do I compensate for holding such beliefs?
5. If authentic, claim ownership of the belief; if socially imposed, consider the costs of holding onto it, and the benefits of disowning it.

"Whose Voice?" offers a number of advantages to SAM. First, identification of a belief or feeling brings it to the foreground, brings it to light, gives it value. Without identification, without a name, the thought or feeling may appear to be benign, yet it can unknowingly initiate and maintain any number of negative effects, including sadness, a sense of inferiority, fear, lethargy, and anxiety.

Second, this invention provides SAM with an opportunity to separate the abused from the abuse—in other words, the self from the subjections of others. SAM learns that he is not the abuse, but one who has the experience of having been abused. Third, doing so empowers SAM to claim what is rightfully his and to strive to disregard what is not. Reclaiming what has been lost or stolen contributes to SAM's evolving sense of self, independent of the abuse. In time, the abuse becomes an event in his history, no longer the dictator of his goals and dreams—his life.

Finally, this intervention brings to light the potency of perception, and the realization that imposed thinking brings with it imposed feelings, namely guilt, shame, a sense of inadequacy, and self-degradation. Such feelings keep SAM forever linked to the sexually abusive experience, whereas his authentic beliefs and feelings, when discovered and expressed, are more likely to promote self-determination and self-efficacy. Full freedom from the experience of CSA is dependent upon these outcomes.

IMPOSITIONS

A thought, in its most basic form, is simply expressed in a series of words. I-am-a-boy: four words composing a thought. A belief is a thought imbued with a point of view: "I am a boy but act like a mistake" or "I am a boy and am proud to be me."

Although SAM is the only "thinker" in his mind, many of his thoughts and beliefs originated during, and in response to, his experience of CSA. Thus, a considerable number of SAM's beliefs, now internalized and experienced as authentic, were at one time socially imposed.

An imposition is a negative message—deceitful, oppressive, and often caustic—inflicted on SAM, intentionally or otherwise. Within the context of CSA, impositions are often employed to enhance subjection, rationalize abuse, enforce concealment, and foster the invalidation of SAM's perceptions and interpretations.

SAM is subjected to these impositions most likely when he is in a traumatic state. As he transfixes on the occurrence of CSA, consciousness constricts him, sensory channels block him, and ego functions segregate him. SAM is hyperaroused, overwhelmed, dissociated, depersonalized, vulnerable, and confused.

A myriad of emotions—for instance, guilt and shame, rage and fear, confusion and desperation—in tandem with sensations such as numbness, "pins and needles," sexual stimulation, and sensory circuit overload, for example, combine to create, unfortunately, ideal conditions for the impositional imbedding of abuse-related messages. Imposers include the perpetrator, family members, peers, the media, social mythology, and SAM himself. In such a traumatic state, and thereafter as well, susceptibility is high and discernment is low.

The most common impositions held by SAM focus on gender and sexuality. By way of illustration, consider the following examples:

1. You want this so bad, boy. You know you do.
2. You are such a pretty boy. God must have been having an off day when He forgot to give you a vagina.
3. You have a boy-pussy, that's what you have.
4. I wish you weren't such a mistake, or I wouldn't have to be teaching you such a lesson.
5. You're such a big boy, a handsome boy, almost a man. Look what you do to me.
6. If you tell anyone, I will die, and you will be the murderer.
7. I love you, son. You just think it hurts.

Once embedded and, consequently, internalized, impositions, once foreign, now seemingly authentic, generalize across SAM's microenvironments and, in a like manner, within his relationships.

Definition

The "Authentic vs. Socially Imposed" intervention, developed on the Gestalt notion of interjection, intends to help SAM distinguish, externalize, and challenge imposed and incorporated aspects of his history.

Description

1. Specify the imposition so that it reflects the message as it was first communicated.
2. Identify the source of the imposition.
3. Help SAM to explore and identify the assumptions generated by holding such an imposition. Do so from the perspective of the boy as he received the message, not from the current chronological perspective.
4. Challenge the validity of the imposition and its assumptions. What indicators exist as to its truthfulness, its falsity?
5. Contemplate and select new positions that reframe, or bring a new perspective to, the imposition. This may involve additional disputation of the original imposition, or it may simply involve replacing it with a more constructive point of view. Both strategies achieve the same outcome: authenticity.
6. Articulate new consequences engendered by holding this new position. Refer to Figure 10.4 to see two examples.

Anticipated Outcomes

1. This intervention helps SAM to discern and differentiate the authentic from the socially imposed. What SAM once viewed as "truths" about himself and his experience of CSA can now be seen as impositions.
2. SAM learns that his self-concept is fluid and dynamic, and that he can continue to build a positive self-concept with authentic, reality-based beliefs about himself.
3. Although SAM is not responsible for the impositions, he can claim responsibility for exploring, identifying, and disputing them as well as generating a new point of view.
4. Even though it is difficult to initiate, let alone master, new ways of thinking, through this process, SAM gains an ability to transform cognitve barriers against self-acceptance.

ANXIETY

Childhood sexual abuse, in this context, is the original stressor, the original fear. Even after the event occurs, anxiety looms: How can I hide this? Who will find out? How can I prevent that from happening? What will they think of me? I will be marked for life. Where can I hide? How can I handle this? Why is he doing this to me? How can she go through with this?

The original fear spawns fear of disclosure. Concealing the abuse 24 hours a day, 7 days a week, overcharges the voluntary and involuntary nervous system and depletes SAM's psychic reservoir. Further, with perpetual concealment comes perpetual fear of disclosure; SAM's psyche, body, and spirit have little, if any, time to rest from fear. Consequently, sensitization results.

Old Impositions and New Positions

IMPOSITION:	You want this so bad, boy. You know you do.
SOURCE:	Perpetrator.
ASSUMPTION(s):	I did not want him to abuse me. I wanted him to love me.
	I am not screwed up. I was a normal boy who experienced something abnormal. I am not the abuse and it is not me.
CONSEQUENCE(s):	He is responsible for the abuse. It doesn't matter if he accepts responsibility or not. I am responsible for how this experience affected me. I am taking care of myself.

IMPOSITION:	You are such a pretty boy. God made a mistake when he forgot to give you a vagina.
SOURCE:	Perpetrator.
ASSUMPTION(s):	Something really is wrong with me.
	I am and always will be a freak.
	I am supposed to be a girl. That must mean I'm gay.
NEW POSITION(s):	I am not a mistake. He made many mistakes at my expense.
	I am a man who happens to be gay. I am not gay because I was abused. Abuse does not create homosexuality.
	As a man who happens to be gay, I can embrace my masculinity, not relinquish it.
CONSEQUENCE(s):	This new perspective reminds me that I am not the abuse, that it was an experience in my life. It reminds me that he had to tell me lies to keep my silence. He had to shame me and guilt me into keeping the secret. I can take pride in taking responsiblity for taking care of me.

FIGURE 10.4. Impositions

Sensitization is a seemingly ceaseless state of psychological, emotional, and physiological arousal. It is chronic, replete with somatic worries, painful introspection, problems with concentration, surges of fear–adrenaline–fear, dissociation, and the list goes on.

Definition

Fear is an affect associated with one's conscious awareness of and response to a recognizable, external, and reality-based event; anxiety, on the other hand, is an intense psychological and physiological state responding to unconscious dynamics such as conflict or the emergence of repressed, or the integration of suppressed, material. Both infiltrate SAM's experience of CSA. Both have cognitive (e.g., rapidity in thinking, pensive and perpetual apprehension), affective (e.g., agitation, frustration, panic), behavioral (e.g., recoiling, startle response, restlessness), and physiological (e.g., palpitations, changes in blood pressure and body temperature) effects.

The "Overcoming Fear and Anxiety" intervention, based on the work of Dr. Claire Weekes, author of *Simple, Effective Treatment of Agoraphobia*, comprises a stepwise strategy toward coping with a habituated stress response cycle.

Description

1. Put anxiety in context. Anxiety, as a function, warns us of danger—potential, threatened, actual or otherwise, and jump-starts the fight-or-flight response.
2. Introduce intervention and detail each step. The four steps are as follows: (1) facing; (2) accepting; (3) floating; and (4) letting time pass.
3. Facing: Facing the fear and the effects of fear can be very challenging—not impossible, not formidable, but challenging. Facing is the first step in surrendering to fear. Running away, shying away, trying to think of anything but the fear are the opposite of facing. Facing asks that SAM fully acknowledge the existence of fear and its effects.
4. Accepting: Acceptance, in this context, asks SAM to move away from the typical fight–flight response pattern. Instead, SAM, in accepting, moves toward, not away from, the symptoms, the palpitations, the panic, the depersonalization. He learns to relax, to let go, to give in. Up to this moment, SAM most likely "white-knuckled" the fear response; accepting asks that he do the polar opposite.
5. Floating with the fear response: Floating, at first, may seem to be impossible to do and, on top of that, insensitive to suggest to SAM. "How can I float," SAM might ask, "when my heart is jumping out of my chest, when my head feels like it's going to blow off my body, and when I know where I am but feel like I've never been there before?" SAM's initial response is usually that of forcing and fighting. Forcing and fighting, ironically, gener-

ate more fear, more adrenaline, and, ultimately, even more fear. If SAM can imagine himself floating on air, like a balloon, like eagle's wings, breathing deeply into the diaphragm, exhaling slowly, through the nose, metered, and measured, he in actuality would release enough tension, thereby relaxing muscles, focusing his mind, and calming the hyperaroused state. Just as SAM's body can heal a wound without direction, so too can breathing, relaxation, and surrender heal his sensitized body.

6. Letting time pass: As the old saying goes, "Time heals everything." Desensitization takes time. While SAM strengthens his capacities toward facing, accepting, and floating, fear diminishes and relaxation increases. Overcoming anxiety and fear becomes a function of repeated experiences of knowing that the stress response is merely a sign of a sensitized body, that the symptoms do not have anything to do with being or becoming crazy, and that when they no longer matter like they used to matter, they abate with time.

7. Help SAM learn each step in progression. Help SAM understand that peacefulness is on the other side of panic, and that it can be his once again. Let him know that there isn't one "right" way to decrease his anxiety. Given his state, SAM is likely to think: "If there is only one right way, then all of the other possibilities are wrong." Help SAM to think in terms of "better" and worse and, moreover, what works for him at any moment in time.

Anticipated Outcomes

As a result of learning this intervention and applying it consistently over time, SAM can experience the following:

1. A greater awareness of his thought, feelings, behaviors, and body before, during, and after a fear or anxiety response.
2. Holistic skills in stress reduction and management.
3. An evolving capacity toward emotional regulation.
4. The ability to prevent or inhibit a full-blown stress response cycle.
5. A decrease in detachment from the body.
6. A sense of empowerment over and control of the generalized fear/anxiety response.

VOICING THE EXPERIENCE

Especially for boys, it is often extremely risky to express intense feelings toward others, about others, or even in the vicinity of others. When feelings such as terror, betrayal, or rage cannot be directed outward toward the appropriate person or object, often they become directed internally. The person, and the feelings attached to that person, are thus introjected in order to deter the honest and unobstructed communication of these powerful feelings.

Introjection actually serves a double purpose—that of protecting SAM from the repercussions such expression might elicit, as well as that of protecting the perpetrator or others who have elicited these emotions. The latter can be seen clearly because, as the person/object is introjected, and the feelings become directed inward, the object then becomes linked with SAM's sense of self—thus preventing it from changing as well as from leaving his life. Meanwhile, the perpetrator, nonoffending caretaker, or other object remains unaffected by these reactions.

Slowly and surely, unexpressed aspects of the abuse internalize: guilt, shame, fear, rage, impositions, and mythology. Consequently, SAM, over time, feels as if he has become, and is, the abuse, having consumed so much of the unexpressed experience. Internalized, these profound feelings have full reign of expression within the self.

As these feelings become directed at the self rather than at the external causative factor, it is not uncommon for SAM to begin experiencing these feelings as belonging to himself. For example, if SAM experiences intense shame, it may often be found that the actual root of the attitude of self-condemnation of the feelings of self-hate are, in reality, the genuine feelings of aversion and disgust that he originally had toward the perpetrator.

Definition

"Voicing the Experience," based loosely on the Gestalt "empty chair" technique, was developed to foster integrated functioning and the acceptance of aspects of oneself that have been invalidated, compensated, or disowned. A line of demarcation exists between the abused self and the compensatory self; both are engaged in a constant struggle toward expression. With this intervention, the introjects, or aspects of others or social expectancies that have been incorporated into the SAM's ego system, can emerge.

Description

"Voicing the Experience" is an experiential and reflective strategy designed to help SAM externalize the multiple layers of his CSA experience. There are five layers in all: the compensatory, the reconciliatory, the invalidated, the concealed, and the authentic.

The compensatory, or surface level, holds the ways in which SAM strives to neutralize or make reparation for the occurrence and effects of his history of CSA. Below the surface is the reconciled truth. Here, SAM attempts to construct a rationale addressing why the abused occurred. Beneath the reconciled layer is the invalidation layer, wherein SAM distorts and minimizes his experience of CSA in order to survive. Concealment lies below. This layer comprises the enforcers of concealment, including those generated by SAM, those imposed by his perpetrator, and those prescribed by social mythology. Finally, in the lowest and most subordinate place of all is the authentic layer, harboring SAM's most genuine, factual, and unadulterated truth vis-à-vis his history of CSA.

To begin, arrange four chairs or mark four spots, side by side. Directly across, set another chair or identify another spot. The four chairs represent "compensation," "reconciliation," "invalidation," and "concealment," respectively; the solitary chair symbolizes SAM's authentic truth.

Instruct SAM to sit in the solitary chair. As much as necessary, assist and support SAM in exploring, identifying, and expressing the authentic truth of his experience, focusing on facts and meaning. At first, he might simply state: "I was sexually abused. I was eight years old. The perpetrator was my mother."

Next, direct SAM to the other side, to the chair indicating "concealment." Guide him in exploring, identifying, and expressing, in as much detail as possible, the enforcers of concealment. Common enforcers include the following: threats against SAM or others important to him, physical violence, SAM's erection and ejaculation, his fear around the reactions of others, and fear of being perceived as gay, feminine, or deviant, among others.

Now, point SAM to the next chair, representing his invalidated truth. Help him to explore, identify, and express statements that indicate the strategies he and others employed to invalidate his experience, as well as consequences of such. For example, such strategies include denial, detachment, body numbing, self-injurious behavior, and compulsions around drinking, drugging, and sexual behaviors, whereas associated consequences encompass decompression, relief, distraction, sense of euphoria, distorted perceptions of reality, emotional delay, psychosomatic symptoms, withdrawal into self, and fear of losing control without the invalidation strategy, among others.

As SAM moves to the "reconciliation" chair, guide him in eliciting the "story" he told himself about the abuse. Pay particular attention to how he reconciled its occurrence, its effects, concealment, and invalidation, and attribution of blame. To illustrate, SAM might convey the following: "I told myself that she was so stressed out, having five kids and all, working two jobs, and my dad gone. Drinking makes people crazy. It's as simple as that. When people drink, they do things and say things they don't mean to do or say. They can't be responsible. We didn't want anyone to find out about the drinking, to think badly of her, so we just kept our mouths shut."

SAM now shifts to the last chair, the one representing "compensation." Just as before, help SAM to explore, identify, and express the various ways he has compensated for the abuse. Perhaps he continues to do so. He may indicate the following: taking on a hypermasculine stance, excessive body building, tattooing, attempts at psychologically "neutering" himself, psychologically aligning with females, relinquishing his masculinity, overachieving to mask his sense of self-degradation, underachieving to confirm its existence, and so on.

After this first cycle, ask SAM to move back and forth, from chair to chair, dialoguing the various perspectives. Throughout this stepwise process, using questions and observations, help SAM to accomplish the following: (1) conveying the essence of each perspective; (2) differentiation of each perspective; (3) illumination of the conflicts between and among the various perspectives, with words or by action; and (4) identification of the consequences of living with such conflicted perspectives.

Anticipated Outcomes

1. This intervention helps SAM to become aware of aspects of himself that he might be denying.
2. Rather than simply talking about the layers of SAM's experience of CSA, SAM's expression of the various perspectives, through words or movement, highlights underlying meaning so that he can eventually experience it more fully.
3. Such an intervention also noninvasively reveals the lines of demarcation between and among the various aspects of SAM and his experience; in turn, the purposes undergirding such barricades can emerge from chair to chair.
4. This strategy fosters congruence among thoughts, feelings, and behaviors within individual perspectives and promotes their differences across perspectives. In this way, the devalued and detached aspects of self, aspects that hold SAM's story and history, can be reclaimed and integrated.
5. SAM has the opportunity to recognize, for example, how invalidation strategies nullify the authentic truth, and how concealed truth forever fosters the compensatory self, until silence is broken and the authentic truth is validated.

REFRAMING

Effects, initial and long-term, positive, neutral, and negative, must be examined in context. Doing so highlights historic/current linkages. Consequently, SAM is presented with an opportunity to view his current behavior, often mediated by dissociation, denial, and depersonalization, as a throwback to the sexually abusive experience or other events occurring at that time, as opposed to "crazy" behavior that seems to emerge and become visible from nowhere. Contextual exploration and analysis also affords SAM the means by which to view effects as natural and creative adaptations to unnatural acts of dereliction, rather than overt, or one-factor indicators of psychopathology.

With the self-perception of a male with a history of CSA who happens to be experiencing an abuse-generated effect, as distinct from an emasculated, inferior, mentally unbalanced sexual abuse victim, SAM has the chance to construct meaning that engenders self-compassion and self-respect. He deserves nothing less.

This new frame of reference, this newly constructed meaning, helps link the present with the past and effects with dynamics. A new understanding is erected over time, one that invites a reconnection with, and not a detachment from, the self.

Definition

Reframing involves the use of communication—words, symbols, and actions—to bring a new and different frame of reference to an experience, be it historic, current, or anticipated. The modification of perspective, and consequent meaning, builds a foundation for attendant action and strategy.

Description

1. Elicit SAM's experience around a particular topic or concern using the fact and meaning method. That is, give emphasis to questions germane to client meaning.
2. Reflect current meaning.
3. Help SAM explore and discern the payoffs and penalties associated with this current perspective.
4. Ask SAM if he would like to explore alternative vantage points, alternative meanings.
5. Brainstorm alternative meanings.
6. Explore and identify potential payoffs and penalties for each, recognizing there may be both for many of the generated perspectives.
7. Select new perspective, and track its process of incorporation.

Anticipated Outcomes

1. This strategy offers SAM the opportunity to systematically explore and examine his conceptualizations of life experiences, and to ascertain the consequences generated by various perspectives.
2. SAM gains awareness of the negative consequences of holding an imposed point of view and awareness of the positive consequences of incorporating a contextually based authentic point of view.
3. Following the notion of reciprocal determinism, when SAM begins to perceive an experience or fact in a new way, his feelings about it change as well as his actions in response to it.
4. Accordingly, SAM can recognize that his thoughts are not "automatic," that they are amenable to change, and that he is not at the mercy of his feelings, as they are generated by his thoughts.
5. Ultimately, SAM learns that perceptions go a long way toward creating reality, and that beliefs can change over time, to create a life SAM looks forward to living.

UNDERSTANDING EMOTIONS

Part I: Experiencing and Naming Emotions

SAM has learned that "big boys don't cry."

He also learned that big boys do play games, and many types of games—basketball, checkers, baseball, and the one wherein you act like you don't need anything but get what you need any way you know how without getting caught. He knows that boys are supposed to run fast, eat fast, think fast, act fast, and when it comes to girls, they better climb higher, race harder, act smarter, and, if necessary, play dumb. He continues to learn how to lift heavy things and how to avoid heavy topics, how to fight, how to start one, how to win one, but not how to avoid one. How to fight bullies is as important as how to fight tears.

Because, in American culture, what's allocated to one gender is denied the other, males quickly learn that they must dominate their feelings by first not having them and, if that doesn't work, by defending against them. However, to defend against feelings is to treat them like the enemy; they must be conquered lest they conquer you. Skills learned along the way include the following: muffling joy, mastering detachment, repressing tears, restricting responsiveness, hiding fear, hindering bliss, controlling laughter, commanding neutrality, and the list goes on.

This socially imposed "curriculum" creates friction and strife for males, in general; for SAM, it serves to further restrict his truth, invalidate his experience, and author his alienation from himself, his gender, and in some cases his life.

As and after SAM is sexually abused, he knows that tears and fears, his feeling confused, overwhelmed, powerless, helpless, hopeless, and alone, are violations of the masculinity code, his core curriculum. In spite of all that is happening to him—physical violations, betrayal, mockery, coercion, premature sexualization, violence—and despite his natural responses to such a horrific event—anxiety, dissociation, depersonalization, derealization, ejaculation in association with pain, trauma—SAM knows in an instant that what he is experiencing cannot be expressed.

DEFINITION

The "Experiencing and Naming Emotions" intervention is designed to help SAM learn to observe and identify feeling states. An intervention focusing on emotional expression follows.

DESCRIPTION

What are feelings? Feelings are, in basic terms, subjective states, which may or may not be experienced consciously, which may or may not be expressed directly, but which convey the meaning associated with all life phenomena.

Feelings are our most direct reaction to what we perceive, and ultimately experience, in the world. Thoughts, feelings, and behaviors are interactive and interconnected.

Thoughts are the primary determinants of emotions. They are symbolic or semantic statements, perhaps inner monologues, that people express within and to themselves. Thinking often becomes the channel for defended feelings.

Emotions follow thought; they are intricate physiological and psychological reactions to conscious and unconscious perceptions of self, others, and anything of this world. Although the terms *emotion* and *feeling* are often used synonymously, the latter, or feeling, is an individual's idiosyncratic experience of a particular emotion.

Thoughts and feelings influence behavior, just as behavior gives rise to thoughts and feelings. A behavior is a physical action that is motivated by, and an expression of, one's thoughts and feelings.

Given the perpetual concealment and invalidation of the facts and meaning associated with SAM's history of CSA, feeling states tend to be foreign to him. For SAM, feelings are obscure, undefinable, except for a few—namely, guilt, shame, anger, and fear. If he becomes aware of certain physiological or somatic sensations, chances are he likens them to symptoms associated with becoming sick or signs indicating a lack of control. Over time, peace, joy, and hope come to be the most foreign of all.

This particular intervention highlights feelings, but in the context of thought and behavior. Guide SAM through the following steps intended to expand his awareness of feelings.

1. Explore broad-based feeling states: sad, mad, glad, and afraid. Attaching a name to something foreign and subjective may, at first, be quite challenging for SAM. However, with time and practice, this entire process will become increasingly familiar. SAM, regardless of his age, may benefit from using a basic feelings list. See Fig. 10.5.
2. Differentiate one feeling state from another. As SAM reflects on a recent feeling state, guide him in answering the following questions:
   • Is there a sense associated with this feeling? An image? A sound? A taste? A smell? A physical sensation in or on the body?
   • Is this feeling state familiar? Foreign? Recent? Historic? Similar to any others?
   • When do you first remember experiencing this sensation? Where were you? What were you doing? How were you doing it? Why were you there?
   • As you reflect on this feeling state, what do you remember thinking prior to noticing it? While or after noticing it, what do you remember doing? What do you remember wanting to do?
   • As you reflect on this feeling state, what would you name it? How might you express this feeling in words?

MY EMOTIONS

What action signs am I experiencing at the moment? **OR**

What action signs did I experience when/on/at _____?

1. _____

2. _____

3. _____

4. _____

What emotion(s) is(are) underlying the signs?

1. _____

2. _____

What can I **SAY** to express _____ directly?

_____

_____

_____

What can I **DO** to express _____ directly?

_____

_____

_____

FIGURE 10.5. Explore broad-based feeling states: sad, mad, glad, and afraid. Attaching a name to something foreign and subjective may, at first, be quite challenging for SAM. However, with time and practice, this entire process will become increasingly familiar. SAM, regardless of his age, may benefit from using a basic feelings list.

The processes of experiencing and naming emotions can be diagrammed as follows and as indicated by the work page later in this chapter.

1. Stop.
2. Identify the situation. I am at _____ with _____.
   The circumstances are: _____.
3. Identify thoughts, behaviors, and sensations.
   I am thinking: _____.
   I am doing: _____.
   I am sensing: _____.
4. The feeling is: _____.
5. I can express this feeling in words, and in this context, by saying: _____.

Part II: Emotional Expression

At the moment SAM was sexually abused, that experience became a fact of his life story. In order for the sexual abuse to continue, and for the perpetrator to remain unaccountable, he or she had to enforce concealment upon SAM. When a fact is concealed, so is its meaning. Feelings create meaning; therefore, SAM's feelings about CSA had to be concealed. Feelings can bring facts to the surface; facts can bring feelings. For SAM, both had to be invalidated and both had to be reconciled in order to foster concealment.

Meaning transforms a fact into an experience. Without feeling, there is no meaning; without meaning, there is no real existence, no authentic awareness of life. SAM needs his feelings to tell the truth. Only when he tells the truth can he know, and can others know, what he feels and what he means.

DESCRIPTION

1. If SAM is fearful of, and defending against, exploring, identifying, and expressing particular feelings, work with the barriers—the fears, the threats, the expectancies. By doing so, SAM has another opportunity to understand the contexts in which he experiences certain feeling states. There are many rules about and injunctions against and implications regarding the existence and expression of feelings.

   1. Big boys don't cry.
   2. Stomach in, chest out.
   3. You have to stay in control.
   4. Don't be emotional. Just don't think about it.
   5. You look sad. What's wrong?
   6. Now, now, it's gonna be all right.
   7. Have a shot, you'll feel better. Chase it with a six-pack.

8. You're not turning sensitive (i.e., queer) on me, are you bud?
9. Look what you're making me feel.
10. A boy never shows signs of weakness.
11. Brush it off. Get back on.
12. Be cool. Don't let them see you sweat.
13. Life separates the men from the boys. What group do you belong in?
14. If you cry, I'll really give you something to cry about.
15. Take it like a man.

Such rules prohibit and inhibit SAM's willingness and ability to tell the truth. To tell the truth is to express meaning; meaning is indicated by feelings; to tell the truth is to know and express feelings. In American culture, and particularly within the male population, the prevailing emotional vocabulary does more to deny, invalidate, and suppress feelings than to encourage direct expression and resolution.

2. If SAM is challenged by a particular emotion or feeling, help him to explore and identify some psychological, physiological, and behavioral signs that convey the indirect expression of emotion. Examples include:
   1. Grinding teeth at night.
   2. Clenched jaw.
   3. Tense muscles/body.
   4. "Nervous" or "upset" stomach.
   5. Acting "as if" one is not feeling anything.
   6. "Trying" to be in control.
   7. Hypervigilant or startle responses.
   8. Monotone, tight and/or off-pitch voice.
   9. Speaking sarcastically; making cynical remarks.
   10. Dreams with violent or aggressive manifest content.
   11. Withdrawing.
   12. Desire or impulse to "press one's buttons."
   13. "Frog" in the throat.
   14. Tears for no apparent reason.
   15. Impulsive or unanticipated expressions of anger.
   16. Self-consciousness.
   17. Feeling "flushed."
   18. Laughing or smiling that is out of sync with current interaction.
   19. Nervous laughter.
   20. Breathlessness.
   21. A sense of "just beneath the surface" irritability.
   22. Procrastination.
   23. Numbing.
   24. Putting others down, talking behind their back, telling jokes at their expense.
   25. "Forgetting."
   26. Habitual lateness.

27. Acting "as if" you don't care.
28. A sense of being "exposed" or "transparent."
29. Rapid heart rate.
30. Negative self-talk.

3. Now, help SAM to discern and define the following:
   What action signs am I experiencing at the moment? _____
   What action signs did I experience when/on/at? _____
   What emotion(s) is(are) underlying the signs? _____
   How might I express this more directly? _____
   I CAN SAY: _____
   I CAN DO: _____

ANTICIPATED OUTCOMES

1. As SAM learns to reflect upon his feelings—that is, experience them, identify their physiological manifestations in his body, and give them a label—he eventually becomes more familiar with them.
2. Releasing the need to defend against foreign and frightening emotions so continuously and vigorously generates a sense of integration of thoughts and feelings, fact and meaning, mind and body, and experience and context.
3. With such skills, SAM now has an opportunity to verify the authenticity of the meanings associated with CSA experience—those imposed by the perpetrator, those imbued with social mythology, those unduly influenced by families and professionals.
4. SAM's developing capacity to identify and express emotions and feelings with words, in turn, enhances his abilities around emotional regulation and control.
5. Emotional expression and emotional regulation diminish the need for SAM's body to circumvent feeling states by means of psychosomatic symptom formation.

STORY GUIDELINES

Perhaps the only way to break the strongholds of concealment, invalidation, reconciliation, and compensation is to tell the story. That SAM tells his story, his history, is more important than how he tells it.

DEFINITION

The "Story Guideline" intervention is simply a set of questions intended to help SAM remember, and give voice to, his history of CSA.

DESCRIPTION

The following questions parallel the SAM model of dynamics and effects. They can be used for both assessment and intervention purposes. Some questions may require modification, depending on SAM's age, vocabulary, developmental needs, and level of comprehension. Be sure not to lead, but to give SAM an opportunity to describe the process.

Preabuse

How did SAM perceive himself before the abuse began? His sense of self? His perceptions of self as a male? As a son? As a brother? As a peer? As a friend? As a child? What was his body image? Gender image?

How did SAM view the perpetrator before the abuse? What was the nature of their relationship? What did he call the perpetrator in terms of name, relation, or role? What did he want most and need most from the perpetrator?

What was his view of those around him, family, friends, neighborhood, community? What was his view of the world? Of his future?

Subjection

When was SAM subjected to CSA? What were the predispositional strategies of the perpetrator: Intrusion? Manipulation? Sexualization? How did SAM, in his mind, define the actions of the perpetrator? How did they effect SAM? What was SAM feeling at the time? What did he anticipate at this time?

SEXUAL ABUSE

When was SAM sexually abused? How is time associated with his memories? Does he associate the sexual abuse with a time of day, season of the year, holiday, special event? How does he mark the time? Where did the first abusive episode take place? Was it indoors or outdoors? What furniture, scenery, or things were part of this place? Ask him to describe the weather, noises in the background, noises in the foreground, the scents of the location, perpetrator, and abuse.

How was SAM sexually abused? An evolving chronology of specific facts is critical. What behaviors were imposed on SAM? What behaviors did SAM have to perform on the perpetrator? What name did SAM give to the sexual acts? What sexual positions were involved? What did the perpetrator say? What emotions did he, she, or they express?

Give SAM an opportunity to depict the physical or bodily sensations that occurred. What was happening within his body during the abuse? How did his body respond? Did he faint? Did he gag? Was he excited? Was he numb? Did his heart race, his hands shake, his body quake? Were his muscles tense? Could he move freely and at will? Did he vomit? What sexual sounds does he remember hearing? What sexual smells were evident to him? What sexual tastes? Does one sense hold primacy over the others? Did he feel pain? Did he feel pleasure? Was there a sensation of "pins and needles"? Did he have an erection? Did he ejaculate? Was there semen? Blood?

What was happening within his mind during the abuse? Was it as if time stopped or slowed down? Was it akin to other experiences? What does SAM remember thinking during the first abusive episode? What did he call this experience?

How did SAM know this first episode was over? What did the perpetrator say and do? What does SAM remember thinking and feeling? What did he do?

What does he remember about later episodes? What was the duration and frequency of the abuse? Was there subsequent abuse by other perpetrators? What feelings does SAM remember experiencing during the abusive episodes? What feelings does SAM experience as he recalls these events?

Concealment

Was the abuse concealed? What aspects of the abusive experience did SAM try hardest to conceal? For how long? How so?

What were the enforcers of concealment? Were they subtle, blatant, verbal, nonverbal? How did SAM understand these to be enforcers? What enforcers were imposed by the perpetrator, by those who knew, by SAM, and by social mythology?

How was disclosure framed by the perpetrator? By SAM? What were the anticipated consequences of disclosure? What were the anticipated consequences of concealment?

Invalidation

What did SAM tell himself while the abuse was occurring? What did he tell himself afterward? What did he experience immediately after the abuse? The next day? Thereafter? How does SAM recall the abuse? What sensory channels were in the foreground (i.e., visual, auditory, olfactory)? What mode of memory is detached? How does SAM experience the memory—like a movie without music, sounds without sight?

What strategies did SAM employ, unconsciously or consciously, intentionally or otherwise, to invalidate the abuse and its effects? Defenses? Denial? Dissociation? Depersonalization? Derealization? Body numbing? Compulsive behaviors? Drugging? Drinking? Gambling? Work?

Reconciliation

How did SAM construct meaning around the abusive events? His role? The role of the perpetrator? The roles of significant others? What did SAM call the abuse? How did he reconcile the effects, given the enforced concealment and his invalidation strategies? What did he tell himself in order to put the abuse in a viable perspective? How did he reconcile its occurrence? Whom or what did he blame?

Compensation

How does SAM describe the inner conflict regarding his experience of CSA? What did he think of himself as a result of the abuse? What were his personal hypotheses about himself, about the perpetrator, about significant others, about the abuse, about the world, and about his future? What did he feel? How did the experience of abuse impact his behavior around others? How did he resolve the conflict within?

How did SAM try to undo the experience? What did he want to project to others?

Initial Effects

What were some of the effects SAM experienced after the abuse first occurred? (If necessary, refer to the Tables 10.1 and 10.2.)

The Cycle Continues

How does SAM continue to conceal, invalidate, reconcile, and compensate for the abuse? How do these defensive, coping, and adaptational strategies manifest within and across his microenvironments? How do they unfold within the domains of peer relations, family relations, dating and partnership relations, community participation, educational endeavors, workplace and career endeavors, and spiritual endeavors, among others?

TABLE 10.1. Common SAM Dynamics

• Pedophilia (Prepubescent attraction)	• Developmentally Discordant Behaviors
• Ephebophilia (Postpubescent attraction)	• Gender Discordant Behaviors
• Perpetrator Fixation	• Graduated Exposure
• Perpetrator Regression	• Boundary Diffusion
• Perpetrator's Distorted Perceptions	• Use of Drugs and Alcohol
• Distorted Rationales	• Exposure to Pornography
• Closed Relational System	• Use of Enemas for Non-Medical Purposes
• Limits Around External Relationships	• Role Confusion
• Age Differential	• Focus on Secondary Sex Characteristics
• Developmental Differential	• Attacking/Enhancing Boy's Gender Integrity
• Physical Differential	
• Role Differential	• Manipulation of Care
• Status Differential	• Oral and Anal Penetration
• Grooming Behaviors	• Penetration of Perpetrator
• Special Gifts and Privileges	• Multiple Episodes
• Coercion	• Concurrent Physical Abuse
• Bribes	• Perpetrator Misattribution
• Intrusion	• Threats to Hurt Boy, Self, Others
• Intimidation	• Threats to Defame Boy
• Force	• Micro and Macro Concealment
• Premature Sexualization	• Social Mythology

Disclosure

Was the abuse disclosed at any point in time? When? To whom? Under what circumstances? Was it accidental, intentional?

Long-Term Effects

What long-term effects are most pressing to SAM? How do they play out within his various relationships across his microenvironments? (If necessary, refer to Tables 10.1 and 10.2.)

ANTICIPATED OUTCOMES

As SAM develops, remembers, and tells his story, the process of doing so noninvasively integrates the past with his present. SAM can now tangibly real-

TABLE 10.2. Common SAM Effects

• Anogenital Injuries	• Academic Problems
• Sexually Transmitted Diseases	• Concentration Difficulties
• Anxiety	• Anticipation of Workplace Failure
• Depression	• Addictive Behaviors
• Intrusion	• Drug and Alcohol Misuse
• Hyperarousal	• Eating Disorders
• Dissociation	• Compulsive Behaviors
• Depersonalization	• Self-Injurious Behaviors
• Derealization	• Developmentally Advanced Sexual
• Denial	Knowledge
• Dysregulated Stress Response	• Self-Concept as "Sex Magnet"
• Dysregulated Circadian Rhythm	• Desperate for Love and Affection
• HPA Axis Dysregulation	• Sexual Abuse Reactivity
• Habituated Panic Response	• Clinging Behavior
• Psychobiological Sensitization	• Interpersonal Sensitivity
• Reduction in Hippocampus Volume	• Fear of Rejection
• Amygiloid Reduction	• Social Introversion
• Hemispheric Incoherence	• Overcompliance
• Corpus Callosum Impairment	• Relational Difficulties
• Indelible Implicit Memories	• Fear of Expressing Care and Affection
• Deficits in Explicit Memory	• Fear of Expressing Anger
• Negative Perceptions of Self	• Somatization
• Sense of Emasculation	• Gagging and Choking Reactions
• Gender Shame	• Pelvic or Joint Paralysis
• Indentity and Role Confusion	• Rectal Discomfort
• Confusion Regarding Sexual Orientation	• Fear of Bathrooms
• Cognitive Dissonance	• Alienation from Body
• Self-Blame	• Sleep Problems
• Diminished Self-Efficacy	• Nightmares and Night Terrors
• Aggression	• Running Away
• Acting Out	• Loss of Spirituality
• Traumatic Rage	• Internalization of Social Mythology

ize that, in telling his story, he is creating a bridge from secrecy to disclosure, from mythology to reality, from fractionation to connection, from fear to action, and from invalidation to reclamation. In retelling the story, time and again, more facts emerge, more meanings arise, and SAM's conviction to his truth grows. Although telling the story does not automatically bring resolution, it does validate the reality of SAM's experience, a reality that disputes the perpetrator's distorted perceptions, impositions, and lies.

The work of constructing the story, and eventually telling it in the first-person present tense (i.e., the boy's perspective as if happening now), serves to integrate fractional aspects of the CSA experience and fractional aspects of SAM. In turn, CSA effects such as hyperarousal, depersonalization, anxiety, and shame diminish, as well as the need for correspondent coping strategies, for instance, invalidation, reconciliation, and compensation.

SELF-MASTERY PROJECT

Just as aftereffects such as guilt and shame have generalized from the abusive experience across many domains of SAM's life, so too can the new skills, acquired during treatment, move from the specific to the general. As SAM develops new skills in the clinical setting and starts to apply them to other areas of his life, his sense of self-mastery will increase as well. This sense of self-mastery further helps to foster an equilibrium in SAM's life between his stressors and the intrapersonal and/or environmental resources available to him for adaptation.

Definition

The self-mastery project, in the clinical setting, is designed to help SAM identify his goals, explore their meaning, set steps for their attainment, and provide recognition for their accomplishment. This progressive format encompasses five points: (1) situation, (2) solutions, (3) selection, (4) steps, and (5) self-praise.

Description

1. *Situation.* This is, perhaps, the most important step of the process. Help SAM to stop long enough to acknowledge the existence of a problematic circumstance. The situation must be identified for it to have meaning. Help SAM to view the circumstance, or target area of change, as independent of interfering emotions as possible.

   What is the situation at hand? Why is it a problem? What meaning does this hold for SAM? What would "change" mean to SAM?

   Help SAM to define the problematic situation as concretely as possible.

What is the problem? What are its cognitive, affective and/or behavioral manifestations? (These are the greatest arenas of personal change—thoughts, feelings, and actions.) When does it happen? Where does it happen? With whom? And, if possible, why does it happen?

To enhance goal attainment, help SAM to: define the goals as accomplishments; define the goals in observable and measurable terms; and define goals that have the potential for achievement.

2. *Solutions.* This, for many, is the most exciting step. It's at the conceptual level, the imaginary level, not requiring commitment to action.

Help SAM to generate as many solutions as possible, without judging them in any way. This is an opportunity to think broadly, no matter how impossible a potential solution may sound.

Because "problems" are typically experienced within the domains of thoughts, feelings, and behaviors, it's best to generate solutions in a like manner. How might I change my thoughts, my feelings, my actions?

In seeking solutions, guide SAM in shaping potential solutions that increase positive human behaviors rather than decrease negative ones.

3. *Selection.* The key here is to stay away from words such as "right" solution or "correct" option. Given SAM's proclivity toward dichotomous thinking, "right" suggests only one viable alternative within an infinite number—that is, every option, aside from the one identified as "right," is identified as "wrong" by default.

It is critical that SAM believe he can accomplish the selected option. The key here, at least in the beginning, is to design and select a strategy that holds the maximum potential for achievement.

Help SAM to explore and experience the meaning associated with each potential solution and outcome. Positive meanings tend to forge the process, even as ambivalence, a sense of inferiority, and frustration emerge. Negative meanings often times indicate obstacles that could potentially inhibit the process of goal attainment. Additionally, it is important that SAM explore and identify the positive and negative consequences associated with each potential solution.

4. *Steps.* The void between the problematic situation and change may appear to be vast. Partialization of strategies, in other words, the generation of stepping-stones to goal attainment, can make this process a less daunting one.

Help SAM to outline a step-by-step process comprised of concrete strategies. Be on the lookout for any steps that may generate fear, concern, and apprehension.

Also, introduce the importance of monitoring as one way to systematically record the goal attainment process. Strategies might include standardized measures, recording logs, critical incident logs, target behavior frequency and duration logs, anecdotal logs, and any others that may facilitate this process for SAM and make it a more viable experience.

Encourage SAM to direct his enthusiasm toward the process, not the outcome.

5. *Self-evaluation.* This is perhaps the most difficult stage. Help SAM to evaluate the goal attainment process, from intention through each partialized step on to outcome. If SAM did not achieve his goal, consider other options designated in the "Solutions" stage, and then begin the process again. If SAM achieved his goal, encourage him to repeat this process with another goal. In either case, introduce the importance of self-reflection and self-praise.

Anticipated Outcomes

1. Given months, perhaps years, of emotional sensitization, a project such as this helps SAM to ground actions in forethought, rather than taking action based simply on emotion.
2. This problem-solving process inhibits dichotomous thinking by generating a number of means to an end.
3. By partializing the "solution" into a set of steps, each with a beginning, middle, and end, SAM has not only the opportunity to experience a sense of achievement during this process, but also the time to assess and adapt along the way.
4. The self-mastery project places SAM in relation to both immediate and long-term consequences, and in relation to others, as he considers various ways those in his microenvironments may be impacted by his choices and changes, and how he may be impacted by their responses.
5. Strategy-based projects such as this promote SAM's ability to generalize acquired knowledge and skills across other domains.

EVALUATION

Given the embryonic status of the sexual abuse treatment field, it is vital to our progress that we advance the knowledge base, develop efficacious interventions, demonstrate accountability, and determine if we are doing what we think we're doing as we determine whether our clients are receiving the best possible services we can provide. In a nutshell, the operating question is: How can we intervene more responsively, more effectively, and more efficiently? The answer, in one word is evaluation. In two words, it is quality enhancement!

Definition

Evaluation, particularly the single-case variety, is a means of answering one of two questions. The first question is this: Did SAM change, as hypothesized, during the course of treatment? The second question is a bit more complex: Did SAM change as a result of treatment? Both questions are important. When we can effectively actualize the first, we can move on to the second; at that point, we can address either one, and build our skill base to answer other questions as well. This intervention is guided and informed by the works of Martin Bloom and Joel Fischer, *Evaluating Practice*, and Richard M. Grinnell, Jr., *Social Work Research and Evaluation*.

Description

1. *Conceptualizing the problem in concrete terms*. Perhaps this is the most vital step, since all other steps emerge from this one. In simple terms, we must conceptualize the "problem"—that is, CSA—or some dynamic and effect of CSA, in concrete terms. Too often we say things like: "SAM has PTSD" (posttraumatic stress disorder), "SAM is shame-based," or "SAM acts out." Such conceptualizations keep us from intervening effectively.

   The problem must be operationalized into concrete terms—terms that define the problem as it is experienced and expressed in the "real world." In other words, we must define the problem in terms of how it is manifested—typically through human action, namely, cognition, affect, behavior, and sensation.

   Stating that "SAM was sexually abused and has PTSD" does not provide us with understanding that can lead to viable intervention. First, there is no universal definition for sexual abuse. Second, PTSD is a concept that is often used to describe sexual abuse effects, but the term, as stated, provides no explanation of the problem. Third, the problem, as stated in abstract terms, does not provide the therapist with a viable understanding of the problem, the location of the problem, and consequently with any viable strategies to intervene effectively and efficiently.

   To foster treatment efficacy, we must conceptualize and operationalize problems so they can be definable, observable, and measurable. For a problem to be definable, we must explain it in terms of concrete dynamics and effects, as experienced by SAM in terms of his cognitions, affect, behavior, and/or sensations. For it to be observable, we must ask: Can we, as therapist and client or collateral, keep track of its occurrences and manifestations? For it to be measurable, can we discern when it occurs, where it occurs, how it occurs, under what conditions, and for what duration?

   Let's take the example, "SAM is shame-based." This term has been widely used over the past decade. How can we operationalize it? Shame is a pervasive sense of defection. After meeting with SAM, we might operationalize shame in this way:

   Cognition: Something is wrong with me. I'm one big mistake. Everyone must think I'm really screwed up. Why would they even want to be with me?

Affect: I feel embarrassed to be me. I feel stupid, ugly, worthless.
Behavior: Hiding, withdrawing, stuttering when speaking.
Sensation: Sick feeling in the pit of my stomach.

In this example, shame is definable. It is observable. Thoughts can be expressed silently, verbally, and in writing. Feelings can be experienced kinesthetically, and expressed in the same way. Actions indicating shame can be noted as well, and it is measurable. SAM can count how many times, within a circumscribed period, he has such thoughts, feelings, or manifestations.

The windows of opportunity for change, for healing, for growth, are not the concepts, but the thoughts, feelings, and behaviors that express the concepts. Shame, sexual addiction, PTSD, anxiety, a sense of inferiority—these concepts are functions of the real-life actions that manifest them; we cannot take action on the concept; the power is in its human expression. We cannot change the fact that SAM was sexually abused. We cannot change "shame-based," for it is a mere abstraction. We can, however, in tandem with SAM, explore, define, observe, and enumerate the problem in concrete terms.

2. *Conceptualizing "change" in concrete terms.* The degree to which we effectively, accurately, and concretely conceptualize the "problem" sets the parameter for the degree to which will be able to conceptualize "change." Just as we identified real-life indicators for the problem, we do the same thing for change. This time, however, we express change in positive terms: that is, in terms of what SAM can and will be doing more of, as opposed to less. A mentality of "lack" is defeating; a mentality of "abundance" is empowering.

To illustrate, rather than decreasing a negative thought, such as "Something is wrong with me. I'm one big mistake," help SAM to increase affirmative thoughts, such as "I am becoming more comfortable with myself" and "I'm under construction. Rome wasn't built in a day." Focusing on the negative maintains a static and retractable connection to the problematic past; focusing on the affirmative expands the possibilities, creates new pathways to goal attainment.

3. *Selecting valid measure congruent with problem and change.* Once the problem and change have been conceptualized using real-world indicators, we can select an outcome measure congruent with the focus at hand. Paper-and-pencil measures and client self-report measures are the most common strategies employed today.

Paper-and-pencil measures are numerous, encompassing a diverse range of human problems and experiences. Additionally, the client can monitor his target actions. Although neither strategy is foolproof, and both strategies are less than ideal in terms of research validity and reliability, the alternative, that of doing nothing, offers more disadvantages and provides no

opportunity for the generation of practice knowledge and practice accountability.

4. *Selecting appropriate interventions conceptualized in terms of definition,
   description, and anticipated outcomes.* In order to select an intervention
   that will help SAM translate the problem into change, we must know what
   it is, how to execute it, and what it's designed to do. In other words, we
   must know the intervention's rationale. Unfortunately, such descriptions
   are few and far between in scholarly, professional, and client-based texts.

   An intervention rationale is composed of three components: (1) definition, (2) description, and (3) anticipated outcomes. The definition answers
   the question, "What is this?" The description address the execution of the
   intervention. The anticipated outcomes answer the question, "Why?" All of
   the interventions in this chapter are presented with a rationale. Please refer
   to them for further information.

5. *Selecting the design.* Single-case designs can help answer the questions posed
   at the beginning of this chapter: Did SAM change during the treatment
   process, and are such changes a function of treatment? Although a detailed
   description of single-case design is beyond the parameters of this book,
   two designs will be briefly addressed: AB and ABAB.

   The AB design is central to most other designs. Comprising a baseline
   observation interval, A, and an intervention interval, B, it answers the question: Did SAM change during the treatment process? Thus, AB presents the
   therapist with an opportunity to compare the extent to which and the ways
   in which the problematic actions were experienced before the intervention
   and after the intervention. It presents the therapist and client with descriptive results.

   The ABAB design is more experimental in nature, addressing the question: Did SAM change as a result of treatment? In other words, this design
   can bring to the foreground cause, effect, and potential mediating factors.
   The first AB is conducted, as described above. In a second A interval, the
   intervention strategy is temporarily suspended, in order to observe and
   generate another baseline period. Then the intervention strategy continues.
   It is postulated that positive changes will occur from the first A to B, and the
   second A to B, whereas a decrease in such changes is anticipated from the
   first B to the second A. The ABAB design offers the therapist and client
   explanatory results.

6. *Implementing evaluation.* The therapist hypothesizes the following: After
   the intervention (i.e., X, or independent variable) is executed, the status of
   the problem will change (i.e., Y, or dependent variable, will increase or
   decrease, depending on direction). The next step is to establish and measure the baseline. This interval must be circumscribed by hour, day, week,
   or in some similar manner. Introduce the intervention. If ABAB, repeat.

7. *Graphically displaying data.* Once the data is recorded, it can be trans-
   ferred to a chart depicting a vertical axis and a horizontal axis. The former

represents the problem and/or the outcome measure, depending on phase; the latter represent times (i.e., hours, days, sessions, weeks, etc.). The phases, ABAB, are demarcated by broken vertical lines. Consult a primer or chapter on single-case research designs for additional information.

8. *Interpreting and employing data.* There are more than a few statistical procedures amenable to single case design. However, visual inspection is an adequate step in many instances. Changes in Y, the dependent variables, over repeated administrations, and charted on the axes, indicate the productivity and efficacy of the intervention protocol.

Anticipated Outcomes

Single-case designs in general, and the ABAB design in particular, offer a number of positive outcomes. To begin, the design fosters purposeful and accountable practice. Such designs, compared to others, demonstrate more conclusively that the intervention protocol, and not some external dynamic, is influencing change. Additionally, the therapist gains knowledge as to what types of interventions produce what types of effects. And this contributes to the therapist's evolving repertoire of effective intervention strategies. The therapist is, in fact, generating practice knowledge rather than simply using practice knowledge. Consequently, therapist confidence, client change, and practice efficacy are enhanced.

Clinical Example

Figure 10.6 presents a graph of a single-case ABAB design employed with Jake. In terms of the particular problem, Jake stated: "Ever since the abuse, I did my best to run away from people. I've been married to Lena now for what—almost thirty two years and been running away from her the whole time. I need to stop running. I want to learn to love my wife how I do in my imagination." In essence, Jake wanted to decrease his detached and avoidant actions and increase his intimate and expressive actions. The intervention was cognitive and behavioral in nature. Avoidant behaviors were indicated by silences, terse responses, disengaging from conversation, isolating, and several others. Expressive actions were operationalized as initiating conversations, focusing on mutual interests, holding hands, and communicating feelings of love, gratitude, or appreciation, among various others. The intervention focused on nonsexual intimacy.

Jake kept daily records of his avoidant actions as well as his intimate actions. A, the first baseline, revealed a significant void between the two. During B, or the first intervention phase, Jake advanced in the direction of intended change. That being the case, the intervention was withdrawn for 1 week during A2, or the second baseline. The purpose was to assess for intervention effects. During this brief phase, Jake's graph evidenced a marked re-

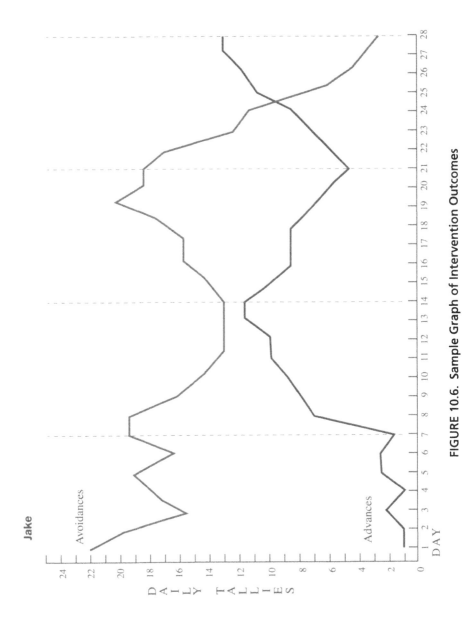

Jake

FIGURE 10.6. Sample Graph of Intervention Outcomes

gression in the direction of pre-baseline behaviors. In response, B, or the second interventive phase, was initiated with the same strategies. This last phase once again demonstrated that Jake was quickly moving in the positive direction of intimacy. The graphed data suggested that the systematic intervention partially explained the increase in target behavior. Other facilitative factors included Jake's readiness, Lena's receptivity, and the support they obtained from other couples in therapy. There were no indications of carryover effects, and the expressed changes could not be assigned to concurrent environmental coincidences.

SUMMARY

This chapter highlighted a number of intervention strategies that can be employed with SAM. All have been utilized with males ranging in age from 5 to 77 and with varying degrees of psychological, cognitive, affective, and developmental capacities. Each intervention was conceptualized in the following way: (1) a definition of the technique; (2) a systematic description of its execution; and (3) its anticipated consequences. This type of interventive conceptualization facilitates practice evaluation. Therapists are encouraged to conceptualize, develop, pilot, evaluate, and refine interventions that may be shared with colleagues in peer consultation groups, at conferences, or through publications.

CHAPTER ELEVEN

FROM SAM

IT'S TRUE THAT SAM is the only one who can take and rightfully claim responsibility for change, for healing. The therapist cannot claim responsibility, but is responsible for conceptualizing CSA within a biopsychosocial perspective, maintaining an awareness of knowledge base developments, intervening purposefully, assuring cultural sensitivity, articulating interventions in terms of rationale and anticipated outcomes, and evaluating and analyzing therapist-based, client-based, strategical, process and outcome variables. This book has attempted to highlight research, introduce a conceptual framework and practice model, and provide some practice pointers and systematic interventions in order to help the therapist render necessary services. This book now leaves the final words to SAM.

This chapter focuses on the perceptions of Nicholas, Kip, Palo, Matt, Victor, Jake, and Ty around some of their experiences in treatment. Nicholas participated in ongoing individual therapy, time-limited group therapy, and collateral therapy with foster parents. Kip engaged in individual therapy conducted in 12-week intervals. After every interval, he would usually take a break for 2 or 3 weeks. Palo and Matt each attended individual therapy sessions and group therapy sessions and participated in a sexual compulsivity support group. Victor and Jake participated in individual therapy, group therapy, and couples counseling. Ty attended individual and group therapy sessions.

NICHOLAS

I wish all little boys like me who got abused could come to therapy. That is one of my wishes. Another wish. I wish all little boys like me who get abused keep tellin' and tellin' and tellin' until somebody helps them.

When there was therapy the first time, the social workers and the case workers made me go with my Mama. She in one room and me in another room but I didn't know what to say or tell 'cause my Mama told me if I tell anything about her and Terry that I was gonna go to Hell and Terry and she was gonna go to jail. So then the social workers and the judge say that I don't have to go anymore. But they didn't know the secret. They didn't know that I was still bein' abused.

When I was in first grade, it was real bad. Terry and my Mama start doing bad things with me and other adult people. I was afraid cause nobody believe me the first time so who was gonna believe me now? One day me and my Mama was going to the bank. We was in one lane and I looked and there was my therapist truck in the next lane. I didn't want my Mama to see him cause she would get real mad at him. She hated the therapist and the social workers. So when Mama was writing stuff for the bank lady, I put my face on the window and looked at my therapist till he looked back at me and just kept saying "Help. Help. Help." I couldn't say it with my voice, just with my mouth. He just smile back at me and I didn't like that. My Mama started pulling away after she was done with the bank lady and I just put my hands like this [in prayer] against the window, hoping he would see that. I didn't think he did.

At that night, when we was eating spaghetti-o's, the social workers came knocking on the door. Mama sent me to my room. When the social workers come in and talk with me, this time I told the truth. They took me to the big office and my therapist was there. Kanga and Roo was there [the pet therapy dogs]. He heard me. He helped me. That's why I want little boys to keep tellin' and tellin' and tellin' till somebody cares. I got a foster Mama and foster Daddy now. I'm in second grade now. And I have a dog named "Boo."

KIP

I really got into the window thing. The exccavat—I can never say that word right. I like the window because I am the one in control. It's interesting to me 'cause sometimes when you look out a window, there are smudges on it and it's hard to see. Sometimes there is a screen and you can't see things as clear as you know is really there. Sometimes you need the screen though 'cause you don't really want to see, maybe save it for next week. And you can make the window big or small or you can look at different parts of the window. When you stand right in front of the window, you can see the horizon. But when you stand far back from the window, you can only see certain things and others are hidden. And what I like most is that it's okay to see whatever you want to see at that time. I got to be in charge of the window, how much I wanted to look, how much I wanted to see. I could even lock it for a week if I wanted and just talk about fun shit.

I also like the painting and the memory box. First, I didn't. I thought it was fag stuff. But every week I would be writing stuff and doing different home-work and writing about my dreams and stuff like that so it got to be a lot of stuff and so I made this thing called a memory box and would keep everything in there so nobody could see and I didn't have to take it back to the projects with me. This was my second memory box, the first one got too small.

This one time, my therapist asked me to take everything out of the box and put it on this big table. I didn't know what was up. But I did. Then he asks me to go outside with him 'cause he wanted to show me something. We go outside and I'm thinkin' this dude must be crazy and he's finally showing his true ways but then he takes me to this window and asks me to look inside. He asks me what I see. It's the window to his office. I saw my clothes, my football that I stopped playing with, the pictures of me when I was a boy, the paintings of me now, all my papers where I wrote about the abuse, my ribbon from the science fair, the clothes I wore that night I was raped, the pictures of me from the doctors from my cutting and stuff. And I had pictures I painted of who I was before, who I was now, and who I wanted to be. I saw my dream journal—I saw me. I was fuckin' lookin' in the window and I saw my life, not just the abuse part but my life. It started raining but I didn't want to go inside. I wanted to keep looking in that window. I was crying, not sad tears but tears because I thought who Kip was and who Kip wants to be got lost. But they didn't. They were right there in the window.

PALO

Therapy to me is like the medicine wheel. The south of the wheel represents innocence, like the innocence of a child. The north of the wheel is wisdom, wisdom of the elders. The west is a place of reflection and the east is about enlightenment. When I came in for therapy, I just wanted a few quick lessons about how to deal with my panic attacks. I didn't even tell the therapist about the abuse. When he asked me about my childhood history, and asked if I had ever experienced physical abuse or sexual abuse, pretty much every kind of abuse, I denied it. I told him what I wanted, just some tools to make the panic attacks go away, and that's where we started. I went to two sessions, learned some things, and that was it.

The panic attacks went away some, but I didn't feel any different. I talked with Morningstar, a Medicine Woman, again, and she said that I must return to therapy and tell the truth. Autumn, my wife, was with me and she really wanted me to go back, too. She wanted to save our marriage.

After a couple more weeks, I went back. Not to therapy. Autumn thought I was going back. I would just go there once a week and walk around the block several times and then go home. I was afraid to see him again. One day, he happened to come out of the building as I was walking by. He said "hello" and I just started crying. Couldn't stop. He asked me if I wanted to come inside. When we got to his office, I cried the entire time. I couldn't even say that I wanted to come back. It was getting late and I finally said, "I lied to you. I lied."

I started going twice a week and after several sessions, I still couldn't get the words out. I had these images in my head of the abuse. I could smell it, taste it, feel it, hear it, and see it but just couldn't speak it. One day he had a bunch of finger paints and paper on the floor. I thought it was for some of the kids he worked with. He said it was for me. He asked me to paint what I couldn't speak. I felt insulted. I thought he thought I was like a child.

I finally agreed to do it and I'm so glad I did. It was amazing to me. When I removed the lids and put my fingers in the paint, I did feel like a boy again. It reminded me of kindergarten, Miss Owl, the playground. I painted one and then another and another—five altogether. After I painted the last one, he asked me to describe them. And I was able to get some words out! We did this for the next two or three sessions. I don't know how or why, but I was able to tell him about my father and my uncles and the neighbor and the trucker, everyone, everything. And what even amazed me more was the panic attacks began to go away. I didn't have those images swimming in my mind all the time when I was studying or working or—I was able to be intimate with Autumn again. And I stopped acting out, stopped the sexual acting out.

So I knew that therapy was medicine for me. I saw how I had to find the innocence of a child in order to tell my story. I saw how contemplating about my past and about the images in my head and about the acting out led to knowledge and understanding. And I gained wisdom, too. I learned how to heal myself. And for that I am grateful.

MATT

I was afraid of myself and afraid for myself. The entire sexual compulsion — voyeurism, exhibitionism, sexual acting out in public—was entirely out of control. If arrests and jail time didn't stop me, I wasn't sure what could. In some ways I think I was a therapist's worst nightmare. Well, maybe not worst, and maybe not nightmare, but certainly a bad dream. I came in with this attitude, "Prove to me that you're safe, that you know what you're doing, that you're not going to hurt me and that you can do something about my past and about my acting out." I remember testing the limits, looking to see when he would falter. When I spoke with the therapist over the phone before the first appointment, I told him that I wanted his licensee number, that I wanted to check to see if he had any complaints registered against him. I told him that I refused to shake hands or hug or be touched in any way. I told him that I had already been to several therapists and that none of them had worked out and that I was aware of the news reports of three therapists in the area who were charged with having sexual relations with their patients. Looking back, if I was a psychotherapist, I would not have scheduled an appointment with me. But he did.

The first session was pretty routine. Lots of questions and answers. At some point, he paused and gently asked if I was aware that I was exposing myself. I was shocked and disgusted. Very inappropriate. He just simply brought it to my attention and all I wanted to do was find the exit. At one point I called him a lecher for doing this work. Lecher—I don't think I ever said that word until that night. I told him to go "fuck himself" and headed for the door. He said to me, "I have an idea about what's going on here. I hope we can talk about this together." I had to leave. He also invited me to come back.

A few days later, he called and left a message, saying that I was welcome to return. I called and scheduled another appointment. During that session, he was really direct about boundaries and what's appropriate. But what we really talked about was what purpose that kind of behavior served in my life. He gave me another chance.

In group therapy, I thought for sure when I told anyone about the incest with my mother, they would flinch, find a way to get out and leave a trail of dust. It still amazes me that people can listen. Then I really thought that once I talked about my compulsions, I would be kicked out. I talked about them in detail—the co-leaders wanted us to talk in details—and was just waiting for the boot, like therapists had done before. In other places, if you are working to stop your sexual compulsions and you tell the therapist that over the weekend you acted out, then they kick you out. But that didn't happen this time.

And then I thought for sure, when they see the kind of thoughts I had in my head, who I really was inside—the pervert, the man who could be a father and husband but instead just does whatever he can to destroy his life, the loser. And all the shame. Just breathing shame. During many sessions I felt like I was contaminating their space, the therapy space. One time I even threw up on the new furniture they just had delivered. But they didn't kick me out.

So, for me, it wasn't any of the projects we worked on, or any particular strategy that helped me, it was just being accepted. Just being heard. Having someone confront the self-loathing in me and cultivate the confidence and promise in me. The psychotherapists treated like I was a human being and not some animal destined for the slaughterhouse.

VICTOR

I had two therapists—well, at one point, three—one for individual, one for group, and eventually one for couples counseling. But in terms of the first two, the individual and the group therapist, that's where trouble started. You see, my individual therapist was this older woman who sat back most of the time, didn't say much, sometimes asked a question or two, and I just laid on her couch and said whatever came to mind. I could count on her to say my name as she came out to the waiting room, and I could count on her to say "Time's up" at the end of the session, and I could count on her to say very little in between, mostly "Uh-huh" and "What do you think about that?" I thought that's what therapy was about. Then one day she refers me to a group for adult males with histories of childhood sexual abuse.

I meet this other therapist, this group therapist, who couldn't be more different. He was alive, active, asked a lot of questions, wanted to know what I remembered, what I thought, how I felt. It was almost like looking in a mirror in a strange way. When I looked at his face, it almost seemed to reflect back what I was feeling inside. When you don't want to see yourself, you hate mirrors.

Anyway, I join this group, and I have this feeling that I have to protect the other members from this therapist. I watched him like a hawk and I criticized just about everything he suggested that we do. The group members started calling me "Watch Dog." If he asked us to do something, I wanted to know why, what was his motive. I sat there waiting sometimes, unable to sit still, almost like I was ready to strike. After a few weeks of this, he confronts me about what I'm doing and suggests that we meet for an individual session. I was afraid at this point because I knew something was up. I didn't know why, but sometimes I even hated this guy. Just hated him.

During the individual session, I see him really trying to understand what's going on, and I really didn't have a clue. He told me what he thought. By the end of the session, I was in tears. You see, with my individual therapist, I knew what to expect from her. I knew what she was going to do, just like I knew how my father was going to rape me on Saturday nights, after he got drunk, and usually with a weapon to my head. I knew that, black and white. With the group therapist, I did not know what to expect. He laughed. He got teary a couple of times. It was okay to be angry, okay to be afraid, okay to just be yourself. I hated that. I hated my mother for that. I hated the fact that she was emotional, that she was alive, that when you thought she was going to yell at you all she did was listen and try to understand. I hated her and I hated him because I never knew what to expect. With my father and with the individual therapist, I could have bet my life on their next action. With my mother and the group therapist, I just never knew, it never was the way I expected. And this is what I learned. And this was a turning point for me, because I realized that I had been categorizing every person I met into one of three categories—wimpy victim, perpetrator, and the person who acts like they care but really doesn't. I didn't have to do that anymore to others. I didn't have to do that to myself.

JAKE

This is not easy to talk about. I'm glad I am in therapy now, but it wasn't my idea. At first, I was only doing it for my wife. She gave me an ultimatum and I didn't want to lose her. I knew that she was a "one in a lifetime" deal and for all that I caused her and did to her, I didn't deserve someone like her. So I came and pretty much hated everything about it.

I want to say first that I'm very uncomfortable bringing this up, but I know other guys out there might relate, and while I'm not a soapbox kind of man, or someone that spent his life helping others, I'm thinking, thinking that facts and the truth are bigger than my shame. The worst part of therapy for me was trying to talk about my past, about the abuse and trying to control my bowels at the same time. Sometimes before therapy I had to vomit in my bathroom and several times I had to pull off onto the side of the road and do it. When I actually got there, there were a few times when I tried talking about the abuse but had to run for the bathroom and there were two times that I just didn't make it. I couldn't control my bowels. But in a strange way, that was a turning point for me.

If somebody can sit with you and be with you while you vomit or lose control of your bowels, mess up their bathroom and office and just respond with understanding and concern—well, that amazed me. And that was my biggest fear. I lived through my biggest fear and was met with compassion. From that point on, I had this resolve to take charge of my past, to stop blaming myself, to forgive myself.

I remember the therapist saying something like, "Jake, if you keep running away or keep trying to control your past, you keep running away from one of the greatest treasures in your life. As a boy, you found a way to live through horrific abuse, the death of your parents, life on the streets and in a group home. You did that on your own. That is your treasure chest—your courage, your fighting spirit, your ability to face obstacles, your faith in God, your willingness to let love in your life after it had been ripped away so many times—that, Jake, is your treasure chest."

In therapy, I learned how to use that treasure chest for the benefit of my marriage, my relationship with my children and grandchildren, my work. When I discovered that treasure chest, and finally gave it a name, my past became part of me. It was no longer Andrew before the abuse and Jake after. Just one man. Just Jake.

TYRONE

The best part of therapy for me is group therapy. We been together for two years now and it's just like a family. I was Tyler when I walked in on the first day, all nervous like, shaking really, acting like I was going to some big gay singles event, thinking more that I might find a boyfriend and thinking hardly nothing about abuse or why we was really there. When I see all the guys there, I just couldn't even open my mouth. It was—there was—like high school, not many guys like me, mostly guys like jocks and brains and all masculine and then me. I didn't want to stay. I called the therapist up after that and said I didn't want to stay. He says to me, "Why don't you make a contract to come one week at a time, and if you decide to leave, all you have to do is come for at least one session after that to let everyone know."

So I kept coming, not saying much, just smiling at every one, laughing when the therapist laughed, looking serious when others was looking serious, watching a lot, listening. Sometimes afterwards some of the guys would go out for coffee or such, and a few times they asked me but I always had an excuse. I couldn't be with these kind of men. I just didn't fit. There was a transvestite in the group and I sort of fit with him but after the evening was over, I always was the first one out the door.

After a couple of months, it was time to tell our stories. I picked last. Kept thinking I would leave before it was my turn. Kept thinking people was not gonna believe me or hate me or beat me up on the way to the subway after the group. But I stayed and I told my story. I don't remember that part, the telling part, but what I remember most is when I stopped talking, there was these nine men—some fathers, a granddaddy, a police man, a sports man, a marine, a artist, a doctor, some gay, some straight, some don't-know-what, black, white, Hispanic, Asian—these nine men and one lady [co-therapist] just looking at me, some crying for me, the granddaddy asking to hug me, the therapist saying he's proud of me. Can you believe it? And as we were leaving, the group gathered around me, and the sports man asked me if I would like to go get something to eat with them. They asked me! And I said, "Yes, Victor!" I said "Yes."

From that time, I started not to feel afraid of men. I started to see that I am a man, just like the therapist been telling me for some time. I started to call myself "Tyrone."

ENDNOTE

Thank you for reading *SAM: The Sexual Abuse of Males—A Model of Theory and Practice.* Thank you for taking an interest in SAM.

REFERENCES

Abel, G. G., Becker, J. V., Mittelman, M., Cunningham-Rather, J., Rouleau, J. L., & Murphy, W. D. (1987). Self-reported sex crimes of nonincarcerated paraphiliacs. *Journal of Interpersonal Violence, 2*, 3–25.

Abracen, J., Looman, J., & Anderson, D. (2000). Alcohol and drug abuse in sexual and nonsexual violent offenders. *Sexual Abuse: A Journal of Research and Treatment, 12*, 263–274.

Abrahams, N., Casey, K., & Daro, D. (1992). Teachers' knowledge, attitudes and beliefs about child abuse and its prevention. *Child Abuse & Neglect, 16*, 229–238.

Ackerman, P. T., Newton, J. E. O., McPherson, W. B., Jones, J. G., & Dykman, R. A. (1998). Prevalence of post traumatic stress disorder and other psychiatric diagnoses in three groups of abused children (sexual, physical, and both). *Child Abuse & Neglect, 22*, 759–774.

Adams-Tucker, C. (1985). Defense mechanisms used by sexually abused children. *Children Today, 29*, 9–34.

Alexander, P. C., Teti, L., & Anderson, C.L. (2000). Child sexual abuse history and role reversal in parenting. *Child Abuse & Neglect, 24*, 829–838.

Allard-Dansereau, C., Haley, N., Hamane, M., & Bernard-Bonnin, A. (1997). Pattern of child sexual abuse by young aggressors. *Child Abuse & Neglect, 21*, 965–974.

Allen, C. M. (1990). Women as perpetrators of child sexual abuse: Recognition barriers. In A. L. Horton, B. L. Johnson, L. M. Roundy, & D. Williams (Eds.), *The incest perpetrator: A family member no one wants to treat* (pp. 108–125). Newbury Park, CA: Sage.

Allen, C. M. (1991). *Women and men who sexually abuse children: A comparative analysis.* Orwell, VT: Safer Society Press.

Allen, L. S., Richey, M. F., Chai, Y. M., & Gorski, R. A. (1991). Sex differences in the corpus callosum of the living human being. *Journal of Neuroscience, 11*, 933–942.

Alpert, J. L., Brown, L. S., Ceci, S. J., Courtois, C. A., Loftus, E. F., & Ornstein, P. A. (Eds.). (1996). *Working group on investigation of memories of childhood abuse: Final report.* Washington, DC: American Psychological Association.

American Humane Association Children's Division. (1993). *AHA fact sheet: Child sexual abuse.* Englewood, CO: AHA.

American Psychiatric Association. (1994). *DSM–IV: Diagnostic and Statistical Manual of Mental Disorders* (4th ed.). Washington, DC: American Psychiatric Association.

Anderson, C. M., Teicher, M. H., Polcari, A., & Renshaw, P. F. (2002). Abnormal T2 relaxation time in the cerebellar vermis of adults sexually abused in childhood: Potential role of the vermis in stress-enhanced risk for drug abuse. *Psychoneuroendocrinology, 27*, 231–244.

Anderson, P. B. (1996). Correlates of college women's self-reports of heterosexual aggression. *Sexual Abuse: A Journal of Research and Treatment, 8*, 121–133.

Antoni, F. A. (2000). Role of pituitary regulation. In G. Fink (Ed.), *Encyclopedia of stress* (Vol. 3, pp. 169–174). San Diego, CA: Academic Press.

Araji, S. K. (1997). *Sexually aggressive children.* Thousand Oaks, CA: Sage.

Armony, J. L., & LeDoux, J. E. (1997). How the brain processes emotional information. In R. Yehuda & A. C. McFarlane (Eds.), *Psychobiology of posttraumatic stress disorder* (pp. 259–270). New York: New York Academy of Science.

Armstrong, L. (1978). *Kiss Daddy goodnight: A speak-out on incest.* New York: Hawthorne Books.

Armstrong, L. (1982). The cradle of sexual politics. In M. Kirkpatrick (Ed.), *Womens sexual experience: Explorations of the dark continent* (pp. 109–125). New York: Plenum Press.

Ashby, L. (1997). *Endangered children: Dependency, neglect, and abuse in American history.* New York: Twayne.

Back, S., & Lips, H. M. (1998). Child sexual abuse: Victim age, victim gender, and observer gender as factors contributing to attributions of responsibility. *Child Abuse & Neglect, 22,* 1239–1252.

Bagley, C. (1988). *Child sexual abuse in Canada: Further analysis of the 1983 National Survey.* Ottawa: Health and Welfare, Canada.

Bagley, C., Wood, M., & Young, L. (1994). Victim to abuser: Mental health and behavioral sequels of child sexual abuse in a community survey of young adult males. *Child Abuse & Neglect, 18,* 683–697.

Baker, A. J., Tabacoff, R., Tornusciolo, G., & Eisenstadt, M. (2001). Calculating number of offenses and victims of juvenile sexual offending: The role of posttreatment disclosures. *Sexual Abuse: A Journal of Research and Treatment, 13,* 79–90.

Bandura, A. (1982). Self-efficacy mechanisms in human agency. *American Psychologist, 37,* 122–147.

Bandura, A. (1986). *Social foundations of thought and action.* Englewood Cliffs, NJ: Prentice-Hall.

Bandura, A. (1990). A perceived self-efficacy in the exercise of personal agency. *Journal of Applied Sports Psychology, 2,* 128–163.

Bartholow, B. N., Doll, L. S., Joy, D., Douglas, J. M., Jr., Bolan, G., Harrison, J. S., Moss, P. M., & McKirnan, D. (1994). Emotional, behavioral and HIV risks associated with sexual abuse among adult homosexual and bisexual men. *Child Abuse & Neglect, 18,* 747–761.

Bass, E., & Davis, L. (1988). *The courage to heal: A guide for women survivors of child abuse.* New York: Harper & Row.

Bauer, P. J., Kroupina, M. G., Schwade, J. A., Dropik, P. L., & Wewerka, S. (1998). If memory serves, will language? Later verbal accessibility of early memories. *Development and Psychopathology, 10,* 655–680.

Bays, J., & Chadwick, D. (1993). Medical diagnosis of the sexually abused child. *Child Abuse & Neglect, 17,* 91–110.

Beck, A. T. (1976). *Cognitive therapy and the emotional disorders.* New York: International Universities Press.

Beck, A. T. (1993). Cognitive therapy: Past, present, and future. *Journal of Consulting and Clinical Psychology, 61,* 194–198.

Beck, A. T., & Emery, G. (1985). *Anxiety disorders and phobias: A cognitive perspective.* New York: Basic Books.

Becker, J. V. (1988). Adolescent sex offenders. *The Behavior Therapist, 11,* 185–187.

Becker, J. V., & Hunter, J. A. (1997). Understanding and treating child and adolescent sexual offenders. *Advances in Clinical Child Psychology, 19,* 177–197.

Beitchman, J. H., Zucker, K. J., Hood, J. E., daCosta, G. A., & Akman, D. (1991). A review of the short-term effects of child sexual abuse. *Child Abuse & Neglect, 15,* 537–556.

Beitchman, J. H., Zucker, K. J., Hood, J. E., daCosta, G. A., Akman, D., & Cassavia, E. (1992). A review of the long-term effects of child sexual abuse. *Child Abuse & Neglect, 16,* 101–118.

Belicki, K., Correy, B., Boucock, A., Cuddy, M., & Dunlop, A. (1994). *Reports of sexual abuse: Facts or fantasies?* St. Catherine's, Ontario: Brock University.

Belsky, J. (1980). Child maltreatment: An ecological integration. *American Psychologist, 35,* 320–335.

Bem, S. L. (1981). Gender schema theory: A cognitive account of sex typing. *Psychological Review, 88*, 354–364.

Bender, L., & Blau, A. (1937). Reactions of children to sexual relations with adults. *American Journal of Orthopsychiatry, 7*, 500–518.

Benedict, L. L. W., & Zautra, A. A. J. (1993). Family environmental characteristics as risk factors for childhood sexual abuse. *Journal of Clinical Child Psychology, 22*, 365–374.

Ben-Porath, Y. S., & Davis, D. L. (2000). *Case studies for interpreting the MMPI-A*. Minneapolis: University of Minnesota Press.

Bera, W. H. (1994). Clinical review of adolescent male sex offenders. In J. C. Gonsiorek, W. H. Bera, & D. LeTourneau (Eds.), *Male sexual abuse: A trilogy of intervention strategies* (pp. 113–144). Thousand Oaks, CA: Sage.

Berkowitz, C. D. (1998). Medical consequences of child sexual abuse. *Child Abuse & Neglect, 22*, 541–550.

Berlin, F., Malin, H. M., & Dean, S. (1991). Effects of statutes requiring psychiatrists to report suspected sexual abuse of children. *American Journal of Psychiatry, 148*, 449–453.

Berliner, L., & Conte, J. R. (1990). The process of victimization: The victims' perspective. *Child Abuse & Neglect, 14*, 29–40.

Berliner, L., & Conte, J. R. (1995). The effects of disclosure and intervention on sexually abused children. *Child Abuse & Neglect, 19*, 371–384.

Bernet, W. (1993). False statements and the differential diagnoses of abuse allegations. *Journal of the American Academy of Child and Adolescent Psychiatry, 32*, 903–910.

Bertalanffy, L. (1968). *General systems theory, human relations*. New York: Braziller.

Black, D. W., Kehrberg, L. L. D., Flumerfelt, D. L., & Schlosser, S. S. (1997). Characteristics of 36 subjects reporting compulsive sexual behavior. *American Journal of Psychiatry, 154*, 243–249.

Black, M., Dubowitz, H., & Harrington, D. (1994). Sexual abuse: Developmental differences in children's behavior and self-perception. *Child Abuse & Neglect, 18*, 85–95.

Blanchard, R., Watson, M. S., Choy, A., Dickey, R., Klassen, P., Kuban, M., & Ferren, D. J. (1999). Pedophiles: Mental retardation, maternal age, and sexual orientation. *Archives of Sexual Behavior, 28*, 111–127.

Blau, L., & Blau, A. (1937). The reactions of children to sexual relationships with adults. *Journal of American Orthopsychiatry, 7*, 500–518.

Blechner, M. J. (1998). Maleness and masculinity. *Contemporary Psychoanalysis, 34*, 597–613.

Block, J., & Block, J. (1980). The role of ego-control and ego-resiliency in the organization of behavior. In W. Collins (Ed.), *Minnesota symposia on child psychiatry; 13. Development of cognition, affect and social relations* (pp. 39–101). Hillsdale, NJ: Lawrence Erlbaum.

Blood, L., & Cornwall, A. (1996). Childhood sexual victimization as a factor in the treatment of substance misusing adolescents. *Substance Use and Misuse, 31*, 1015–1039.

Bloom, F. E. (1983). Endorphins: Cellular and molecular aspects for addictive phenomena. In P. K. Levinson, D. R. Gerstein, & D. R. McLoff (Eds.), *Commonalities in substance abuse and habitual behavior*. Lexington, MA: D. C. Heath.

Bloom, M., Fischer, J., & Orme, J. G. (1995). *Evaluating practice: Guidelines for the accountable professional*. Boston: Allyn & Bacon.

Bolger, K. E., & Patterson, C. J. (2001). Developmental pathways from child maltreatment to peer rejection. *Child Development, 72*, 549–568.

Bolton, F. G., Jr., Morris, L. A., & MacEachron, A. E. (1989). *Building a new life: The pathways to recovery. Males at risk: The other side of child sexual abuse*. Newbury Park, CA: Sage.

Boney-McCoy, S., & Finkelhor, D. (1995a). Psychosocial sequelae of violent victimization in a national youth sample. *Journal of Consulting and Clinical Psychology, 63*, 726–736.

Boney-McCoy, S., & Finkelhor, D. (1995b). Prior victimization: A risk factor for child sexual abuse and for PTSD-related symptomatology among abused youth. *Child Abuse & Neglect, 19*, 1401–1421.

Boney-McCoy, S., & Finkelhor, D. (1996). Is youth victimization related to trauma symptoms and depression after controlling for prior symptoms and family relationships? A longitudinal, prospective study. *Journal of Consulting and Clinical Psychology, 64,* 1406–1416.

Boon, F. (1991). Letter to the editor: John F. McDermott, Jr., MD. *Journal of Psychiatric Treatment and Evaluation, 4,* 117–124.

Botash, A. (2000). *Evaluating the sexually abused child: Education manual for medical professionals.* Baltimore: Johns Hopkins University Press.

Bottoms, B., & Goodman, G. S. (1994). Perceptions of children's credibility in sexual assault cases. *Journal of Applied Social Psychology, 24,* 702–732.

Bowen, K., & Aldous, M. B. (1999). Medical evaluation of sexual abuse in children without disclosed or witnessed abuse. *Archives of Pediatrics and Adolescent Medicine, 153,* 1160–1164.

Bower, B. (1994, October 22). Stress hormones hike emotional memories. *Science News, 146,* 262.

Bower, G. H., & Sivers, H. (1998). Cognitive impact of traumatic events. *Development and Psychopathology, 10,* 625–654.

Bowlby, J. (1973). *Attachment and loss: Vol. 2. Separation: Anxiety and anger.* New York: Basic Books.

Bowlby, J. (1980). *Attachment and loss: Vol. 3. Loss.* New York: Basic Books.

Bowlby, J. (1982). *Attachment and loss : Vol. 1. Attachment* (2nd ed.). New York: Basic Books.

Bowlby, J. (1984). Psychoanalysis as a natural science. *Psychoanalytic Psychology, 1,* 7–21.

Bowlby, J. (1988). *A secure base.* New York: Basic Books.

Bradley, A. R., & Wood, J. M. (1996). How do children tell? The disclosure process in child sexual abuse. *Child Abuse & Neglect, 20,* 881–891.

Brannon, J. M., Larson, B., & Doggett, M. (1991). Peer counseling strategies: Facilitating self-disclosure among sexually victimized juvenile offenders. *Journal of Addictions and Offender Counseling, 11,* 51–58.

Braun B. G., & Sachs, R. G. (1985). The development of multiple personality disorder: Predisposing, precipitating and perpetuating factors. In R. P. Kluft (Ed.), *Childhood antecedents of multiple personalities* (pp. 37–64). Washington, DC: American Psychiatric Press.

Bremner, J. D. (1999). Acute and chronic responses to psychological trauma: Where do we go from here? *American Journal of Psychiatry, 156,* 349–351.

Bremner, J. D. (2002). *Does stress damage the brain? Understanding trauma-related disorders from a mind–body perspective.* New York: W. W. Norton.

Bremner, J. D., Krystal, J. H., Southwick, S. M., & Charney, D. S. (1996a). Noradrenergic mechanisms in stress and anxiety: I. Preclinical studies. *Synapse, 23,* 28–38.

Bremner, J. D., Krystal, J. H., Southwick, S. M., & Charney, D. S. (1996b). Noradrenergic mechanisms in stress and anxiety: II. Clinical studies. *Synapse, 23,* 39–51.

Bremner, J. D., Licinio, J., Darnell, A., Krystal, J. H., Owens, M. J., Southwick, S. M., Nemeroff, C. B., & Charney, D. S. (1997). Elevated CSF corticotropin-releasing factor concentrations in posttraumatic stress disorder. *American Journal of Psychiatry, 154,* 624–629.

Bremner, J. D., & Narayan, M. (1998). The effects of stress on memory and the hippocampus throughout the life cycle: Implications for childhood development and aging. *Developmental Psychopathology, 10,* 871–886.

Bremner, J. D., Randall, P. R., Capelli, S., Scott, T., McCarthy, G., & Charney, D. S. (1995). Deficits in short-term memory in adult survivors of childhood abuse. *Psychiatry Research, 59,* 97–107.

Bremner, J. D., Randall, P., Vermetten, E., Staib, L., Bronen, R. A., Mazure, C., Capelli, S., McCarthy, G., Innis, R. B., & Charney, D. S. (1997). Magnetic resonance imaging-based measurement of hippocampal volume in posttraumatic stress disorder related to childhood physical and sexual abuse—A preliminary report. *Biological Psychiatry, 41,* 23–32.

Bremner, J. D., Southwick, S. M., & Charney, D. S. (1999). The neurobiology of posttraumatic stress disorder: An integration of animal and human research. In P. A. Saigh & J. D. Bremner

(Eds.), *Posttraumatic stress disorder: A comprehensive text* (pp. 103–143). Needham Heights, MA: Allyn & Bacon.

Brenner, C. (1986). *The mind in conflict.* Madison, CT: International Universities Press.

Bretherton, I. (1993). From dialogue to internal working models: The co-construction of self in relationships. In C. A. Nelson (Ed.), *Minnesota symposia on child psychology: Vol. 26. Memory and affect in development* (pp. 237–264). Hillsdale, NJ: Lawrence Erlbaum.

Briere, J. (1992). Methodological issues in the study of sexual abuse effects. *Journal of Consulting and Clinical Psychology, 60,* 196–203.

Briere, J. (1995). *Psychometric properties of the TSI: Professional manual.* Odessa, FL: Psychological Assessment Resources.

Briere, J. (1996b). Treatment outcome research with abused children: Methodological considerations in three studies. *Child Maltreatment, 1,* 348–352.

Briere, J., & Runtz, M. (1987). Post-sexual abuse trauma: Data and implications for clinical practice. *Journal of Interpersonal Violence, 2,* 367–379.

Briere, J., & Conte, J. R. (1993). Self-reported amnesia for abuse in adults molested as childhood. *Journal of Traumatic Stress, 6,* 21–31.

Briere, J., & Elliott, D. M. (1994). Immediate and long-term impacts of child sexual abuse. *Future of Children, 4,* 54–69.

Briere, J., Elliott, D. M., Harris, K., & Cotman, A. (1995). Trauma symptom inventory: Psychometrics and association with childhood and adult victimization in clinical samples. *Journal of Interpersonal Violence, 10,* 387–401.

Briere, J., Evans, D., Runtz, M., & Wall, T. (1988). Symptomatology in men who were molested as children: A comparison study. *American Journal of Orthopsychiatry, 58,* 457–461.

Briere, J., & Runtz, M. (1990). Differential adult symptomology associated with three types of child abuse histories. *Child Abuse & Neglect, 14,* 357–364.

Briere, J., Smiljanich, K., & Henschel, D. (1994). Sexual fantasies, gender, and molestation history. *Child Abuse & Neglect, 18,* 131–137.

Briggs, F., & Hawkins, R. M. F. (1996). A comparison of childhood experiences of convicted male child molesters and men who were sexually abused in childhood and claimed to be nonoffenders. *Child Abuse & Neglect, 20,* 221–233.

Brinton, R. D., & Berger, T. W. (2000). Hippocampal neurons. In G. Fink (Ed.), *Encyclopedia of stress* (Vol. 2, pp. 364–371). San Diego, CA: Academic Press.

Brodsky, B. S., Oquendo, M., Ellis, S. P., Haas, G. L., Malone, K. M., & Mann, J. J. (2001). The relationship of childhood abuse to impulsivity and suicidal behavior in adults with major depression. *American Journal of Psychiatry, 158,* 1871–1877.

Bronfenbrenner, U. (1977). Toward an experimental ecology of human development. *American Psychologist, 32,* 513–531.

Bronfenbrenner, U. (1979). *The ecology of human development: Experiments by nature and design.* Cambridge, MA: Harvard University Press.

Brongersma, E. (1988). A defense of sexual liberty for all age groups. *The Howard Journal of Reform, 27,* 32–43.

Broussard, S. D., & Wagner, W. G. (1988). Child sexual abuse: Who is to blame? *Child Abuse & Neglect, 12,* 563–569.

Broussard, S. D., Wagner, W. G., & Kazelskis, R. (1991). Undergraduate students' perceptions of child sexual abuse: The impact of victim sex, perpetrator sex, respondent sex, and victim response. *Journal of Family Violence, 6,* 267–278.

Brower, A. M., & Nurius, P. S. (1993). *Social cognition and individual change: Current theory and counseling guidelines.* Newbury Park, CA: Sage.

Brown, D., Scheflin, A. W., & Hammond, D. C. (1998). *Memory, trauma, treatment, and the law: An essential reference on memory for clinicians, researchers, attorneys, and judges.* New York: W. W. Norton.

Brown, G. R., & Anderson, B. (1991). Psychiatric morbidity in adult inpatients with childhood histories of sexual and physical abuse. *American Journal of Psychiatry, 148,* 55–61.

Brown, J., Cohen, P., Johnson, J. G., & Salzinger, S. (1998). A longitudinal analysis of risk factors for child maltreatment: Findings of a 17-year prospective study of officially recorded and self-reported child abuse and neglect. *Child Abuse & Neglect, 22*, 1065–1078.

Brown, L. K., Kessel, S. M., Lourie, K. J., Ford, H. H., & Lipsitt, L. P. (1997). Influence of sexual abuse on HIV-related attitudes and behaviors in adolescent psychiatric inpatients. *Journal of the American Academy of Child and Adolescent Psychiatry, 36*, 316–322.

Brown, L. K., Lourie, K. J., Zlotnick, C., & Cohn, J. (2000). Impact of sexual abuse in the HIV-risk-related behavior of adolescents in intensive psychiatric treatment. *American Journal of Psychiatry, 157*, 1413–1415.

Brown, S. (1988). *Treating adult children of alcoholics: A developmental perspective.* New York: John Wiley & Sons.

Brown, S. C., & Craik, F. I. M. (2000). Encoding and retrieval of information. In E. Tulving & F. I. M. Craik (Eds.), *The Oxford handbook of memory* (pp. 93–107). New York: Oxford University Press.

Browne, A., & Finkelhor, D. (1986). Impact of child sexual abuse: A review of the research. *Psychological Bulletin, 99*, 66–77.

Brownmiller, S. (1975). *Against our will: Men, women and rape.* New York: Simon & Schuster.

Bruckner, D. F., & Johnson, P. E. (1987). Treatment for adult male victims of childhood sexual abuse. *Social Casework: The Journal of Contemporary Social Work, 68*, 81–87.

Budin, L. E., & Johnson, C. F. (1989). Sex abuse prevention programs: Offenders' attitudes about their efficacy. *Child Abuse & Neglect, 13*, 77–87.

Burgess, A. W., Hartman, C. R., & Baker, T. (1995). Memory presentations of childhood sexual abuse. *Journal of Psychosocial Nursing, 131*, 981–986.

Burgess, A. W., Hartman, C., McCausland, M., & Powers, P. (1984). Response patterns in children and adolescents exploited through sex rings and pornography. *American Journal of Psychiatry, 141*, 656–662.

Burgess, A. W., Hartman, C., & McCormack, A. (1987). Abused to abuser: Antecedents or socially deviant behaviors. *American Journal of Psychiatry, 144*, 1431–1436.

Burgess, A. W., & Holmstrom, L. L. (1974). Rape trauma syndrome. *American Journal of Psychiatry, 131*, 981–986.

Burgess, A. W., & Holmstrom, L. L. (1979). Rape: Sexual disruption and recovery. *American Journal of Orthopsychiatry, 49*, 648–657.

Burkhardt, S., & Rotatori, A. F. (1995). *Treatment and prevention of childhood sexual abuse.* Washington, DC: Taylor & Francis.

Burton, D. L. (2000). Were adolescent sexual offenders children with sexual behavior problems? *Sexual Abuse: A Journal of Research and Treatment, 12*, 37–48.

Butler, L. D., & Spiegel, D. (1997). Trauma and memory. In L. J. Dickson, M. B. Riba, & J. M. Oldham (Series Eds.) and D. Spiegel (Vol. Ed.), Section II of the American Psychiatric Press review of psychiatry: Volume 16. *Repressed memories* (pp. 13–54). Washington, DC: American Psychiatric Press.

Cahill, L. (1997). The neurobiology of emotionally influenced memory. In R. Yehuda & A. C. McFarlane (Eds.), *Psychobiology of posttraumatic stress disorder.* Annals of the New York Academy of Sciences (Vol. 821, pp. 238–246). New York: New York Academy of Sciences.

Calam, R., Horne, L., Glasgow, D., & Cox, A. (1998). Psychological disturbance and child sexual abuse: A follow-up study. *Child Abuse & Neglect, 22*, 901–913.

Calvert, J. F., Jr., & Munsie-Benson, M. (1999). Public opinion and knowledge about childhood sexual abuse in a rural community. *Child Abuse & Neglect, 23*, 671–682.

Campbell, J. A., & Carlson, K. (1995). Training and knowledge of professionals on specific topics in child sexual abuse. *Journal of Child Sexual Abuse, 4*, 75–86.

Campis, L. B., Hebden-Curtis, J., & Demaso, D. R. (1993). Developmental differences in detection and disclosure of sexual abuse. *Journal of the American Academy of Child and Adolescent Psychiatry, 32*, 920–924.

Cappelleri, J. C., Eckenrode, J., & Powers, J. L. (1993). The epidemiology of child abuse: Findings from the second national incidence and prevalence study of child abuse and neglect. *American Journal of Public Health, 83,* 1622–1624.

Carballo-Dieguez, A., & Dolezal, C. (1995). Association between history of childhood sexual abuse and adult HIV-risk sexual behavior in Puerto Rican men who have sex with men. *Child Abuse & Neglect, 19,* 595–605.

Carlat, D. J., & Camargo, C. A., Jr. (1991). Review of bulimia nervosa in males. *American Journal of Psychiatry, 148,* 831–843.

Carlat, D. J., Carmargo, C. A., Jr., & Herzog, D. B. (1997). Eating disorders in males: A report on 135 patients. *American Journal of Psychiatry, 154,* 1127–1132.

Carmen, E. J., Rieker, P. P., & Mills, T. (1984). Victims of violence and psychiatric illness. *American Journal of Psychiatry, 141,* 378–383.

Carnes, P. (1983). *Out of the shadows: Understanding sexual addiction.* Minneapolis, MN: CompCare.

Cavaiola, A. A., & Schiff, M. (1988). Behavioral sequelae of physical and/or sexual abuse in adolescents. *Child Abuse and Neglect, 12,* 181–188.

Cazenave, N. A. (1984). Race, socioeconomic status and age: The social context of American masculinity. *Sex Roles, 11,* 639–656.

Centers for Disease Control. (1997, August 29). Perceptions of child sexual abuse as a public health problem: Vermont, September 1995. *Morbidity and Mortality Weekly Report, 46,* 801–803.

Chandy, J. M., Blum, R. W., & Resnick, M. D. (1997). Sexually abused male adolescents: How vulnerable are they? *Journal of Child Sexual Abuse, 6,* 1–16.

Chapman, J. R., & Smith, B. E. (1987). *Child sexual abuse: An analysis of case processing.* Washington, DC: American Bar Association.

Charney, D. S., Deutch, A. Y., Krystal, J. H., Southwick, S. M., & Davis, M. (1993). Psychobiologic mechanisms of posttraumatic stress disorder. *Archives of General Psychiatry, 50,* 295–305.

Cheit, R. E., & Goldschmidt, E. B. (1997). Child molesters in the criminal justice system: A comprehensive case-flow analysis of the Rhode Island docket (1985–1993). *Criminal and Civil Confinement, 23,* 267–301.

Child Trauma Academy. (2002). *Brain organization and function: A brief overview.* Retrieved June 30, 2002, from www.childtraumaacademy.com.

Christianson, S. A. (1992). *The handbook of emotion and memory.* Hilllsdale, NJ: Lawrence Erlbaum.

Christianson, S. A., & Safer, M. A. (1996). Emotional events and emotions in autobiographical memories. In D. C. Rubin (Ed.), *Remembering our past: Studies in autobiographical memory* (pp. 218–241). New York: Cambridge University Press.

Chu, J. A. (1998). *Rebuilding shattered lives: The responsible treatment of complex posttraumatic and dissociative disorders.* New York: John Wiley & Sons.

Chu, J. A., & Dill, D. L. (1990). Dissociative symptoms in relation to childhood physical and sexual abuse. *American Journal of Psychiatry, 147,* 887–892.

Chu, J. A., Frey, L. M., Ganzel, B. L., & Matthews, J. A. (1999). Memories of childhood abuse: Dissociation, amnesia, and corroboration. *American Journal of Psychiatry, 156,* 749–755.

Chu, J. A., Matthews, J. A., Frey, L. M., & Ganzel, B. (1996). The nature of traumatic memories of childhood abuse. *Dissociation, 9,* 2–17.

Cicchetti, D., Rogosch, M. L., & Holt, K. D. (1993). Resilience in maltreated children: Processes leading to adaptive outcome. *Development and Psychopathology, 5,* 626–647.

Cincinnati Children's Hospital Medical Center. (2000, May 8). *Children's testimony more reliable than physical exams.* Retrieved August 5, 2002, from www.cchmc.org/about-us/news-media/news-releases/2000/5_00-08-abuse.html.

Clark, D. B., Lesnick, L., & Hegedus, A. M. (1997). Trauma and other adverse life events in adolescents with alcohol abuse and dependence. *Journal of the American Academy of Child and Adolescent Psychiatry, 36,* 1744–1751.

Claytor, R. N., Barth, K. L., & Shubin, C. I. (1989). Evaluating child sexual abuse: Observations regarding ano-genital injury. *Pediatrics, 28,* 419–422.

Cochran, S. D., & Peplau, L. A. (1991). Sexual risk reduction behaviors among young heterosexual adults. *Social Science & Medicine, 33,* 25–36.

Cohen, L. J., Gans, S. N., McGeoch, P. G., Pozansky, O., Itskovich, Y., Murphy, S., Klein, E., Cullen, K., & Galynker, I. I. (2002). Impulsive personality traits in male pedophiles versus healthy controls: Is pedophilia an impulsive-aggressive disorder? *Comprehensive Psychiatry, 43,* 127–134.

Cohen, P., Brown, J., & Smaile, E. (2001). Child abuse and neglect and the development of mental disorders in the general population. *Development and Psychopathology, 13,* 981–999.

Cole, C. H., & Barney, E. E. (1987). Safeguards and the therapeutic window: A group treatment strategy for adult incest survivors. *American Journal of Orthopsychiatry, 57,* 601–609.

Cole, P. M., & Putnam, F. W. (1992). Effect of incest on self and social functioning: A developmental psychopathology perspective. *Journal of Consulting and Clinical Psychology, 60,* 174–184.

Collings, S. J. (1995). The long-term effects of contact and noncontact forms of child sexual abuse in a sample of university men. *Child Abuse & Neglect, 19,* 1–6.

Collins, M. E. (1996). Parents' perceptions of the risk of CSA and their protective behavior: Findings from a qualitative study. *Child Maltreatment, 1,* 53–64.

Comas-Diaz, L. (1995). Puerto Rican and sexual child abuse. In L. A. Fontes (Ed.), *Sexual abuse in nine North American cultures: Treatment and prevention* (pp. 31–66). Thousand Oaks, CA: Sage.

Commission on Obscenity and Pornography. (1970). *The Report of the Commission on Obscenity and Pornography.* Washington, DC: U.S. Government Printing Office.

Conte, J. R. (1990). The incest offender: An overview and introduction. In A. L. Horton, B. L. Johnson, L. M. Roundy, & D. Williams, (Eds.), *The incest perpetrator: A family member no one wants to treat,* (pp. 19–27). Newbury Park, CA: Sage.

Conte, J. R., Fogarty, L., & Collins, M. E. (1991). National survey of professional practice in child sexual abuse. *Journal of Family Violence, 6,* 149–166.

Conte, J. R., & Schuerman, J. R. (1987). Factors associated with an increased impact of child sexual abuse. *Child Abuse and Neglect, 11,* 201–211.

Conte, J. R., Wolfe, S., & Smith, T. (1989). What sexual offenders tell us about prevention strategies. *Child Abuse & Neglect, 13,* 293–301.

Convoy, H., Weiss, P., & Zverina, J. (1995). Sexual abuse experiences of psychiatric patients. *Medicine and Law, 14,* 283–292.

Cornell, W. F., & Olio, K. A. (1991). Integrating affect in treatment with adult survivors of physical and sexual abuse. *American Journal of Orthopsychiatry, 6,* 59–69.

Cortoni, F., & Marshall, W. L. (2001). Sex as a coping strategy and its relationship to juvenile sexual history and intimacy in sexual offenders. *Sexual Abuse: A Journal of Research and Treatment, 13,* 27–43.

Costin, L. Karger, H., & Stoez, D. (1996). *The politics of child abuse in America.* New York: Oxford University Press.

Courtois, C. A. (1988). *Healing the incest wound: Adult survivors in therapy.* New York: W. W. Norton.

Courtois, C. A. (1999). *Recollections of sexual abuse: Treatment principles and guidelines.* New York: W. W. Norton.

Crabtree, A. (1992). Dissociation and memory: A two-hundred year perspective. *Dissociation, 5,* 150–154.

Crenshaw, W., Crenshaw, L., & Lichtenberg, J. (1995). When educators confront child abuse: An analysis of the decision to report. *Child Abuse & Neglect, 19,* 1095–1113.

Crittenden, P. M. (1992). Treatment of anxious attachment in infancy and early childhood. *Development and Psychopathology, 4,* 575–602.

Crooks, R., & Baur, K. (1993). *Our sexuality* (5th ed.). Redwood City, CA: Benjamin/Cummings.

Cross, T. P., Whitcomb, D., & De Vos, E. (1995). Criminal justice outcomes of prosecution of child sexual abuse: A case flow analysis. *Child Abuse & Neglect, 19*, 1431–1422.

Crowder, A. F. (1995). *Opening the door: A treatment model for therapy with male survivors of sexual abuse.* New York: Brunner/Mazel.

Crowley, M. J., O'Callaghan, M. G., & Ball, P. G. (1994). The judicial impact of psychological expert testimony in a simulated child sexual abuse trial. *Law and Human Behavior, 18*, 89–105.

Cullen, B. J., Smith, P. H., Funk, J. B., & Haaf, R.A . (2000). A matched cohort comparison of a criminal justice system's response to child sexual abuse: A profile of perpetrators. *Child Abuse & Neglect, 24*, 569–577.

Cunningham, R. M., Stiffman, A. R., & Dore, P., & Earls, F. (1994). The association of physical and sexual abuse with HIV risk behaviors in adolescence and young adulthood: Implications for public health. *Child Abuse & Neglect, 18*, 233–245.

Cupoli, J. M., & Sewell, P. M. (1988). One thousand fifty-nine children with a chief complaint of sexual abuse. *Child Abuse & Neglect, 12*, 151–162.

Dale, P., & Allen, J. (1998). On memories of childhood abuse: A phenomenological study. *Child Abuse & Neglect, 22*, 799–812.

Dalenberg, C. J. (1996). Accuracy, time and circumstances of disclosure in therapy of recovered and continuous memories of abuse. *Journal of Psychiatry and Law, 24*, 229–275.

Dallam, S. D. (2001). Science or propaganda? An examination of Rind, Tromovitch and Bauserman (1998). *Journal of Child Sexual Abuse, 9*, 109–134.

Damasio, A. R. (1994). *Descartes' error: Emotion and the human brain.* New York: Grosset/Putnam.

Davies, J. M., & Frawley, M. G. (1994). *Treating the adult survivor of childhood sexual abuse: A psychoanalytic perspective.* New York: Basic Books.

Davis, L. L. (1986). The role of the teacher in preventing child sexual abuse. In M. Nelson & K. Clark (Eds.), *The educator's guide to preventing child sexual abuse* (pp.). Santa Cruz, CA: Network Publications.

Davies, M. G. (1995). Parental distress and ability to cope following disclosure of extra-familial sexual abuse. *Child Abuse & Neglect, 19*, 399–408.

Deaux, K., & Major, B. (1987). Putting gender into context: An interactive model of gender related behavior. *Psychological Review, 94*, 369–389.

De Bellis, M. D. (2001). Developmental traumatology: The psychobiological development of maltreated children and its implications for research, treatment, and policy. *Development and Psychopathology, 13*, 539–564.

De Bellis, M. D., Baum, A. S., Birmaher, B., Keshavan, M. S., Eccard, C. H., Boring, A. M., Jenkins, F. J., & Ryan, N. D. (1999). Developmental traumatology part I: Biological stress systems. *Biological Psychiatry, 45*, 1259–1270.

De Bellis, M. D., Broussard, E. R., Herring, D. J., Wexler, S., Moritz, G., & Benitez, J. G. (2001). Psychiatric co-morbidity in caregivers and children involved in maltreatment: A pilot research study with policy implications. *Child Abuse & Neglect, 25*, 923–944.

De Bellis, M. D., Chrousos, G. P., Dorn, L. D., Burke, L. Helmers, K., Kling, M. A., Trickett, P. K., & Putnam, F. W. (1994). Hypothalamic-pituitary-adrenal axis dysregulation in sexually abused girls. *Journal of Clinical Endocrinology and Metabolism, 78*, 249–255.

De Bellis, M. D., Hall, J., Boring, A., Frustaci, K., & Moritz, G. (2001). A pilot longitudinal study of hippocampal volumes in pediatric maltreatment-related posttraumatic stress disorder. *Biological Psychiatry, 50*, 305–309.

De Bellis, M. D., Keshavan, M. S., Beers, S. R., Hall, J., Frustaci, K., Masalehdan, A., Noll, J., & Borin, J. M. (2001). Sex differences in brain maturation during childhood and adolescence. *Cerebral Cortex, 11*, 552–557.

De Bellis, M. D., Keshavan, M. S., Clark, D. B., Casey, B. J., Giedd, J. N., Boring, A. M., Frustaci, K., & Ryan, N. D. (1999). Developmental traumatology part II; Brain development. *Biological Psychiatry, 45*, 1271–1284.

De Bellis, M. D., & Putnam, F. W. (1994). The psychobiology of childhood maltreatment. *Child and Adolescent Psychiatric Clinics of North America, 3,* 663–677.

Deblinger, E., & Heflin, A. H. (1996). *Treating sexually abused children and their non-offending parents: A cognitive-behavioral approach.* Thousand Oaks, CA: Sage.

Deblinger, E., McLeer, S. V., Atkins, M. S., Ralphe, D., & Foa, E. (1989). Post-traumatic stress in sexually abused, physically abused, and nonabused children. *Child Abuse and Neglect, 13,* 403–408.

DeBruyn, L., Lujan, C., & May, P. (1992). A comparative study of abused and neglected American Indian children in the southwest. *Social Science and Medicine, 35,* 305–315.

DeJong, A. R., Emmett, G. A., & Hervada, A. R. (1982). Sexual abuse of children: Sex-, race-, and age-dependent variables. *American Journal of Diseases of Childhood, 136,* 129–134.

DeJong, A. R., Hervada, A. R., & Emmett, G. A. (1983). Epidemiologic variations in CSA. *Child Abuse and Neglect, 7,* 155–162.

de Lacoste, M. C., Adesanya, T., & Woodward, D. J. (1990). Measures of gender differences in the human brain and their relationships to brain weight. *Biological Psychiatry, 28,* 931–942.

Denney, N. W., & Quadagno, D. (1992). *Human sexuality* (2nd ed.). St. Louis, MO: Mosby Year Book.

Dersch, C. A., & Munsch, J. (1999). Male victims of sexual abuse: An analysis of substantiation of child protective services reports. *Journal of Child Sexual Abuse, 8,* 27–48.

Desenclos, J. C., Garrity, D., & Wroten, J. (1992). Pediatric gonococcal infection, Florida, 1984 to 1988. *American Journal of Public Health, 82,* 426–428.

DeVoe, E. R., & Faller, K. C. (1999). The characteristics of disclosure among children who have been sexually abused. *Child Maltreatment, 4,* 217–227.

Deykin, E. Y., Buka, S. L., & Zeena, T.H. (1992). Depressive illness among chemically dependent adolescents. *American Journal of Psychiatry, 149,* 1341–1347.

de Young, M. (1989). The world according to NAMBLA: Accounting for deviance. *Journal of Sociology & Social Welfare, 16,* 111–126.

Dhabhar, F. S. (2000). Stress-induced enhancement of immune function. In G. Fink (Ed.), *Encyclopedia of stress* (Vol. 2, pp. 515–522). San Diego, CA: Academic Press.

Dhaliwal, G. K., Gauzas, L., Antonowicz, D. H., & Ross, R. R. (1996). Adult male survivors of childhood sexual abuse: Prevalence, sexual abuse characteristics, and long-term effects. *Clinical Psychology Review, 16,* 619–639.

Dhawan, S., & Marshall, W. L. (1996). Sexual abuse histories of sexual offenders. *Sexual Abuse: A Journal of Research and Treatment, 8,* 7–15.

Dhooper, S. S., Royce, D. D., & Wolfe, L. C. (1991). A statewide study of the public attitudes toward child abuse. *Child Abuse & Neglect, 15,* 37–44.

Diamond, M., & Karlen, A. (1980). *Sexual decisions.* Boston: Little, Brown.

DiIorio, C., Hartwell, T., & Hansen, N. (2002). Childhood sexual abuse and risk behaviors among men at high risk for HIV infection. *American Journal of Public Health, 92,* 214–219.

Dimock, P. T. (1988). Adult males sexually abused as children: Characteristics and implications for treatment. *Journal of Interpersonal Violence, 3,* 203–221.

DiPietro, E. K., Runyan, D. K., & Frederickson, D. D. (1997). Predictors of disclosure during medical evaluation for suspected sexual abuse. *Journal of Child Sexual Abuse, 6,* 133–142.

Disorbio, J. M., & Bruns, D. (1998). *Psychological profiles of rehabilitation patients reporting childhood sexual abuse.* Paper presented at the Annual Meeting of the American Psychological Association. Available online: www.healthpsych.com.

Doll, L. S., Joy, D., Bartholow, B. N., Harrison, J. S., Bolan, G., Douglas, J. M., Saltzman, L. E., Moss, P. M., & Delgado, W. (1992). Self-reported childhood and adolescent sexual abuse among adult homosexual and bisexual men. *Child Abuse & Neglect, 16,* 855–864.

Donaldson, S. (1990). Rape of males. In W. R. Dynes (Ed.), *Encyclopedia of homosexuality* (Vol. 2, pp. 1094–1098). New York: Garland.

Donaldson, S. (1993, December 29). The rape crisis behind bars. *The New York Times,* A11.

Draijer, N., & Langeland, W. (1999). Childhood trauma and perceived parental dysfunction in the etiology of dissociative symptoms in psychiatric inpatients. *American Journal of Psychiatry,* *156*, 379–385.

Draucker, C. B. (1992). *Counselling survivors of childhood sexual abuse.* London: Sage.

Dube, R., & Hebert, M. (1988). Sexual abuse children under 12 years of age: A review of 511 cases. *Child Abuse & Neglect, 12*, 321–330.

Dubowitz, H., Black, M., Harrington, D., & Verschoore, A. (1993). A follow-up study of behavior problems associated with child sexual abuse. *Child Abuse & Neglect, 17*, 743–754.

Duncan, L. E., Peterson, B. E., & Winter, D. G. (1997). Authoritarianism and gender roles: Toward a psychological analysis of hegemonic relationships. *Personality and Social Psychology Bulletin, 23*, 41–49.

Duncan, L. E., & Williams, L. M. (1998). Gender role socialization and male-on-male vs. female-on-male child sexual abuse. *Sex Roles, 39*, 765–785.

Dunn, G. E., Ryan, J. J., Paolo, A. M., & Van Fleet, J. (1995). Comorbidity of dissociative disorders among patients with substance use disorders. *Psychiatric Services, 46*, 153–156.

Dziuba-Leatherman, J., & Finkelhor, D. (1994). How does receiving information about sexual abuse influence boys' perceptions of their risk? *Child Abuse & Neglect, 18*, 557–568.

Eckenrode, J., Laird, M., & Doris, J. (1993). School performance and disciplinary problems among abused and neglected children. *Developmental Psychology, 29*, 53–62.

Eckenrode, J., Munsch, J., Powers, J., & Doris, J. (1988). The nature and substantiation of official sexual abuse reports. *Child Abuse & Neglect, 12*, 311–319.

Edwards, E., Harkins, K., Wright, G., & Menn, F. (1990). Effects of bilateral adrenalectomy on the induction of learned helplessness behavior. *Neuropsychopharmacology, 3*, 109–114.

Egeland, B., Carson, E., & Stroufe, L. A. (1993). Resilience as process. *Development and Psychopathology, 5*, 517–528.

Egeland, B., & Jacobvitz, D. (1988). Breaking the cycle of abuse. *Child Development, 59*, 1080–1088.

Eisenberg, N., Owens, R. G., & Dewey, M. E. (1987). Attitudes of health professionals to child sexual abuse and incest. *Child Abuse & Neglect, 11*, 109–116.

Ellason, J. W., Ross, C. A., Sainton, K., & Mayran, L. W. (1996). Axis I and II comorbidity and childhood trauma in chemical dependency. *Bulletin of the Meninger Clinic, 60*, 39–51.

Elliott, A., & Peterson, L. (1993). Maternal sexual abuse of children: When to suspect it and how to uncover it. *Postgraduate Medicine, 94*, 169–180.

Elliott, D. M. (1997). Traumatic events: Prevalence and delayed recall in the general population. *Journal of Counseling and Clinical Psychology, 65*, 811–820.

Elliott, D. M., & Briere, J. (1994). Forensic sexual abuse evaluations in older children: Disclosures and symptomatology. *Behavioral Sciences and the Law, 12*, 261–277.

Elliott, D. M., & Briere, J. (1995). Poststraumatic stress associated with delayed recall of sexual abuse: A general population study. *Journal of Traumatic Stress, 8*, 629–647.

Elliott, D. M., & Fox, B. (1994, November). *Child abuse and amnesia: Prevalence and triggers to memory recovery.* Paper presented at the Annual Meeting of the International Society of Traumatic Stress Studies, Chicago.

Elliott, M. (Ed.). (1994). *Female sexual abuse of children.* New York: Guilford Press.

Elliott, M., Browne, K., & Kilcoyne, J. (1995). Child sexual abuse prevention: What offenders tell us. *Child Abuse & Neglect, 19*, 579–594.

Ellis, A. (1995). Rational emotive behavior therapy. In R. J. Corsini & D. Wedding (Eds.), *Current psychotherapies* (5th ed., pp. 162–196). Itasca, IL: F. E. Peacock.

Elwell, M. E., & Ephross, P. E. (1987). Initial reactions of sexually abused children. *Social Casework: The Journal of Contemporary Social Work, 68*, 109–116.

Epstein, M. A., & Bottoms, B. L. (1998). Memories of childhood sexual abuse: A survey of young adults. *Child Abuse & Neglect, 22*, 1217–1238.

Erikson, E. H. (1963). *Childhood and society* (2nd ed.). New York: W. W. Norton.

Estes, L. S., & Tidwell, R. (2002). Sexually abused children's behaviors: Impact of gender and mother's experience of intra- and extra-familial sexual abuse. *Family Practice, 19*, 36–44.

Estes, R., & Weiner, N. A. (2001). *The commercial exploitation of children in the U.S., Canada and Mexico.* Washington, DC: United States Department of Justice, National Institute of Justice.

Etherington, K. (1997). Maternal sexual abuse of males. *Child Abuse Review, 6,* 107–117.

Fairbairn, W. R. D. (1994). *From instinct to self: Selected papers of W.R.D. Fairbairn* (Vols. 1–2, E. F. Birtles & D. E. Scharff, Eds.). Northvale, NJ: Aronson Press.

Faller, K. C. (1987). Women who sexually abuse children. *Violence and Victims, 2,* 263–276.

Faller, K. C. (1988). *Child sexual abuse: An interdisciplinary manual for diagnosis, case management, and treatment.* New York: Columbia University Press.

Faller, K. C. (1989). Characteristics of a clinical sample of sexually abused children: How boy and girl victims differ. *Child Abuse & Neglect, 13,* 281–291.

Faller, K. C. (1990). Sexual abuse by paternal caretakers: A comparison of abusers who are biological fathers in intact families, stepfathers, and noncustodial fathers. In A. L. Horton, B. L. Johnson, L. M. Roundy, & D. Williams (Eds.), *The incest perpetrator: A family member no one wants to treat* (pp. 65–73). Newbury Park, CA: Sage.

Faller, K. C. (1995). A clinical sample of women who have sexually abused children. *Journal of Child Sexual Abuse, 4,* 13–30.

Faller, K. C., & Henry, J. (2000). Child sexual abuse: A case study in community collaboration. *Child Abuse & Neglect, 24,* 1215–1225.

Fanselow, M. S., & Gale, G. D. (2000). Amygdala. In G. Fink (Ed.), *Encyclopedia of stress* (Vol. 1, pp. 178–182). San Diego, CA: Academic Press.

Famularo, R., Fenton, T., Kinscherff, R., & Augustyn, M. (1996). Psychiatric comorbidity in childhood posttraumatic stress disorder. *Child Abuse & Neglect, 20,* 953–961.

Farber, E. D., Showers, J., Johnson, C. F., Joseph, J. A., Oshins, L. (1984). The sexual abuse of children: A comparison of male and female victims. *Journal of Clinical Psychology, 13,* 294–297.

Faust, J., Runyon, M., & Kenny, M. (1995). Family variables associated with the onset and impact of intrafamilial childhood sexual abuse. *Clinical Psychological Review, 15,* 443–456.

Federal Bureau of Investigation. (1999). *FBI uniform crime reporting definitions. CIUS 99 Section II: Forcible rape.* Retrieved October 13, 2002, from www.fbi.gov/ucr.cius_99/99crime/99c2_04.pdf

Fehrenbach, P., & Monastersky, C. (1988). Characteristics of female adolescent sex offenders. *American Journal of Orthopsychiatry, 58,* 148–151.

Fehrenbach, P., Smith, W., Monastersky, C., & Deischer, R. (1986). Adolescent sexual offenders: Offender and offense characteristics. *American Journal of Orthopsychiatry, 56,* 225–233.

Feiring, C., Taska, L., & Chen, K. (2002). Trying to understand why horrible things happen: Attribution, shame, and symptom development following sexual abuse. *Child Maltreatment, 7,* 26–41.

Feiring, C., Taska, L., & Lewis, M. (1996). A process model for understanding adaptation to sexual abuse: The role of shame in defining stigmatization. *Child Abuse & Neglect, 20,* 767–782.

Feiring, C., Taska, L., & Lewis, M. (1999). Age and gender differences in children's and adolescents' adaptation to sexual abuse. *Child Abuse & Neglect, 23,* 115–128.

Feldman-Summers, S., & Pope, K. S. (1994). The experience of "forgetting" childhood abuse: A national survey of psychologists. *Journal of Consulting and Clinical Psychology, 62,* 636–639.

Ferenczi, S. (1949). Confusion of tongues between the adult and the child: The language of tenderness and passion. *International Journal of Psychoanalysis, 30,* 225–230. (Original work published 1932)

Fergusson, D. M., Linskey, M. T., & Horwood, L. J. (1996a). Childhood sexual abuse and psychiatric disorder in young adulthood: I. Prevalence of sexual abuse and factors associated with sexual abuse. *Journal of the American Academy of Child & Adolescent Psychiatry, 35,* 1355–1364.

Fergusson, D. M., Linskey, M. T., & Horwood, L. J. (1996b). Childhood sexual abuse and psychiatric disorder in young adulthood: II. Psychiatric outcomes of childhood sexual abuse. *Journal of the American Academy of Child & Adolescent Psychiatry, 35*, 1365–1374.

Ferrara, M. L., & McDonald, S. (1996). *Treatment of the juvenile sexual offender: Neurological and psychiatric impairments.* Northvale, NJ: Jason Aronson.

Festinger, L. (1964). *Conflict, decision and dissonance.* Stanford, CA: Stanford University Press.

Figley, C. R. (Ed.). (1995). *Compassion fatigue: Coping with secondary traumatic stress disorder in those who treat the traumatized.* New York: Brunner/Mazel.

Finkelhor, D. (1981). The sexual abuse of boys. *Victimology: An International Journal, 6*, 76–84.

Finkelhor, D. (1984). *Child sexual abuse: New theory and research.* New York: Free Press.

Finkelhor, D. (Ed.). (1986). *A sourcebook on child sexual abuse.* Beverly Hills, CA: Sage.

Finkelhor, D. (1987). The sexual abuse of children: Current research reviewed. *Psychiatric Annals, 17*, 233–241.

Finkelhor, D. (1988). The trauma of child sexual abuse: Two models. In G. E. Wyatt & G. J. Powell (Eds.), *Lasting effects of child sexual abuse* (pp. 61–82). Newbury Park, CA: Sage.

Finkelhor, D. (1990). Early and long-term effects of child sexual abuse: An update. *Professional Psychology: Research and Practice, 21*, 325–330.

Finkelhor, D. (1994). Current information on the scope and nature of child sexual abuse. *The Future of Children, 4*, 31–53.

Finkelhor, D. (1995). The victimization of children: A developmental perspective. *American Journal of Orthopsychiatry, 65*, 177–193.

Finkelhor, D., Asdigian, N., & Dziuba-Leatherman, J. (1995). The effectiveness of victimization prevention instruction: An evaluation of children's responses to actual threats and assaults. *Child Abuse & Neglect, 19*, 141–153.

Finkelhor, D., & Browne, A. (1985). The traumatic impact of child sexual abuse: A conceptualization. *American Journal of Orthopsychiatry, 55*, 530–541.

Finkelhor, D., & Dziuba-Leatherman, J. (1995). Victimization prevention programs: A national survey of children's exposure and reactions. *Child Abuse & Neglect, 19*, 129–139.

Finkelhor, D., Hotaling, G., Lewis, I. A., & Smith, C. (1990). Sexual abuse in a national survey of adult men and women: Prevalence, characteristics, and risk factors. *Child Abuse & Neglect, 14*, 19–28.

Finkelhor, D., Mitchell, K., & Wolak, J. (2001). *Highlights of the youth Internet safety survey.* Washington, DC: United States Department of Justice, Office of Juvenile Justice and Delinquency Prevention.

Finkelhor, D., Moore, D., Hamby, S. L., & Straus, M. A. (1997). Sexually abused children in a national survey of parents: Methodological issues. *Child Abuse & Neglect, 21*, 1–9.

Finkelhor, D., & Ormrod, R. (2001). *Child abuse reported to the police.* Washington, DC: United States Department of Justice, Office of Juvenile Justice and Delinquency Prevention.

Finkelhor, D., & Russell, D. E. H. (1984). Women as perpetrators. In D. Finkelhor (Ed.), *Child sexual abuse: New theory and research* (pp. 181–185). New York: Free Press.

Finkelhor, D., Williams, L. M., & Burns, N. (1988). *Nursery crimes: Sexual abuse in day care.* Newbury Park, CA: Sage.

Finkelhor, D., Williams, L., Burns, N., & Kalinowski, M. (1988). *Nursery crimes: Sexual abuse in day care.* Newbury Park, CA: Sage.

Finlayson, L. M., & Koocher, G. P. (1991). Professional judgment and child abuse reporting in sexual abuse cases. *Professional Psychology Research & Practice, 22*, 464–472.

Firestone, P., Bradford, J. M., McCoy, M., Greenberg, D. M., & Curry, S. (1999). Prediction of recidivism in incest offenders. *Journal of Interpersonal Violence, 14*, 511–531.

Firestone, P., Bradford, J. M., McCoy, M., Greenberg, D. M., Curry, S., & Larose, M. R. (2000). Prediction of recidivism in extrafamilial child molesters based on court related assessments. *Sexual Abuse: A Journal of Research and Treatment, 12*, 203–222.

Fischer, D. G., & McDonald, W. L. (1998). Characteristics of intrafamilial and extrafamilial child sexual abuse. *Child Abuse & Neglect, 22,* 915–929.

Fish, V., & Scott, C. G. (1999). Childhood abuse recollections in a nonclinical population: Forgetting and secrecy. *Child Abuse & Neglect, 23,* 791–802.

Fivush, R. (1998). Children's recollections of traumatic and nontraumatic events. *Development and Psychopathology, 10,* 699–716.

Fivush, R., & Schwarzmueller, A. (1995). Say it once again: Effects of repeated questions on children's event recall. *Journal of Traumatic Stress, 8,* 555–580.

Flavell, J. H. (1985). *Cognitive development* (2nd ed.). Englewood Cliffs, NJ: Prentice-Hall.

Fletcher, K. E. (1996). Child posttraumatic stress disorder. In E. J. Mash & R. A. Barkley (Eds.), *Child psychopathology* (pp. 242–276). New York: Guilford.

Foa, E. B., Steketee, G., & Rothbaum, B. O. (1989). Behavioral/cognitive conceptualizations of post-traumatic stress disorder. *Behavior Therapy, 20,* 155–176.

Fondacaro, K. M., Holt, J. C., & Powell, T. A. (1999). Psychological impact of childhood sexual abuse on male inmates: The importance of perception. *Child Abuse & Neglect, 23,* 361–369.

Fontanella, C., Harrington, D., & Zuravin, S.J. (2000). Gender differences in the characteristics and outcomes of sexually abused preschoolers. *Journal of Child Sexual Abuse, 9,* 21–40.

Forbey, J. D., Ben-Porath, Y. S., & Davis, D. L. (2000). A comparison of sexually abused and nonsexually abused adolescents in a clinical treatment facility using the MMPI-A. *Child Abuse & Neglect, 24,* 557–568.

Fortune, M. M. (1988). Reporting child abuse. In A L. Horton & J. A. Williamson (Eds.), *Abuse and religion* (pp. 189–197). Lexington, MA: Lexington Books.

Freud, A. (1936). *The ego and mechanisms of defense.* London: Hogarth Press.

Freud, A. (1965). *Normality and pathology in childhood: Assessments of development.* New York: International Universities Press.

Freud, A. (1967). Comments on psychic trauma. In *The writings of Anna Freud* (Vol. V, pp. 221–241). New York: International Universities Press.

Freud, S. (1962). The aetiology of hysteria. In J. Strachey (Ed. and Trans.), *The standardized edition of the complete psychological works of Sigmund Freud* (Vol. 3., pp. 189–224). London: Hogarth Press. (Original work published 1896)

Freund, K., Watson, R., & Dickey, R. (1990). Does sexual abuse in childhood cause pedophilia: An exploratory study. *Archives of Sexual Behavior, 19,* 557–568.

Freyd, J. J. (1996). *Betrayal trauma: The logic of forgetting childhood abuse.* Cambridge, MA: Harvard University Press.

Freyd, J. J., DePrince, A. P., & Zurbriggen, E. L. (2001). Self-reported memory for abuse depends upon victim-perpetrator relationship. *Journal of Trauma & Dissociation, 2,* 5–16.

Friedman, S., Smith, L., Fogel, D., Paradis, C., Viswanathan, R., Ackerman, R., & Trappler, B. (2002). The incidence and influence of early traumatic life events in patients with panic disorder: A comparison with other psychiatric outpatients. *Anxiety Disorders, 16,* 259–272.

Friedrich, W. N. (1996). Clinical considerations of empirical treatment studies of abused children. *Child Maltreatment, 1,* 343–347.

Friedrich, W. N., Beilke, R. L., & Urquiza, A. J. (1988). Behavior problems in young sexually abused boys: A comparison study. *Journal of Interpersonal Violence, 3,* 21–28.

Friedrich, W. N., Gerber, P. N., Koplin, B., Davis, M., Giese, J., Mykelbust, C., et al.. (2001). Multimodal assessment of dissociation in adolescence: Inpatients and juvenile sex offenders. *Sexual Abuse: A Journal of Research and Treatment, 13,* 167–177.

Friedrich, W. N., & Luecke, W. J. (1988). Young school-age sexually aggressive children. *Professional Psychology: Research and Practice, 19,* 155–164.

Friedrich, W. N., Urquiza, A. J., & Beilke, R. L. (1986). Behavior problems in sexually abused young children. *Journal of Pediatric Psychology, 11,* 47–57.

Fromm-Reichman, F. (1950). *Principles of intensive psychotherapy.* Chicago: University of Chicago Press.

Fromuth, M. E., & Burkhart, B. R. (1987). Childhood sexual victimization among college men: Definitional and methodological issues. *Violence and Victims, 2,* 241–253.

Fromuth, M. E., & Burkhart, B. R. (1989). Long-term psychological correlates of childhood sexual abuse in two samples of college men. *Child Abuse and Neglect, 13,* 533–542.

Froum, A. G., & Kendall-Tackett, K. A. (1998). Law enforcement officers' approaches to evaluations of child sexual abuse. *Child Abuse & Neglect, 22,* 939–942.

Furniss, T. (1991). *The multi-professional handbook of child sexual abuse: Integrated management, therapy and legal intervention.* London: Routledge Press.

Gale, J., Thompson, R. J., Moran, T., & Sack, W. H. (1988). Sexual abuse in young children: Its clinical presentation and characteristic patterns. *Child Abuse and Neglect, 12,* 163–170.

Garbarino, J. (1977). The human ecology of child maltreatment: A conceptual model for research. *Journal of Marriage and the Family, 39,* 721–735.

Garbarino, J. (1981). *Selected readings on adolescent maltreatment.* DHHS# 81-30301. Washington, DC: National Center on Child Abuse and Neglect.

Garbarino, J. (1986). Can we measure success in preventing child abuse? Issues in policy, programming and research. *Child Abuse & Neglect, 10,* 143–156.

Garbarino, J., & Eckenrode, J. (1997). *Understanding abusive families: An ecological approach to theory and practice.* Baltimore, MD: Brookes.

Garfinkel, P. E., Lin, E., Goering, P., Spegg, C., Goldbloom, D.S ., Kennedy, S., et al. (1995). Bulimia nervosa in a Canadian community sample: Prevalence and comparison subgroups. *American Journal of Psychiatry, 152,* 1052–1058.

Garland, R. J. & Dougler, M. J. (1990). The abused/abuser hypothesis of child sexual abuse: A critical review of theory and research. In J. R. Feierman (Ed.), *Pedophilia: Biosocial dimensions* (pp. 488–509). New York: Springer-Verlag.

Garnefski, N., & Diekstra, R. F. W. (1997). Child sexual abuse and emotional and behavioral problems in adolescence: Gender differences. *Journal of the American Academy of Child and Adolescent Psychiatry, 36,* 323–329.

Gartner, R. B. (1999). *Betrayed as boys: Psychodynamic treatment of sexually abused men.* New York: Guilford Press.

Gay, P. (1988). *Freud: A life of our time.* New York: W. W. Norton.

Gellert, G. A., Durfee, M. J., Berkowitz, C. D., Higgins, K. V., & Tubiolo, V. C. (1993). Situational and sociodemographic characteristics of children infected with human immunodeficiency virus from pediatric sexual abuse. *Pediatrics, 91,* 39–44.

Germain, C. B., & Gitterman, A. (1996). *The life model of social work practice.* New York: Columbia University Press.

Gil, E., & Johnson, T. C. (1993). *Sexualized children: Assessment and treatment of sexualized children and children who molest.* Rockville, MD: Launch Press.

Gilgun, J. F., & Reiser, E. (1990). The development of sexual identity among men sexually abused as children. *Families in Society: The Journal of Contemporary Human Services, 71,* 515–523.

Gill, M., & Tutty, L. M. (1997). Sexual identity for male survivors of childhood sexual abuse: A qualitative study. *Journal of Child Sexual Abuse, 6,* 31–47.

Gill, M., & Tutty, L. M. (1999). Male survivors of childhood sexual abuse: A qualitative study and issues for clinical consideration. *Journal of Child Sexual Abuse, 7,* 19–33,

Gilligan, C. (1982). *In a different voice.* Cambridge, MA: Harvard University Press.

Glod, C. A., & Teicher, M. H. (1996). Relationship between early abuse, posttraumatic stress disorder, and activity levels in prepubertal children. *Journal of the American Academy of Child and Adolescent Psychiatry, 35,* 1384–1393.

Glod, C. A., Teicher, M. H., Hartman, C. R., & Harakal, T. (1997). Increased nocturnal activity and impaired sleep maintenance in abused children. *Journal of the American Academy of Child and Adolescent Psychiatry,. 36,* 1236–1243.

Glover, N. M., Janikowski, T. P., & Benshoff, J. J. (1995). The incidence of incest histories among clients receiving substance abuse treatment. *Journal of Counseling and Development, 73,* 475–480.

Gold, S. N., Elhai, J. D., Lucenko, B. A., & Swingle, J. M. (1998). Abuse characteristics among childhood sexual abuse survivors in therapy: A gender comparison. *Child Abuse & Neglect, 22,* 1005–1012.

Gold, S. N., Elhai, J. D., Lucenko, B,. Swingle, J. M., & Hughes, D. M. (1997, June). *A comparison of abuse characteristics among men and women survivors of childhood sexual abuse.* Paper presented at the Fifth International Family Violence Research Conference. Durham, NH.

Gold, S. N., Hughes, D., & Hohnecker, L. (1994). Degrees of repression of sexual abuse memories. *American Psychologist, 49,* 441–442.

Golding, J. M., Sanchez, R. P., & Sego, S. A. (1997). The believability of hearsay testimony in a child sexual abuse assault trial. *Law and Human Behavior, 21,* 299–325.

Goldman, R. L. (1994). Children and youth with intellectual disabilities: Targets for sexual abuse. *International Journal of Disability, Development and Education, 41,* 89–102.

Goldstein, E. G. (1984). *Ego psychology and social work practice.* New York: Free Press.

Goldstein, E. G. (1995). *Ego psychology and social work practice* (2nd ed.). New York: Free Press.

Goldstein, H. (1982). Cognitive approaches to direct practice. *Social Service Review, 56,* 539–555.

Gomes-Schwartz, B., Horowitz, J. M., & Cardarelli, A. P. (1990). *Child sexual abuse: The initial effects.* Newbury Park, CA: Sage.

Gomes-Schwartz, B., Horowitz, J. M., Cardarelli, A. P., & Sauzier, M. (1990). The aftermath of child sexual abuse: 18 Months later. In B. Gomes-Schwartz, J. M. Horowitz, & A. P. Cardarelli (Eds.), *Child sexual abuse: The initial effects* (pp. 132–184). Newbury Park, CA: Sage.

Gomes-Schwartz, B., Horowitz, J. M., & Sauzier, M. (1985). Severity of emotional distress among sexually abused preschool, school-age, and adolescent children. *Hospital and Community Psychiatry, 36,* 503–508.

Gonsiorek, J. C. (1994). Assessment of and treatment planning and individual psychotherapy for sexually abused adolescent males. In J. C. Gonsiorek, W. H. Bera & D. LeTourneau (Eds.), *Male sexual abuse: A trilogy of intervention strategies* (pp. 3–110). Thousand Oaks, CA: Sage.

Gonsiorek, J. C., Bera, W. H., & LeTourneau, D. (1994). *Male sexual abuse: A trilogy of intervention strategies.* Thousand Oaks, CA: Sage.

Gonzalez, L. S., Waterman, J., & Kelly, R. J., McCord, J., & Oliveri, M. K. (1993). Children's patterns of disclosures and recantations of sexual and ritualistic abuse allegations in psychotherapy. *Child Abuse & Neglect, 17,* 281–289.

Goodman, G. S., Taub, E. P., Jones, D. P. H., England, P., Port, L. K., Rudy, L., & Prado, L. (1992). Testifying in criminal court. *Monographs of the Society for Research in Child Development, 57,* (Serial No. 229). Chicago: University of Chicago Press.

Gordon, M. (1990). Males and females as victims of childhood sexual abuse: An examination of the gender effect. *Journal of Family Violence, 5,* 321–332.

Gore-Felton, C., Arnow, B., Koopman, C., Thoresen, C., & Spiegel, D. (1999). Psychologists' beliefs about the prevalence of childhood sexual abuse: The influence of sexual abuse history, gender, and theoretical orientation. *Child Abuse & Neglect, 23,* 803–811.

Grassian, S., & Holtzen, D. (1996, July). *Memory of sexual abuse by a parish priest.* Paper presented at Trauma and Memory: An International Research Conference. Durham, NH.

Gray, A., Busconi, A., Houchens, P., & Pithers, W. D. (1997). Children with sexual behavior problems and their caregivers: Demographics, functioning and clinical patterns. *Sexual Abuse: A Journal of Research and Treatment, 9,* 267–290.

Gray, A. S., & Pithers, W. D. (1993). Relapse prevention with sexually aggressive adolescents and children: Expanding treatment and supervision. In H. E. Barbaree, W. L. Marshall, & S. Hudson (Eds.), *The juvenile sex offender* (pp. 289–319). New York: Guilford Press.

Gray, A., Pithers, W. D., Busconi, A., & Houchens, P. (1999). Developmental and etiological characteristics of children with sexual behavior problems: Treatment implications. *Child Abuse & Neglect, 23,* 601–621.

Gray, E. (1993). *Unequal justice.* New York: Free Press.

Greenberg, D. M., Bradford, J. M. W., & Curry, S. (1993). A comparison of sexual victimization in the childhoods of pedophiles and hebephiles. *Journal of Forensic Sciences, 38,* 432–436.

Greenberg, D., Bradford, J., Firestone, P., & Curry, S. (2000). Recidivism of child molesters: A study of victim relationship with the perpetrator. *Child Abuse & Neglect, 24,* 1485–1494.

Greene, R. R., & Ephross, P. H. (1991). *Human behavior theory and social work practice.* Hawthorne, NY: Aldine De Gruyter.

Grice, D. E., Brady, K. T., Dustan, L. R., Malcolm, R., & Kilpatrick, D. G. (1995). Sexual and physical assault history and posttraumatic stress disorder in substance dependent individuals. *American Journal on Addictions, 4,* 297–305.

Gries, L. T., Goh, D. S., & Cavanaugh, J. (1996). Factors associated with disclosure during child sexual abuse assessment. *Journal of Child Sexual Abuse, 5,* 1–19.

Grilo, C. M., Sanislow, C., Fehon, D. C., Martino, S., & McGlashan, T. H. (1999). Psychological and behavioral functioning in adolescent psychiatric inpatients who report histories of childhood abuse. *American Journal of Psychiatry, 156,* 538–543.

Grossoehme, D. H. (1998). Child abuse reporting: Clergy perceptions. *Child Abuse & Neglect, 22,* 743–747.

Groth, A. N., & Birnbaum, H. J. (1978). Adult sexual orientation and attraction to underage persons. *Archives of Sexual Behavior, 7,* 175–181.

Groth, A. N., & Burgess, A. W. (1980). Male rape: Offenders and victims. *American Journal of Psychiatry, 137,* 806–810.

Groth, A. N., Hobson, W. F., & Gary, T. S. (1982). The child molester: Clinical observations. In J. Conte & D. Shore (Eds.), *Social Work and child sexual abuse.* New York: Haworth.

Grotstein, J. S. (1985). *Splitting and projective identification.* Northvale, NJ: Jason Aronson.

Grunberg, N. E., & Baum, A. (1985). Biological commonalities of stress and substance abuse. In S. Shiffman & T. A. Wills (Eds.), *Coping and substance abuse* (pp. 25–62). New York: Academic Press.

Guidano, V. F., & Liotti, G. (1985). *A constructivistic foundation for cognitive therapy.* New York: Plenum Press.

Gully, K. J., Hansen, K., Britton, H., Langley, M., & McBride, K. K. (2000). The child sexual abuse experience and the child sexual abuse medical examination: Knowing what correlations exist. *Journal of Child Sexual Abuse, 9,* 15–27.

Gutierres, S. E., Russo, N. F., & Urbanski, L. (1994). Sociocultural and psychological factors in American Indian drug use: Implications for treatment. *International Journal of the Addictions, 29,* 1761–1786.

Gutman, L. T., St. Claire, K. K., Weedy, C., Herman-Giddens, M. E., Lane, B., Niemeyer, J. G., & McKinney, R. E. (1991). Human immunodeficiency virus transmission by child sexual abuse. *American Journal of Diseases of Childhood, 145,* 137–141.

Gutman, L. T., Herman-Giddens, M., & McKinney, R. E., Jr. (1993). Pediatric AIDS: Barriers to recognizing the role of child sexual abuse. *American Journal of Diseases of Childhood, 147,* 775–780.

Hall, D. K., Mathews, F., & Pearce, J. (1998). Factors associated with sexual behavior problems in young sexually abused children. *Child Abuse & Neglect, 22,* 1045–1063.

Hall, D. K., Mathews, F., & Pearce, J. (2002). Sexual behavior problems in sexually abused children: A preliminary typology. *Child Abuse & Neglect, 26,* 289–312.

Hammerschlag, M. R. (1998). The transmissibility of sexually transmitted diseases in sexually abused children. *Child Abuse & Neglect, 22,* 623–635.

Hamner, M. B., & Arana, G. W. (2000). Beta-Endorphin. In G. Fink (Ed.), *Encyclopedia of stress* (Vol. 1, pp. 321–323). San Diego, CA: Academic Press.

Hanson, R. K. (1990). Characteristics of sex offenders who were sexually abused as children. In R. Langevin (Ed.), *Sex offenders and their victims* (pp. 77–85). Oakville, Ontario, Canada: Juniper Press.

Hanson, R. K., & Bussière, M. T. (1998). Predicting relapse: A meta-analysis of sexual offender recidivism studies. *Journal of Consulting and Clinical Psychology, 66*, 348–362.

Hanson, R. K., & Slater, S. (1988). Sexual victimization in the history of sexual abusers: A review. *Annals of Sex Research, 1*, 485–499.

Harber, K. D., & Pennebaker, J. W. 1992). Overcoming traumatic memories. In S. Christianson (Ed.), *The handbook of emotion and memory: Research and theory* (pp. 359–387). Hillsdale, NJ: Lawrence Erlbaum.

Harrison, P. A., Fulkerson, J. A., & Beebe, T. J. (1997). Multiple substance abuse among adolescent physical and sexual abuse victims. *Child Abuse & Neglect, 21*, 529–539.

Harrison, P. A., Hoffman, N. G., & Edwall, G. E. (1989). Sexual abuse correlates: Similarities between male and female adolescents in chemical dependency treatment. *Journal of Adolescent Research, 4*, 385–399.

Hart, J., Gunnar, M., & Cicchetti, D. (1995). Salivary cortisol in maltreated children: Evidence of relations between neuro-endocrine activity and social competence. *Development & Psychopathology, 7*, 11–26.

Hart, J., Gunnar, M., & Cicchetti, D. (1996). Altered neuro-endocrine activity in children related to symptoms of depression, *Development & Psychopathology, 8*, 201–214.

Harter, S. (1983). Developmental perspectives on the self-system. In P. Mussen & E. M. Hetherington (Eds.), *Handbook of child psychology* (pp. 275–385). New York: John Wiley & Sons.

Hartman, C. R., & Burgess, A. W. (1993). Information processing of trauma. *Child Abuse & Neglect, 17*, 47–58.

Hartmann, H. (1964). *Essays on ego psychology.* New York: International Universities Press.

Harvey, M. R. (1996). An ecological view of psychological trauma and trauma recovery. *Journal of Traumatic Stress, 9*, 3–23.

Harvey, M. R., & Herman, J. L. (1994). Amnesia, partial amnesia, and delayed recall among adult survivors of childhood trauma. *Consciousness and Cognition, 4, 295–306.*

Haskett, M. E., Wayland, K., Hutcheson, T., & Tavana, J. (1995). Substantiation of sexual abuse allegations: Decision making process of child protection investigations. *Journal of Child Sexual Abuse, 4*, 19–47.

Hastie, R. (1980). Memory for behavioral information that confirms or contradicts a personality impression. In R. Hastie, T. M. Ostrom, E. B. Ebbesen, R. S. Wyer, Jr., D. L. Hamilton, & D. E. Carlston (Eds.), *Person memory: The cognitive basis for social perception* (pp. 155–178). Hillsdale, NJ: Lawrence Erlbaum.

Haywood, T. W., Kravitz, H. M., Wasyliw, O. E., Goldberg, J., & Cavanaugh, J. L., Jr. (1996). Cycle of abuse and psychopathology in cleric and noncleric molesters of children and adolescents. *Child Abuse & Neglect, 20*, 1233–1243.

Hecht, D. A., & Hansen, D. J. (1999). Adolescent victims and intergenerational issues in sexual abuse. In V. B. Van Hasselt & M. Hersen (Eds.), *Handbook of psychological approaches with violent criminal offenders: Contemporary strategies and issues* (pp. 303–328). New York: Plenum Press.

Heller, S. S., Larrieu, J. A., D'Imperio, R., & Boris, N. W. (1999). Research on resilience to child maltreatment: Empirical considerations. *Child Abuse & Neglect, 23*, 321–338.

Herman, J. L. (1981). *Father-daughter incest.* Cambridge, MA: Harvard University Press.

Herman, J. L. (1992). *Trauma and recovery.* New York: Basic Books.

Herman, J. L. (1995). Crime and memory. *Bulletin of the American Academy of Psychiatry and the Law, 23*, 5–17.

Hernandez, J. (1995). The concurrence of eating disorders with histories of child abuse among adolescents. *Journal of Child Sexual Abuse, 4*, 73–85.

Herrenkohl, E. C., Herrenkohl, R. R., & Egolf, B. (1994). Resilient early school-age children from maltreating homes: Outcomes in late adolescence. *American Journal of Orthopsychiatry, 64*, 301–309.

Hetherton, J., & Beardsall, L. (1998). Decisions and attitudes concerning child sexual abuse:

Does the gender of the perpetrator make a difference to child protection professionals? *Child Abuse & Neglect, 22,* 1265–1283.

Hibbard, R. A., & Hartman, G. L. (1992). Behavioral problems in alleged sexual abuse victims. *Child Abuse & Neglect, 16,* 755–762.

Hibbard, R. A., Ingersoll, G. M., & Orr, D. P. (1990). Behavioral risk, emotional risk, and child abuse among adolescents in a nonclinical setting. *Pediatrics, 86,* 896–901.

Hibbard, R. A., & Zollinger, T. W. (1990). Patterns of child sexual knowledge among professionals. *Child Abuse & Neglect, 14,* 347–355.

Hibbard, R. A., & Zollinger, T. W. (1992). Medical evaluation referral patterns for sexual abuse victims. *Child Abuse & Neglect, 16,* 533–540.

Hindman, J. (1988). Research disputes assumptions about child molesters. *National District Attorneys Association Bulletin* (July/August), pp. 1–3.

Hislop, J. (2001). *Female sex offenders: What therapists, law enforcement, and child protective services need to know.* Ravensdale, WA: Issues Press.

Hobbs, G. F., Hobbs, C. J., & Wynne, J. M. (1999). Abuse of children in foster and residential care. *Child Abuse & Neglect, 23,* 1239–1252.

Hobbs, G. F., & Wynne, J. M. (1989). Sexual abuse of English boys and girls: The importance of anal examination. *Child Abuse & Neglect, 13,* 195.

Holder, W. M., & Corey, M. (1993). *Child protective services risk management: A decision making handbook* (Rev. ed.). Charlotte, NC: ACTION for Child Protection.

Hollis, F., & Woods, M. (1981). *Casework: A psychosocial therapy* (3rd ed.). New York: Random House.

Holmes, G. R., & Offen, L. (1996). Clinicians' hypotheses regarding clients' problems: Are they less likely to hypothesize sexual abuse in male compared to female clients? *Child Abuse & Neglect, 20,* 493–501.

Holmes, G. R., Offen, L., & Waller, G. (1997). See no evil, hear no evil, speak no evil: Why do relatively few male victims of childhood sexual abuse receive help for abuse-related issues in adulthood? *Clinical Psychology Review, 17,* 69–88.

Holmes, W.C . (1997). Association between a history of childhood sexual abuse and subsequent, adolescent psychoactive substance use disorder in a sample of HIV seropositive men. *Journal of Adolescent Health, 20,* 414–419.

Holmes, W. C., & Slap, G. B. (1998). Sexual abuse of boys: Definition, prevalence, correlates, sequelae, and management. *Journal of the American Medical Association, 280,* 1855–1862.

Hopper, J. W., & van der Kolk, B. A. (2001). Retrieving, assessing, and classifying traumatic memories: A preliminary report on three case studies of a new standardized method. *Journal of Aggression, Maltreatment, and Trauma, 4,* 33–71.

Hornstein, N. D., & Putnam, F. W. (1992). Clinical phenomenology of child and adolescent dissociative disorders. *Journal of the American Academy of Child and Adolescent Psychiatry, 31,* 1077–1085.

Horowitz, M. J. (1986). Stress response syndromes: A review of post-traumatic and adjustment disorders. *Hospital and Community Psychiatry, 37,* 241–249.

Horowitz, M. J. (2001). *Stress response syndromes* (3rd ed.). New York: Jason Aronson.

House Report Number 103-393. Retrieved October 1, 2002, from www.ojjdp.ncjrs.org/pubs/guidelines.

Hunter, J. A., Jr. (1991). A comparison of the psychosocial maladjustment of adult males and females sexually molested as children. *Journal of Interpersonal Violence, 6,* 205–217.

Hunter, J. A., Jr., & Becker, J. V. (1994). The role of deviant sexual arousal in juvenile sexual offending: Etiology, evaluation, and treatment. *Criminal Justice and Behavior, 21,* 132–149.

Hunter, M. (1990a). *The sexually abused male: Prevalence, impact, and treatment* (Vol. 1). Lexington, MA: Lexington Books.

Hunter, M. (1990b). *The sexually abused male: Application of treatment strategies* (Vol. 2). Lexington, MA: Lexington Books.

Hunter, M. (1995). Uncovering the relationship between a client's adult compulsive sexual behavior and childhood sexual abuse. In M. Hunter (Ed.), *Adult survivors of sexual abuse: Treatment innovations*, (pp. 56–79). Thousand Oaks, CA: Sage.

Hussey, D. L., Strom, G., & Singer, M. (1992). Male victims of sexual abuse: An analysis of adolescent psychiatric inpatients. *Child and Adolescent Social Work Journal, 9*, 491–503.

Huston, R. L., Parra, J. M., Prihoda, T. J., & Foulds, D. M. (1995). Characteristics of childhood sexual abuse in a predominately Mexican-American population. *Child Abuse & Neglect, 19*, 165–176.

Huston, R. L., Prihoda, T. J., Parra, J. M., & Foulds, D. M. (1997). Factors associated with report of penetration in child sexual abuse cases. *Journal of Child Sexual Abuse, 6*, 63–74.

Hutchings, P. S., & Dutton, M. A. (1993). Sexual assault history in a community mental health center clinical population. *Community Mental Health Journal, 29*, 59–63.

Hyde, J. S. (2000). *Understanding human sexuality* (7th ed.). New York: McGraw Hill.

Ingram, D. L., Everett, D., Lyna, P. R., White, S. T., & Rockwell, L. A. (1992). Epidemiology of adult sexually transmitted disease agents in children being evaluated for sexual abuse. *Pediatric Infectious Diseases, 11*, 945–950.

Isquith, P. K., Levine, M., & Scheiner, J. (1993). Blaming the child: Attributions of responsibility to victims of child sexual abuse. In G. S. Goodman & B. L. Bottoms (Eds.), *Child victims, child witnesses: Understanding and improving testimony* (pp. 203–228). New York: Guilford Press.

Ito, Y., Teicher, M. H., Glod, C. A., & Ackerman, E. (1998). Preliminary evidence for aberrant cortical development in abused children: A quantitative EEG study. *Journal of Neuropsychiatry and Clinical Neurosciences, 10*, 298–307.

Ito, Y., Teicher, M. H., Glod, C. A., Harper, D., Magnus, E., & Gelbard, H. A. (1993). Increased prevalence of electrophysiological abnormalities in children with psychological, physical, and sexual abuse. *Journal of Neuropsychiatry and Clinical Neurosciences, 5*, 401–408.

Jackson, H., & Nutall, R. (1993). Clinician responses to sexual abuse allegations. *Child Abuse & Neglect, 17*, 127–143.

Jacobs, J. E., Hashima, P. Y., & Kenning, M. (1995). Children's perceptions of the risk of sexual abuse. *Child Abuse & Neglect, 19*, 1443–1456.

Jacobson, A., & Richardson, B. (1987). Assault experiences of 100 psychiatric inpatients: Evidence of the need for routine inquiry. *American Journal of Psychiatry, 144*, 908–913.

Janoff-Bulman, R. (1989). Assumptive worlds and the stress of traumatic events: Applications of the schema construct. *Social Cognition, 7*, 113–136.

Janoff-Bulman, R. (1992). *Shattered assumptions: Towards a new psychology of trauma*. New York: Free Press.

Janoff-Bulman, R., & Frieze, I. H. (1983). A theoretical perspective for understanding reactions to victimization. *Journal of Social Issues, 39*, 1–17.

Janus, M. D., Burgess, A. W., & McCormack, A. (1987). Histories of sexual abuse in adolescent male runaways. *Adolescence, 22*, 405–417.

Jenkins, P. (2001). *Pedophiles and priests: Anatomy of a contemporary crisis*. New York: Oxford University Press.

Jenny, C., & Roesler, T. A., & Poyer, K. L. (1994). Are children at risk for sexual abuse by homosexuals? *Pediatrics, 94*, 41–44.

Johnson, R. L., & Shrier, D. K. (1985). Sexual victimization of boys: Experience at an adolescent medicine clinic. *Journal of Adolescent Health Care, 6*, 372–376.

Johnson, R. L., & Shrier, D. (1987). Past sexual victimization by females by male patients in an adolescent medicine clinic population. *American Journal of Psychiatry, 144*, 650–652.

Johnson, T. C. (1989). Female child perpetrators: Children who molest other children. *Child Abuse & Neglect, 13*, 571–585.

Johnson, T. C. (1991). Identification and treatment approaches for children who molest other children. *The APSAC Advisor, 4*, 9–11, 23.

Johnson, T. C. (1999). Development of sexual behavior problems in childhood. In J. A. Shaw (Ed.), *Sexual aggression* (pp. 41–74). Washington, DC: American Psychiatric Press.

Jones, D. P. H., & McGraw, J. M. (1987). Reliable and fictitious accounts of sexual abuse in children. *Journal of Interpersonal Violence, 2*, 27–45.

Joseph, R. (1999). The neurology of traumatic "dissociative" amnesia: Commentary and literature review. *Child Abuse & Neglect, 23*, 715–727.

Jumper, S. A. (1995). A meta-analysis of the relationship of child sexual abuse to adult psychological adjustment. *Child Abuse & Neglect, 19*, 715–728.

Kahn, T. J., & Chambers, H. J. (1991). Assessing reoffense risk with juvenile sex offenders. *Bulletin of the Child Welfare League of America, 70*, 333–345.

Kalichman, S. C. (1992). Clinician's attributions of responsibility for sexual and physical child abuse: An investigation of case-specific influences. *Journal of Child Sexual Abuse, 1*, 33–47.

Kalichman, S. C., Craig, M. E., & Follingstad, D. R. (1990). Professionals' adherence to mandatory child abuse reporting laws: Effects of responsibility attribution, confidence ratings, and situational factors. *Child Abuse & Neglect, 14*, 69–77.

Kaplan, H. I., & Sadock, B. J. (1998). *Synopsis of psychiatry: Behavioral sciences/clinical psychiatry* (8th ed.). Philadelphia: Lippincott, Williams & Wilkins.

Kaplan, H. I., & Sadock, B. J. (1999). *Comprehensive textbook of psychiatry* (7th ed.). Baltimore: Lippincott, Williams & Wilkins.

Karp, C. L., Butler, T. L., & Bergstrom, S. C. (1998). *Treatment strategies for abused adolescents: From victim to survivor.* Thousand Oaks, CA: Sage.

Kasl, C. D. (1990). Female perpetrators of sexual abuse: A feminist view. In M. Hunter (Ed.), *The sexually abused male: Vol. 1. Prevalence, impact, and treatment* (pp. 259–274). Lexington, MA: D. C. Heath.

Kaufman, K. L., Hilliker, D. R., & Daleiden, E. (1996). Subgroup differences in the modus operandi of adolescent sexual offenders. *Child Maltreatment, 1*, 17–24.

Keary, K., & Fitzpatrick, C. (1994). Children's disclosure of sexual abuse during formal investigation. *Child Abuse & Neglect, 18*, 543–548.

Kelley, S. J. (1990). Parental stress response to sexual abuse and ritualistic abuse of children in daycare centers. *Nursing Research, 39*, 25–29.

Kelley, S. J., Brant, R., & Waterman, J. (1993). Sexual abuse of children in day care centers. *Child Abuse & Neglect, 17*, 71–89.

Kellogg, N. D. & Hoffman, T. J. (1995). Unwanted and illegal sexual experiences in childhood and adolescence. *Child Abuse & Neglect, 19*, 1457-1468.

Kellogg, N. D., & Hoffman, T. J. (1997). Child sexual revictimization by multiple perpetrators. *Child Abuse & Neglect, 21*, 953–964.

Kellogg, N. D., Parra, J. M., & Menard, S. (1998). Children with anogenital symptoms and signs referred for sexual abuse evaluators. *Archives of Pediatrics and Adolescent Medicine, 152*, 634–641.

Kelly, R. J., Wood, J. J., Gonzalez, L. S., MacDonald, V., & Waterman, J. (2002). Effects of mother-son incest and positive perceptions of sexual abuse experiences on the psychosocial adjustment of clinic-referred men. *Child Abuse & Neglect, 26*, 425–441.

Kempe, C. H., Silverman, F. N., Steele, B. F., Droegemiller, W., & Silver, H. K. (1962). The battered child syndrome. *Journal of the American Medical Association, 181*, 17–24.

Kendall, P. C., & Hollon, S. D. (1981). *Assessment strategies for cognitive-behavioral interventions.* New York: Academic Press.

Kendall-Tackett, K. A., & Simon, A. F. (1992). A comparison of the abuse experiences of male and female adults molested as children. *Journal of Family Violence, 7*, 57–62.

Kendall-Tackett, K. A., & Watson, M. W. (1991). Factors that influence professionals' perceptions of behavioral indicators of child sexual abuse. *Journal of Interpersonal Violence, 6*, 385–395.

Kendall-Tackett, K. A., Williams, L. M., & Finkelhor, D. (1993). Impact of sexual abuse on children: A review and synthesis of recent empirical studies. *Psychological Bulletin, 113*, 164–180.

Kenny, M. C. (2001). Child abuse reporting: Teachers' perceived deterrents. *Child Abuse & Neglect, 25*, 81–92.

Kernberg, O. F. (1976). *Object relations theory and clinical psychoanalysis*. New York: Jason Aronson.

Kernberg, O. (1980). *Internal world and external reality*. New York: Jason Aronson.

Kessler, R. C., Sonnega, A., Bromet, E., Hughes, M., & Nelson, C. B. (1995). Post-traumatic stress disorder in the National Comorbidity Survey. *Archives of General Psychiatry, 52*, 1048–1060.

Kilpatrick, D. G., & Saunders, B. E. (1997). *The prevalence and consequences of child victimization: Results from the National Survey of Adolescents* (Final Report - 181028). Washington, DC: United States Department of Justice, National Institute of Justice, Office of Justice Programs.

Kinard, E. M. (2001). Perceived and actual academic competence in maltreated children. *Child Abuse & Neglect, 25*, 33–45.

Kinsey, A. C., Pomeroy, W. B., Martin, C. E., & Gebhard, P. H. (1953). *Sexual behavior in the human female*. Philadelphia: Saunders.

Kipke, M. D., Unger, J. B., O'Connor, S., Palmer, R. F. & LaFrance, S. R. (1997). Street youth, their peer group affiliation and differences according to residential status, subsistence patterns, and use of services. *Adolescence, 32*, 265–291.

Kirby, J. S., Chu, J. A., & Dill, D. L. (1993). Correlates of dissociative symptomatology in patients with physical and sexual histories. *Comprehensive Psychiatry, 34*, 258–263.

Kirschbaum, L., Wust, S., & Hellhammer, D. (1992). Consistent sex differences in cortisol responses to psychological stress. *Psychosomatic Medicine, 54*, 648–657.

Kiser, L. J., Ackerman, B. J., Brown, E., Edwards, N. B., McColgan, E., Pugh, R., & Pruitt, D. B. (1988). Post-traumatic stress disorder in young children: A reaction to purported sexual abuse. *Journal of the American Academy of Child and Adolescent Psychiatry, 27*, 645–649.

Kisiel, C. L., & Lyons, J. S. (2001). Dissociation as a mediator of psychopathology among sexually abused children and adolescents. *American Journal of Psychiatry, 158*, 1034–1039.

Klein, I., & Janoff-Bulman, R. (1996). Trauma history and personal narratives: Some clues to coping among survivors of child abuse. *Child Abuse & Neglect, 20*, 45–54.

Knight, R. A., & Prentsky, R. A. (1993). Exploring characteristics for classifying juvenile sex offenders. In H. E. Barbaree, W. L. Marshall, & S. M. Hudson (Eds.), *The juvenile sex offender* (pp. 45–83). New York: Guilford Press.

Knopp, F. H., & Lackey, L. B. (1987). *Female sexual abusers: A summary of data from 44 treatment providers*. Orwell, VT: Safer Society Press.

Kobayashi, J. (1995). Perceived parental deviance, parent-child bonding, child abuse and child sexual aggression. *Sexual Abuse: A Journal of Research and Treatment, 7*, 25–44.

Kohlberg, L. (1966). A cognitive-developmental analysis of children's sex-role concepts and attitudes. In E. E. Maccoby (Ed.), *The development of sex differences* (pp. 82–173). Stanford, CA: Stanford University Press.

Kohut, H. (1959). Introspection, empathy and psychoanalysis. *Journal of the American Psychoanalytic Association, 7*, 459–483.

Kohut, H. (1977). *The restoration of the self*. New York: International Universities Press.

Kohut, H. (1984). *How does analysis cure?* Chicago: University of Chicago Press.

Kolko, D. J., Moser, J. T., & Weldy, S. R. (1988). Behavioral/emotional indicators of sexual abuse in child psychiatric inpatients: A controlled comparison with physical abuse. *Child Abuse and Neglect, 12*, 529–541.

Kolko, D. J., Selelyo, F., & Brown, E. J. (1999). The treatment histories and service involvement of physically and sexually abusive families: Description, correspondence, and clinical correlates. *Child Abuse & Neglect, 23*, 459–476.

Kollack-Walker, S., Day, H. E. W., & Akil, H. (2000). Central stress neurocircuits. In G. Fink (Ed.), *Encyclopedia of stress* (Vol. 1, pp. 414–422). San Diego, CA: Academic Press.

Korbin, J. E., Coulton, C. J., Lindstrom-Ufuti, H., & Spilsbury, J. (2000). Neighborhood views on the definition and etiology of child maltreatment. *Child Abuse & Neglect, 24*, 1509–1527.

Kornheiser, T. (1998, January 8). Kennedy's story is a profile in courage. *The Washington Post*, D1, D2.

Krivacska, J. J. (1990). *Designing child sexual abuse prevention programs: Current approaches and a proposal for the prevention, reduction and identification of sexual misuse.* Springfield, IL: Charles C. Thomas.

Krug, R. (1989). Adult male report of sexual abuse by mothers: Case descriptions, motivations and long-term consequences. *Child Abuse and Neglect, 13,* 111–119.

Krystal, H. (1978). Trauma and effects. *Psychoanalytic Study of the Child, 33,* 81–116.

Krystal, H. (1988). *Integration and self healing.* Hillsdale, NJ: Analytic Press.

Krystal, J. H., Kosten, T. R., Southwick, S., Mason, J. W., Perry, B. D., & Giller, E. L. (1989). Neurobiological aspects of PTSD: Review of clinical and preclinical studies. *Behavior Therapy, 20,* 177–198.

Krystal, J. H., Southwick, S. M., & Charney, D. S. (1995). Post traumatic stress disorder: Psychological mechanisms of traumatic remembrance. In D. L. Schacter (Ed.), *Memory distortion: How minds, brains, and societies reconstruct the past* (pp. 150–172). Cambridge, MA: Harvard University Press.

Lab, D. D., Feigenbaum, J. D., & De Silva, P. (2000). Mental health professionals' attitudes and practices toward male childhood sexual abuse. *Child Abuse & Neglect, 24,* 391–409.

Lamb, S. (1986). Treating sexually abused children: Issues of blame and responsibility. *American Journal of Orthopsychiatry, 56,* 303–463.

Lamb, S., & Edgar-Smith, S. (1994). Aspects of disclosure: Mediators of outcome of childhood sexual abuse. *Journal of Interpersonal Violence, 9,* 307–326.

Lambert, J. D. C. (2000). GABA (Gamma aminobutyric acid). In G. Fink (Ed.). *Encyclopedia of stress* (Vol. 2, pp. 177–190). San Diego, CA: Academic Press.

Lambie, I., Seymour, F., Lee, A., & Adams, P. (2002). Resiliency in the victim-offender cycle in male sexual abuse. *Sexual Abuse: A Journal of Research and Treatment, 14,* 31–48.

Lanktree, C., Briere, J., & Zaidi, L. (1991). Incidence and impact of sexual abuse in a child outpatient sample: The role of direct inquiry. *Child Abuse & Neglect, 15,* 447–453.

Lauer, R., & Handel, W. (1983). *Social psychology: The theory and application of social interaction* (2nd ed.). Boston: Houghton Mifflin.

Lawson, C. (1993). Mother-son sexual abuse: Rare or underreported? A critique of the research. *Child Abuse & Neglect, 17,* 261–269.

Lawson, L. & Chaffin, M. (1992). False negatives in sexual abuse disclosure interviews: Incidence and influence of caretaker's belief in abuse in cases of accidental abuse discovery by diagnosis of STD. *Journal of Interpersonal Violence, 7,* 532–542.

Lebowitz, L., Harvey, M. R., & Herman, J. L. (1993). A stage-by-dimension model of recovery from sexual trauma. *Journal of Interpersonal Violence, 8,* 378–391.

LeDoux, J. E. (1992). Emotion as memory: Anatomical systems underlying indelible neural traces. In S. A. Christianson (Ed.), *Handbook of emotion and memory* (pp. 269–288). Hillsdale, NJ: Lawrence Erlbaum.

LeDoux, J. E. (1994). Emotion, memory and the brain. *Scientific American, 270,* 50–57.

LeDoux, J. E. (1995). Emotion: Clues from the brain. *Annual Review of Psychology, 46,* 209–235.

LeDoux, J. E. (1996). *The emotional brain: The mysterious underpinning of emotional life.* New York: Simon & Schuster.

LeDoux. J. E., Romanski, L., & Xagoraris, A. (1991). Indelibilitiy of subcortical emotional memories. *Journal of Cognitive Neuroscience, 1,* 238–243.

Lee, J. D. P., Jackson, H. J., Pattison, P., & Ward, T. (2002). Developmental risk factors for sexual offending. *Child Abuse & Neglect, 26,* 73–92.

Leserman, J., Drossman, D. A., Li, Z., Toomey, T. C., Nachman, G., & Glogau, L. (1996). Sexual and physical abuse history in gastroenterology practice: How types of abuse impact health status. *Psychosomatic Medicine, 58,* 4–15

Leverich, G. S., McElroy, S. L., Suppes, T., Keck, P. E., Jr., Denicoff, K. D., Nolen, W. A., Altshuler, L. L., Rush, A. J., Kupka, R., Frye, M. A., Autio, K. A., & Post, R. M. (2002). Early physical and sexual abuse associated with an adverse course of bipolar illness. *Biological Psychiatry, 51,* 288–297.

Levesque, R. J. R. (1994). Sex differences in the experience of child sexual victimization. *Journal of Family Violence, 9,* 357–369.

Levitan, R. D., Parikh, S. V., Lesage, A. D., Megadoren, K. M., Adams, M., Kennedy, S. H., & Goering, P. N. (1998). Major depression in individuals with a history of childhood physical or sexual abuse: Relationship to neurovegetative features, mania, and gender. *American Journal of Psychiatry, 155,* 1746–1752.

Levy, M. S. (1998). A helpful way to conceptualize and understand reenactments. *Journal of Psychotherapy Practice and Research, 7,* 227–235.

Lew, M. (1988). *Victims no longer: Men recovering from incest and other sexual child abuse.* New York: Nevraumont.

Lew, M. (1990). *Victims no longer: Men recovering from incest and other sexual abuse* (2nd ed.). New York: Harper & Row.

Lewis, D. O., Yeager, C. A., Swica, Y., Pincus, J. H., & Lewis, M. (1997). Objective documentation of child abuse and dissociation in 12 murderers with dissociative identity disorder. *American Journal of Psychiatry, 154,* 1703–1710.

Lichtenberg, J., Bornstein, M., & Silver, D. (Eds.). (1984). *Empathy I.* Hillsdale, NJ: Analytic Press.

Liggan, D. Y., & Kay, J. (1999). Some neurobiological aspects of psychotherapy. *Journal of Psychotherapy Practice and Research, 8,* 103–114.

Lindegren, M. L., Hanson, I. C., Hammett, T. A., Beil, J., Fleming, P. L., & Ward, J. W. (1998). Sexual abuse of children: Intersection with HIV epidemic. *Pediatrics, 102,* 46. Available online: www.pediatrics.org/cqi/content/full/102/4/e46.

Lindsay, D., & Embree, J. (1992). Sexually transmitted diseases: A significant complication of childhood sexual abuse. *Canadian Journal of Infectious Diseases, 3,* 122–128.

Linton, S. J. (1997). A population-based study of the relationship between sexual abuse and back pain: Establishing a link. *Pain, 73,* 47–53.

Lipshires, L. (1994). Female perpetration of child sexual abuse: An overview of the problem. *Moving Forward Newsjournal, 2.* Available online: www.movingforward.org/v2n6-cover.html.

Lisak, D. (1994a). The psychological impact of sexual abuse: Content analysis of interviews with male survivors. *Journal of Traumatic Stress, 7,* 525–548

Lisak, D. (1994b). Subjective assessment of relationships with parents by sexually aggressive and nonaggressive men. *Journal of Interpersonal Violence, 9,* 399–411.

Lisak, D. (1995). Integrating a critique of gender in the treatment of male survivors of childhood abuse. *Psychopathology, 32,* 258–269.

Lisak, D., & Luster, L. (1994). Educational, occupational, and relationship histories of men who were sexually and/or physically abused as children. *Journal of Traumatic Stress, 4,* 507–523.

Lister, E. (1982). Forced silence: A neglected dimension of trauma. *American Journal of Psychiatry, 139,* 872–876.

Little, L., & Hamby, S.L. (2001). Memory of childhood sexual abuse among clinicians: Characteristics, outcomes, and current therapy attitudes. *Sexual Abuse: A Journal of Research and Treatment, 13,* 233–248.

Livingston, R., Lawson, L., & Jones, J. J. (1993). Predictors of self-reported psychopathology in children abused repeatedly by a parent. *Journal of the American Academy of Child and Adolescent Psychiatry, 32,* 948–953.

Locke, G. R., III. (1996). The epidemiology of functional gastrointestinal disorders in North America. *Gastroenterology Clinics of North America, 25,* 1–19.

Lodico, M. A., Gruber, E., & DiClemente, R. J. (1996). Childhood sexual abuse and coercive sex among school-based adolescents in a midwestern state. *Journal of Adolescent Health, 18,* 211–217.

Lofland, J., & Lofland, L. (1995). *Analyzing social settings: A guide to qualitative observation and analysis* (3rd ed.). Belmont, CA: Wadsworth.

Loftus, E. F., & Ketcham, K. (1994). *The myth of repressed memory: False memories and allegations of sexual abuse.* New York: St. Martin's Press.

Longstreth, G. F., & Wolde-Tsadik, G. (1993). Irritable bowel-type symptoms in HOM examinees:

Prevalence, demographics, and clinical correlates. *Digestive Diseases and Sciences, 38,* 1581–1589.

Lott, D. A. (1998). Brain development, attachment and impact on psychic vulnerability. *Psychiatric Times, 15,* 1–6.

Lovallo, W. R., & Sollers, J. J., III. (2000). Autonomic nervous system. In G. Fink (Ed.)., *Encyclopedia of stress* (Vol. 1, pp. 275–284). San Diego, CA: Academic Press.

Lowman, J. (1987). Taking young prostitutes seriously. *Canadian Review of Sociology and Anthropology, 24,* 103.

Lundberg, U. (2000). Catecholamines. In G. Fink (Ed.), *Encyclopedia of stress* (Vol. 1, pp. 408–413). San Diego, CA: Academic Press.

Luster, T., & Small, S. A. (1994). Factors associated with sexual risk-taking behaviors among adolescents. *Journal of Marriage and the Family, 56,* 622–632.

Lynch, D. L., Stern, A. E., Oates, K., & O'Toole, B. I. (1993). Who participates in child sexual abuse research? *Journal of Child Psychology and Psychiatry, 34,* 935–944.

Lynskey, M. T., & Fergusson, D. M. (1997). Factors protecting against the development of adjustment difficulties in young adults exposed to childhood sexual abuse. *Child Abuse & Neglect, 21,* 1177–1190.

Macfie, J., Cicchetti, D., & Toth, S.L. (2001). Dissociation in maltreated versus nonmaltreated preschool-aged children. *Child Abuse & Neglect, 25,* 1253–1267.

MacMillan, H. L., Fleming, J. E., Streiner, D. L., Lin, E., Boyle, M. H., Jamieson, E., Duku, E. K., Walsh, C.A., Wong, M. Y. Y., & Beardslee, W. R. (2001). Childhood abuse and lifetime psychopathology in a community sample. *American Journal of Psychiatry, 158,* 1878–1883.

MacMillan, R. (2000). Adolescent victimization and income deficits in adulthood: Rethinking the costs of criminal violence from a life course perspective. *Criminology, 38,* 553–588.

MacMillan, R. (2001). Violence and the life course: The consequences of victimization for personal and social development. *Annual Reviews in Sociology, 27,* 1–22.

Maes, M., De Vos, N., Van Hunsel, F., Van West, D., Westenberg, H., Cosyns, P., & Neels, H. (2001). Pedophilia is accompanied by increased plasma concentrations of catecholamines, in particular epinephrine. *Psychiatry Research, 103,* 43–49.

Maes, M., De Vos, N., Westenberg, H., Van Hunsel, F., Hendriks, D., Cosyns, P., & Scharpé, S. (2001). Lower baseline plasma cortisol and prolactin with increased body temperature and higher mCPP-induced cortisol responses in men with pedophilia. *Neuropsychopharmocology, 26,* 17–26.

Mahoney, D., & Faulkner, M. (1997). *The boylove manifesto.* Retrieved September 2, 2002, from www.healthyplace.com/communities/abuse/socum/articles/pedophiles.htm.

Mahoney, M. J. (1974). *Cognition and behavioral modification.* Cambridge, MA: Ballinger.

Marlatt, G. A., & Gordon, J. R. (1985). *Relapse prevention: Maintenance strategies in the treatment of addictive behaviors.* New York: Guilford Press.

Marmar, C. R., Foy, D., Kagan, B., & Pynoos, R. S. (1994). An integrated approach for treating poststraumatic stress. In R. Pynoos (Ed.), *Posttraumatic stress disorder: A clinical review* (pp. 99–132). Lutherville, MD: Sidran Press.

Marshall, W. L. (1993). The role of attachments, intimacy, and loneliness in the etiology and maintenance of sexual offending. *Sexual and Marital Therapy, 8,* 109–121.

Marshall, W. L., Hamilton, K., & Fernandez, Y.M. (2001). Empathy deficits and cognitive distortions in child molesters. *Sexual Abuse: A Journal of Research and Treatment, 13,* 123–130.

Marshall, W. L., & Mazzucco, A. (1995). Self-esteem and parental attachments in child molesters. *Sexual Abuse: A Journal of Research and Treatment, 7,* 279–285.

Marshall, W. L., Serran, G. A., & Cortoni, F. A. (2000). Childhood attachments, sexual abuse, and their relationship to adult coping in child molesters. *Sexual Abuse: A Journal of Research and Treatment, 12,* 17–26.

Marshall, W. N., & Locke, C., Jr. (1997). Statewide survey of physician attitudes to controversies about child abuse. *Child Abuse & Neglect, 21,* 171–179.

Mason, W. A., Zimmerman, L., & Evans, W. (1998). Sexual and physical abuse among incarcerated youth: Implications for sexual behavior, contraceptive use, and teenage pregnancy. *Child Abuse & Neglect, 22,* 987–995.

Masson, J.M. (1984). *The assault on truth.* New York: Farrar, Straus & Giroux.

Masten, A. S., Best, K. M., & Garmezy, N. (1990). Resilience and development: Contributions from the study of children who overcame adversity. *Development and Psychopathology, 2,* 425–444.

Mathews, R. (1989). *Female sexual offenders: An exploratory study.* Brandon, VT: Safer Society Press.

Mathew, S. J., Coplan, J. D., Smith, E. L. P., Schoepp, D. D., Rosenblum, L. A., & Gorman, J. M. (2001). Glutamate-hypothalamic-pituitary-adrenal axis interactions: Implications for mood and anxiety disorders. *CNS Spectrums, 6,* 656–572.

Matthews, J. K. (1994). Working with female sexual abusers. In M. Elliott (Ed.), *Female sexual abuse of children* (pp. 57–73). New York: Guilford Press.

Matthews, J., Matthews, R., & Speltz, K. (1991). Female sexual offenders: A typology. In M.Q. Patton (Ed.), *Family sexual abuse: Frontline research and evaluation* (pp. 199–219). Newbury Park, CA: Sage.

Matthews, R., Hunter, J. A., & Vuz, J. (1997). Juvenile female sexual offenders: Clinical characteristics and treatment issues. *Sexual Abuse: A Journal of Research and Treatment, 9,* 187–199.

May, R., & Yalom, I. (1995). Existential psychotherapy. In R.J. Corsini & D. Wedding (Eds.), *Current psychotherapies* (5th ed., pp. 262–292). Itasca, IL: F. E. Peacock.

Mayer, A. (1992). *Women sex offenders: Treatment and dynamics.* Holmes Beach, FL: Learning Publications.

McCann, I. L., & Pearlman, L. A. (1990). Vicarious traumatization: A framework for understanding the psychological effects of working with victims. *Journal of Traumatic Stress, 3,* 131–149.

McCann, J., Reay, D., Siebert, J., Stephens, B. G., & Wirtz, S. (1996). Postmortem perianal findings in children. *American Journal of Forensic Medicine and Pathology, 17,* 289–298.

McCann, J., & Voris, J. (1993). Perianal injuries resulting from sexual abuse: A longitudinal study. *Pediatrics, 91,* 390–397.

McCarty, L. (1986). Mother-child incest: Characteristics of the offender. *Child Welfare, 65,* 447–458.

McCauley, M. R., & Parker, J. F. (2001). When will a child be believed? The impact of the victim's age and juror's gender on children's credibility and verdict in a sexual-abuse case. *Child Abuse & Neglect, 25,* 523–539.

McClellan, J., Adams, J., Douglas, D., McCurry, C., & Storck, M. (1995). Clinical characteristics related to severity of sexual abuse: A study of seriously mentally ill youth. *Child Abuse & Neglect, 19,* 1245–1254.

McClellan, J., McCurry, C., Ronnei, M., Adams, J., Storck, M., Eisner, A., & Smith, C. (1997). Relationship between sexual abuse, gender, and sexually inappropriate behaviors in seriously mentally ill youths. *Journal of the American Academy of Child and Adolescent Psychiatry, 36,* 959–965.

McEwen, B. (2000a). Allostasis and allostatic load: Implications for neuropsychopharmacology. *Neuropsychopharmacology, 22,* 108–124.

McEwen, B. (2000b). Effects of adversive experiences for brain structure and function. *Biological Psychiatry, 48,* 721–731.

McGaugh, J. L. (1992). Affect, neuromodulatory systems, and memory storage. In S. A. Christianson (Ed.), *Handbook on emotion and memory* (pp. 245–268). Hillsdale, NJ: Lawrence Erlbaum.

McGee, R. A., Wolfe, D. A., & Wilson, S. K. (1997). Multiple maltreatment experiences and adolescent behavior problems: Adolescents' problems. *Development and Psychopathology, 9,* 131–149.

McKelvey, R. S., & Webb, J. A. (1995). A pilot study of abuse among Vietnamese Amerasians. *Child Abuse & Neglect, 19,* 545–553.

McKibben, A., Proulx, J., & Lussier, P. (2001). Sexual aggressors' perceptions of effectiveness of strategies to cope with negative emotions and deviant sexual fantasies. *Sexual Abuse: A Journal of Research and Treatment, 13*, 257–273.

McLeer, S. V., Callaghan, M., Henry, D., & Wallen, J. (1994). Psychiatric disorders in sexually abused children. *Journal of the American Academy of Child and Adolescent Psychiatry, 33*, 313–319.

McLeer, S. V., Deblinger, E., Henry, D., & Orvaschel, H. (1992). Sexually abused children at high risk for post traumatic stress disorder. *Journal of the American Academy of Child and Adolescent Psychiatry, 31*, 875–879.

McLeer, S. V., Dixon, J. F., Henry, D., Ruggiero, K., Escovitz, K., Niedda, T., & Scholle, R. (1998). Psychopathology in non-clinically referred sexually abused children. *Journal of the American Academy of Child and Adolescent Psychiatry, 37*, 1326–1333.

Meiselman, K. (1979). *Incest: A psychological study of causes and effects with treatment recommendations.* San Francisco: Jossey-Bass.

Meiselman, K. (1990). *Resolving the trauma of incest: Reintegration therapy with survivors.* San Francisco: Jossey-Bass.

Melchert, T. P. (1996). Childhood memory and a history of different forms of abuse. *Professional Psychology: Research and Practice, 27*, 438–446.

Melchert, T. P. (1998). Family of origin history, psychological distress, quality of childhood memory, and content of first and recovered childhood memories. *Child Abuse & Neglect, 22*, 1203–1216.

Melchert, T. P., & Parker, R. L. (1997). Different forms of child abuse and memory. *Child Abuse & Neglect, 21*, 125–135.

Mendel, M. P. (1995). *The male survivor: The impact of sexual abuse.* Beverly Hills, CA: Sage.

Merry, S., & Andrews, L. (1994). Psychiatric status of sexually abused children 12 months after disclosure of abuse. *Journal of the American Association of Child and Adolescent Psychiatry, 33*, 939–944.

Meyer, C. (Ed.). (1983). *Clinical social work in the eco-systems perspective.* New York: Columbia University Press.

Meyerson, L. A., Long, P. J., Miranda, R., Jr., & Marx, B. P. (2002). The influence of childhood sexual abuse, physical abuse, family environment and gender on the psychological adjustment of adolescents. *Child Abuse & Neglect, 26*, 387–405.

Mian, M., Wehrspann, W., Klajner-Diamond, H., LeBaron, D., & Winder, C. (1986). Review of one hundred and twenty-five children six years of age and under who were sexually abused. *Child Abuse and Neglect, 10*, 223–229.

Mills, A. (1993). Helping male victims of sexual abuse. *Nursing Standard, 7*, 36–39.

Miner, M. H., & Crimmins, C. L. S. (1995). Adolescent sex offenders: Issues of etiology and risk factors. In B. K. Schwartz & H. R. Cellini (Eds.), *The sexual offender: Vol. 1. Corrections, treatment, and legal practice* (pp. 9.1–9.15). Kingston, NJ: Civic Research Institute.

Miner, M. H., Siekert, G. P., & Ackland, M. A. (1997). *Evaluation: Juvenile sex offender treatment programs, Minnesota Correctional Facility—Sauk Centre, Final Report, Biennium 1995–1997.* Minneapolis: University of Minnesota, Department of Family Practice and Community Health, Program in Human Sexuality.

Moisan, P. A., Sanders-Phillips, K., & Moisan, P. M. (1997). Ethnic differences in circumstances of abuse and symptoms of depression and anger among sexually abused black and latino boys. *Child Abuse & Neglect, 21*, 473–488.

Molnar, B. E., Berkman, L. F., & Buka, S. L. (2001). Psychopathology, childhood sexual abuse and other childhood adversities: Relative links to subsequent suicidal behavior in the United States. *Psychological Medicine, 31*, 965–977.

Money, J. (1987). Sin, sickness or status? Homosexual and gender identity and psychoneuroendocrinology. *American Psychologist, 42*, 384–399.

Money, J., & Wiedeking, C. (1980). Gender identity/role: Normal differentiation and its transitions. In B. B. Wolman & J. Money (Eds.), *Handbook of human sexuality* (pp. 269–284). Englewood Cliff, NJ: Prentice Hall.

Moore, B. E., & Fine, B. D. (1990). *Psychoanalytic terms and concepts.* Binghamton, NY: Vail-Ballow Press.

Moore. (1992).

Morgan, C. A., Hazlett, G., Want, S., Richardson, E. G., Jr., Schnurr, P., & Southwick, S. M. (2001). Symptoms of dissociation in humans experiencing acute, uncontrollable stress: A prospective investigation. *American Journal of Psychiatry, 158*, 1239–1427.

Morrell, B., Mendel, M., & Fischer, L. (2001). Object relations disturbances in sexually abused males. *Journal of Interpersonal Violence, 16*, 851–864.

Morrow, J., Yeager, C. A., & Lewis, D. O. (1997). Encopresis and sexual abuse in a sample of boys in residential treatment. *Child Abuse & Neglect, 21*, 11–18.

Mraovich, L. R., & Wilson, J. F. (1999). Patterns of child abuse and neglect associated with chronological age of children living in a midwestern county. *Child Abuse & Neglect, 23*, 899–903.

Mulder, R. T., Beautrais, A. L., Joyce, P. R., & Fergusson, D. M. (1998). Relationship between dissociation, childhood sexual abuse, childhood physical abuse, and mental illness in a general population sample. *American Journal of Psychiatry, 155*, 806–811.

Murphy, W. D., & Peters, J. M. (1992). Profiling child sexual abusers: Psychological considerations. *Criminal Justice and Behavior, 19*, 24–37.

Murphy, W. D., & Smith, T. A. (1996). Sex offenders against children: Empirical and clinical issues. In J. Briere, L. Berliner, J. A. Bulkley, C. Jenny, & T. Reid (Eds.), *The APSAC handbook on child maltreatment* (pp. 175–191). Thousands Oaks, CA: Sage.

Myers, J. E. B. (1994). *The backlash: Child protection under fire.* Thousand Oaks, CA: Sage.

Myers, J. E. B. (1995). New era of skepticism regarding children's credibility. Special theme: Suggestibility of child witnesses: The social science amicus brief in State of New Jersey vs. Margaret Kelly Michaels. *Psychology, Public Policy, and Law, 1*, 387–398.

Nagel, D. E., Putnam, F. W., Noll, J. G., & Trickett, P. K. (1997). Disclosure patterns of sexual abuse and psychological functioning at a 1-year follow-up. *Child Abuse & Neglect, 19*, 137–147.

Nagy, S., Adcock, A. G., & Nagy, M. C. (1994). A comparison of risky health behaviors of sexually active, sexually abused, and abstaining adolescents. *Pediatrics, 93*, 570–575.

Nasjleti, M. (1980). Suffering in silence: The male incest victim. *Child Welfare, 59*, 269–275.

National Center for Victims of Crime. (1995a). *FYI: Male rape.* Arlington, VA.

National Center for Victims of Crime. (1995b). *FYI: Sexual assault legislation.* Arlington, VA.

National Center on Child Abuse and Neglect. (1989). *Study findings: Study of the national incidence and prevalence of child abuse and neglect (NIS-2).* Washington, DC: U. S. Department of Health and Human Services.

National Center on Child Abuse and Neglect. (1994). *Child maltreatment 1992: Reports from the States to the National Child Abuse and Neglect Data System.* Washington, DC: U.S. Department of Health and Human Services.

National Center on Child Abuse and Neglect. (1998). *Child maltreatment 1996: Reports from the States to the National Child Abuse and Neglect Data System.* Washington, DC: U.S. Government Printing Office.

National Committee to Prevent Child Abuse. (2002). *Web page information.* Retrieved/October 18, 2002, from www.childabuse.org.

National Research Council. (1993). *Understanding child abuse and neglect.* Washington, DC: National Academy Press.

National Task Force on Juvenile Sexual Offending. (1993). *Final report.* Boulder, CO: National Adolescent Perpetrator Network, C.H. Kempe National Center, University of Colorado Health Services Center.

Neisen, J. H., & Sandall, H. (1990). Alcohol and other drug abuse in a gay/lesbian population: Related to victimization? *Journal of Psychology and Human Services, 3*, 151–168.

Nelson, E. C., Heath, A. C., Madden, P. A. F., Cooper, M. L., Dinwiddie, S. H., Bucholz, K. K.,

Glowinski, A., McLaughlin, T., Dunne, M. P., Statham, D. J., & Martin, N. G. (2002). Association between self-reported childhood sexual abuse and adverse psychosocial outcomes: Results from a twin study. *Archives of General Psychiatry, 59*, 139–145.

Nemeroff, C., Heim, C., Owens, M., Newport, J., Miller, A., & Plotsky, P. (1999). *Neurochemical mechanisms underlying depression and anxiety disorders: The influence of early trauma.* New Developments in Understanding Depression and Its Treatment. Monograph. Wyeth-Ayerst Laboratories.

Neumark-Sztainer, D., & Hannan, P. J. (2000). Weight-related behaviors among adolescent boys and girls: Results from a national survey. *Archives of Pediatric and Adolescent Medicine, 154*, 569–577.

Newberger, C. M., Gremy, I. M., Waternauz, C. M., & Newberger, E. H. (1993). Mothers of sexually abused children: Trauma and repair in longitudinal perspective. *American Journal of Orthopsychiatry, 63*, 92–102.

Nutt, D.J. (2000). The psychobiology of posttraumatic stress disorder. *Journal of Clinical Psychiatry, 61*(Suppl. 5), 24–29.

Nutall, R., & Jackson, H. (1994). Personal history of childhood abuse among clinicians. *Child Abuse & Neglect, 18*, 455–472.

O'Brien, M. J. (1991). Taking sibling-incest seriously. In M. Q. Patton (Ed.), *Family sexual abuse: Frontline research and evaluation* (pp. 75–92). Newbury Park, CA: Sage.

Ochberg, F. M. (Ed.). (1988). *Post-traumatic therapy and victims of violence.* New York: Brunner/Mazel.

O'Donohue, W., & O'Hare, E. (1997). The credibility of sexual abuse allegations: Child sexual abuse, adult rape and sexual harassment. *Journal of Psychopathology and Behavioral Assessment, 19*, 273–279.

Ogawa, J. R., Stroufe, L. A., Weinfield, N. S., Carlson, E. A., & Egeland, B. (1997). Development and the fragmented self: A longitudinal study of dissociative symptomatology in a normative sample. *Development and Psychopathology, 9*, 855–879.

Öhman, A. (2000). Fear. In G. Fink (Ed.), *Encyclopedia of stress* (Vol. 2, pp. 111–115). San Diego, CA: Academic Press.

Okamura, A., Heras, P., & Wong-Kernberg, L. (1995). Asians, Pacific Island and Filipino Americans and sexual child abuse. In L. Fontes (Ed.), *Sexual abuse in nine North American cultures* (pp. 67–96). Thousand Oaks, CA: Sage.

Olson, P. E. (1990). The sexual abuse of boys: A study of long-term psychological effects. In M. Hunter (Ed.), *The sexually abused male: Prevalence, impact and treatment* (pp. 137–152). Lexington, MA: Lexington Books.

O'Toole, R., Webster, S. W., O'Toole, A. W., & Lucal, B. (1999). Teachers' recognition and reporting of child abuse: A factorial survey. *Child Abuse & Neglect, 23*, 1083–1101.

Paine, M. L., & Hansen, D. J. (2002). Factors influencing children to self-disclosure sexual abuse. *Clinical Psychology Review, 22*, 271–295.

Paradise, J. E. (2001). Current concepts in preventing sexual abuse. *Current Opinions in Pediatrics, 13*, 402–407.

Paul, J. P., Catania, J., Pollack, L., & Stall, R. (2001). Understanding childhood sexual abuse as a predictor of sexual risk-taking among men who have sex with men: The Urban Men's Health Study. *Child Abuse & Neglect, 25*, 557–584.

Pearce, J. W., & Pezzot-Pearce, T. D. (1997). *Psychotherapy of abused and neglected children.* New York: Guilford Press.

Pearlman, L. A., & Saakvitne, K. W. (1995). *Trauma and the therapist: Countertransference and vicarious traumatization in psychotherapy with incest survivors.* New York: W. W. Norton.

Pennebaker, J. W. (1993). Putting stress into words: Health, linguistic, and therapeutic implications. *Behavioral Research and Therapy, 31*, 539–548.

Pennebaker, J. W., Kiecolt-Glaser, J. K., & Glaser, R. (1988) Disclosure of traumas and immune function: Health implications for psychotherapy. *Journal of Consulting and Clinical Psychology, 56*, 239–245.

Perez, C., & Widom, C. (1994). Childhood victimization and long-term intellectual and academic outcomes. *Child Abuse & Neglect, 18,* 617–633.

Perry, B. D. (1997). Incubated in terror: Neurodevelopmental factors in the "cycle of violence." In J. Osofsky (Ed.), *Children, youth and violence: The search for solutions* (pp. 124–149). New York: Guilford Press.

Perry, B. D. (1999). The memories of states: How the brain stores and retrieves traumatic experience. In J. Goodwin & R. Attias, (Eds.), *Splintered reflections: Images of the body in trauma* (pp. 9–38). New York: Basic Books.

Perry, B. D. (2000). *The neuroarcheology of child maltreatment: The neurodevelopmental costs of adverse childhood events.* Retrieved April 15, 2002, from www.childtrauma.org/neuroarcheology.htm.

Perry, B. D. (2001). Violence and childhood: How persisting fear can alter the developing child's brain. In D. Schetky & E. Benedek (Eds.), *Textbook of child and adolescent forensic psychiatry* (pp. 221–238). Washington, DC: American Psychiatric Press.

Perry, B. D., & Pollard, R. (1998). Homeostasis, stress, trauma and adaptation: A neurodevelopmental view of childhood trauma. *Child and Adolescent Psychiatric Clinics of North America, 7,* 33–51.

Perry, B. D., Pollard, R. A., Blakely, T. L., Baker, W. L., & Vigilante, D. (1995). Childhood trauma, the neurobiology of adaptation, and "use-dependent" development of the brain: How states become traits. *Infant Mental Health Journal, 16,* 271–291.

Pescosolido, F. J. (1989). Sexual abuse of boys by males: Theoretical and treatment implications. In S. Sgroi (Ed.), *Vulnerable populations: Sexual abuse treatment for children, adult survivors, offenders, and persons with mental retardation.* Lexington, MA: D. C. Heath.

Peters, D. K., & Range, L. M. (1995). Childhood sexual abuse and current suicidality in college women and men. *Child Abuse & Neglect, 19,* 335–341.

Phillips, R. G., & LeDoux, J. E. (1992). Differential contribution of amygdala and hippocampus to cued and contextual fear conditioning. *Behavioral Neuroscience, 106,* 274–285.

Piaget, J., & Inhelder, B. (1969). *The psychology of the child.* New York: Basic Books.

Pierce, R., & Pierce, L. H. (1985). The sexually abused child: A comparison of male and female victims. *Child Abuse & Neglect, 9,* 191–199.

Pierce, L. H., & Pierce, R. L. (1990). Adolescent/sibling incest perpetrators. In A. L. Horton, B. L. Johnson, L. M. Roundy, & D. Williams, (Eds.), *The incest perpetrator: A family member no one wants to treat* (pp. 99–107). Newbury Park, CA: Sage Publications.

Pithers, W. D., & Gray, A. (1998). The other half of the story: Children with sexual behavioral problems. *Psychology, Public Policy and the Law, 4,* 200–217.

Pillemer, D. B., & White, S. H. (1989). Childhood events recalled by children and adults. In H. W. Reese (Ed.), *Advances in child development and behavior* (Vol. 21, pp. 297–340). San Diego, CA: Academic Press.

Pintello, D., & Zuravin, S. (2001). Intrafamilial child sexual abuse: Predictors of postdisclosure maternal belief and protective action. *Child Maltreatment, 6,* 344–352.

Pipe, M. E. & Goodman, G. S. (1991). Elements of secrecy: Implications for children's testimony. *Behavioral Sciences and the Law, 9,* 33–41.

Pithers, W. D., Gray, A., Busconi, A., & Houchens, P. (1998). Children with sexual behavior problems: Identification of five distinct child types and related treatment considerations. *Child Maltreatment, 3,* 384–406.

Pleck, J. H. (1981). *The myth of masculinity.* Cambridge, MA: MIT Press.

Pleck, J. H. (1987). The theory of male sex-role identification: Its rise and fall, 1936 to the present. In H. Brod (Ed.), *The making of masculinities: The new men's studies* (pp. 21–38). New York: Nash Publishing.

Plummer, C. A. (2001). Prevention of child sexual abuse: A survey of 87 programs. *Violence and Victims, 16,* 575–588.

Pollack, W. (1999). *Real boys: Rescuing our sons from the myths of boyhood.* New York: Henry Holt.

Pollard, T. (2000). Adrenaline. In G. Fink (Ed.), *Encyclopedia of stress* (Vol. 1, pp. 52–57). San Diego, CA: Academic Press.

Polusny, M. A., & Follette, V. M. (1996). Remembering childhood sexual abuse: A national survey of psychologists' clinical practices, beliefs, and personal experiences. *Professional Psychology: Research and Practice, 27,* 41–52.

Prentsky, R. A., & Knight, R. A. (1993). Age of onset of sexual assault: Criminal and life history correlates. In G. W. Hall, R. Hirschman, J. Graham, & M. Zaragoza (Eds.), *Sexual aggression: Issues in Etiology, Assessment and Treatment.* London: Taylor & Francis.

Prentsky, R. A., Knight, R. A., & Lee, A. F. (1996). *Child sexual molestation: Research issues.* Washington, DC: U.S. Department of Justice, Office of Justice Programs.

Prentsky, R. A., Knight, R. A., & Lee, A. F. S. (1997). Risk factors associated with recidivism among extrafamilial child molesters. *Journal of Consulting and Clinical Psychology, 65,* 141–149.

Prentsky, R. A., Lee, A. F., Knight, R. A., & Cerce, D. (1997). Recidivism rates among child molesters and rapists: A methodological analysis. *Law and Human Behavior, 21,* 635–659.

Priest, R. (1992). Child sexual abuse histories among African-American college students: A preliminary study. *American Journal of Orthopsychiatry, 62,* 475–476.

Proulx, J., McKibben, A., & Lusignan, R. (1996). Relationships between affective components and sexual behaviors in sexual aggressors. *Sexual Abuse: A Journal of Research and Treatment, 8,* 279–289.

Proulx, J., Pellerrin, B., Paradis, Y., McKibben, A., Aubut, J., & Quimet, M. (1997). Aesthetic and dynamic predictors of recidivism in sexual aggressors. *Sexual Abuse: A Journal of Research and Treatment, 9,* 7–28.

Putnam, F. W. (1995). Development of dissociative disorders. In D. Cicchetti & D.J. Cohen (Eds.), *Developmental psychopathology: Vol. 2. Risk, disorder and adaptation* (pp. 581–608). New York: John Wiley & Sons.

Putnam, F. W., & Trickett, P. K. (1993). Child sexual abuse: A model of chronic trauma. In D. Reiss, J. E. Richter, & M. Radke-Yarrow (Eds.), *Children and violence* (pp. 82–95). New York: Guilford Press.

Pynoos, R. S., & Eth, S. (1985). Developmental perspective on psychic trauma in children. In C. R. Figley (Ed.), *Trauma and its wake: The study and treatment of posttraumatic stress disorder* (pp. 36–52). New York: Brunner/Mazel.

Pynoos, R. S., Steinberg, A. M., & Wraith, R. (1995). A developmental model of childhood traumatic stress. In D. Cicchetti & D. J. Cohen (Eds.), *Developmental psychopathology: Vol. 2. Risk disorder and adaptation* (pp. 72–93). New York: John Wiley & Sons.

Pynoos, R. S., Steinberg, A. M., & Aronson, L. (1997). Traumatic experiences: The early organization of memory in school-age children and adolescents. In P. Appelbaum, P. M. Elin, & L. Uyehara (Eds.), *Trauma and memory: Clinical and legal controversies* (pp. 272–288). New York: Oxford University Press.

Quayle, E., & Taylor, M. (2001). Child seduction and self-representation on the Internet. *Cyberpsychology & Behavior: The Impact of the Internet, Multimedia and Virtual Reality on Behavior and Society, 4,* 597–608.

Rachman, S. (1980). Emotional processing. *Behavior, Research and Therapy, 18,* 51–60.

Raj, A., Silverman, J. G., & Amaro, H. (2000). The relationship between sexual abuse and sexual risk among high school students: Findings from the 1997 Massachusetts Youth Risk Behavior Survey. *Maternal and Child Health Journal, 4,* 125–134.

Ramsey-Klawsnik, H. (1990, November). *Sexually abused boys: Indicators, abusers and impact of trauma.* Paper presented at the Third National Conference on the Male Survivor, Tuscon, AZ.

Rank, O. (1952). *The trauma of birth.* New York: Alfred A. Knopf.

Rascovsky, M., & Rascovsky, A. (1950). On consumated incest. *International Journal of Psychoanalysis, 31,* 42–47.

Rasmussen, L. A. (1999). The trauma outcome process: An integrated model for guiding clinical practice with children with sexually abusive behavior problems. *Journal of Child Sexual Abuse, 8,* 3–33.

Ratner, P. A., Johnson, J. L., Shoveller, J. A., Chan, K., Martindale, S. L., Schilder, A. J., et al. (In press). Non-consensual sex experienced by men who have sex with men: Prevalence and association with mental health. *Patient Education and Counseling.*

Rauch, S., van der Kolk, B. A., Fisler, R., Alpert, N. M., Orr, S. P., Savage, C. R., Fischman, A. J., Jenike, M. A., & Pitman, R. K. (1996). A symptom provocation study of posttraumatic stress disorder using positron emission tomography and script-driven imagery. *Archives of General Psychiatry, 53,* 380–387.

Ray, S. L. (1996). Adult male survivors of incest: An exploratory study. *Journal of Child Sexual Abuse, 5,* 103–114.

Ray, J. A., & English, D. J. (1995). Comparison of female and male children with sexual behavior problems. *Journal of Youth and Adolescence, 24,* 439–451.

Raymond, N. C., Coleman, E., Ohlerking, F., Christenson, G. A., & Miner, M. (1999). Psychiatric comorbidity in pedophilic sex offenders. *American Journal of Psychiatry, 156,* 786–788.

Reinhart, M. A. (1987). Sexually abused boys. *Child Abuse and Neglect, 11,* 229–235.

Reinger, A., Robison, E., & McHugh, M. (1995). Mandated training of professionals: A means for improving reporting of suspected child abuse. *Child Abuse & Neglect, 19,* 63–69.

Rew, L., Esparza, D., & Sands, D. (1991). A comparative study among college students of sexual abuse in childhood. *Archives of Psychiatric Nursing, 5,* 331–340.

Rew, L., Taylor-Seehafer, M., & Fitzgerald, M. L. (2001). Sexual abuse, alcohol and other drug use, and suicidal behaviors in homeless adolescents. *Issues in Comprehensive Pediatric Nursing, 24,* 225–240.

Richardson, M. F., Meredith, W. H., & Abbot, D. A. (1993). Sexual self concept in male adolescent sexual abuse survivors. *Journal of Family Violence, 8,* 89–100.

Richey-Suttles, S., & Remer, R. (1997). Psychologists' attitudes toward adult male survivors of sexual abuse. *Journal of Child Sexual Abuse, 6,* 43–61.

Riegel, D. (2000). *Understanding loved boys and boy lovers.* Philadelphia: SafeHaven Foundation Press.

Rieker, P. P., & Carmen, E. H. (1986). The victim-to-patient process: The disconfirmation and transformation of abuse. *American Journal of Orthopsychiatry, 56,* 360–370.

Rimsza, M. E. (1993). Words too terrible to hear: Sexual transmission of human immunodeficiency virus to children. *American Journal of Diseases of Childhood, 147,* 711–712.

Rimsza, M., & Niggemann, E. (1982). Medical evaluation of sexually abused children: A review of 311 cases. *Pediatrics, 69,* 8–13.

Rind, B., Trimovitch, P., & Bauserman, R. (1998). A meta-analytic examination of assumed properties of child sexual abuse using college samples. *Psychological Bulletin, 124,* 22–53.

Risin, L. I., & Koss, M. P. (1987). The sexual abuse of boys: Prevalence and descriptive characteristics of childhood victimization. *Journal of Interpersonal Violence, 2,* 309–323.

Roane, T. H. (1992). Male victims of sexual abuse: A case review within a child protective team. *Child Welfare, 71,* 231–239.

Robin, R. W., Chester, B., Rasmussen, J. K., Jaranson, J. M., & Goldman, D. (1997). Prevalence, characteristics, and impact of childhood sexual abuse in a southwestern American Indian tribe. *Child Abuse & Neglect, 21,* 769–787.

Rodgers, C. (1987). Sex roles in education. In D. Hargraves & A. Colley (Eds.), *The psychology of sex roles.* New York: Hemisphere.

Roesler, T. A., & McKenzie, N. (1994). Effects of childhood trauma on psychological functioning in adults sexually abused as children. *Journal of Nervous and Mental Disease, 182,* 145–150.

Roesler, T. A., & Wind, T. W. (1994). Telling the secret: Adult women describe their disclosures of incest. *Journal of Interpersonal Violence, 9,* 327–338.

Rogeness, G., Amrung, S., Macedo, C., & Harris, W. (1986). Psychopathology in abused and neglected children. *Journal of the American Academy of Child Psychiatry, 25,* 659–665.

Rohsenow, D. J., Corbett, R., & Devine, D. (1988). Molested as children: A hidden contribution to substance abuse? *Journal of Substance Abuse Treatment, 5,* 13–18.

Romano, E., & De Luca, R. V. (1996). Characteristics of perpetrators with histories of sexual abuse. *International Journal of Offender Therapy and Comparative Criminology, 40,* 147–156.

Roozendaal, B., Quirarte, G. L., & McGaugh, J. L. (1997). Stress-activated hormonal systems and the regulation of memory storage. In R. Yehuda & A. C. McFarlane (Eds.), *Psychobiology of posttraumatic stress disorder* (pp. 247–258). New York: New York Academy of Sciences.

Rossetti, S. J. (1995). The impact of child sexual abuse on attitudes toward God and the Catholic Church. *Child Abuse & Neglect, 19,* 1469-1481.

Roth, S., & Friedman, M.J. (1998). Childhood trauma remembered: A report on the current scientific knowledge base and its applications. *Journal of Child Sexual Abuse, 7,* 83–109.

Rotheram-Borus, M. J., Meyer-Bahlburg, H. F. L., Koopman, C., Rosario, M., Exner, T.M., Henderson, R., Matthieu, M., & Gruen, R. S. (1992). Lifetime sexual behaviors among runaway males and females. *Journal of Sex Research, 29,* 15–29.

Rothschild, B. (2000). *The body remembers: The psychophysiology of trauma and trauma treatment.* New York: W. W. Norton.

Rowan, A. B., & Foy, D. W. (1993). Post-traumatic stress disorder in child sexual abuse survivors: A literature review. *Journal of Traumatic Stress, 6,* 3–20.

Rowan, E. L., Rowan, J. B., & Langelier, P. (1990). Women who molest children. *Bulletin of the American Academy of Psychiatry and the Law, 18,* 79–83.

Rowe, E., & Eckenrode, J. (1999). The timing of academic difficulties among maltreated and nonmaltreated children. *Child Abuse & Neglect, 23,* 813–832.

Roy, A. (2002). Urinary free cortisol and childhood trauma in cocaine dependent adults. *Journal of Psychiatric Research, 36,* 173–177.

Rubinstein, M., Yeager, C. A., Goodstein, C. & Lewis, D. O. (1993). Sexually assaultive male juveniles: A follow-up. *American Journal of Psychiatry, 150,* 262–265.

Ruchkin, V. V., Eisemann, M., & Hägglöf, B. (1998). Juvenile male rape victims: Is the level of post-traumatic stress related to personality and parenting? *Child Abuse & Neglect, 22,* 889–899.

Rudin, M. M., Zalewski, C., & Bodmer-Turner, J. (1995). Characteristics of child sexual abuse victims according to perpetrator gender. *Child Abuse & Neglect, 19,* 963–973.

Ruggiero, K. J., McLeer, S. V., & Dixon, J. F. (2000). Sexual abuse characteristics associated with survivor psychopathology. *Child Abuse & Neglect, 24,* 951–964.

Rush, F. (1980). *The best kept secret: Sexual abuse of children.* New York: McGraw-Hill.

Russell, D. E. H. (1986). *The secret trauma: Incest in the lives of girls and women.* New York: Basic Books.

Russell, J. A., & Douglas, A. J. (2000). Opioids. In G. Fink (Ed.), *Encyclopedia of stress* (Vol. 2, pp. 87–98). San Diego, CA: Academic Press.

Rutter, M. (1987). Psychosocial resilience and protective mechanisms. *American Journal of Orthopsychiatry, 57,* 316–331.

Ryan, G. (1995, November). *Treatment of sexually abusive youth: The evolving consensus.* Paper presented at the International Experts Conference. Utrecht, the Netherlands.

Ryan, G. (1996). The sexual abuser. In E. Helfer &. R. Kempe (Eds.), *The battered child* (5th ed.) (pp. 329–346). Chicago: University of Chicago Press.

Ryan, G., & Lane, S. (Eds.). (1997). *Juvenile sexual offending: Causes, consequences, and correction* (Revised ed.). San Francisco: Jossey-Bass.

Ryan, G., Miyoshi, T. J., Metzner, J. L., Krugman, R. D., & Fryer, G. E. (1996). Trends in a national sample of sexually abusive youths. *Journal of the American Academy of Child and Adolescent Psychiatry, 35,* 17–25.

Ryan, K. D., Kilmer, R. P., Cauce, A. M., Watanabe, H., & Hoyt, D. R. (2000). Psychological consequences of child maltreatment in homeless adolescents: Untangling the unique effects of maltreatment and family environment. *Child Abuse & Neglect, 24,* 333–352.

Sabotta, E. E., & Davis, R. L. (1992). Fatality after report to a child abuse registry in Washington State, 1973–1986. *Child Abuse & Neglect, 16*, 627–635.

Sadeh, A., Hayden, R., McGuire, J., Sachs, H., & Civita, R. (1994). Somatic, cognitive, and emotional characteristics of abused children in a psychiatric hospital. *Child Psychology and Human Development, 24*, 191–200.

Saleeby, D. (Ed.). (1992). *The strengths perspective in social work practice.* New York: Longman Press.

Salmon, P., & Calderbank, S. (1996). The relationship of childhood physical and sexual abuse to adult illness behavior. *Journal of Psychosomatic Research, 40*, 329–336.

Salter, A. C. (1992). Epidemiology of child sexual abuse. In W. O'Donohue & J. H. Geer (Eds.), *Sexual abuse of children: Vol. 1. Theory and research* (pp. 108–138). Hillsdale, NJ: Lawrence Erlbaum.

Salter, A. C. (1995). *Transforming trauma: A guide to understanding and treating adult survivors of child sexual abuse.* Thousand Oaks, CA: Sage.

Sanders, B., & Giolas, M. H. (1991). Dissociation and childhood trauma in psychologically disturbed adolescents. *American Journal of Psychiatry, 148*, 50–54.

Sandfort, T., Brongersma, E., & van Naerssen, A. (1990). Man-boy relationships: Different concepts for a diversity of phenomena. *Journal of Homosexuality, 20*, 5–12.

Sansone, R. A., Gaither, G. A., & Songer, D. A. (2001). Reporting of weight history: Sexually abused versus nonabused males. *Eating Behaviors, 2*, 85–86.

Sansonnet-Hayden, H., Haley, G., Marriage, K., & Fine, S. (1987). Sexual abuse and psychopathology in hospitalized adolescents. *Journal of the American Academy of Child and Adolescent Psychiatry, 26*, 753–757.

Saplonsky, R. M. (1993). Potential behavior modification of glucocorticoid damage to the hippocampus. *Behavioral Brain Research, 57*, 175–182.

Saradjian, J. (1996). *Women who sexually abuse children: From research to clinical practice.* Chichester, UK: John Wiley & Sons.

Sarlin, C. N. (1962). Depersonalization and derealization. *Journal of the American Psychoanalytic Association, 10*, 784–804.

Sarwer, D. B., Crawford, I., & Durlak, J. A. (1997). The relationship between childhood sexual abuse and adult male sexual dysfunction. *Child Abuse & Neglect, 21*, 649–655.

Sass, K. J., Spencer, D. D, Kim, J. H., Westerveld, M., Novelly, R. A., & Lencz, T. (1990). Verbal memory impairment correlates with hippocampal pyramidal cell density. *Neurology, 40*, 1694–1697.

Saxe, G., & Wolfe, J. (1999). Gender and posttraumatic stress disorder. In P. A. Saigh & J. D. Bremner (Eds.), *Posttraumatic stress disorder: A comprehensive text* (pp. 160–179). Boston: Allyn & Bacon.

Schaaf, K. K., & McCanne, T. R. (1998). Relationship of childhood sexual, physical, and combined sexual and physical abuse to adult victimization and posttraumatic stress disorder. *Child Abuse & Neglect, 22*, 1119–1133.

Schacter, D. L. (1995). Memory distortion: History and current status. In D. L. Schacter, J. T. Coyle, G. D. Fishbach, M. M. Mesulam, & L. E. Sullivan (Eds.), *Memory distortion: How minds, brains, and societies reconstruct the past* (pp. 1–43). Cambridge, MA: Harvard University Press.

Schacter, D. L. (1996). *Searching for memory: The brain, the mind, and the past.* New York: Basic Books.

Scheflin, A. W., & Brown, D. (1996). Repressed memory or dissociative amnesia: What the science says. *Journal of Psychiatry & Law, 24*, 143–187.

Schiffer, F., Teicher, M. H., & Papanicolaou, A. C. (1995). Evoked potential evidence for right brain activity during the recall of traumatic memories. *Journal of Neuropsychiatry and Clinical Neurosciences, 7*, 169–175.

Schore, A. N. (1994). *Affect regulation and the origin of the self.* Hillsdale, NJ: Lawrence Erlbaum.

Schore, A. N. (1996). *Affect regulation and the origin of the self: The neurobiology of emotional development.* Hillsdale, NJ: Lawrence Erlbaum.

Schore, A. N. (2001). The effects of early relational trauma on right brain development, affect regulation, and infant mental health. *Infant Mental Health Journal, 22,* 201–269.

Schwartz, M. (1994). Negative impact of sexual abuse on adult male gender: Issues and strategies for intervention. *Child and Adolescent Social Work Journal, 11,* 179–194.

Schwarz, J. (1999, June 2). *Women, men view and judge childhood sexual abuse cases differently.* Press release, University of Washington, Seattle.

Sebold, J. (1987). Indicators of child sexual abuse in males. *Social Casework: The Journal of Contemporary Social Work, 68,* 75–80.

Sedlak, A .J., & Broadhurst, D. D. (1996). *Executive summary of the Third National Incidence Study of Child Abuse and Neglect.* Washington, DC: United States Department of Health and Human Services, Administration for Children, Youth and Families, National Center of Child Abuse and Neglect.

Sedney, M. (1987). Development of androgyny: Parental influences. *Psychology Womens Quarterly, 11,* 311–326.

Sgroi, S. M. (1989). Stages of recovery for adult survivors of child sexual abuse. In S. M. Sgroi (Ed.), *Vulnerable populations: Sexual abuse treatment for children, adult survivors, offenders, and persons with mental retardation* (pp. 111–130). Lexington, MA: D. C. Heath.

Sgroi, S. M. (1992). Foreword. In S. Shapiro & G. M. Dominiak (Eds.), *Sexual trauma and psychopathology: Clinical intervention with adult survivors.* New York: Lexington Books.

Sgroi, S. M., Blick, L. C., & Porter, F. S. (1982). A conceptual framework for child sexual abuse. In S. M. Sgroi (Ed.), *Handbook of clinical intervention in child sexual abuse* (pp. 9–37). Lexington, MA: D. C. Heath.

Shaw, J. A., Lewis, J. E., Loeb, A., Rosado, J., & Rodriguez, R. A. (2000). Child on child sexual abuse: Psychological perspectives. *Child Abuse & Neglect, 24,* 1591–1600.

Siegel, D. J. (1995). Memory, trauma, and psychotherapy: A cognitive science view. *Journal of Psychotherapy Practice and Research, 4,* 93–122.

Siegel, D. J. (1996). Cognition, memory and dissociation. *Child and Adolescent Psychiatric Clinics of North America, 5,* 509–536.

Siegel, D. J. (1997). An overview of cognitive processes, childhood memory and trauma. In C. Prozan (Ed.), *Construction and reconstruction of memory: Dilemmas of childhood sexual abuse* (pp. 39–70). New York: Jason Aronson.

Siegel, D. J. (1999). *The developing mind: Toward a neurobiology of interpersonal experience.* New York: Guilford Press.

Siegel, D. J. (2001). Memory: An overview, with emphasis on development, interpersonal, and neurobiological aspects. *Journal of the American Academy of Child and Adolescent Psychiatry, 40,* 997–1011.

Sigmon, S. T., Greene, M. P., Rohan, K. J., & Nichols, J. E. (1996). Coping and adjustment in male and female survivors of childhood sexual abuse. *Journal of Child Sexual Abuse, 5,* 57–75.

Silverman, A. B., Reinherz, H. Z., & Giaconia, R. M. (1996). The long-term sequelae of child and adolescent abuse: A longitudinal community study. *Child Abuse & Neglect, 20,* 709–723.

Simpson, T. L., & Miller, W. R. (2002). Concomitance between childhood sexual and physical abuse and substance use problems: A review. *Clinical Psychology Review, 22,* 27–77.

Simpson, T. L., Westerberg, V. S., Little, L. M., & Trujillo, M. (1994). The effect of systematic screening on the reporting rates of childhood sexual and physical abuse among out-patient substance abusers. *Journal of Substance Abuse Treatment, 11,* 347–358.

Sipe, R., Jensen, E. L., & Everett, R. S. (1998). Adolescent sexual offenders grown up: Recidivism in young adulthood. *Criminal Justice Behavior, 25,* 109–124.

Sirles, E. A., Smith, J. A., & Kusama, H. (1989). Psychiatric status of intrafamilial child sexual abuse victims. *Journal of the American Academy of Child and Adolescent Psychiatry, 28,* 225–229.

Sjöberg, R. L., & Lindblad, F. (2002). Limited disclosure of sexual abuse of children whose experiences were documented by videotape. *American Journal of Psychiatry, 159,* 312–314.

Skuse, D., Bentovim, A., Hodges, J., Stevenson, J., Andreou, C., Lanyado, M., New, M., Williams, B., & McMillan, D. (1998). Risk factors for development of sexually abusive behavior in sexually victimized adolescent boys: Cross sectional study. *British Medical Journal, 317,* 175–179.

Sloan, P., & Karpinski, E. (1942). Effects of incest on participants. *American Journal of Orthopsychiatry, 12,* 666–673.

Slusser, M. M. (1995). Manifestations of sexual abuse in preschool-aged children. *Issues in Mental Health Nursing, 16,* 481–491.

Smallborne, S. W., & Dadds, M. R. (2000). Attachment and coercive sexual behavior. *Sexual Abuse: A Journal of Research and Treatment, 12,* 3–15.

Smith, B. E., & Elstein, S. G. (1993). *The prosecution of child sexual and physical abuse cases.* Washington, DC: American Bar Association.

Smith, D. W., & Saunders, B. (1995). Personality characteristics of father/perpetrators and nonoffending mothers in incest families: Individual and dyadic analyses. *Child Abuse & Neglect, 19,* 607–617.

Smith, H., & Israel, E. (1987). Sibling incest: A study of the dynamics of 25 cases. *Child Abuse & Neglect, 11,* 101–108.

Smith, H. D., Fromuth, M. E., & Morris, C. C. (1997). Effects of gender on perceptions of child sexual abuse. *Journal of Child Sexual Abuse, 6,* 51–63.

Smolak, L., & Murnen, S. K. (2002). A meta-analytic examination of the relationship between child sexual abuse and eating disorders. *The International Journal of Eating Disorders, 31,* 136–150.

Snow, B., & Sorenson, T. (1990). Ritualistic child abuse in a neighborhood setting. *Journal of Interpersonal Violence, 5,* 474–487.

Sobsey, D., Randall, W., & Parrila, R. K. (1997). Gender differences in abused children with and without disabilities. *Child Abuse & Neglect, 21,* 707–720.

Sorenson, T., & Snow, B. (1991). How children tell: The process of disclosure in child sexual abuse. *Child Welfare, 70,* 3–15.

Southwick, S. S., Yehuda, R., & Wang, S. (1998). Neuroendocrine alterations in posttraumatic stress disorder. *Psychiatric Annals, 28,* 436–442.

Spaccarelli, S. (1994). Stress, appraisal, and coping in child sexual abuse: A theoretical and empirical review. *Psychological Bulletin, 116,* 340–362.

Spencer, M. J., & Dunklee, P. (1986). Sexual abuse of boys. *Pediatrics, 78,* 133–138.

Spencer, T. D., & Tan, J. C. H. (1999). Undergraduate students' reactions to analogue male disclosure of sexual abuse. *Journal of Child Sexual Abuse, 8,* 73–90.

Spiegel, D. (1986). Dissociation, double binds, and posttraumatic stress in multiple personality disorder. In B. G. Braun (Ed.), *Treatment of multiple personality disorder* (pp. 61–78). Washington, DC: American Psychiatric Press.

Spiegel, D., & Cardena, E. (1991). Disintegrated experience: The dissociative disorders revisited. *Journal of Abnormal Psychology, 100,* 366–378.

Spiegel, J. (1995). The sexual abuse of males: A structural equation model of dynamics and effects. (Doctoral dissertation, Florida State University, August, 1995). *Dissertation Abstracts International, 58,* 5708A.

Spiegel, J. (1997, June). *The sexual abuse of males (SAM): A national study.* Paper presented at the Fifth International Conference on Family Violence Research, Portsmouth, NH.

Spiegel, J. (1998, June). *The sexual abuse of males: A model of treatment.* Paper presented at the Sixth International Conference on Family Violence Research, Portsmouth, NH.

Squire, L. R. (1995). Biological foundations of accuracy and inaccuracy in memory. In D. L. Schacter (Ed.), *Memory distortion: How minds and societies reconstruct the past* (pp. 197–254). Cambridge, MA: Harvard University Press.

Squire, L. R., & Kandel, E. R. (2000). *Memory: From mind to molecules.* New York: Scientific American Library.

Squire, L. R., & Zola, S. (1998). Episodic memory, semantic memory, and amnesia. *Hippocampus, 8,* 205–211.

Stanwood, G. D., & Zigmond, M. J. (2000). Dopamine, central. In G. Fink (Ed.)., *Encyclopedia of stress* (Vol. 1, pp. 739–745). San Diego, CA: Academic Press.

Stein, J. A., Golding, J. N., Siegel, J. M., Burnam, M. A., & Sorenson, S. B. (1988). Longterm psychological sequelae of child sexual abuse: The Los Angeles Epidemiological Catchment Area Study. In G. E. Wyatt & E. J. Powell (Eds.), *Lasting effects of child sexual abuse* (pp. 135-156). Beverly Hills, CA: Sage.

Stein, M. B., Walker, J. R., Hazen, A. L., & Forde, D. R. (1997). Full and partial posttraumatic stress disorder: Findings from a community survey. *American Journal of Psychiatry, 154,* 1114–1119.

Stevens, J. (1992). *Applied multivariate statistics for the social sciences* (2nd ed.). Hillsdale, NJ: Lawrence Erlbaum.

Strathdee, S. A., Hogg, R. S., Martindale, S. L., Cornelisse, P. G. A., Craib, K., Schilder, A., Montaner, J. S. G., O'Shaughnessy, M. V., & Schechter, M. T. (1996, July). *Sexual abuse is an independent predictor of sexual risk-taking among young HIV-negative men: Results from a prospective study at baseline.* Paper presented at the Eleventh International Conference on AIDS, Vancouver, BC.

Straus, M., & Smith, C. (1990). Family patterns and child abuse. In M. Straus & R. Gelles (Eds.), *Physical violence in American families: Risk factors and adaptations to violence in 8,145 families* (pp. 145–165). New Brunswick, NJ: Transaction Press.

Strauss, A. L. (1987). *Qualitative analysis for social scientists.* New York: Cambridge University Press.

Stroud, D. D. (1999). Familial support as perceived by adult victims of childhood sexual abuse. *Sexual Abuse: A Journal of Research and Treatment, 11,* 159–175.

Stroud, D. D., Martens, S. L., & Barker, J. (2000). Criminal investigation of child sexual abuse: A comparison of cases referred to the prosecutor to those not referred. *Child Abuse & Neglect, 24,* 689–700.

Strupp, H. H. (1992). Humanism and psychotherapy: A personal statement of the therapist's essential values. In R. B. Miller (Ed.), *The restoration of dialogue: Readings in the philosophy of clinical* (530–568). Washington, DC: American Psychological Association.

Strupp, H., & Binder, J. L. (1985). *Psychotherapy in a new key: A guide to time-limited dynamic psychotherapy.* New York: Basic Books.

Struve, J. (1990). Dancing with the patriarchy: The politics of sexual abuse. In M. Hunter (Ed.), *The sexually abused male: Vol. 1. Prevalence, impact and treatment* (pp. 3–45). Lexington, MA: Lexington Books.

Styron, T., & Janoff-Bulman, R. (1997). Childhood attachment and abuse: Long-term effects on adult attachment, depression, and conflict resolution. *Child Abuse & Neglect, 21,* 1015–1023.

Sullivan, H. S. (1953). *The interpersonal theory of psychiatry.* New York: W. W. Norton.

Sullivan, H. S. (1968). *The interpersonal theory of psychiatry* (2nd ed.). New York: W. W. Norton.

Sullivan, P. M., & Knutson, J.F. (2000a). Maltreatment and disabilities: A population-based epidemiological study. *Child Abuse & Neglect, 24,* 1257–1273.

Sullivan, P. M., & Knutson, J. F. (2000b). The prevalence of disabilities and maltreatment among runaway children. *Child Abuse & Neglect, 24,* 1275–1288.

Summit, R. (1983). The child sexual abuse accommodation syndrome. *Child Abuse and Neglect, 7,* 177–193.

Sutherland, S. M., & Davidson, J. R. (1999). Pharmacological treatment of PTSD. In P. A. Saigh & J. D. Bremner (Eds.), *Posttraumatic stress disorder: A comprehensive text* (pp. 103–143). Needham Heights, MA: Allyn & Bacon.

Swanston, H. Y., Parkinson, P. N., Oates, K., O'Toole, Plunkett, A. M., & Shrimpton, S. (2002). Further abuse of sexually abused children. *Child Abuse & Neglect, 26,* 115–127.

Swett, C., Jr., Surrey, J., & Cohen, C. (1990). Sexual and physical abuse histories and psychiatric symptoms among male psychiatric outpatients. *American Journal of Psychiatry, 147,* 632–636.

Talley, N. J., Fett, S. L., Zinsmeister, A. R., & Melton, L. J. (1994). Gastrointestinal tract symptoms and self-reported abuse: A population-based study. *Gastroenterology, 107,* 1040–1049.

Tardif, M., & Van Gijseghem, H. (2001). Do pedophiles have a weaker identity structure compared with nonsexual offenders? *Child Abuse & Neglect, 25,* 1381–1394.

Tavris, C., & Wade, C. (1984). *The longest war: Sex differences in perspective.* New York: Harcourt Brace Jovanovich.

Teicher, M. H. (1997). Preliminary evidence for abnormal cortical development in physically and sexually abused children using EEG coherence and MRI. *Annals of the New York Academy of Sciences, 821,* 160–175.

Teicher, M. H. (2000). Wounds that time wouldn't heal: The neurobiology of childhood abuse. *Cerebrum, 2,* 50–67.

Teicher, M. H., Andersen, S.L., Polcari, A., Anderson, C.M., & Navalta, P. (2002). Developmental neurobiology of childhood stress and trauma. *The Psychiatric Clinics of North America, 25,* 397–426.

Teicher, M. H., Glod, C. A., Surrey, J., & Swett, C., Jr. (1993). Early childhood abuse and limbic system ratings in adult psychiatric outpatients. *Journal of Neuropsychiatry and Clinical Neurosciences, 5,* 301–306.

Teicher, M. H., Ito, Y., Glod, C. A., Andersen, S. L., Dumont, N., & Ackerman, E. (1997). Preliminary evidence for abnormal cortical development in physically and sexually abused children using EEG coherence and MRI. *Annals of the New York Academy of Sciences, 821,* 160–175.

Terr, L. (1988). What happens to early memories of trauma? A study of twenty children under age five at the time of documented traumatic events. *Journal of the American Academy of Child and Adolescent Psychiatry, 27,* 96–104.

Terr, L. C. (1991). Childhood traumas: An outline and overview. *American Journal of Psychiatry, 148,* 10–20.

Terr, L. C. (1996). True memories of childhood trauma: Flaws, absences, and returns. In K. Pezdek & W.P. Banks (Eds.), *The recovered memory/false memory debate* (pp. 69–80). New York: Academic Press.

Thomlinson, B., Stephens, M., Cunes, J. W., & Grinnell, R. M. (1991). Characteristics of male and female child sexual abuse victims. *Journal of Child & Youth Care,* (Special Issue), 65–76.

Thompson, C. W. (2002, March 19). FBI cracks child porn ring based on Internet. *Washington Post,* A2.

Thorstad, D. (1991). Man/boy love and the American gay movement. *Journal of Homosexuality, 20,* 251–274.

Tilelli, J. A., Turek, D., & Jaffe, A.C. (1980). Sexual abuse of children: Clinical findings and implications for management. *New England Journal of Medicine, 302,* 319–323.

Timnick, L. (1985, August 25). 22% in survey were child abuse victims. *Los Angeles Times,* p. 1.

Tjaden, P. G., & Thoennes, N. (1992). Predictors of legal intervention in child maltreatment cases. *Child Abuse & Neglect, 16,* 807–821.

Toth, S. L. & Cicchetti, D. (1996). Patterns of relatedness, depressive symptomatology, and perceived competence in maltreated children. *Journal of Consulting and Clinical Psychology, 64,* 32–41.

Travin, S., Cullen, K., & Protter, B. (1990). Female sex offenders: Severe victims and victimizers. *Journal of Forensic Sciences, 35,* 140–150.

Trute, B., Adkins, E., & MacDonald, G. (1992). Professional attitudes regarding the sexual abuse of children: Comparing police, child welfare and community mental health. *Child Abuse & Neglect, 16,* 359–368.

Tulving, E., & Craik, F. I. M. (2000). *The Oxford handbook of memory.* New York: Oxford University Press.

Tulving, E., & Pearlstone, Z. (1966). Availability versus accessibility of information in memory for words. *Journal of Verbal Learning and Verbal Behavior, 5*, 381–391.

Tulving, E., & Schacter, D. L. (1990). Priming and human memory systems. *Science, 247*, 301–306.

Tyler, K. A., Hoyt, D. R., Whitbeck, L. B., & Cauce, A. M. (2001). The impact of childhood sexual abuse on later sexual victimization among runaway youth. *Journal of Research on Adolescence, 11*, 151–176.

Tzeng, O., & Schwarzin, H. (1990). Gender and race differences in child sexual abuse correlates. *International Journal of Intercultural Relations, 14*, 135–161.

Urquiza, A. J., & Capra, M. (1990). The impact of sexual abuse: Initial and long-term effects. In M. Hunter (Ed.), *The sexually abused male: Prevalence, impact and treatment* (Vol. 1, pp. 105–135). Lexington, MA: Lexington Books.

Urquiza, A. J., & Crowley, C. (1986, May). *Sex differences in the survivors of CSA.* Paper presented at the Fourth National Conference on the Sexual Victimization of Children, New Orleans, LA.

U.S. Congress, House. (1993, 1st session). National Child Protection Act of 1993 (House Report No. 103-393). Washington, DC: U.S. Congress.

U.S. Department of Health and Human Services. (1999). *Children's bureau, child maltreatment 1996: Reports from the states to the national child abuse and neglect data system.* Washington, DC: U.S. Government Printing Office.

U.S. Department of Justice. (1996). *Child victimizers: Violent offenders and their victims.* (NCJ-153258). Washington, DC: U.S. Government Printing Office.

U.S. Department of Justice. (1997a). *Child sexual molestation: Research issues.* (NCJ-163390). Washington, DC: U.S. Government Printing Office.

U.S. Department of Justice. (1997b). *Sex offenses and offenders.* (NCJ-163392). Washington, DC: U.S. Government Printing Office.

U.S. Department of Justice. (2000). *Sexual assault of young children as reported to law enforcement: Victim, incident, and offender characteristics.* Washington, DC: Department of Justice, Office of Justice Programs.

Vaillant, G. E. (1992). *Ego mechanisms of defense: A guide for clinicians and researchers.* Washington, DC: American Psychiatric Press.

van der Hart, O., & Nijenhuis, E. R. S. (1999). Bearing witness to uncorroborated trauma: The clinician's development of reflective belief. *Professional Psychology: Research and Practice, 30*, 37–44.

van der Hart, O., Steele, K., Boon, S., & Brown, P. (1993). The treatment of traumatic memories: Synthesis, realization, and integration. *Dissociation, 6*, 162–180.

van der Kolk, B. A. (1987). *Psychological trauma.* Washington, DC: American Psychiatric Press.

van der Kolk, B. A. (1989). The compulsion to repeat the trauma: Re-enactment, revictimization and masochism. *Psychiatric Clinics of North America, 12*, 385–411.

van der Kolk, B. A. (1994). The body keeps score: Memory and the evolving psychobiology of posttraumatic stress. *Harvard Review of Psychiatry, 1*, 253–265.

van der Kolk, B. A. (1996). Trauma and memory. In B. A. van der Kolk, A. C. McFarlane, & L. Weisaeth (Eds.), *Traumatic stress* (pp. 279–302). New York: Guilford Press.

van der Kolk, B.A., & Fisler, R. (1995). Dissociation and the fragmentary nature of traumatic memories: overview and exploratory study. *Journal of Traumatic Stress, 8*, 505–525.

van der Kolk, B. A., McFarlane, A. C., & van der Hart, O. (1996). A general approach to treatment of posttraumatic stress disorder. In B. A. van der Kolk, A. C. McFarlane & L. Weisaeth (Eds.), *Traumatic stress: The effects of overwhelming experience on mind, body, and society* (pp. 417–440). New York: Guilford Press.

van der Kolk, B. A., McFarlane, A. C. & Weisaeth, L. (Eds.). (1996). *Traumatic stress: The effects of overwhelming experience on mind, body, and society.* New York: Guilford Press.

van der Kolk, B. A., Pelcovitz, D., Roth, S., Mandel, F. S., McFarlane, A., & Herman, J. L. (1996).

Dissociation, somatization, and affect regulation: The complexity of adaptation to trauma. *American Journal of Psychiatry, 153*, 83–93.

van der Kolk, B. A., Perry, J. C., & Herman, J. L. (1991). Childhood origins of self-destructive behavior. *American Journal of Psychiatry, 148*, 1665–1671.

van der Kolk, B. A. & Saporta, J. (1993). The biological response to psychic trauma: Mechanisms and treatment of intrusion and numbing. *Anxiety Research, 4*, 199–212.

van der Kolk, B. A., & van der Hart, O. (1989). Pierre Janet and the breakdown of adaptation in psychological trauma. *American Journal of Psychiatry, 146*, 1530–1540.

van der Kolk, B. A., & van der Hart, O. (1995). The intrusive past: The flexibility of memory and the engraving of trauma. In C. Caruth (Ed.), *Trauma: Explorations in memory* (pp. 158–182). Baltimore: Johns Hopkins University Press.

Violato, C., & Genuis, M. (1993). Factors which differentiate sexually abused from nonabused males: An exploratory study. *Psychological Reports, 72*, 767–770.

Vulliamy, A. P., & Sullivan, R. (2000). Reporting child abuse: Pediatricians' experiences with the child protection system. *Child Abuse & Neglect, 24*, 1461–1470.

Wagner, W. G., Aucoin, R., & Johnson, J. T. (1993). Psychologists' attitudes concerning child sexual abuse: The impact of sex of perpetrator, sex of victim, age of victim, and victim response. *Journal of Child Sexual Abuse, 2*, 61–74.

Walker, E. A., Gelfand, A. N., Gelfand, M. D., & Katon, W. J. (1995). Psychiatric diagnoses, sexual and physical victimization, and disability in patients with irritable bowel syndrome or inflammatory bowel disease. *Psychosomatic Medicine, 25*, 1259–1267.

Walker, E. A., Katon, W. J., Roy-Bryne, P. P., Jemelka, R. P., & Russo, J. (1993). Histories of sexual victimization in patients with irritable bowel syndrome or inflammatory bowel disease. *American Journal of Psychiatry, 150*, 1502–1506.

Wallen, J., & Berman, K. (1992). Possible indicators of childhood sexual abuse for individuals in substance abuse treatment. *Journal of Child Sexual Abuse, 1*, 63–74.

Waller, N. G., Putnam, F. W., & Carlson, E. B. (1996). Types of dissociation and dissociative types: A taxometric analysis of dissociative experiences. *Psychological Methods, 1*, 320–321.

Wallerstein, R. (1983). Defenses, defense mechanisms and the structure of the mind. *Journal of the American Psychoanalytic Association*, 31, 201–225.

Ward, T., Hudson, S. M., & Marshall, W. L. (1995). Cognitive distortions and affective deficits in sexual offenders: A cognitive deconstructionist interpretation. *Sexual Abuse: A Journal of Research and Treatment, 7*, 67–83.

Waterman, C. K., & Foss-Goodman, D. (1984). Child molesting: Variables relating to attribution of fault to victims, offenders, and nonparticipating parents. *Journal of Sex Research, 20*, 329–349.

Waterman, J., Kelly, R., Oliveri, M. K., & McCord, J. (1993). *Beyond the playground walls: Sexual abuse in preschools.* New York: Guilford Press.

Watkins, B., & Bentovim, A. (1992). The sexual abuse of males children and adolescents: A review of current research. *Journal of Child Psychology and Psychiatry, 33*, 197–248.

Watts, A. G. (2000). Anatomy of the hypothalamo-pituitary-adrenal axis. In G. Fink (Ed.)., *Encyclopedia of stress* (Vol. 2, pp. 477–483). San Diego, CA: Academic Press.

Weekes, C. (1976). *Simple, effective treatment of agoraphobia.* New York: Hawthorn Books.

Weeks, R., & Widom, C. (1998). Self-reports of early victimization among incarcerated adult male felons. *Journal of Interpersonal Violence, 13*, 346–361.

Weihe, V. R. (1990). *Sibling abuse: Hidden physical, emotional and sexual trauma.* Lexington, MA: D. C. Heath.

Wells, R., McCann, J., Adams, J., Voris, J., & Ensign, J. (1995). Emotional, behavioral and physical symptoms reported by parents of sexually abused, non-abused and allegedly abused prepubescent females. *Child Abuse & Neglect, 19*, 155–163.

Weinberg, S. K. (1955). *Incest behavior.* New York: Citadel Press.

Weinstein, B., Levine, M., Kogan, N., Harkavy-Friedman, J., & Miller, J. M. (2000). Mental health professionals' experiences reporting suspected child abuse and maltreatment. *Child Abuse & Neglect, 24,* 1317–1328.

Weinstein, D., Staffelbach, D., & Biaggio, M. (2000). Attention-deficit hyperactivity disorder and posttraumatic stress disorder: Differential diagnosis in childhood sexual abuse. *Clinical Psychology Review, 20,* 359–378.

Weir, I., & Wheatcroft, M. (1995). Allegations of children's involvement in ritual sexual abuse: Clinical experience of 20 cases. *Child Abuse & Neglect, 19,* 491–505.

Wellman, M. M. (1993). Child sexual abuse and gender differences: Attitudes and prevalence. *Child Abuse & Neglect, 17,* 539–547.

Wells, R., McCann, J., Adams, J., Voris, J., & Dahl, B. (1997). A validational study of the structured interview of symptoms associated with sexual abuse (SASA) using three samples of sexually abused, allegedly abused, and nonabused boys. *Child Abuse & Neglect, 21,* 1159–1167.

Wheeler, M. A., Stuss, D. T., & Tulving, E. (1997). Toward a theory of episodic memory: The frontal lobes and autonoetic consciousness. *Psychological Bulletin, 121,* 331–354.

Wherry, J. N., Jolly, J. B., Feldman, J., Balkozar, A., & Manjanatha, S. (1994). The Child Dissociative Checklist: Preliminary findings of a screening measure. *Journal of Child Sexual Abuse, 3,* 51–66.

Whitfield, C. L. (1995). *Memory and abuse: Remembering and healing the effects of trauma.* Deerfield Beach, FL: Health Communications.

Widom, C. S. (1995). Victims of childhood sexual abuse: Later criminal consequences. *National Institute of Justice: Research in brief.* Washington, DC: National Institute of Justice.

Widom, C. S. (1999). Posttraumatic stress disorder in abused and neglected children grown up. *American Journal of Psychiatry, 156,* 1223–1229.

Widom, C. S., & Ames, M. A. (1994). Criminal consequences of childhood sexual victimization. *Child Abuse & Neglect, 18,* 303–318.

Widom, C. S., & Morris, S. (1997). Accuracy of adult recollections of childhood victimization: Part 2. Childhood sexual abuse. *Psychological Assessment, 9,* 34–46.

Wilson, J. P., & Lindy, J. (Eds.). (1994). *Countertransference in the treatment of PTSD.* New York: Guilford Press.

Wilson, R. J. (1999). Emotional congruence in sexual offenders against children. *Sexual Abuse: A Journal of Research and Treatment, 11,* 33–47.

Windle, M., Windle, R. C., Scheidt, D. M., & Miller, G. B. (1995). Physical and sexual abuse and associated mental disorders among alcoholic inpatients. *American Journal of Psychiatry, 152,* 1322–1328.

Winnicott, D. W. (1965). Ego distortion in terms of the true self and false self. In *Maturational processes and the facilitating environment* (pp. 179–192). Madison, CT: International Universities Press. (Original work published 1962)

Winnicott, D. W. (1965). Ego integration and child development. In *Maturational processes and the facilitating environment* (pp. 148–152). Madison, CT: International Universities Press. (Original work published 1962)

Winnicott, D. W. (1965). *Maturational process and the facilitating environment.* New York: International Universities Press.

Wolfe, D. A., Sas, L., & Wekerle, C. (1994/3). Factors associated with the development of posttraumatic stress disorder among child victims of sexual abuse. *Child Abuse & Neglect, 18,* 37–50.

Wolfe, F. A. (1985, March). *Twelve female sexual offenders.* Paper presented at the conference, Next Steps in Research on the Assessment and Treatment of Sexually Aggressive Persons. St. Louis, MO.

Wolpe, J. (1990). *The practice of behavior therapy* (4th ed.). Elmsford, NY: Pergamon Press.

Woods, S. C., & Dean, K. S. (1985). *Sexual abuse of males research project.* Washington, DC: Department of Health and Human Services Administration for Children, Youth and Families Children's Bureau National Center on Child Abuse and Neglect.

Worling, J. R. (1995). Adolescent sibling-incest offenders: Differences in family and individual functioning when compared to adolescent nonsibling sex offenders. *Child Abuse & Neglect, 19*, 633–643.

Wurtele, S. K., Kaplan, G. M., & Keairnes, M. (1990). Childhood sexual abuse among chronic pain patients. *Clinical Journal of Pain, 6*, 110–113.

Wurtele, S. K., & Miller-Perrin, C. L. (1992). *Preventing child sexual abuse: Sharing the responsibility*. Lincoln: University of Nebraska Press.

Yates, J. L., & Nasby, W. (1993). Dissociation, affect, and network models of memory: An integrative proposal. *Journal of Traumatic Stress, 6*, 305–326.

Young, R. E., Bergandi, T. A., & Titus, T. G. (1994). Comparison of the effects of sexual abuse on male and female latency-aged children. *Journal of Interpersonal Violence, 9*, 291–306.

Zellman, G. (1990a). Child abuse reporting and failure to report among mandated reporters. *Journal of Interpersonal Violence, 5*, 3–22.

Zellman, G. (1990b). Linking schools and social services: The case of child abuse reporting. *Education Evaluation and Policy Analysis, 12*, 41–45.

Zellman, G., & Bell, K. (1989). *The role of professional background, case characteristics and protective agency response in mandated child abuse reporting*. Santa Monica, CA: Rand Corporation.

Zierler, S., Feingold, L., Laufer, D., Velentgas, P., Kantrowitz-Gordon, I., & Mayer, K. (1991). Adult survivors of childhood sexual abuse and subsequent risk of HIV infection. *American Journal of Public Health, 81*, 572–575.

Zlotnick, C., Begin, A., Shea, T., Pearlstein, T., Simpson, E., & Costello, E. (1994). The relationship between characteristics of sexual abuse and dissociative experiences. *Comprehensive Psychiatry, 35*, 465–470.

Zlotnick, C., Zimmerman, M., Wolfsdorf, B. A., & Mattia, J. I. (2001). Gender differences in patients with posttraumatic stress disorder in a general psychiatric practice. *American Journal of Psychiatry, 158*, 1923–1925.

Zoellner, L. A., Sacks, M. B., & Foa, E. B. (2001). Stability of emotions for traumatic memories in acute and chronic PTSD. *Behaviour Research and Therapy, 39*, 697–711.

Zola, S. M. (1998). Memory, amnesia and the issue of recovered memory: Neurobiological aspects. *Clinical Psychology Review, 18*, 915–932.

ADDITIONAL RESOURCES

Albany Times Union. (1996, June 29). Sex group loses tax exempt status. *Albany Times Union,* A6.

Alexander, P. C. (1992). Application of attachment theory to the study of sexual abuse. *Journal of Consulting and Clinical Psychology, 60,* 185–195.

Alexander, P. C. (1993). The differential effects of abuse characteristics and attachment in the prediction of long-term effects of sexual abuse. *Journal of Interpersonal Violence, 8,* 346–362.

Allers, C. T., Benjack, K. J., White, J., & Rousey, J. T. (1993). HIV vulnerability and the adult survivor of childhood sexual abuse. *Child Abuse & Neglect, 17,* 291–298.

Allers, C. T., White, J. F., & Mullis, F. (1997). The treatment of dissociation in an HIV-infected, sexually abused adolescent male. *Psychotherapy, 34,* 201–206.

American Academy of Child and Adolescent Psychiatry. (1988). Practice parameters for the assessment and evaluation of children and adolescents with posttraumatic stress disorder. *Journal of the American Academy of Child and Adolescent Psychiatry, 37,* 4–26.

Americans for a Society Free from Age Restrictions. (2002). *Home page.* Retrieved October 10, 2002, from www.asfar.org.

Ames, M. A., & Houston, D. A. (1990). Legal, social, and biological definitions of pedophilia. *Archives of Sexual Behavior, 19,* 333–342.

Arata, C. M. (1998). To tell or not to tell: Current functioning of child sexual abuse survivors who disclosed their victimization. *Child Maltreatment, 3,* 63–71.

Ashton, V. (1999). Worker judgments of seriousness about and reporting of suspected child maltreatment. *Child Abuse & Neglect, 23,* 539–548.

Bagley, C., & King, K. (1990). *Child sexual abuse: The search for healing.* New York: Routledge, Chapman and Hall.

Bagley, C., & Mallick, K. (1999). *Child sexual abuse and adult offenders: New theory and research.* Aldershot, UK: Ashgate.

Ballard, D. T., Blair, G. D., Devereaux, S., Valentine, L. K., Horton, A. L., & Johnson, B. L. (1990). A comparative profile of the incest perpetrator: Background characteristics, abuse history, and use of social skills. In A. L. Horton, B. L. Johnson, L. M. Roundy, & D. Williams (Eds.), *The incest perpetrator: The family member no one wants to treat* (pp. 43–64). Newbury Park, CA: Sage.

Bandura, A. (1977). Self-efficacy: Toward unifying theory of behavioral change. *Psychological Review, 84,* 191–215.

Bandura, A. (1993). Perceived self-efficacy in cognitive development and functioning. *Educational Psychologist, 28,* 117–148.

Bass, C., Bond, A., Gill, D., & Sharpe, M. (1999). Frequent attenders without organic disease in a gastroenterology clinic: Patient characteristics and health care use. *General Hospital Psychiatry, 21,* 30–38.

Beck, A. T., & Weishaar, M. E. (1995). Cognitive therapy. In R. J. Corsini & D. Wedding (Eds.), *Current psychotherapies* (5th ed., pp. 229-261). Itasca, IL: F. E. Peacock.

Becker, J. V., Cunningham-Rathner, J., & Kaplan, M. S. (1985, November). *The adolescent sexual perpetrator: Demographics, criminal history, victims, sexual behavior and recommendations for reducing future offenses.* Paper presented at the 7th National Conference on Child Abuse & Neglect, Chicago.

Bell, D., & Belicki, K. (1998). A community-based study of well-being in adults reporting childhood abuse. *Child Abuse & Neglect, 22,* 681–685.

Belsky, J. (1993). Etiology of child maltreatment: A developmental-ecological analysis. *Psychological Bulletin, 114,* 413–434.

Benjamin, J. (1997). *On boys and lovers.* Retrieved May 11, 2002, from www.fpc.net/pages/boymuse/report.html.

Berenson, A. B. (1998). Normal anogenital anatomy. *Child Abuse & Neglect, 22,* 589–596.

Berliner, L. (1991). Reporting child abuse: Helping or hurting? *Journal of Interpersonal Violence, 6,* 110–118.

Berliner, L., & Saunders, B. (1996). Treating fear and anxiety in sexually abused children: Results of a controlled two-year follow-up study. *Child Maltreatment, 1,* 294–309.

Bertalanffy, L. (1974). The unified theory for psychiatry and behavioral sciences. In S. Feinstein & P. Giovacchini (Eds.), *Adolescent psychiatry* (Vol. 3, pp. 43-49). New York: Basic Books.

Bishop, S. J., Murphy, J. M., Hicks, R., Quinn, D. Lewis, P. J., Grace, M., & Jellinek, M. S. (2000). What progress has been made in meeting the needs of seriously maltreated children? The course of 200 cases through the Boston Juvenile Court. *Child Abuse & Neglect, 24,* 599–610.

Blanchard, R., Watson, M. S., Choy, A., Dickey, R., Klassen, P., Kuban, M., & Ferren, D.J. (1999). Pedophiles: Mental retardation, maternal age, and sexual orientation. *Archives of Sexual Behavior, 28,* 111–127.

Blanck, G., & Blanck, R. (1974). *Ego psychology: Theory and practice.* New York: Columbia University Press.

Blum, H. P., & Goodman, W. H. (1995). Countertransference. In B. E. Moore, & B. D. Fine (Eds.), *Psychoanalysis: The major concepts* (pp. 121–129). New Haven, CT: Yale University Press.

Blumenthal, S., Gudjonsson, G., & Burns, J. (1999) Cognitive distortions and blame attribution in sex offenders against adults and children. *Child Abuse & Neglect, 23,* 129–143.

Bradley, R. G., & Follingstad, D. R. (2001). Utilizing disclosure in the treatment of the sequelae of childhood sexual abuse: A theoretical and empirical review. *Clinical Psychology Review, 21,* 1–32.

Bremner, J. D., Krystal, J. H., Putnam, F. W., Southwick, S. M., Marmar, C., Charney, D. S., & Mazure, C. M. (1998). Measurement of dissociative states with the Clinician-Administered Dissociative States Scale (CADSS). *Journal of Traumatic Stress, 11,* 125–136.

Brett, E. A., & Ostroff, R. (1985). Imagery and posttraumatic stress disorder: An overview. *American Journal of Psychiatry, 142,* 417–424.

Briere, J. (1996a). *Therapy for adults molested as children: Beyond survival* (2nd ed.). New York: Springer.

Briere, J., & Runtz, M. (1988). Symptomatology associated with childhood sexual victimization in a non-clinical adult sample. *Child Abuse & Neglect, 12,* 51–59.

Briere, J., & Runtz, M. (1989). The Trauma Symptom Checklist (TSC-33): Early data on a new scale. *Journal of Interpersonal Violence, 4,* 151–163.

Briere, J., & Runtz, M. (1993). Childhood sexual abuse: Long-term sequelae and implications for psychological assessment. *Journal of Interpersonal Violence, 8,* 312–330.

Britton, G., & Lumpkin, M. (1984). Battle to imprint for the 21st century. *Reading Teacher, 37,* 724–733.

Brown, D. (1995). Pseudomemories: The standard of science and the standard of care in trauma treatment. *American Journal of Clinical Hypnosis, 37,* 1–24.

Brown, J. (1990). The treatment of male victims with mixed-gender, short-term group psychotherapy. In M. Hunter, (Ed.), *The sexually abused male: Application of treatment strategies* (Vol. 2, pp. 137–169). Lexington, MA: Lexington Books.

Bryant, R. A., Sackville, T., Dant, S. T., Moulds, M., & Guthrie, R. (1999). Treating acute stress disorder: An evaluation of cognitive behavior therapy and supportive counseling techniques. *American Journal of Psychiatry, 156,* 17801–1786.

Burgess, A. W. (1985). *The sexual victimization of adolescents.* Washington, DC: National Institute of Mental Health, DHHS Publication Number (ADM) 85-1382.

Burgess, A. W., & Holmstrom, L. L. (1975). Sexual trauma of children and adolescents. *Nursing Clinics of America, 10,* 551–563.

Burgess, E. S., & Wurtele, S. K. (1998). Enhancing parent-child communication about sexual abuse: A pilot study. *Child Abuse & Neglect, 22,* 1167–1175.

Bussey, K., & Grimbeek, E. J. (1995). Disclosure processes: Issues for child sexual abuse victims. In K. J. Rotenberg (Ed.), *Disclosure processes in children and adolescents* (pp. 166–203). Cambridge, UK: Cambridge University Press.

Butts, J. A., & Snyder, H. N. (1997). The youngest delinquents: Offenders under age 15. *Juvenile Justice Bulletin,* 1–11.

Carrion, V. G., & Steiner, H. (2000). Trauma and dissociation in delinquent adolescents. *Psychosomatic Medicine, 62,* 26–32.

Celano, M. P. (1992). A developmental model of victims' internal attributions of responsibility for sexual abuse. *Journal of Interpersonal Violence, 7,* 57–69.

Chard, K. M., Weaver, T. L., & Resnick, P. A. (1997). Adaptive cognitive processing therapy for child sexual abuse survivors. *Cognitive and Behavioral Practice, 4,* 31–52.

Chertoff, J. (1998). Psychodynamic assessment and treatment of traumatized patients. *Journal of Psychotherapy Practice and Research, 7,* 35–46.

Christian, R., Dwyer, S., Shumm, W. R., & Coulson, L.A . (1988). Prevention of sexual abuse for preschoolers: Evaluation of a pilot program. *Psychological Reports, 62,* 387–396.

Cicchetti, D., & Toth, S. L. (1995). A developmental psychopathology perspective on child abuse and neglect. *Journal of the American Academy of Child and Adolescent Psychiatry, 34,* 541–565.

Coffey, P., Leitenberg, H., Henning, K., Turner, T., & Bennett, R. T. (1996). Mediators of the long-term impact of child sexual abuse: Perceived stigma, betrayal, powerlessness, and self-blame. *Child Abuse & Neglect, 20,* 447–455.

Cohen, J. A., & Mannarino, A. P. (1993). A treatment model for sexually abused preschoolers. *Journal of Interpersonal Violence, 8,* 115–131.

Cohen, J. A., & Mannarino, A. P. (1996). A treatment outcome study for sexually abused preschool children: Initial findings. *Journal of the American Academy of Child and Adolescent Psychiatry, 35,* 42–50.

Cohen, J. A., & Mannarino, A. P. (1997). A treatment study for sexually abused preschool children: Outcome during a one-year follow-up. *Journal of the American Academy of Child and Adolescent Psychiatry, 36,* 1228–1235.

Cohen, J. A., & Mannarino, A. P. (1997). Interventions for sexually abused children: Initial treatment outcome findings. *Child Maltreatment, 3,* 17–26.

Cohen, J. A., & Mannarino, A. P. (2000). Predictors of treatment outcome in sexually abused children. *Child Abuse & Neglect, 24,* 983–994.

Cohen, J. A., Mannarino, A. P., & Rogal, S. (2001). Treatment practices for childhood posttraumatic stress disorder. *Child Abuse & Neglect, 25,* 123–135.

Conte, J. R. (1985). The effects of sexual abuse on children: A critique and suggestions for future research. *Victimology: An International Journal, 10,* 110–130.

Conway, M. A. (1990). *Autobiographical memory: An introduction.* Philadelphia: Open University Press.

Conway, M. A. (1992). *Autobiographical memory: An introduction.* Philadelphia: Open University Press.

Conway, M. A. (1997). *Recovered memories and false memories: Debates in psychology.* Oxford: Oxford University Press.

Coons, P. M. (1998). The dissociative disorders: Rarely considered and underdiagnosed. *Psychiatric Clinics of North America, 21,* 637–648.

Corwin, D. L., & Olafson, E. (1993). Overview: Clinical identification of sexually abused children. *Child Abuse & Neglect, 17,* 3–5.

Courtois, C. A. (1997). Guidelines for the treatment of adults abused or possibly abused as children. *American Journal of Psychotherapy, 51,* 497–510.

Crawford, S. L. (1999). Intrafamilial sexual abuse: What we think we know about mothers, and implications for intervention. *Journal of Child Sexual Abuse, 7,* 55–74.

Crenshaw, D. A., Rudy, C., Triemer, D., & Zingaro, J. (1986). Psychotherapy with sexually abused children: Breaking the silent bond. *Residential Group Care & Treatment, 3,* 25–38.

Crimes Against Children Research Center. (1998). Fact sheet. Retrieved July 7, 2002, from www.unh.edu/ccrx/factsheet.html.

Crivillé, A. (1990). Child physical and sexual abuse: The roles of sadism and sexuality. *Child Abuse & Neglect, 14,* 121–127.

Cunningham, R. M., Stiffman, A. R., Dore, P., & Earls, F. (1994). The association of physical and sexual abuse and HIV infection: Implications for public health. *Child Abuse & Neglect, 18,* 233–245.

Daldin, H. (1988). The fate of the sexually abused child. *Clinical Social Work Journal, 16,* 22–31.

Daro, D. (1991). Child sexual abuse prevention: Separating fact from fiction. *Child Abuse & Neglect, 15,* 1–4.

Deblinger, E., Lippmann, J., & Steer, R. (1996). Sexually abused children suffering posttraumatic stress symptoms: Initial treatment outcome findings. *Child Maltreatment, 1,* 310-321.

Deblinger, E., McLeer, S. V., & Henry, D. (1990). Cognitive behavioral treatment for sexually abused children suffering post-traumatic stress: Preliminary findings. *Journal of the American Academy of Child and Adolescent Psychiatry, 29,* 747–752.

Deblinger, E., Steer, R. A., & Lippmann, J. (1999). Two-year follow-up study of cognitive behavioral therapy for sexually abused children suffering post-traumatic stress symptoms. *Child Abuse & Neglect, 23,* 1371–1378.

deMause, L. (1990). The history of child assault. *Journal of Psychohistory, 18,* 1–29.

de Young, M. (1982). Self-injurious behavior in incest victims: A research note. *Child Welfare, 61,* 577–584.

DiTomasso, M. J., & Routh, D. K. (1993). Recall of abuse in childhood and three measures of dissociation. *Child Abuse & Neglect, 17,* 477–485.

Dixon, K. N., Arnold, L. E., & Calestro, K. (1978). Father-son incest: Underreported psychiatric problem? *American Journal of Psychiatry, 135,* 835–838.

Douglas, A., Coghill, D., & Will, D. (1996). A survey of the first five years' work of a child sexual abuse team. *Child Abuse Review, 5,* 227–238.

Downs, W. R. (1993). Developmental considerations of the effects of childhood sexual abuse. *Journal of Interpersonal Violence, 8,* 331–345.

Draucker, C. B. (1995). A coping model for adult survivors of childhood sexual abuse. *Journal of Interpersonal Violence, 10,* 159–175.

Drews, J. R., & Bradley, T. T. (1989). Group treatment for adults molested as children: An educational and therapeutic approach. *Social Work with Groups, 12,* 57–75.

Egeland, B., Carlson, E., & Stroufe, L. A. (1993). Resilience as process. *Development & Psychopathology, 5,* 517–528.

Eichenbaum, H. (1997). Declarative memory: Insights from cognitive neurobiology. *Annual Reviews in Psychology, 48,* 547–572.

Eisenberg, N., Owens, R. G., & Dewey, M. E. (1987). Attitudes of health professionals to child sexual abuse and incest. *Child Abuse & Neglect, 11,* 109–116.

Elliott, A. N., & Carnes, C. N. (2001). Reactions of nonoffending parents to the sexual abuse of their child: A review of the literature. *Child Maltreatment, 6,* 314–331.

Elliott, D. M., & Briere, J. (1992). The sexually abused boy: Problems in manhood. *Medical Aspects of Human Sexuality, 26*, 68–71.

Engle, P. (1997). Art therapy and dissociative disorders. *Art Therapy: Journal of the American Art Therapy Association, 14*, 246–254.

Erikson, E. H. (1982). *The life cycle completed.* New York: W. W. Norton.

Esser-Stuart, J. E., & Skibinski, G. J. (1998). Child sexual abuse intervention: An exploratory study of policy concerns and implications for program development. *Journal of Child Sexual Abuse, 7*, 87–103.

Etherington, K. (1995). Adult male survivors of childhood sexual abuse. *Counselling Psychology Quarterly, 8*, 233–241.

Everson, M. D., & Boat, B. W. (1989). False allegations of sexual abuse by children and adolescents. *Journal of the American Academy of Child and Adolescent Psychiatry, 28*, 230–240.

Faller, K. C., & Corwin, D. L. (1995). Children' interview statements and behaviors: Role in identifying sexually abused children. *Child Abuse & Neglect, 19*, 71–82.

Federal Bureau of Investigation. (1998). *Implementing the National Incident-Based Reporting System.* Retrieved October 3, 2002, from www.nibrs.search.org/frmain.htm.

Fergusson, D. M., Horwood, L. J., & Woodward, L. J. (2000). The stability of child abuse reports: A longitudinal study of the reporting behavior of young adults. *Psychological Medicine, 30*, 529–544.

Fergusson, D. M., & Mullen, P. E. (1999). *Childhood sexual abuse: An evidence based perspective.* Thousand Oaks, CA: Sage.

Finkelhor, D. (1987). The trauma of child sexual abuse: Two models. *Journal of Interpersonal Violence, 2*, 348–366.

Finkelhor, D., & Berliner, L. (1995). Research on the treatment of sexually abused children: A review and recommendations. *Journal of the American Academy of Child and Adolescent Psychiatry, 34*, 1408–1423.

Finkelhor, D., & Murphy, L. (2001, April). Offenders incarcerated for crimes against juveniles. *Juvenile Justice Bulletin.* Washington, DC: U.S. Department of Justice, Office of Justice and Delinquency Programs.

Firestone, P., Bradford, J. M., Greenberg, D. M., & Nunes, K. L. (2000). Differentiation of homicidal child molesters, nonhomicidal child molesters, and nonoffenders by phallometry. *American Journal of Psychiatry, 157*, 1847–1850.

Flathman, M. (1999). Trauma and delayed memory: A review of the "repressed memories" literature. *Journal of Child Sexual Abuse, 8*, 1–23.

Flavell, J. H., Miller, P. H., & Miller, S. A. (1993). *Cognitive development* (3rd ed.). Englewood Cliffs, NJ: Prentice Hall.

Foa, E. B., & Meadows, E. A. (1997). Psychosocial treatments for posttraumatic stress disorder: A critical review. *Annual Reviews in Psychology, 48*, 449–480.

Foa, E. B., Molnar, C., & Cashman, L. (1995). Change in rape narratives during exposure therapy for posttraumatic stress disorder. *Journal of Traumatic Stress, 8*, 675–690.

Freedman, A. M., Kaplan, H. I., & Sadock, B. (Eds.). (1975). *Comprehensive textbook on psychiatry* (2nd ed.) Baltimore: Williams & Wilkins.

Freeman-Longo, R. E. (1986). The impact of sexual victimization on males. *Child Abuse & Neglect, 10*, 411–414.

Freshwater, K., Leach, C., & Aldridge, J. (2001). Personal constructs, childhood sexual abuse and revictimization. *British Journal of Medical Psychology, 74*, 379–397.

Freund, K., & Blanchard, R. (1989). Phallometric diagnosis of pedophilia. *Journal of Consulting and Clinical Psychology, 57*, 100–105.

Freyd, J. J. (1994). Betrayal trauma: Traumatic amnesia as an adaptive response to childhood abuse. *Ethics & Behavior, 4*, 307–329.

Friedman, S., Smith, L., Fogel, D., Paradis, C., Viswanathan, R., Ackerman, R., et al. (2002). The incidence and influence of early traumatic life events in patients with panic disorder: A comparison with other psychiatric outpatients. *Journal of Anxiety Disorders, 16*, 259–272.

Friedrich, W. N. (1990a). *Psychotherapy of sexually abused children and their families.* New York: W. W. Norton.

Friedrich, W. N. (1990b). The person of the therapist. *Psychotherapy of sexually abused children and their families,* (pp. 268–280). New York: W. W. Norton.

Friedrich, W. N. (1993). Sexual victimization and sexual behavior in children: A review of recent literature. *Child Abuse & Neglect, 17,* 59–66.

Friedrich, W. N. (1995). *Psychotherapy with sexually abused boys: An integrated approach.* Thousand Oaks, CA: Sage.

Friedrich, W. N., Grambsch, P., Damon, L., Hewitt, S. K., Koverola, C., Lang, R. A., Wolfe, V., & Broughton, D. (1992). Child sexual behavior inventory: Normative and clinical comparisons. *Psychological Assessment, 4,* 303–311.

Friedrich, W. N., Luecke, W. J., Beilke, R. L., & Place, V. (1992). Psychotherapy outcome of sexually abused boys: An agency study. *Journal of Interpersonal Violence, 7,* 386–409.

Friedrich, W. N., Luecke, W. J., Beilke, R. L., & Place, V. (1992). Psychotherapy outcome of sexually abused boys. *Journal of Interpersonal Violence, 7,* 396–409.

Fritz, G. S., Stoll, K., & Wagner, N. N. (1981). A comparison of males and females who were sexually molested as children. *Journal of Sex & Marital Therapy, 7,* 54–59.

Fromm-Reichmann, F. (1975). *Frieda Fromm-Reichmann: Psychoanalysis and psychotherapy, selected papers.* Chicago: University of Chicago Press.

Fromuth, M. E., Burkhart, B. R., & Jones, C. W. (1991). Hidden child molestation: An investigation of adolescent perpetrators in a nonclinical sample. *Journal of Interpersonal Violence, 6,* 376–384.

Futterman, D., Hein, K., Reuben, N., Dell, R., & Shaffer, N. (1993). Human immunodeficiency virus-infected adolescents: The first 50 patients in a New York City program. *Pediatrics, 91,* 730–735.

Gabriele, J. D. E. (1998). Cognitive neuroscience of human memory. *Annual Reviews in Psychology, 49,* 87–115.

Gambrill, E. D. (1983). Behavioral intervention with child abuse and neglect. *Progress in Behavior Modification, 15,* 1–56.

Gershuny, B. S., & Thayer, J. F. (1999). Relations among psychological trauma, dissociative phenomena, and trauma-related distress: A review and integration. *Clinical Psychology Review, 19,* 631–657.

Giarretto, H. (1982). A comprehensive child sexual abuse treatment program. *Child Abuse & Neglect, 6,* 263–278.

Gibson, L. E., & Leitenberg, H. (2000). Child sexual abuse prevention programs: Do they decrease the occurrence of child sexual abuse? *Child Abuse & Neglect, 24,* 1115–1125.

Gil, T., Calev, A., Greenberg, D., Kugelmass, S., & Lerer, B. (1990). Cognitive functioning in post-traumatic stress disorder. *Journal of Traumatic Stress, 3,* 29–46.

Gluck, M. A., & Myers, C. E. (1997). Psychobiological models of hippocampal function in learning and memory. *Annual Reviews in Psychology, 48,* 481–514.

Gold, E. R. (1986). Long-term effects of sexual victimization in childhood: An attributional approach. *Journal of Consulting and Clinical Psychology, 54,* 471–475.

Gold, S. N., Lucenko, B. A., Elhai, J. D., Swingle, J. M., & Sellers, A. H. (1999). A comparison of psychological/psychiatric symptomatology of women and men sexually abused as children. *Child Abuse & Neglect, 23,* 683–692.

Golding, J. M., Cooper, M. L., & George, L. K. (1997). Sexual assault history and health perceptions: seven general populations studies. *Health Psychology, 16,* 417–425.

Goldstein, D. S. (2000). Sympathetic nervous system. In G. Fink (Ed.), *Encyclopedia of stress* (Vol. 3, pp. 558–565). San Diego, CA: Academic Press.

Goodman, A. (1998). *Sexual addiction: An integrated approach.* Madison, CT: International Universities Press.

Goodman, G. S., Quas, J. A., Bottoms, B. L., Qin, J., Shaver, P. R., Orcutt, H., & Shapiro, C. (1997).

Children's religious knowledge: Implications for understanding satanic ritual abuse allegations. *Child Abuse & Neglect, 21,* 1111–1130.

Gordon, L. (1986). Incest and resistance: Patterns of father-daughter incest, 1880-1930. *Social Problems,* 37, 253–267.

Gothard, J. S., & Ivker, N. A. C. (2000). The evolving law of alleged delayed memories of childhood sexual abuse. *Child Maltreatment, 5,* 176–189.

Gothard, S., & Heinrich, T. (1999). *Does treatment work? Administrative and research findings from a treatment outcome program.* Paper presented at the Conference on Responding to Child Maltreatment, San Diego, CA.

Grayston, A. D., & De Luca, R. V. (1995). Group therapy for boys who have experienced sexual abuse: Is it the treatment of choice? *Journal of Child and Adolescent Group Therapy, 5,* 57–82.

Grayston, A. D., & De Luca, R. V. (1996). Social validity of group treatment for sexually abused boys. *Child & Family Behavior Therapy, 18,* 1–11.

Green, A. H. (1993). Child sexual abuse: Immediate and long-term effects and intervention. *Journal of the American Academy of Child and Adolescent Psychiatry,* 32, 890–902.

Gries, L. T., Goh, D. S., Andrews, M. B., Gilbert, J., Praver, F., & Stelzer, D. N. (2000). Positive reaction to disclosure and recovery from child sexual abuse. *Journal of Child Sexual Abuse, 9,* 29–51.

Grocke, M., Smith, M., & Graham, P. (1995). Sexually abused and nonabused mothers' discussions about sex and their children's sexual knowledge. *Child Abuse & Neglect, 19,* 985–996.

Gully, K. J., Britton, H., Hanse, K., Goodwill, K., & Nope, J. L. (1999) A new measure for distress during child sexual abuse examinations: The genital examination distress scale. *Child Abuse & Neglect, 23,* 61–70.

Guthrie, R., & Bryant, R. (1999). Attempting suppression of traumatic memories over extended periods in acute stress disorder. *Behaviour Research and Therapy, 38,* 899–907.

Hack, T. F., Osachuk, T. A. G., & De Luca, R. V. (1994). Group treatment for sexually abused preadolescent boys. *Families in Society: The Journal of Contemporary Human Services, 75,* 217–228.

Hall-Marley, S., & Damon, L. (1993). Impact of structured group therapy on young victims of sexual abuse. *Journal of Child and Adolescent Group Therapy, 3,* 41–48.

Hanson, R. F., Resnick, H. S., Saunders, B. E., Kilpatrick, D. G., & Best, C. (1999). Factors related to the reporting of childhood rape. *Child Abuse & Neglect, 23,* 559–569.

Hanson, R. K., & Bussiere, M. T. (1998). Predicting relapse: A meta-analysis of sexual offender recidivism studies. *Journal of Consulting and Clinical Psychology, 66,* 348–362.

Harper, J. (1993). Prepubertal male victims of incest: A clinical study. *Child Abuse & Neglect, 17,* 419–421.

Hartman, C. R., & Burgess, A. W. (1993). Treatment of victims of rape trauma. In J. P. Wilson & B. Raphael (Eds.), *International book of traumatic stress syndromes* (pp. 507–516). New York: Plenum Press.

Hartmann, H. (1958). *Ego psychology and the problem of adaptation.* New York: International Universities Press.

Haskett, M. E., Nowlan, N. P., Hutcheson, J. S., & Whitworth, J. M. (1991). Factors associated with successful entry into therapy in child sexual abuse cases. *Child Abuse & Neglect, 15,* 467–476.

Haugaard, J. J., & Emery, R. E. (1989). Methodological issues in child sexual abuse research. *Child Abuse & Neglect, 13,* 89–100.

Hazzard, A., Webb, C., Kleemeier, C., Angert, L., & Pohl, J. (1991). Child sexual abuse prevention: Evaluation and one-year follow-up. *Child Abuse & Neglect, 15,* 123–138.

Heim, C., Newport, D. J., Bonsall, R., Miller, A. H., & Nemeroff, C. B. (2001). Altered pituitary-adrenal axis responses to provocative challenge tests in adult survivors of childhood abuse. *American Journal of Psychiatry, 154,* 575–581.

Herman, J. L., & Harvey, M. R. (1993, April). The false memory debate: Social science or social backlash? *The Harvard Mental Health Letter, 9,* 4–6.

Herman, J. L., & Harvey, M. F. (1997). Adult memories of childhood trauma: A naturalistic clinical study. *Journal of Traumatic Stress, 10,* 557–571.

Hetherton, J. (1999). The idealization of women: Its role in the minimization of child sexual abuse by females. *Child Abuse & Neglect, 23,* 161–174.

Hill, C. E., & Alexander, P .C. (1993). Process research in the treatment of adult victims of childhood sexual abuse. *Journal of Interpersonal Violence, 8,* 415–427.

Hill, S. Y., De Bellis, M. D., Keshavan, M. S., Lowers, L., Shen, S., Hall, J., & Pitts, T. (2001). Right amygdala volume in adolescent and young adult offspring from families at high risk for developing alcoholism. *Biological Psychiatry, 49,* 894–905.

Honing, R. G., Grace, M. C., Lindy, J. D., Newman, C. J., & Titchener, J. L. (1999). Assessing long-term effects of trauma: Diagnosing symptoms of avoidance and numbing. *American Journal of Psychiatry, 156,* 483–485.

Horowitz, M. J., & Reidbord, S. P. (1992). Memory, emotion, and response to trauma. In S. A. Christianson (Ed.), *Handbook of emotion and memory* (pp. 343–358). Hillsdale, NJ: Lawrence Erlbaum.

Horton, C. B., & Cruise, T. K. (1997). Clinical assessment of child victims and adult survivors of child maltreatment. *Journal of Counseling & Development, 76,* 94–104.

House Con. Res. 107. Retrieved October 1, 2002, from www.legistative.noaa.gov.

Howe, M. L. (1998). Individual differences in factors that modulate storage and retrieval of traumatic memories. *Development and Psychopathology, 10,* 681–698.

Howing, P. T., Wodarski, J. S., Gaudin, J. M., Jr., & Kurtz, P. D. (1989). Effective interventions to ameliorate the incidence of child maltreatment: The empirical base. *Social Work, 34,* 330–338.

Irwin, H. J. (1994). Proneness to dissociation and traumatic childhood events. *Journal of Nervous and Mental Disease, 182,* 456–460.

Isely, P. J. (1992). A time-limited group therapy model for men sexually abused as children. *Group, 16,* 233–246.

Isely, P. J. (in press). Child sexual abuse and the catholic church: An historical and contemporary review. *Pastoral Psychology.*

Isely, P. J., & Isely, P. (1990). The sexual abuse of male children by church personnel: Intervention and prevention. *Pastoral Psychology, 39,* 85–99.

Jackson, S., Thompson, R. A., Christiansen, E. H., Colman, R. A., Wyatt, J., Buckendahl, C. W., Wilcox, B. L., & Peterson, R. (1999). Predicting abuse-prone parental attitudes and discipline practices in a nationally representative sample. *Child Abuse & Neglect, 23,* 15–29.

Jackson, T. L., & Ferguson, W. P. (1983). Attribution of blame in incest. *American Journal of Community Psychology, 11,* 313–322.

Jacobs, W. J., Laurance, H. E., Thomas, K. G. F., Luzcak, S. E., & Nadel, L. (1996). On the veracity and variability of traumatic memory. *Tramatology 2,* 2. Available: www.rdz.stjohns.edu/trauma/art3v2i2.html.

Jehu, D., Klassen, C., & Gazan, M. (1986). Cognitive restructuring of distorted beliefs associated with childhood sexual abuse. *Journal of Social Work and Human Sexuality, 4,* 49–69.

Jennings, K. T. (1993). Female child molesters: A review of the literature. In M. Elliott (Ed.), *Female sexual abuse of children* (pp. 219–234). New York: Guilford Press.

Johnson, T. C. (1988). Child perpetrators—children who molest other children: Preliminary findings. *Child Abuse & Neglect, 12,* 219–229.

Jones, D. P. H. 1999. Editorial: Children with sexual behavior problems. *Child Abuse & Neglect, 23,* 597–599.

Kaufman, K. L., Hilliker, D. R., & Daleiden, E. L. (1996). Subgroup differences in the modus operandi of adolescent sexual offenders. *Child Management, 1,* 17–24.

Kellogg, N. D., & Hoffman, T. J. (1997). Child sexual revictimization by multiple perpetrators. *Child Abuse & Neglect, 21,* 953–964.

Kempe, C. H. (1978). Sexual abuse, another hidden pediatric problem: The 1977 C. Anderson Aldrich Lecture. *Pediatrics, 62,* 382–389.

Kendall, P. C. (1991). *Child and adolescent psychotherapy: Cognitive behavioral procedures.* New York: Guilford Press.

Kendall-Tackett, K. A. (1991). Characteristics of abuse that influence when adults molested as children seek treatment. *Journal of Interpersonal Violence, 6,* 486–493.

Kendall-Tackett, K. A., & Simon, A. F. (1987). Perpetrators and their acts: Data from 365 adults molested as children. *Child Abuse & Neglect, 11,* 217–245.

Kenny, M. S., & McEachern, A. G. (2000). Racial, ethnic, and cultural factors of childhood sexual abuse: A selected review of the literature. *Clinical Psychology Review, 20,* 905–922.

Kercher, G. A., & McShane, M. (1984). The prevalence of child sexual abuse victimization in an adult sample of Texas residents. *Child Abuse & Neglect, 8,* 495–501.

Kerns, D. L. (1998). Triage and referrals for child sexual abuse medical examinations: Which children are likely to have positive medical findings? *Child Abuse & Neglect, 22,* 515–518.

King, J. A., Mandansky, D., King, S., Fletcher, K. E., & Brewer, J. (2001). Early sexual abuse and low cortisol. *Psychiatry and Clinical Neurosciences, 55,* 71–74.

King, N. J., Tonge, B. J., Mullen, P., Myerson, N., Heyne, D., Rollings, S., Martin, R., & Ollendick, T. H. (2000). Treating sexually abused children with posttraumatic stress symptoms: A randomized clinical trial. *Journal of the American Academy of Child and Adolescent Psychiatry, 39,* 1347–1355.

Kinnard, E. M. (2001). Perceived and actual academic competence in maltreated children. *Child Abuse & Neglect, 25,* 33–45.

Kinzl, J. F., Traweger, C., Guenther, V., & Biebl, W. (1994). Family background and sexual abuse associated with eating disorders. *American Journal of Psychiatry, 151,* 1127–1131.

Kite, M. E. (1992). Individual differences in males' reactions to gay males and lesbians. *Journal of Applied Social Psychology, 22,* 1122–1239.

Knapp, S., & VandeCreek, L. (1996). Risk management for psychologists: Treating patients who recover lost memories of childhood abuse. *Professional Psychology: Research and Practice, 27,* 452–459.

Knight, R. A., & Prentsky, R. A. (1993). Exploring characteristics for classifying juvenile sex offenders. In H. E. Barbaree, W. L. Marshall, & S. M. Hudson (Eds.), *The juvenile sex offender* (pp. 45–83). New York: Guilford Press.

Kobayashi, J., Sales, B. D., Becker, J. V., Figueredo, A. J., & Kaplan, M. S. (1995). Perceived parental deviance, parent child bonding, child abuse and child sexual aggression. *Sexual Abuse: A Journal of Research and Treatment, 7,* 25–44.

Koenigsberg, H. W., & Siever, L. J. (2000). Borderline personality disorder. In G. Fink (Ed.), *Encyclopedia of stress* (Vol. 1, pp. 339–341). San Diego, CA: Academic Press.

Kraizer, S. K. (1986). Rethinking prevention. *Child Abuse & Neglect, 10,* 259–261.

Kruczek, T., & Vitanza, S. (1999). Treatment effects with an adolescent abuse survivor's group. *Child Abuse & Neglect, 23,* 477–485.

Ku, L., Sonnenstein, F. L., & Pleck, J. H. (1992). Patterns of HIV risk and preventive behaviors among teenage men. *Public Health Reports, 107,* 131–138.

Kuhn, T. S. (1970). *The structure of scientific revolutions* (2nd ed.). Chicago: University of Chicago Press.

Lamb, M. E., Sternberg, K. J., & Esplin, P. W. (1998). Conducting investigative interviews of alleged sexual abuse victims. *Child Abuse & Neglect, 22,* 813–823.

Langsley, D. G., Schwartz, M. N., & Fairbairn, R. H. (1968). Father–son incest. *Comprehensive Psychiatry, 9,* 218–226.

Lanktree, C. B., & Briere, J. (1995). Outcome of therapy for sexually abused children: A repeated measures study. *Child Abuse & Neglect, 19,* 1145–1155.

Larzelere, R. E., Collins, L., & Collins, R. A. (1993, October). *During and post-treatment effects of group therapy for sexual victimizations.* Paper presented at the annual Conference on Responding to Child Maltreatment, San Diego, CA.

Leberg, E. (1997). *Understanding child molesters: Taking charge.* Thousand Oaks, CA: Sage.

LeDoux, J. E. (1993). Emotional memory systems in the brain. *Behavior and Brain Research, 58,* 69–79.

Leitenberg, H., Greenwald, E., & Cado, S. (1992). A retrospective study of long-term methods of coping with having been sexually abused during childhood. *Child Abuse & Neglect, 16,* 399–407.

Leitenberg, H., Greenwald, E., & Tarran, M. J. (1989). The relation between sexual activity among children during preadolescence and/or early adolescence and sexual behavior and sexual adjustment in young adulthood. *Archives of Sexual Behavior, 18,* 299–313.

Lev-Wiesel, R. (2000). Quality of life in adult survivors of childhood sexual abuse who have undergone therapy. *Journal of Child Sexual Abuse, 9,* 1–13.

Levendosky, A. A., & Buttenheim, M. (2000). A multi-method treatment for child survivors of sexual abuse: An intervention informed by relational and trauma theories. *Journal of Child Sexual Abuse, 9,* 1–19.

Leventhal, J. M. (1998). Epidemiology of sexual abuse of children: Old problems, new directions. *Child Abuse & Neglect, 22,* 481–491.

Levin, F. M. (1995). Psychoanalysis and the brain. In B. E. Moore & B. D. Fine (Eds.), *Psychoanalysis: The major concepts* (pp. 537–552). New Haven, CT: Yale University Press.

Liem, J. H., & Boudewyn, A. C. (1999). Contextualizing the effects of childhood sexual abuse on adult self and social functioning: An attachment theory perspective. *Child Abuse & Neglect, 23,* 1141–1157.

Lindsay, D. Stephen, & Read, J. D. (1994). Psychotherapy and memories of childhood sexual abuse: A cognitive perspective. *Applied Cognitive Psychology, 8,* 281–338.

Lipovsky, J. A., Saunders, B. E., & Murphy, S. M. (1989). Depression, anxiety, and behavior problems among victims of father–child sexual assault and nonabused siblings. *Journal of Interpersonal Violence, 4,* 452–468.

Lipovsky, J. A., Swenson, C. C., Ralston, M. E., & Saunders, B. E. (1998). The abuse clarification process in the treatment of intrafamilial child abuse. *Child Abuse & Neglect, 22,* 729–741.

Lisak, D. (1993). Men as victims: Challenging cultural myths. (Commentary). *Journal of Traumatic Stress, 6,* 577–580.

Lisak, D., & Ivan, C. (1995). Deficits in intimacy and empathy in sexually aggressive men. *Journal of Interpersonal Violence, 10,* 296–308.

Linton, S. J. (2002). A prospective study of the effects of sexual or physical abuse on back pain. *Pain, 96,* 347–351.

Llewlyn, S. P. (1997). Therapeutic approaches for survivors of childhood sexual abuse: A review. *Clinical Psychology and Psychotherapy, 4,* 32–41.

Lomonaco, S., Scheidlinger, S., & Aronson, S. (2000). Five decades of children's group treatment: An overview. *Journal of Child and Adolescent Group Therapy, 10,* 77–96.

Lowman, J. (1987). Taking prostitutes seriously. *Canadian Review of Sociology and Anthropology, 24,* 99–116.

Lyon, T. (1996). The effect of threats on children's disclosure of sexual abuse. *The APSAC Advisor, 9,* 9–15.

MacMillan, R. (2001, August 8). *Bill aims to hammer net child molesters.* Newsbytes. Retrieved August 10, 2002, from www.inforwar.com.

Maes, M., van West, D., De Vos, N., Westenberg, H., Van Hunsel, F., Hendriks, D., et al. (2001). Lower baseline plasma cortisol and prolactin and increased body temperature, and higher mCPP-induced cortisol responses in men with pedophilia. *Neuropsychopharmacology, 24,* 37–46.

Mahoney, M. J. (1991). *Human change process: The scientific foundations of psychotherapy.* New York: Basic Books.

Mahoney, M. J. (1991). *Human change processes: The scientific foundations of psychotherapy.* San Francisco: Jossey-Bass.

Marmar, C. R., Weiss, D. S., Schlenger, W. E., Fairbank, J. A., Jordan, B. K., Kulka, R. A., & Hough,

R. L. (1994). Peritraumatic dissociation and posttraumatic stress in male Vietnam theater veterans. *American Journal of Psychiatry, 151,* 902–907.

Marshall, R. D., Spitzer, R., & Liebowitz, M. R. (1999). Review and critique of the new *DSM–IV* diagnosis of acute stress disorder. *American Journal of Psychiatry, 156,* 1677–1685.

McCann, I. L., Sakheim, D. K., & Abrahamson, D. J. (1988). Trauma and victimization: A model of psychological adaptation. *Counseling Psychologist, 16,* 531–594.

McCann, I. L., & Pearlman, L. A. (1990). *Psychological trauma and the adult survivor: Theory, therapy and transformation.* New York: Brunner/Mazel.

McCann, J. (1998). The appearance of acute, healing, and healed anogenital trauma. *Child Abuse & Neglect, 22,* 605–615.

McCarroll, J. E., Newby, J. H., Thayer, L. E., Ursano, R. J., Norwood, A. E., & Fullerton, C. S. (1999). Trends in child maltreatment in the US Army, 1975–1997. *Child Abuse & Neglect, 23,* 855–861.

McLeer, S. V., Deblinger, E., Atkins, M. S., Foa, E. B., & Ralphe, D. L. (1988). Post-traumatic stress disorder in sexually abused children. *Journal of the American Academy of Child and Adolescent Psychiatry, 27,* 650–654.

McNulty, C., & Wardle, J. (1994). Adult disclosure of sexual abuse: A primary cause of psychological distress? *Child Abuse & Neglect, 18,* 549–555.

Meadows, E. A., & Foa, E. B. (1999). Cognitive-behavioral treatment of traumatized adults. In P. A. Saigh, & J. D. Bremner (Eds.), *Posttraumatic stress disorder: A comprehensive text* (pp. 376–390). Boston: Allyn & Bacon.

Millar, G. M., & Stermac, L. (2000). Substance abuse and childhood maltreatment: Conceptualizing the recovery process. *Journal of Substance Abuse Treatment, 10,* 175–182.

Miller, D. T, & Porter, C. A. (1983). Self-blame in victims of violence. *Journal of Social Issues, 39,* 139–152.

Miller-Perrin, C. L., Wurtele, S. K., & Kondrick, P. A. (1990). Sexually abused and nonabused children's conceptions of personal body safety. *Child Abuse & Neglect, 14,* 99–112.

Miltenburg, R., & Singer, E. (1997). A theory and support method for adult sexual abuse survivors living in an abusive world. *Journal of Child Sexual Abuse, 6,* 39–63.

Morrissette, P. J. (1999). Post-traumatic stress disorder in childhood sexual abuse: A synthesis and analysis of theoretical models. *Child and Adolescent Social Work Journal, 16,* 77–97.

Mullen, P. E., Martin, J. L., Anderson, J. C., Romans, S. E., & Herbison, G. P. (1996). The long-term impact of physical, emotional, and sexual abuse of children: A community study. *Child Abuse & Neglect, 20,* 7–21.

Muller, R. T., Caldwell, R. A., & Hunter, J. E. (1993). Child provocativeness and gender as factors contributing to the blaming of victims of physical child abuse. *Child Abuse & Neglect, 17,* 249–260.

Myers, M. F. (1989). Men sexually assaulted as adults and sexually abused as boys. *Archives of Sexual Behavior, 18,* 203–215.

Narang, D. S., & Contreras, J. M. (2000). Dissociation as a mediator between child abuse history and adult abuse potential. *Child Abuse & Neglect, 24,* 653–665.

Nash, M. R., Hulsey, T. L., Sexton, M. C., Harralson, T. L., & Lambert, W. (1993). Long-term sequelae of childhood sexual abuse: Perceived family environment, psychopathology, and dissociation. *Journal of Consulting and Clinical Psychology, 61,* 276–283.

National Center on Child Abuse and Neglect. (1988). *Study findings: National incidence and prevalence of child abuse and neglect.* Washington, DC: Westat, Inc.

National Center on Child Abuse and Neglect. (1989). *Study findings: Study of the national incidence and prevalence of child abuse and neglect (NIS-2).* Washington, DC: U.S. Department of Health and Human Services.

National Organization on Male Sexual Victimization. (2002). *Web page information.* Retrieved October 25, 2002, from www.malesurvivor.org.

National Resource Center on Child Sexual Abuse. (1992). *NRCCSA News*, (Vol. 1, May/June).

Newton, D. E. (1978). Homosexual behavior and child molestation: A review of the evidence. *Adolescence, 13*, 29–43.

Oates, R. K., Tebbutt, J., Swanston, H., Lynch, D. L., & O'Toole, B. I. (1998). Prior childhood sexual abuse in mothers of sexually abused children. *Child Abuse & Neglect, 22*, 1113–1118.

O'Donohue, W. T., & Elliott, A. N. (1992). Treatment of the sexually abused child: A review. *Journal of Clinical Child Psychology, 21*, 218–228.

O'Donohue, W., & Geer, J. H. (Eds.). (1992). *The sexual abuse of children: Theory and research*. Hillsdale, NJ: Lawrence Erlbaum.

O'Donohue, W., & Geer, J. H. (Eds.). (1992). *The sexual abuse of children: Clinical issues*. Hillsdale, NJ: Lawrence Erlbaum.

Okami, P. (1991). Self-reports of "positive" childhood and adolescent sexual contacts with older persons: An exploratory study. *Archives of Sexual Behavior, 20*, 437–457.

Olafson, E., Corwin, D. L., & Summit, R. C. (1993). Modern history of child sexual abuse awareness: Cycles of discovery and suppression. *Child Abuse & Neglect, 17*, 7–24.

Olivardia, R., Pope, H. G, Jr., Mangweth, B., & Hudson, J. I. (1995). Eating disorders in college men. *American Journal of Psychiatry, 152*, 1279–1285.

Orbach, Y., Lamb, M. E., Sternberg, K. J., Williams, J. M. G., & Dawud-Noursi, S. (2001). The effect of being a victim or witness of family violence on the retrieval of autobiographical memories. *Child Abuse & Neglect, 25*, 1427–1437.

Orenchuk-Tomiuk, N., Matthey, G., & Christensen, C. P. (1990). The resolution model: A comprehensive treatment framework in sexual abuse. *Child Welfare, 69*, 417–431.

Palm, K. M., & Gibson, P. (1998). Recovered memories of childhood sexual abuse: Clinicians' practices and beliefs. *Professional Psychology: Research and Practice, 29*, 257–261.

Paris, J. (1997). Childhood trauma as an etiological factor in the personality disorders. *Journal of Personality Disorders, 11*, 34–49.

Patton, M. Q. (1991). *Family sexual abuse: Frontline research and evaluation*. Newbury Park, CA: Sage.

Paivio, S. C., & Bahr, L. (1998). Interpersonal problems, working alliances, and outcomes in short-term experiential therapy. *Psychotherapy Research, 8*, 392–407.

Pennebaker, J. W. (1997). Writing about emotional experiences as a therapeutic process. *Psychological Science, 8*, 162–166.

Perry, B. D. (1993). Neurodevelopment and the neurophysiology of trauma I: Conceptual considerations for clinical work with maltreated children. *APSAC Advisor, 6*, 1–18.

Perry, B. D. (1994). Neurobiological sequelae of childhood trauma: Post-traumatic stress disorders in children. In M. Murburg (Ed.), *Catecholamine function in post traumatic stress disorder: Emerging concepts* (pp. 253–276). Washington, DC: American Psychiatric Press.

Pescosolido, F. J. (1993). Clinical considerations related to victimization dynamics and post-traumatic stress in the group treatment of sexually abused boys. *Journal of Child and Adolescent Group Therapy, 3*, 49–73.

Peterson, R. F., Basta, S. M., & Dykstra, T. A. (1993). Mothers of molested children: Some comparisons of personality characteristics. *Child Abuse & Neglect, 17*, 409–418.

Pilkonis, P. A. (1993). Studying the effects of treatment in victims of childhood sexual abuse. *Journal of Interpersonal Violence, 8*, 392–401.

Pithers, W. D., Gray, A., Busconi, A., & Houchens, P. (1998). Caregivers of children with sexual behavior problems: Psychological and family functioning. *Child Abuse & Neglect, 22*, 129–141.

Pleck, J. H. (1995). The gender role strain paradigm: An update. In R. F. Levant & W. S. Pollack (Eds.), *A new psychology of men* (pp. 11–32). New York: Basic Books.

Pleck, J. H. (1995). The gender role strain: An update. In R. F. Lavant & W. S. Pollack (Eds.), *A new psychology of men* (pp. 1–32). New York: Basic Books.

Prentsky, R. M., Knight, R. A., & Lee, A. F. S. (1995). A rationale for the treatment of sex offenders: Pro bono publico. In J. McGuire (Ed.), *What works: Reducing reoffending guidelines from research and practice* (pp. 153–170). New York: John Wiley & Sons.

Price, J. L., Hilsenroth, M. J., Petretic-Jackson, P. A., & Bonge, D. (2001). A review of individual psychotherapy outcomes for adult survivors of childhood sexual abuse. *Clinical Psychology Review, 21,* 1095–1121.

Pruitt, J. A., & Kappius, R. E. (1992). Routine inquiry into sexual victimization: A survey of therapists' practices. *Professional Psychology: Research and Practice, 23,* 474–479.

Putnam, F. W. (1991). Dissociative disorders in children and adolescents: A developmental perspective. *Psychiatric Clinics of North America, 14,* 519–531.

Putnam, F. W. (1992). Using hypnosis for therapeutic abreactions. *Psychiatric Medicine, 10,* 51–65.

Putnam, F. W. (1997). *Dissociation in children and adolescents: A developmental perspective.* New York: Guilford Press.

Putnam, F. W., Carlson, E. B., Ross, C. A., Anderson, G., Clark, P. Torem, M., Bowman, E. S., Coons, P., Chu, J. A., Dill, D. L., Loewenstein, R. J., & Braun, B. G. (1996). Patterns of dissociation in clinical and nonclinical samples. *Journal of Nervous and Mental Disease, 184,* 673–679.

Pynoos, R. S., Steinberg, A. M., Ornitz, E. M., & Goenjian, A. K. (1997). Issues in the developmental neurobiology of traumatic stress. In R. Yehuda & A. C. McFarlane (Eds.), *Psychobiology of posttraumatic stress disorder* (pp. 176–193). New York: New York Academy of Science.

Raiha, N. K., & Soman, D. J. (1997). Victims of child abuse and neglect in the U.S. army. *Child Abuse & Neglect, 21,* 759–768.

Rassin, E., Merckelbach, H., & Muris, P. (2001). Thought suppression and traumatic intrusions in undergraduate students: A correlational study. *Personality and Individual Differences, 31,* 485–493.

Ray, J. A., & English, D. J. (1995). Comparison of female and male children with sexual behavioral problems. *Journal of Youth and Adolescence, 24,* 439–451.

Reeker, J., Ensing, D., & Elliott, R. (1997). A meta-analytic investigation of group treatment outcomes for sexually abused children. *Child Abuse & Neglect, 21,* 669–680.

Reidy, T. J., & Hochstadt, N. J. (1993). Attribution of blame in incest cases: A comparison of mental health professionals. *Child Abuse & Neglect, 17,* 371–381.

Resnick, M. D., & Blum, R. W. (1994). The association of consensual sexual intercourse during childhood with adolescent health risk and behaviors. *Pediatrics, 94,* 907–913.

Rimsza, M. E., & Berg, R. A. (1988). Sexual abuse: Somatic and emotional reactions. *Child Abuse & Neglect, 12,* 201–208.

Rodriguez, N., Ryan, S. W., Rowan, A. B., & Foy, D. W. (1996). Posttraumatic stress disorder in a clinical sample of adult survivors of childhood sexual abuse. *Child Abuse & Neglect, 20,* 943–952.

Rodriguez, N., Vande Kemp, H., & Foy, D. W. (1998). Posttraumatic stress disorder in childhood sexual abuse and physical abuse: A critical review of the empirical research. *Journal of Child Sexual Abuse, 7,* 17–45.

Rodriguez-Srednicki, O., & Twaite, J. A. (1999). Attitudes toward victims of child sexual abuse among adults from four ethnic/cultural groups. *Journal of Child Sexual Abuse, 8,* 1–24.

Rogers, M. L. (1995). Factors influencing recall of childhood sexual abuse. *Journal of Traumatic Stress, 8,* 691–716.

Rolls, E. T. (2000). Memory systems in the brain. *Annual Reviews in Psychology, 51,* 599–630.

Rosenzweig, M.R. (1996). Aspects of the search for neural mechanisms of memory. *Annual Review in Psychology, 47,* 1–32.

Roth, S., & Lebowitz, L. (1988). The experience of sexual trauma. *Journal of Traumatic Stress, 1,* 79–107.

Roth, S., & Newman, E. (1991). The process of coping with sexual trauma. *Journal of Traumatic Stress, 4,* 279–297.

Ruiz, M. A., Pincus, A. L., & Ray, W. J. (1999). The relationship between dissociation and personality. *Personality and Individual Differences, 27,* 239–249.

Ryan, G., & Lane, S. (1991). *Juvenile sexual offending* (2nd ed.). San Francisco: Jossey-Bass.

Ryan, G., Lane, S., Davis, J., & Isaac, C. (1987). Juvenile sex offenders: Development and correction. *Child Abuse & Neglect, 11,* 385–395.

Sarrel, P. M., & Masters, W. H. (1982). Sexual molestation of men by women. *Archives of Sexual Behavior, 11,* 117–131.

Saunders, R., Colton, M., & Roberts, S. (1999). Child abuse fatalities and cases of extreme concern: Lessons from reviews. *Child Abuse & Neglect, 23,* 257–268.

Saywitz, K. J., Mannarino, A. P., Berliner, L., & Cohen, J. A. (2000). Treatment for sexually abused children and adolescents. *American Psychologist, 55,* 1040–1049.

Schacht, A. J., Kerlinsky, D., & Carlson, C. (1990). Group therapy with sexually abused boys: Leadership, projective identification, and countertransference issues. *International Journal of Group Psychotherapy, 40,* 401–417.

Schoenewolf, G. (1991). The feminist myth about sexual abuse. *Journal of Psychohistory, 18,* 331–343.

Schooler, J. W., & Eich, E. (2000). Memory for emotional events. In E. Tulving & F. I. M. Craik (Eds.), *The Oxford handbook of memory* (pp. 379–392). New York: Oxford University Press.

Schwartz, D., & Dodge, K. A. (1993). The emergence of chronic peer victimization in boys' play groups. *Child Development, 64,* 1755–1772.

Schwartz, M. F., Galperin, L. D., & Masters, W. H. (1995). Sexual trauma within the context of traumatic and inescapable stress, neglect, and poisonous pedagogy. In M. Hunter (Ed.), *Adult survivors of sexual abuse: Treatment innovations* (pp. 1–17). Thousand Oaks, CA: Sage.

Schwartz, M. F., Galperin, L. D., & Masters, W. H. (1995). Dissociation and treatment of compulsive reenactment of trauma. In M. Hunter (Ed.), *Adult survivors of sexual abuse: Treatment innovations* (pp. 42–55). Thousand Oaks, CA: Sage.

Scott, K. D. (1992). Childhood sexual abuse: Impact on a community's mental health status. *Child Abuse & Neglect, 16,* 285–295.

Scott, W. (1992). Group therapy with sexually abused boys: Notes toward managing behavior. *Clinical Social Work Journal, 20,* 395–409.

Sgroi, S. M. (Ed.). (1982). *Handbook of clinical intervention in child sexual abuse.* Lexington, MA: Lexington Books.

Shapiro, J. P., Dorman, R. L., Burkey, W. M., & Welker, C. J. (1999). Predictors of job satisfaction and burnout in child abuse professionals: Coping, cognition, and victimization history. *Journal of Child Sexual Abuse, 7,* 23–42.

Shapiro, S. (1992). Suicidality and the sequelae of childhood victimization. In S. Shapiro & G. M. Dominiak (Eds.), *Sexual trauma and psychopathology: Clinical intervention with adult survivors* (pp. 1–79). New York: Lexington Books.

Shin, L. M., McNally, R. J., Kosslyn, S. M., Thompson, W. L., Rauch, S. L., Alpert, N. M., Metzger, L. J., Lasko, N. B., Orr, S. P., & Pitman, R. K. (1999). Regional cerebral blood flow during script-driven imagery in childhood sexual abuse-related PTSD: A PET investigation. *American Journal of Psychiatry, 156,* 575–584.

Siegel, D. J. (1997). Working with memories of trauma. In B. S. Monk & J. A. Incorvaia (Eds.), *Psychotherapy with children and adolescents,* (pp 221–278). New York: Jason Aronson.

Silbert, M. H., & Pines, A. M. (1981). Sexual child abuse as an antecedent to prostitution. *Child Abuse & Neglect, 5,* 407–411.

Silver, R. L., Boon, C., & Stones, M. H. (1983). Searching for meaning in misfortune: Sense of incest. *Journal of Social Issues, 39,* 81–102.

Simari, C. G., & Baskin, D. (1982). Incestuous experiences within homosexual populations: A preliminary study. *Archives of Sexual Behavior, 11,* 329–344.

Simeon, D., Guralnik, O., Schmeidler, J., Sirof, B., & Knutelska, M. (2001). The role of childhood interpersonal trauma in depersonalization disorder. *American Journal of Psychiatry, 158,* 1027–1033.

Simon, J. M. (1995). The highly misleading truth and responsibility in mental health practices act: The "false memory" movement's remedy for a nonexistent problem. *Moving Forward, 3*(1), 12–21.

Simon-Roper, L. (1996). Victim's response cycle: A model for understanding the incestuous victim-offender relationship. *Journal of Child Sexual Abuse, 5,* 59–79.

Simrel, K. O., Lloyd, D. W., & Kanda, M. (1980). *Medical corroborating evidence in child sexual abuse/assault cases.* Washington, DC: Children's Hospital National Medical Center.

Singer, K. I. (1989). Group work with men who experienced incest in childhood. *American Journal of Orthopsychiatry, 59,* 468–472.

Singer, M. I., Hussey, D., & Strom, K. J. (1992). Grooming the victim: An analysis of a perpetrator's seduction letter. *Child Abuse & Neglect, 16,* 877–886.

Smith, D., Pearce, L., Pringle, M., & Caplan, R. (1995). Adults with a history of child sexual abuse: Evaluation of a pilot therapy service. *British Medical Journal, 310,* 1175–1178.

SNAP: Survivors Network of those Abused by Priests. (2002). *Home page.* Retrieved February 1, 2003, from www/survivorsnetwork.org./

Spiegel, D. (Ed.). (1994). *Dissociation: Culture, mind, and body.* Washington, DC: American Psychiatric Press.

Spiegel, J. (1996, November). *The sexual abuse of males: A theoretical model.* Invited presenter. Special Program, Boston University School of Social Work. North Dartmouth, MA.

Spiegel, J. (1997, March). *The sexual abuse of males: A structural equation model of dynamics and effects.* Paper presented at the Quantitative Methods Symposium, Council on Social Work Education, 43rd Annual Program Meeting. Chicago.

Spiegel, J. (1998a, March). *Sexual self-concept: Early data on a new scale.* Paper presented at the Quantitative Methods Symposium, Council on Social Work Education, 44rd Annual Program Meeting. Orlando, FL.

Spiegel, J. (1998b, July). *Intervention development for and outcomes of males with histories of childhood sexual abuse.* Paper presented at the Program Evaluation and Family Violence Research: An International Conference. Durham, NH.

Spiegel, J. (2000, May). *The sexual abuse of males: Treatment goals, objectives, interventions and outcomes.* Invited presenter. Paper and workshop presented at the Twelfth Annual Prevent Child Abuse—Orange County Conference. Anaheim, CA.

Spiegel, S. (1989). *An interpersonal approach to child therapy: The treatment of children and adolescents from an interpersonal point of view.* New York: Columbia University Press.

Stauffer, L. B., & Deblinger, E. (1996). Cognitive behavioral groups for nonoffending mothers and their young sexually abused children: A preliminary treatment outcome study. *Child Maltreatment, 1,* 65–76.

Steele, K., & Colrain, J. (1990). Abreactive work with sexual abuse survivors: Concepts and techniques. In M. Hunter (Ed.), *The sexually abused male: Vol. 2. Application of treatment strategies,* (pp. 1–55). Lexington, MA: D. C. Heath.

Stein, M. B., Walker, J. R., Anderson, G., Hazen, A. L., Ross, C. A., Eldridge, G., & Forde, D. R. (1996). Childhood physical and sexual abuse in patients with anxiety disorders and in a community sample. *American Journal of Psychiatry, 153,* 275–277.

Stevenson, M. R. (2000). Public policy, homosexuality, and the sexual coercion of children. *Journal of Psychiatry and Human Sexuality, 12,* 1–19.

Stiffman, A. R. (1989). Physical and sexual abuse in runaway youths. *Child Abuse & Neglect, 13,* 417–426.

Stocks, J. T. (1998). Recovered memory therapy: A dubious practice technique. *Social Work, 43,* 423–436.

Stout-Miller, R., Miller, L. S., & Langenbrunner, M. R. (1997). Religiosity and child sexual abuse: A risk factor assessment. *Journal of Child Sexual Abuse, 6,* 15–34.

Straker, G., & Waks, B. (1997). Limit setting in regard to self-damaging acts: The patient's perspective. *Psychotherapy, 34,* 192–200.

Strauss, A. L., & Corbin, J. (1990). *Basics of qualitative research: Grounded theory procedures and techniques.* Newbury Park, CA: Sage.

Stuss, D. T., & Levine, B. (2002). Adult clinical neuropsychology: Lessons from studies of the frontal lobes. *Annual Reviews in Psychology, 53,* 401–433.

Sullivan, P. M., Scanlon, J. M., Brookhouser, P. E., & Schulte, L. E. (1992). The effects of psychotherapy on behavior problems of sexually abused deaf children. *Child Abuse & Neglect, 16,* 297–307.

Sutherland, S. M. (1999). The neurobiology of poststraumatic stress disorder: An integration of animal and human research. In P. A. Saigh & J. D. Bremner (Eds.), *Posttraumatic stress disorder: A comprehensive text* (pp. 103–143). Needham Heights, MA: Allyn & Bacon.

Taubman, S. (1984). Incest in context. *Social Work, 29,* 35–40.

Timnick, L. (1985, August 25). 22% in survey were child abuse victims. *Los Angeles Times,* A1.

Tingus, K. D., Heger, A. H., Foy, D. W., & Leskin, G. A. (1996). Factors associated with entry into therapy in children evaluated for sexual abuse. *Child Abuse & Neglect, 20,* 63–68.

Tobias, B. A., Kihlstrom, J. F., & Schacter, D. L. (1992). Emotion and implicit memory. In S.A. Christianson (Ed.), *Handbook of emotion and memory,* (pp. 67–92). Hillsdale, NJ: Lawrence Erlbaum.

Tong, L., Oates, K., & McDowell, M. (1987). Personality development following sexual abuse. *Child Abuse & Neglect, 11,* 371–183.

Tulving, E. (2002). Episodic memory: From mind to brain. *Annual Reviews in Psychology, 52,* 1–25.

Turner, S. W., McFarlane, A. C., & van der Kolk, B. A. (1996). The therapeutic environment and new explorations in the treatment of posttraumatic stress disorder. In B. A. van der Kolk, A. C. McFarlane, & L. Weisaeth (Eds.), *Traumatic stress: The effects of overwhelming experience on mind, body, and society* (pp. 537–558). New York: Guilford Press.

Ullman, S. E. (1997). Attributions, world assumptions, and recovery from sexual assault. *Journal of Child Sexual Abuse, 6,* 1–19.

Urquiza, A. J., Wyatt, G. E., & Goodlin-Jones, B. L. (1997). Clinical interviewing with trauma victims: Managing interviewer risk. *Journal of Interpersonal Violence, 12,* 759–772.

U.S. Department of Health and Human Services, National Center on Child Abuse and Neglect. (1996a). *Child maltreatment 1994: Reports from the States to the National Center on Child Abuse and Neglect.* Washington, DC: U.S. Government Printing Office.

U.S. Department of Health and Human Services, National Center on Child Abuse and Neglect. (1996b). *The National Incidence Study of Child Abuse and Neglect (NIS-3).* Washington, DC: U.S. Government Printing Office.

U.S. Department of Health and Human Services. (1998). *Child maltreatment 1996: Reports from the states to the National Child Abuse and Neglect Data System.* Washington, DC: U.S. Government Printing Office.

U.S. Department of Health and Human Services. (1999). *Child maltreatment, 1999: Reports from the States to the National Child Abuse and Neglect Data System.* Washington, DC: U.S. Government Printing Office.

van der Hart, O., & Friedman, B. (1989). A reader's guide to Pierre Janet: A neglected intellectual heritage. *Dissociation, 2,* 3–16.

van der Kolk, B. A. (1988). The trauma spectrum: The interaction of biological and social events in the genesis of the trauma response. *Journal of Traumatic Stress, 1,* 273–290.

van der Kolk, B. A., Burbridge, J. A., & Suzuki, J. (1997). The psychobiology of traumatic memory: Clinical implications of neuroimaging studies. In R. Yehuda & A. C. McFarlane (Eds.), *Psychobiology of posttraumatic stress disorder* (pp. 99–113). New York: New York Academy of Science.

Vander Mey, B. J. (1988). The sexual victimization of male children: A review of previous research. *Child Abuse & Neglect, 12,* 61–72.

Vander Mey, B. J., & Neff, R. L. (1984). Adult-child incest: A sample of substantiated cases. *Family Relations, 33,* 549–557.

Verduyn, C., & Calam, R. (1999) Cognitive behavioral interventions with maltreated children and adolescents. *Child Abuse & Neglect, 23,* 197–207.

Waterman, J. (1986a). Developmental considerations. In K. MacFarlane, J. Waterman, S. Conerly, L. Damon, M. Durfee, & S. Long (Eds.), *Sexual abuse of young children,* (pp. 15–29). New York: Guilford Press.

Waterman, J. (1986b). Family dynamics of incest with young children. In K. MacFarlane, J. Waterman, S. Conerly, L. Damon, M. Durfee, & S. Long (Eds.), *Sexual abuse of young children,* (pp. 204–219). New York: Guilford Press.

Weinrott, M. (1996). *Juvenile sexual aggression: A critical review.* Boulder: University of Colorado, Center for the Study and Prevention of Violence.

Weisz, J. R., Weiss, B., Han, S. S., Granger, D. A., & Morton, T. (1995). Effects of psychotherapy with children and adolescents revisited: A meta-analysis of treatment outcome studies. *Psychological Bulletin, 17,* 450–468.

Wells, M., Glickauf-Hughes, C., & Beaudoin, P. (1995). An ego-object relations approach to treating childhood sexual abuse survivors. *Psychotherapy, 32,* 416–429.

Westbury, E., & Tutty, L. M. (1999). The efficacy of group treatment for survivors of childhood abuse. *Child Abuse & Neglect, 23,* 31–44.

White, E. (1982). *A boy's own story.* New York: Random House.

White, E. (1988). *The beautiful room is empty.* New York: Random House.

White, E. (1998). *The farewell symphony.* New York: Random House.

White, M. T., & Weinter, M. B. (1986). *The theory and practice of self psychology.* New York: Brunner/Mazel.

Winkelspecht, S. M., & Singg, S. (1998). Therapists' self-reported training and success rates in treating clients with childhood sexual abuse. *Psychological Reports, 82,* 579–582.

Wright, R. C., & Schneider, S. L. (1999). Motivated self-deception in child molesters. *Journal of Child Sexual Abuse, 8,* 89–111.

Wyatt, G. E., Loeb, T. B., Solis, B., Carmona, J. V., & Romero, G. (1999). The prevalence and circumstances of child sexual abuse: Changes across a decade. *Child Abuse & Neglect, 23,* 45–60.

Yapko, M. D. (1994). Suggestibility and repressed memories of abuse: A survey of psychotherapists' beliefs. *American Journal of Clinical Hypnosis, 36,* 163–171.

Yehuda, R. (2000). Biology of posttraumatic stress disorder. *Journal of Clinical Psychiatry, 61*(Suppl.), 14–21.

Yehuda, R., Teicher, M. H., Levengood, R. A., Trestman, R. L., & Siever, L. J. (1994). Circadian regulation of basal cortisol levels in posttraumatic stress disorder. *Annals of the New York Academy of Sciences, 746,* 378–380.

Yehuda, R., Teicher, M. H., Trestman, R. L., Levengood, R. A., & Siever, L. J. (1996). Cortisol regulation in posttraumatic stress disorder and major depression: A chronobiological analysis. *Biological Psychiatry, 40,* 79–88.

Yorukoglu, A., & Kemph, J. P. (1966). Children not severely damaged by incest with a parent. *Journal of the Academy of Child Psychiatry, 5,* 111–124.

Young, L. (1992). Sexual abuse as the problem of embodiment. *Child Abuse & Neglect, 16,* 89–100.

Young, M. B., & Erickson, C. A. (1988). Cultural impediments to recovery: PTSD in contemporary America. *Journal of Traumatic Stress, 1,* 431–443.

Zamanian, K., & Adams, C. (1997). Group psychotherapy with sexually abused boys: Dynamics and interventions. *International Journal of Group Psychotherapy, 47,* 109–126.

INDEX

Abbot, D. A., 33–34, 39, 46–47, 84, 147, 165, 211, 235
Abel, G. G., 26, 28, 140, 142
Abracen, J., 45
Abrahams, N., 55, 59
Abuse. excuse," 54
Abuse reactivity, 97–99, 212–216, 443
Abuse-related stimuli, 368–370
Academic effects of abuse, 84–85, 228–239, 443
Accommodation, 21–22, 323
Acetycholine, 162
Ackerman, B. J., 44, 52, 67, 72–73, 76–78, 81, 86, 88, 92, 94, 96–97, 99, 178, 180, 186, 212
Ackerman, E., 71, 215, 335
Ackerman, P. T., 75–77, 84, 134
Ackerman, R., 73–75
Ackland, M. A., 30
Acknowledging abuse, 366–367
Acting out, 116, 344–346, 377, 443
Action connection, 414–418
    anticipated outcomes, 415–416
    clinical example, 416–418
    definition, 415
    description, 415
Adams, J., 16, 24–25, 33–34, 46, 69, 82–86, 88, 93–94, 25, 42, 72–73, 76, 78, 81, 94, 98, 147, 176, 210, 334, 354
Adams, M., 74
Adams, P., 28, 140, 213
Adams-Tucker, C., 54, 73–74, 78, 83–84, 86, 88, 92, 94–95, 97, 145, 184, 203, 228, 234
Adcock, A. G., 82, 93
Addiction. *See* Compulsive behaviors; Substance abuse
Adesanya, T., 214
Adkins, E., 62
Adolescent Sexual Concerns Questionnaire, 67
Adolescents
    abuse-related effects, 64–99

abused, 65–66
    anxiety, 72
    depression, 73
    eating disorders, 82
    neurological effects of abuse, 71–72
    offenders, 30–31
    psychiatric diagnosis, 75
    relational effects, 86
    self-image, 83
    sexuality effects of abuse, 87–88
    suicidality, 74
Adults abused as children
    abuse-related effects, 64–99
    anxiety, 72–73
    depression, 73–74
    eating disorders, 82
    neurological effects of abuse, 71–72
    psychiatric diagnosis, 75–76
    relational effects of abuse, 86–87
    self-image, 83–84
    sexuality effects of abuse, 89–90
    suicidality, 74–75
"Age of Denial," 6–7
"Age of Validation," 7
Age
    at abuse onset, 39–40
    at evaluation, 40
    differential, 41, 442
    of abuse termination, 40
    perpetrator's, 40
Aggression, 15, 164, 443
    after abuse, 92–93
Akil, H., 117, 149, 154
Akman, D., 102
Alcohol abuse. *See* Substance abuse
Aldous, M. B., 68, 335
Alexander, P. C., 143
Alienation from body, 443 (*See also* Body numbing and

Depersonalization)
Allard-Dansereau, C., 11, 38, 42, 46, 64, 69, 82, 147
Allen, C. M., 12, 32–33, 144, 177
Allen, J., 80–81
Allen, L. S., 214
Allers, C. T., 91
Alpert, J. L., 129
Alpert, N. M., 214–215, 329
Altshuler, L. L., 11, 15, 38, 42, 66, 74–76, 145, 374
Amaro, H., 88–89
Ambivalence, 371–379
American Academy of Child and Adolescent Psychiatry, 404
American Humane Association, 37
American Psychiatric Association, 27, 29, 134, 148, 187, 218, 331
American Psychological Association, 331–332
Americans for a Society Free from Age Restrictions, 11
Ames, M. A., 97
Amnesia, 79–81, 188–189, 218–227
Amrung, S., 84
Amygdala, 71, 120, 121–122, 124, 128, 130, 152–156, 162–163, 170, 183, 200–202, 215–216, 219–22-, 259, 313, 377, 390
Andersen, S. L., 71, 215, 335
Anderson, B., 25, 33, 67–68, 74, 76, 95, 148, 218, 357
Anderson, C. L., 143
Anderson, C. M., 70–71
Anderson, D., 45
Anderson, P. B., 32
Andreou, C., 213
Andrews, L., 85
Anger. *See also* Rage
    fear of expressing, 443
    identifying, 399
Anogenital injuries, 68–69, 443
Antoni, F. A., 152

Antonowicz, D. H., 48
Anxiety, 72–73, 164, 281, 287, 311,
  323, 376, 414, 426–429, 443
  accepting, 428
  anticipated outcomes, 429
  assessing, 371
  brainstem and, 119
  definition, 428
  description, 428–429
  disorders, 25, 29
  externalizing, 279
  facing, 428
  floating, 428–429
  lessening, 444
  letting time pace, 428–429
  reducing, 368–370
Araji, S. K., 7, 30–31
Arana, G. W., 158
Armony, J. L., 170, 201
Armstrong, L., 6–7
Arnow, B., 11, 62–63
Aronson, L., 228
Arousal continuum, 149, 150, 152
Asdigian, N., 177
Ashby, L., 3, 5
Association of Family Conciliation Courts, 52
Assumptions. See also Perceptions; Perspectives
  biophysical subsystem, 116–117
  boy's perspective, 317, 329–
    330
  brain basics, 117–123
  cognitive-perceptual system,
    113–114
  conceptual perspective, 317,
    323–324
  developmental perspective,
    317, 324–325
  dynamics and effects perspec-
    tive, 317, 327–328
  ecosystems perspective, 317–
    320
  facts and meaning perspec-
    tive, 317, 328–329
  intrapsychic subsystem, 115–
    116
  memory, 124–131
  multisystemic, multitemporal
    determinism, 317, 320–321
  of SAM Model, 109–135, 317–
    332
  parallel processes perspective,
    317, 321–322
  philosophical, 317–332
  relational perspective, 317,
    325–327
  self-determinative perspective,
    317, 330

self-system, 111–114
sex, gender, and schemas,
  131–135
strengths perspective, 317, 331
theoretical perspective, 317,
  322–323
Atkins, M. S., 34, 78, 88
Attachment, 253, 255–256
Attention deficit/hyperactivity
  disorder, 85
Aubut, J., 29
Aucoin, R., 61
Augustyn, M., 84–85
Authentic vs. socially imposed
  intervention, 424–426
Authentication, 388–392
Autio, K. A., 11, 15, 38, 42, 66,
  74–76, 145, 374
Avoidance, 350–351
  reducing, 368–370
Avoidant personality disorder, 76

Babysitting, 30
Back, S., 60–62, 206, 233–234
Bagley, C. 25–27, 38–39, 52, 67,
  73–74, 76, 78, 85, 92, 180,
  222, 230, 334
Bahr, L., 403
Baker, A. J., 27, 30, 142
Baker, T., 79–81, 224
Baker, W. L., 118, 127, 131, 164,
  170, 189, 216, 329
Balkozar, A., 78
Ball, P. G., 60
Bandura, A., 111, 113, 209, 321,
  364
Barker, J., 56–57
Barney, E. E., 355–356, 379
Baron, L., 7
Barr, B., 10
Barth, K. L., 69
Bartholow, B. N., 25, 33–35, 37,
  39–42, 44, 46, 64, 67, 75, 81,
  87–89, 91–92, 142, 146, 167,
  176, 212, 238
Basal ganglia, 120, 122, 125, 130
Bass, E., 7–8
Battered child syndrome, 5
Bauer, P. J., 126, 222, 329
Baum, A. S., 69–71, 160, 164,
  193–194
Baur, K., 131
Bauserman, R., 3, 9
Bays, J., 68–69
Beardsall, L., 54–55, 57–58, 61, 177
Beardslee, W. R., 42, 82, 146
Beautrais, A. L., 76, 78, 134
Beck, A. T., 114, 202, 321, 364,
  387

Becker, J. V., 26–27, 28, 30, 140,
  142
Beebe, T. J., 14, 47, 146, 196, 199
Beers, S. R., 69, 71–72
Begin, A., 78
Behavioral problems, 92
Beil, J., 91
Beilke, R. L., 15, 44, 72–73, 84,
  86, 88, 92–93, 95, 210, 228,
  403
Beitchman, J. H., 102
Belicki, K., 80
Beliefs. See also Perceptions
  generated by defenses, 386
  imposed by CSA, 386–387
  imposed by perpetrator, 386
  social mythology, 247, 255,
    257, 267, 275, 280, 290, 297,
    319, 378, 385–386, 441–442
Bell, K., 61
Belsky, J., 110–111
Bem, S. L., 110, 131–133
Bender, L., 5
Benedict, L. L. W., 102
Benitez, J. G., 25–26, 42, 72–74
Benjack, K. J., 91
Ben-Porath, Y. S., 73, 76, 86, 134,
  145
Benshoff, J. J., 38
Bentovim, A., 24, 213, 334
Bera, W. H., 97, 212, 343
Bergandi, T. A., 39, 73, 86, 88,
  92–93
Berger, T. W., 201
Bergstrom, S. C., 342
Berkman, L. F., 74
Berkowitz, C. D., 24–25, 27, 33,
  37, 42, 46, 49, 57, 67, 69,
  91, 164
Berlin, F., 59
Berliner, L., , 28, 43–45, 46, 50,
  52, 102, 139, 146–147, 178–
  179, 206, 403–404
Berman, K., 39
Bernard-Bonnin, A., 11, 38, 42,
  46, 64, 69, 82, 147
Bernet, W., 80
Bertalanffy, L., 321
Best, K. M., 103
Betrayal, 22–23, 95, 243
Biaggio, M., 85
Binder, J. L., 333
Biophysical system, 116–117 (See
  also Psychobiology)
Birmaher, B., 69–71, 160, 164
Birnbaum, H. J., 38, 139–140
Black, D. W., 198
Black, M., 15, 64–65, 67, 82, 84,
  86, 89, 92–95, 228

Blakley, T. L., 118, 127, 131, 164, 170, 189, 216, 329
Blame. *See* Self-blame; Responsibility
Blanchard, R., 29
Blanck, G., 116
Blanck, R., 116
Blau, A., 5
Blechner, M. J., 233
Blick, L. C., 46, 139, 146
Block, J., 103–104
Block, J., 103–104
Blood, L., 39
Bloom, F. E., 193–194
Bloom, M., 322, 447
Blum, R. W., 15, 74, 82, 89, 93–94, 96, 210
Boat, B. W., 52
Bodmer-Turner, J., 32, 38, 141
Body numbing, 192–193, 441
Bolan, G., 25, 33–35, 37, 39–42, 44, 46, 64, 67, 75, 81, 87–89, 91–92, 142, 146, 167, 176, 212, 238
Bolger, K. E., 207
Bolton, F. G.., Jr., 340–341, 343, 367, 371, 384
Boney-McCoy, S., 3, 47–48, 66, 73, 76–77, 84, 102, 164, 210
Bonge, D., 403
Boon, F., 82
Boon, S., 329, 363, 381
Borderline personality disorder, 76
Borin, J. M., 69, 71–72
Boring, A. M., 69–73, 76, 78, 92, 148, 160, 164, 214
Boris, N. W., 104
Bornstein, M., 333
Botash, A., 90
Bottoms, B. L., 60, 222
Boucock, A., 80
Boundaries
  diffusion of, 139–146, 243, 272–273, 442
  in therapy, 353–354
Bowen, K., 68, 335
Bower, B., 170
Bower, G. H., 166
Bowlby, J., 111–112, 115, 126, 333, 336–337, 364
Boyle, M. H., 42, 82, 146
"Boylove Manifesto," 9
Boys
  abuse-related effects, 64–99
  aggression, 92–93
  anxiety, 72
  depression, 73
  effects across time, 65–66

encopresis/enuresis, 82–83
expectancies, 357–360
histories, 453–460
neurological effects of abuse, 69–71
perspective of, 317, 329–330, 368–370
physical findings, 68–69
preabuse perceptions, 440
psychiatric diagnosis, 75
relational effects, 86
self-image, 83
sexuality effects, 87
suicidality, 74
Bradford, J. M. W., 28–29
Bradley, A. R., 33, 49, 51, 143
Brady, K. T., 39
Brain, 318–319
  acetycholine, 162
  amygdala, 121–122
  basal ganglia, 122
  basics, 117–123
  brainstem, 119, 151–152
  catecholamines, 158–159
  cerebrum, 122–123
  cortex, 122–123, 155–157
  diencephalon, 119–120, 152, 200–202
  disremembering and, 219–220
  effects of sexual abuse, 213–216
  glial cells, 117–118
  hippocampus, 120–121
  limbic system, 120, 152–155
  memory, 129–131
  neurons, 117–118
  response to threat, 150–157
  traumatic memory, 200–202
Brainstem, 119, 200–202
  response to threat, 151–152
Brannon, J. M., 50
Brant, R., 32
Braun, B. G., 221
Bremner, J. D., 10, 15, 70–71, 79–80, 118–119, 121, 127, 129–130, 149–150, 155, 158–159, 161, 163–164, 170, 175, 185, 189, 200, 214–216, 219–220, 319, 329
Brenner, C., 321
Bretherton, I., 124
Bribes, 35, 43–44, 442
Briere, J., 38–42, 44, 46, 50, 52–53, 65–67, 73–74, 76–80, 86, 90, 94–95, 105, 164, 184, 210, 212, 220–222, 227, 329–330, 339–341, 343, 346, 351, 354–356, 365, 368, 371, 377–379, 381, 384, 387, 390, 396, 402–403

Briggs, F., 27, 65
Brinton, R. D., 201
Britton, H., 15, 33, 42, 44–46, 53, 55, 68–69, 131, 147–148, 164, 334, 335
Broadhurst, D. D., 39, 54
Brodsky, B. S., 74, 93, 210
Bromet, E., 76–77
Bronen, R. A., 80
Bronfenbrenner, U., 110, 318, 321, 364
Brongersma, E., 8
Brookhouser, P. E., 403
Broussard, E. R., 25–26, 42, 72–74
Broussard, S. D., 60–61, 110, 318, 321, 364
Brower, A. M., 112–113, 129, 312, 364
Brown, D., 79–80, 102, 121, 124–126, 188, 219, 223, 395
Brown, E. J., 58
Brown, E., 44, 52, 67, 72–73, 76–78, 81, 86, 88, 92, 94, 96–97, 99, 178, 180, 186, 212
Brown, G. R., 25, 33, 67–68, 74, 76, 95, 148, 218, 357
Brown, J., 16, 65–66, 101
Brown, L. K., 76, 88, 91–92, 134
Brown, L. S., 129
Brown, P., 329, 363, 381
Brown, S. C., 127
Brown, S., 203
Browne, A., 7, 15, 20, 22–23, 103–104, 364
Browne, K., 26, 28, 33, 35, 37, 43, 45, 47, 141–142, 147, 177–178, 206
Brownmiller, S., 11
Bruckner, D. F., 89–90, 240
Bruns, D., 82, 95
Bucholz, K. K., 25, 74–75, 82, 87
Budin, L. E., 35, 142
Buka, S. L., 39, 74, 82
Burbridge, J. A., 150, 214, 319, 381
Burgess, A. W., 20, 24–26, 34–35, 43, 51, 53–54, 67, 69, 73–74, 77–89, 92–98, 105, 139, 142, 144–145, 148, 157, 170–171, 175, 178, 181, 185, 205, 212, 218, 224, 228, 230, 233, 236, 354, 381
Burke, L., 71
Burkhardt, S., 102
Burkhart, B. R., 37, 65, 146
Burnam, M. A., 39, 67, 72–73, 76, 89, 93, 96, 106, 212
Burns, N., 32–33, 36

Burton, D. L., 30
Busconi, A., 32, 37, 39–41, 56, 97–98, 143–144, 213
Bussière, M. T., 29, 143
Butler, L. D., 171–172
Butler, T. L., 342

Cahill, L., 166, 201
Calam, R., 66, 148, 212
Calderbank, S., 26, 96
Callaghan, M., 85
Calvert, J. F., Jr., 54, 60
Camargo, C. A., Jr., 82
Camouflaging, 184
Campbell, J. A., 12
Campis, L. B., 48
Capelli, S., 80
Caplan, R., 403
Cappelleri, J. C., 26
Capra, M., 24, 146
Carballo-Dieguez, A., 50, 52, 64, 92, 168, 180, 222, 319
Cardarelli, A. P., 42, 48–50, 52–53, 66
Cardena, E., 187
Carlat, D. J., 82
Carlson, E. A., 78
Carlson, E. B., 187
Carlson, E., 103–104
Carlson, K., 12
Carmen, E. H., 7, 165, 181–182, 199, 208, 206, 355, 365, 382, 389
Carmen, E. J., 67
Carnes, P., 195
Carpenter, D. R., 30
Carrion, V. G., 79
Case examples, 453–460
    action connection, 416–418
    change chart, 413–414
    compensation, 293–302
    concealment, 266–274
    cycle continuation, 303–314
    evaluation, 450–452
    facts and meaning, 421
    introduction to, 138–139
    invalidation, 274–283
    reconciliation, 283–293
    sexual abuse, 256–265
    subjection, 245–256
Case illustrations
    Jake, 252–254, 263–264, 272–273, 281–282, 290–291, 299–300, 311–313, 458–460
    Kip, 246–247, 257–258, 266–267, 275–276, 284–285, 294–295, 303–304, 454–455
    Matt, 249–251, 259–261, 269–

270, 278–279, 287–288, 297–298, 307–309, 456–457.
    Nicholas, 245–246, 256, 266, 274–275, 283–284, 293, 303, 453–454
    Palo, 247–249, 258–259, 267–269, 277–278, 285–286, 295–297, 304–307, 455–456
    Ty, 254–256, 264–265, 273–274, 282–283, 291–293, 301–302, 313–314, 459–460
    Victor, 251–252, 261–263, 270–272, 279–280, 288–289, 298–299, 309–311, 457–458
Casey, B. J., 71–73, 76, 78, 92, 214
Casey, K., 55, 59
Cassavia, E., 102
Catania, J., 11–12, 38, 41, 44–46, 89, 147, 238, 334, 374
Catecholamines, 158–159
Cauce, A. M., 14, 25–26, 38–40, 47, 73–74, 85, 94–95, 164, 228
Cavaiola, A. A., 27, 45, 50, 67, 73–74, 88, 92–94, 96, 106, 145–146, 205
Cavanaugh, J. L., Jr., 27
Cavanaugh, J., 51, 164, 179, 357
Cazenave, N. A., 232
Ceci, S. J., 129
Centers for Disease Control, 60
Cerce, D., 29
Cerebrum, 122–123
Chadwick, D., 68–69
Chaffin, M., 48–50, 179
Chai, Y. M., 214
Chambers, H. J., 30
Chan, K., 11, 33, 38, 45, 74, 82, 148, 176, 374
Chandy, J. M., 15, 74, 82, 89, 93–94, 96, 210
Change chart intervention, 371, 411–414
    anticipated outcomes, 412–414
    clinical example, 413–414
    definition, 411
    description, 412
Chapman, J. R., 56
Chard, K. M., 403
Charney, D. S., 15, 71, 79–80, 118–119, 121, 123, 129–130, 150, 155, 158–159, 161, 163–164, 169–170, 172, 174–175, 200, 214–216, 219, 329
Cheit, R. E., 56, 144
Chen, K., 207

Chester, B., , 25, 33, 34, 38–39, 44–47, 52, 74–76, 84–88, 93–94, 96, 102, 146, 168, 176, 188, 210, 228
Child Abuse Prevention and Treatment Act, 6
Child Behavior Checklist, 67
Child offenders, 31–32
Child sexual abuse
    abuse reactivity, 97–99, 212–213
    academic effects, 84–85, 228–229, 443
    accommodation syndrome, 7, 20–22
    acknowledging, 366–367
    ADHD, 85
    adolescent offenders, 30–31
    age at evaluation, 40
    age at onset, 39–40
    age at termination, 40
    age difference, 41
    aggression after, 92–93
    amnesia, 218–227
    anxiety, 72–73
    arousal continuum, 150
    behavioral problems after, 92
    beliefs imposed by, 386–387
    body numbing, 192–193
    brain's response, 150–157
    bribes, 43
    case examples, 138–139, 453–460
    child offenders, 31–32
    co-abuse, 41
    coercion, 43–44
    compensation, 207–217, 293–302
    compulsive behavior, 193–196
    concealment, 47, 165–180, 266–274
    concurrent abuse, 42–43
    coping after, 96–97
    criminality after, 96
    cycle continuation, 217–227, 303–314
    defenses, 185–199
    denial, 186
    depersonalization, 191–192
    depression, 73–74
    derealization, 191–192
    diagnosis, 133–135
    dichotomous relating, 240–241
    dichotomous thinking, 202–207
    disabled children, 102–103
    disclosure, 48–51
    dissociation, 78–79, 186–190

duration, 41–42
dynamics of, 24–63 , 139–148
eating disorders, 82
effects of, 64–99, 139–242, 414, 443
encopresis, 82–83
enuresis, 82–83
false allegations, 52
family dynamics, 24–26
family responses, 52–54
feelings after, 95
female perpetrators, 32–33
force, 44–45
frequency, 41
gender differences, 99–101
gender identity confusion, 239
historic abuse, 42–43
history of research, 3–10
HIV/AIDS, 91–92
homophobia, 90
hyperarousal, 189–190
invalidation, 180–199, 274–283
isolation, 186, 239–240
lack of training on, 12–13
literature on abuse of males, 23–64
multiple episodes, 42
neurological effects, 69–72
neurotransmitters responding, 157–166
nondisclosure, 51–52
of girls, 14
overresponsibility, 240
pedophiles, 29–30
perceptions of, 64–65
perpetrator drug/alcohol abuse, 45
perpetrator/boy relationship, 33–34
perpetrators, 26–29, 37–38, 45
personality disorders, 76
physical effects, 68–72, 294
pornography exposure, 43
posttraumatic stress disorder, 76–77
prevalence, 38–39
processing, 392–395
professional perceptions, 61–63
protective factors, 103–104
psychiatric effects, 75–81
rape trauma syndrome, 20–21, 23
reactions to, 64
reconciliation, 200–207, 283–293
recovered memories, 79–81
reenactments, 57, 225–226, 231

regression after, 93
relational effects, 228–242
relational effects, 86–88
repression, 190
risk factors, 101–103
risk of death, 96
ritual abuse, 35–36
role of the Internet, 36–37
running away, 94
selection criteria, 34–35
self-blame, 94–95
self-image, 83–84
self-injurious behavior, 81
sexuality effects, 88–90, 230–242
sexually abusive acts, 46–47
sexually transmitted diseases, 90–92
sibling offenders, 31
social intervention, 54–59
social perceptions, 60–61
social responses, 54
somatic complaints after, 95–96
statistics, 8, 14, 146
story guidelines, 439–444
strangers, 34
stress response psychobiology, 149–150, 157–164
subjection, 139–146, 245–256
subsequent abuse, 47
substance abuse, 81–82
suicidality, 74–75
suppression, 186
tandem perpetrators, 33
theoretical models, 20–23
trauma symptoms, 77–78
traumagenic dynamics model, 20
traumatic memories, 166–180, 200–207
treatment history, 67–68
triggers for effects, 414–418
workplace effects, 85, 228–230
Child Trauma Academy, 118
Childhood Sensuality Circle, 6
Choking reactions, 443
Choy, A., 29
Christenson, G. A., 27, 29
Christianson, S. A., 81, 219, 221
Chrousos, G. P., 71
Chu, J. A., 78–79, 158, 160, 164, 167, 170, 172, 174, 190, 199, 220–221, 329–330, 338, 343, 346–347, 352, 354–355, 363, 368, 372, 377, 403
Cicchetti, D., 70, 78, 103–104
Cincinnati Children's Hospital Medical Center, 52

Circle sex, 36
Civita, R., 84
Clark, D. B., 39, 71–73, 76,78, 82, 92, 214
Claytor, R. N., 69
Client
  expectations, 16, 357–360
  role of, 338–339
Client–therapist relationship. See Therapeutic alliance
Clinical notes
  compensation, 294–302
  concealment, 266–274
  cycle continuation, 303–314
  invalidation, 274–283
  reconciliation, 283–293
  sexual abuse, 256–265
  subjection, 245–256
Clinton, W. J., 8
Co-abuse, 16, 41
Cochran, S. D., 61
Coercion, 35, 43–44, 442
  emotional, 43–44
  physical, 44
Cognitive dissonance, 443
Cognitive-behavioral interventions, 369–370
Cognitive-perceptual system, 113–114
Cohen, C., 75
Cohen, J. A., 403–404
Cohen, L. J., 29
Cohen, P., 15, 65–66, 101
Cohn, J., 76, 91, 134
Cole, C. H., 355–356, 379
Cole, P. M., 111–113
Coleman, E., 27, 29
Collings, S. J., 50, 73–75, 86, 93
Collins, L., 403
Collins, M. E., 12, 61, 147
Collins, R. A., 403
Comas-Diaz, L., 233
Comorbid symptoms
  reducing, 368–370
Compensation, 137, 207–217, 243
  abuse reactivity, 212–216
  case examples, 293–302
  clinical notes, 294–302
  defenses and, 216–217
  definition, 293
  story guidelines, 442
Compulsive behaviors, 89–90, 193–196, 231, 308–309, 441, 443
  identifying, 398–399
  reducing, 368–370
Concealment, 21, 47, 137, 167–180, 243, 269, 442

Concealment (*continued*)
case examples, 266–274
clinical notes, 266–274
definition, 266
hyperarousal, 173–180
impositions, 424–426
story guidelines, 441
traumatic memories, 168–173
Concentration difficulties, 443
Conceptual perspective, 317, 323–324
Concurrent abuse, 42–43
Conte, J. R., 12, 24, 28, 34–35, 43–46, 50, 52, 61, 65, 72, 83, 86, 88, 92, 98, 102, 106, 139–140, 142, 146–147, 178–179, 206–207, 212, 220–221, 234
Continuous memory, 79–80, 222–224
Control issues, 236–237, 294, 384
Convoy, H., 39, 218
Cooper, M. L., 25, 74–75, 82, 87
Coplan, J. D., 162
Corbett, R., 38, 82
Corey, M., 58
Cornelisse, P. G. A., 89, 234
Cornell, W. F., 381, 401
Cornwall, A., 39
Corpus callosum, 71–72, 118, 214, 443
Correy, B., 80
Cortex, 122–123, 200–202, 214, 219
response to threat, 155–157
Cortoni, F. A., 27, 141
Costello, E., 78
Costin, L., 4
Cosyns, P., 30
Cotman, A., 371
Coulton, C. J., 11, 60
Countertransference, 16, 346–361
traumatic, 348–354
Courtois, C. A., 7, 129, 148, 181, 218, 227, 317, 325, 329, 331, 336–340, 343–344, 349–350, 352–355, 358, 363–365, 367–368, 371–373, 378–380, 388, 393–398, 402, 404
Cox, A., 66, 148, 212
Crabtree, A., 170
Craib, K., 89, 234
Craig, M. E., 61
Craik, F. I. M., 127–129, 214
Crawford, I., 39, 44, 46
Crenshaw, L., 59
Crenshaw, W., 59
Crimes Against Children Research Center, 28

Criminal prosecution, 55–57
Criminality, 96
Crimmins, C. L. S., 31
Crittenden, P. M., 125–126
Crooks, R., 131
Cross, T. P., 56–57, 143
Crowder, A. F., 177, 338, 340–341, 343, 353–355, 358, 363–365, 372, 377, 380, 385, 388, 394, 398, 403
Crowley, C., 25, 37, 65, 67, 74–75, 88–89, 93, 72, 106, 145
Crowley, M. J., 60
Cuddy, M., 80
Cullen, B. J., 26, 56, 58, 144
Cullen, K., 29, 32–33, 141
Cunes, J. W., 33, 40
Cunningham, R. M., 92
Cunningham-Rather, J., 26, 28, 140, 142
Cupoli, J. M., 33, 39–40, 46, 54–55, 69
Curry, S., 28–29
Cybermolesters Enforcement Act, 10
Cycle continuation, 137, 217–227
amnesia, 218–227
case examples, 303–314
clinical notes, 303–314
definition, 303
response cycle, 243
story guidelines, 442

D'Imperio, R., 104
daCosta, G. A., 102
Dadds, M. R., 27
Dahl, B., 24, 33–34, 46, 69, 82–86, 88, 94, 147, 176, 210, 334, 354
Daldin, H., 188, 207, 210
Dale, P., 80–81
Daleiden, E., 44, 178
Dalenberg, C. J., 79, 224
Dallam, S. D., 9
Damasio, A. R., 201
Damon, L., 403
Darnell, A., 15, 71
Daro, D., 55, 59
Davidson, J. R., 151, 159–161, 163
Davies, J. M., 187, 195, 203, 221, 226, 236, 329, 337, 343–344, 347, 350, 354, 368, 403
Davies, M. G., 53, 233, 354
Davis, D. L., 73, 76, 86, 134, 145
Davis, L. L., 7–8, 234
Davis, M., 123, 163, 197
Davis, R. L., 96
Day, H. E. W., 117, 149, 154

De Bellis, M. D., 3, 25–26, 42, 69–74, 76, 78, 92, 133, 135, 146, 148–149, 151, 158–161, 163–164, 214–216, 364
de Lacoste, M. C., 214
De Luca, R. V., 26, 37, 102, 403
De Silva, P., 11–13, 62–63, 234
De Vos, E., 56–57, 143
De Vos, N., 30
de Young, M., 6
Dean, K. S., 16, 26, 33–34, 37, 41–43, 46–47, 49–50, 52, 64, 83, 86–87, 89, 94–95, 147, 165, 180, 212, 222, 235, 319
Dean, S., 59
Deaux, K., 110
Deblinger, E., 34, 47, 78, 88, 322, 346, 363, 387, 403
DeBruyn, L., 38
Defense mechanisms, 115–116, 185–196, 380–381, 441
amnesia, 79–81, 188–189, 218–227
and social environment, 221–222
beliefs generated by, 386
body numbing, 192–193
compensation and, 216–217
compulsive behaviors, 89–90, 193–196, 231, 308–309, 368–370, 398–399, 441, 443
contextualizing, 432–433
delayed recall, 223–224
denial, 186, 432–433, 441, 443
depersonalization, 191–192, 268–270, 282, 291, 307, 313, 441, 432–433, 443–444
derealization, 191–192, 260, 268–270, 282, 291, 313, 441, 443
dichotomous thinking, 202–207, 210–211, 230, 243, 277, 286, 291, 393
disremembering, 219–222
dissociation, 78–79, 115, 164, 186–190, 219–221, 243, 262, 268–270, 275, 313, 319, 322, 373, 441, 443
fractionation, 226–227, 265, 292, 365
integration, 226–227
isolation, 186
numbing, 192–193, 224–225, 287, 262, 309, 323, 368–370, 426, 438, 441
peridissociation, 78–79
reenactment, 57, 225–226, 231
repression, 115, 190, 267, 323

respecting, 372–373
suppression, 115, 186, 223
Deischer, R., 30
DeJong, A. R., 27, 34, 37, 39–40, 42, 44–47, 68, 144
Delayed disclosure, 22
Delayed recall, 223–224
Delgado, W., 33–35, 37, 39–42, 44, 46, 64, 142, 146, 167
Demaso, D. R., 48
Denial, 186, 441, 443
contextualizing, 432–433
Denicoff, K. D., 11, 15, 38, 42, 66, 74–76, 145, 374
Denney, N. W., 131
Depersonalization, 191–192, 268–270, 282, 291, 307, 313, 441, 443
contextualizing, 432–433
lessening, 444
Depression, 73–74, 164, 279, 443
assessing, 371
DePrince, A. P., 80
Derealization, 191–192, 260, 268–270, 282, 291, 313, 441, 443
Dersch, C. A., 49, 55–56, 175, 177
Desenclos, J. C., 90
Deutch, A. Y., 123 163
Developmental perspective, 317, 324–325
Developmentally discordant behaviors, 442
Devine, D., 38, 82
DeVoe, E. R., 51
Dewey, M. E., 61–62, 132
Deykin, E. Y., 39, 82
Dhabhar, F. S., 149
Dhaliwal, G. K., 48
Dhawan, S., 26
Dhooper, S. S., 60
Diamond, M., 131
Dichotomous relating, 240–241
Dichotomous thinking, 202–207, 210–211, 243, 277, 286, 291, 393
effects on career, 230
Dickey, R., 29, 97, 212
DiClemente, R. J., 33, 89
Diekstra, R. F. W., 15, 42, 64, 67, 74, 93, 96
Diencephalon, 119–120, 200–202
response to threat, 152
DiIorio, C., 11, 38, 82, 88–89, 238, 335
Dill, D. L., 78–79, 221
Dimock, P. T., 15, 33, 37, 82–83, 87, 89, 105, 145, 165, 175, 210, 212, 233, 235–237

Dinwiddie, S. H., 25, 74–75, 82, 87
Disabled children, 102–103
Disclosure, 48–51
delayed, 22
dodging, 184
family responses, 52–54
indirect, 49
social responses to, 54
story guidelines, 443
Disorbio, J. M., 82, 95
Disorganized attachment, 246–247
Disremembering
and the brain, 219–220
and the mind, 220–221
and the social environment, 221–222
Dissociation, 78–79, 115, 164, 186–190, 219–221, 243, 262, 268–270, 275, 313, 319, 322, 373, 441, 443
assessing, 371
contextualizing, 432–433
depersonalization, 191–192, 268–270, 282, 291, 307, 313, 432–433, 441, 443–444
derealization, 191–192, 260, 268–270, 282, 291, 313, 441, 443
reducing, 368–370
state-dependent psychobiology, 189–190
Distorting reality, 139–146, 442
Dixon, J. F., 14, 33–34, 40, 46, 65, 72–73, 76–78, 85–86, 90, 134, 143, 147, 168, 212, 334
Doggett, M., 50
Dolezal, C., 50, 52, 64, 92, 168, 180, 222, 319
Doll, L. S., 25, 33–35, 37, 39–42, 44, 46, 64, 67, 75, 81, 87–89, 91–92, 142, 146, 167, 176, 212, 238
Domestic violence, 25, 42–43, 306
Donaldson, S., 233
Dopaminergic neuronal system, 160–161
Doré, P., 92
Doris, J., 55, 84, 228
Dorn, L. D., 71
Douglas, A. J., 163
Douglas, J. M., 33–35, 37, 39–42, 44, 46, 64, 142, 146, 167
Douglas, J. M., Jr., 25, 37, 39, 67, 75, 81, 87–89, 91–92, 176, 212, 238

Dougler, M. J., 27
Doyle, T., 7
Draijer, N., 78
Draucker, C. B., 343
Droegmueller, W., 5
Dropik, P. L., 126, 222, 329
Drossman, D. A., 69
Drug abuse. See Substance abuse
Dubé, R., 37–38, 43–46, 55, 68, 102
Dubowitz, H., 15, 64–65, 67, 82, 84, 86, 89, 92–95, 228
Duka, E. K., 42, 82, 146
Dumont, N., 71, 215, 335
Duncan, L. E., 14, 37–38, 47, 64, 87–88, 90, 110, 132, 147, 165, 181, 208, 210, 232, 234, 236–237, 239
Dunklee, P., 24, 27, 33, 38, 40–42, 46, 68, 75, 83, 91, 93–95, 143
Dunlop, A., 80
Dunn, G. E., 39
Dunne, M. P., 25, 74–75, 82, 87
Durfee, M. J., 24–25, 27, 33, 37, 42, 46, 49, 57, 67, 91, 164
Durlak, J. A., 39, 44, 46
Dustan, L. R., 39
Dutton, M. A., 33, 38, 41–42, 47, 64
Dyadic perpetration, 33
Dykman, R. A., 75–77, 84, 134
Dynamics and effects perspective, 317, 327–328
Dynamics, 24–63, 139–148, 231
abuse reactivity, 212–213
academic effects, 228–229
adolescent offenders, 30–31
age and, 39–41
amnesia, 218–227
arousal continuum, 150
body numbing, 192–193
brain's response, 150–157
case examples, 138–139
child offenders, 31–32
co-abuse, 41
coercion, 43–44
common, 442
compensation, 207–217
compulsive behavior, 193–196
concealment, 165–180
concurrent abuse, 42–43
continuing the cycle, 217–226
defenses, 185–199
denial, 186
depersonalization, 191–192
derealization, 191–192
dichotomous relating, 240–241

Dynamics (*continued*)
dichotomous thinking, 202–207
disclosure, 48–51
dissociation, 186–190
duration, 41–42
effects of, 139–242
false allegations, 52
family, 24–26, 52–54
female perpetrators, 32–33
force, 44–45
frequency, 41
gender identity confusion, 239
historic abuse, 42–43
hyperarousal, 189–190
invalidation, 180–199
isolation, 186, 239–240
multiple episodes, 42
neurotransmitters responding, 157–166
nondisclosure, 51–52
overresponsibility, 240
pedophiles, 29–30
perpetrator concealment, 47
perpetrator drug/alcohol abuse, 45
perpetrator gender, 37–38
perpetrator rationales, 45
perpetrator sexual orientation, 38
perpetrator/boy relationship, 33–34
perpetrators, 26–29
pornography exposure, 43
prevalence, 38–39
professional perceptions, 61–63
reconciliation, 200–207
reenactments, 57, 225–226, 231
repression, 190
ritual abuse, 35–36
role of the Internet, 36–37
SAM Model, 139–148
selection criteria, 34–35
sexuality effects, 230–242
sexually abusive acts, 46–47
sibling offenders, 31
social intervention, 54–59
social perceptions, 60–61
social responses, 54
stress response psychobiology, 149–150, 157–164
subjection, 139–146
subsequent abuse, 47
suppression, 186
tandem perpetrators, 33
threats, 44
traumatic memories, 166–180, 200–207

Dziuba-Leatherman, J., 12, 144, 147–148, 154, 176–177, 183, 208

Earls, F., 92
Eastmen, B., 30
Eating disorders, 82, 294, 443
Eccard, C. H., 69–71, 160, 164
Eckenrode, J., 26, 55, 84, 228, 364
Ecosystems perspective, 317–320, 364
Edgar-Smith, S., 48, 48, 49–52, 178–180, 233, 334, 357
Edwall, G. E., 39, 82
Edwards, E., 160
Edwards, N. B., 44, 52, 67, 72–73, 76–78, 81, 86, 88, 92, 94, 96–97, 99, 178, 180, 186, 212
Effects of abuse, 64–99, 414, 438–439, 443
abuse reactivity, 97–99, 212–213
academic, 84–85, 228–239, 443
acting out, 116, 344–347, 377, 443
ADHD, 85
aggression, 92–93
amnesia, 218–227
anxiety, 72–73
arousal continuum, 150
behavioral problems, 92
body numbing, 192–193
brain's response, 150–157
case examples, 138–139
compensation, 207–217
compulsive behavior, 193–196
concealment, 165–180
continuing the cycle, 217–226
coping, 96–97
criminality, 96
defenses, 185–199
denial, 186
depersonalization, 191–192
depression, 73–74
derealization, 191–192
dichotomous relating, 240–241
dichotomous thinking, 202–207
dissociation, 78–79, 186–190
dynamics, 139–148
eating disorders, 82
encopresis, 82–83
enuresis, 82–83
feelings, 95
flashbacks, 279, 293, 300, 312, 323, 376–378
flooding, 323, 377–378
gastrointestinal, 69
gender identity confusion, 239

guilt, 83, 95, 289, 294, 299, 319, 384, 426, 430
headaches, 69
HIV/AIDS, 91–92
homophobia, 90
hyperarousal, 164, 167, 173–180, 189–190, 243, 268, 275, 281, 294, 306–307, 368–370, 373, 443–444
hypervigilance, 260, 288, 438
intrusive thinking, 224–225, 277–278, 287, 294, 368–370, 377–378
invalidation, 180–199
isolation, 186, 239–240
neurological, 69–72, 157–166
normalizing, 367–370, 372
overresponsibility, 240
panic attacks, 414, 443
perceptions, 64–65
perfectionism, 228–229
personality disorders, 76
perspective, 317, 327–328
physical, 68–72, 443
posttraumatic stress disorder, 76–77
powerlessness, 23, 236–237, 387
psychiatric, 75–81
reactions, 64
reconciliation, 200–207
recovered memories, 79–81
regression, 93, 115
relational, 86–88, 228–242
repression, 190
running away, 94
SAM Model, 139–148
self-blame, 94–95
self-image, 83–84
self-injurious behavior, 81
self-legitimacy, 99
sexuality, 88–90, 230–242
sexually transmitted diseases, 90–92
shame, 16, 51–52, 83, 95, 252, 265, 270, 273–274, 293–294, 300, 304, 309, 319, 353–354, 368, 379, 384, 387, 426, 430, 443–444
sleep disturbances, 94
smoking, 81–82
somatization, 95–96, 115, 198, 443
stress, 149–150, 157–164, 268, 281–282, 304, 323, 440, 424–426, 443
subjection, 139–146

substance abuse, 81–82, 368–370, 377, 441
suicidality, 74–75
suppression, 186
trauma symptoms, 77–78
traumatic memories, 166–180, 200–207
treatment history, 67–68
triggers for, 414–418
workplace, 85, 228–230, 443
Egeland, B., 78, 103–104
Ego, 115–116
Egolf, B., 104, 228
Eisemann, M., 233
Eisenberg, N., 61–62, 132
Eisenstadt, M., 27, 30, 142
Eisner, A., 98
Elhai, J. D., 11, 14, 25, 33–34, 37, 39–43, 45–47, 68, 87, 146, 147–148, 178, 357
Ellason, J. W., 38
Elliott, A., 69, 82, 142
Elliott, D. M., 52–53, 66, 79–81, 221–222, 224, 371
Elliott, M., 26, 28, 33, 35, 37, 43, 45, 47, 141–142, 147, 177–178, 206, 218, 223
Elliott, R., 403
Ellis, A., 322, 387
Ellis, S. P., 74, 93, 210
Elstein, S. G., 56
Elwell, M. E., 26
Emasculation, 443
Embree, J., 90
Emery, G., 202
Emmett, G. A., 27, 34, 37, 40, 42, 47, 68, 144
Emotional connection, 383–385
Emotional seduction, 250
Emotions
  amygdala and, 121–122
  connecting to, 383–385
  expressing, 436–439
  identifying, 399–400
  naming, 434–436
  understanding, 434–439
Empathy. See Preparatory empathy; Therapeutic alliance
Empty chair technique, 430–432
Encopresis, 82–83
Endogenous opioids, 163
Enemas, 442
England, P., 56
English, D. J., 24–26, 32, 42, 53, 57, 98, 139, 178, 354
Ensign, J., 69, 84, 403
Entrapment, 21–22
Enuresis, 82–83

Ephebophilia, 442
Ephross, P. E., 25
Ephross, P. H., 208
Epstein, M. A., 222
Erikson, E. H., 111, 113, 229, 364
Escovitz, K., 14, 33–34, 40, 46, 65, 72–73, 7678, 85–86, 90, 134, 143, 147, 168, 212, 334
Esparza, D., 38, 48, 72, 84, 93, 95–96, 175, 210, 218
Estes, L. S., 25, 98
Estes, R., 10
Eth, S., 65
Etherington, K., 46, 84
Evading, 184
Evaluation, 446–452
  anticipated outcomes, 450
  clinical example, 450–452
  definition, 446–447
  description, 447–450
Evans, D., 39–40, 67, 73–74, 76–78, 94–95, 105, 184, 212
Evans, W., 89
Everett, D., 90
Everett, R. S., 29
Everson, M. D., 52
Existential anguish, 395–396
Exner, T. M., 93
Explicit memory, 129–131 201–202, 373
  deficits, 443

Facts and meaning intervention, 317, 328–329, 418–422
  anticipated outcomes, 420–421
  clinical example, 421–422
  definition, 419
  description, 419–420
Facts and meaning perspective, 317, 328–329
Fairbairn, W. R. D., 111
Fall River (Mass.) diocese, 8
Faller, K. C., 11, 32–34, 36, 38, 41, 51, 53, 55–58, 141–144, 233, 339, 346, 371
False allegations, 52
False memory dispute, 7–9
Family dynamics, 24–26, 271
  co-abused siblings, 41
  gender differences, 100
  protecting siblings, 250, 298–299
  protective factors, 103–104
  responses to abuse, 52–54
  risk factors, 101–103
  sibling offenders, 31
Family systems theory, 6
Famularo, R., 84–85

Fanselow, M. S., 120, 152
Farber, E. D., 41
Faulkner, M., 9, 11
Faust, J., 104
Fear, 83, 231, 243, 387, 426, 430
  brainstem and, 119
  of bathrooms, 443
  of expressing affection, 443
  of expressing anger, 443
  of failure, 228–229
  of rejection, 443
Federal Bureau of Investigation, 10, 177
Feelings. See Emotions
Fehon, D. C., 73–74, 82, 93, 148
Fehrenbach, P., 26, 30, 32–33, 57, 141, 144
Feigenbaum, J. D., 11–13, 62–63, 234
Feingold, L., 38, 82, 89, 91, 238
Feiring, C., 14, 24, 26, 33–34, 41–42, 44, 46, 48, 143, 146, 164, 207
Feldman, J., 78
Feldman-Summers, S., 38, 79–80, 221–222
Female perpetrators, 26, 32–34, 36–38, 41, 44, 47, 55, 57–58, 60–61, 84, 87, 90, 140–141, 144–145, 147, 159, 176–177, 233, 236
Feminism, 6, 14
Fenton, T., 84–85
Ferenczi, S., 4
Fergusson, D. M., 66, 76, 78, 102–104, 134
Fernandez, Y. M., 45
Ferren, D. J., 29
Ferrera, M. L., 30
Festinger, L., 208
Fett, S. L., 69
Figley, C. R., 349, 364
Fine, B. D., 187, 191
Fine, S., 25, 73, 37, 39, 42, 47, 74–75, 92, 97, 146, 212
Finkelhor, D., 3, 7–8, 11–13, 15, 20, 22–23, 25, 28, 32–34, 36–37, 38–41, 44–45, 47–48, 50–51, 56, 66–67, 73, 76–77, 84, 88, 99, 102–106, 134, 143–144, 146–148, 151, 154, 164–165, 167, 175–179, 183, 208, 210, 233, 328, 334, 364, 404
Finlayson, L. M., 59
Firestone, P., 28–29
Fischer, D. G., 40, 42, 45, 164
Fischer, J., 332, 447
Fischer, L., 334

Fischman, A. J., 214–215, 329
Fish, V., 80
Fisler, R., 15, 70–71, 78–81, 117, 148, 168–172, 191, 193–194, 214–215, 220, 223, 225, 329
Fitzgerald, M. L., 94
Fitzpatrick, C., 51, 179, 357
Fivush, R., 222, 329
Flashback Media Group, 11
Flashbacks, 77, 159, 172, 202, 215, 239, 279, 293, 300, 312, 323, 376–377, 379
  regulating reactions, 376–378
Flavell, J. H., 113–114, 182
Fleming, J. E., 42, 82, 146
Fleming, P. L., 91
Fletcher, K. E., 76
Flooding, 205, 215, 323, 377–378
Flumerfelt, D. L., 198
Foa, E. B., 34, 78, 81, 88, 390
Fogarty, L., 12, 61
Fogel, D., 73–75
Follette, V. M., 80, 222
Follingstad, D. R., 62
Fondacaro, K. M., 14, 34, 39–41, 64–65, 73–74, 76, 146, 335
Fontanella, C., 14, 25, 39, 48, 55, 72, 78, 82, 88, 93–94, 102, 177, 179, 334
Forbey, J. D., 73, 76, 86, 134
Force, 44–45, 442
Ford, H. H., 88, 91–92
Forde, D. R., 65, 77
Forms
  action connection, 417
  change chart, 413
  evaluation graph, 451
  facts and meaning, 422
  impositions, 427
  my emotions, 440
  whose voice?, 422
Fortune, M. M., 59
Foss-Goodman, D., 60, 62, 206
Foulds, D. M., 14, 33–34, 38–39, 46–47, 55, 68
Fox, B., 80–81, 222, 224
Foy, D. W., 85, 401
Fractionation, 226–227, 265, 292, 365
Frawley, M. G., 187, 195, 203, 221, 226, 236, 329, 337, 343–344, 347, 350, 354, 368, 403
Freedman, A. M., 6
Freud, A., 113, 115–116, 149, 157, 321, 349, 364
Freud, S., 3–4
  rejects Ferenczi, 4
Freund, K., 97, 212

Frey, L. M., 79, 158, 160, 164, 170, 172, 190, 220
Freyd, J. J., 80, 127
Friedman, M. J., 124
Friedman, S., 73–75
Friedrich, W. N., 15, 25–26, 44, 46, 53, 72–73, 84, 86, 88, 92–93, 95, 97–98, 145, 148, 197, 210, 228, 233, 338, 343, 346, 401, 403
Frieze, I. H., 102
Fromm-Reichmann, F., 349
Fromuth, M. E., 37, 63, 65, 146, 234
Froum, A. G., 55
Frustaci, K., 69–73, 76, 78, 92, 148, 160, 164, 214
Frye, M. A., 11, 15, 38, 42, 66, 74–76, 145, 374
Fryer, G. E., 26, 31, 213
Fulkerson, J. A., 14, 47, 146, 196, 199
Funk, J. B., 26, 56, 58, 144
Furniss, T., 44, 178

GABA pathways, 161–162
Gagging reactions, 443
Gaither, G. A., 82
Gale, G. D., 120, 152
Gale, J., 25, 33–34, 40, 42, 67, 72–73, 86, 88, 92–93, 98, 145
Galynker, I. I., 29
Game playing, 44, 256
  to reinforce concealment, 47
Gans, S. N., 29
Ganzel, B. L., 79, 158, 160, 164, 170, 172, 190, 220
Garbarino, J., 109, 318, 321, 364
Garfinkel, P. E., 82
Garland, R. J., 27
Garmezy, N., 103
Garnefski, N., 15, 42, 64, 67, 74, 93, 96
Garrity, D., 90
Gartner, R. B., 3, 210, 235–236, 238, 242, 319, 334, 336, 338, 340, 343, 347–350, 352, 354–356, 368
Gary, T. S., 38, 139–140
Gastrointestinal problems, 69
Gauthe, G., 7
Gauzas, L., 48
Gay, P., 4
Gebhard, P. H., 5
Gelbard, H. A., 71, 214–215
Gelfand, A. N., 69
Gelfand, M. D., 69

Gellert, G. A., 24–25, 27, 33, 37, 42, 46, 49, 57, 67, 91, 164
Gender
  differences, 99–101
  female perpetrators, 32–33
  of perpetrators, 37–38
Gender roles, 180–184, 210, 247, 253, 275, 289, 294
  and emotions, 434, 436–438
  and schemas, 131–135
  conflict, 251–252, 262, 302
  confusion, 16, 83, 145–146, 231, 239, 254–255, 271, 307, 442–443
  development of, 131–135
  different from sex, 131–135
  discordant behaviors, 442
  sexual self-concept, 232–235
  socialization, 14–15
Generalized stress response, 66, 78, 85–86, 95, 371
Genuis, M., 26, 37–38, 47
Georgia Supreme Court, 4
Gerber, P. N., 197
Germain, C. B., 318, 364
Giaconia, R. M., 65
Giaretto, H., 6
Giedd, J. N., 71–73, 76, 78, 92, 214
Giese, J., 197
Gifts, 442
Gil, E., 338
Gilgun, J. F., 64, 87, 230
Gill, M., 14, 53, 64, 78, 83, 85–87, 89–90, 139, 168, 178–179, 181, 185, 206, 210, 212, 230, 232, 235–238, 240, 335, 349, 354
Giller, E. L., 151, 159–160, 165
Gilligan, C., 132
Giolas, M. H., 78
Gitterman, A., 318, 364
Glaser, R., 402
Glasgow, D., 66, 147, 212
Glial cells, 117–118
Glod, C. A., 70–71, 94, 213–215, 335
Glogau, L., 69
Glover, N. M., 38
Glowinski, A., 25, 74–75, 82, 87
Glutamatergic system, 161–162
Goering, P. N., 74, 82
Goh, D. S., 51, 164, 179, 357
Gold, S. N., 11, 14, 25, 33–34, 37, 39–43, 45–47, 68, 80, 87, 146–148, 178, 357
Goldberg, J., 27
Goldbloom, D. S., 82
Golding, J. M., 60

Golding, J. N., 39, 67, 72–73, 76, 89, 93, 96, 106, 212
Goldman, D., 25, 33, 34, 38–39, 44–47, 52, 74–76, 84–88, 93–94, 96, 102, 146, 168, 176, 188, 210, 228
Goldman, R. L., 103
Goldschmidt, E. B., 56, 144
Goldstein, E. G., 112–113, 115, 117, 184, 187, 196
Gomes-Schwartz, B., 42, 46, 48–50, 52–53, 66, 72, 75, 78, 83, 86, 92–93, 106, 212
Gonorrhea, 89–90
Gonsiorek, J. C., 99, 343, 373
Gonzalez, L. S., 33, 51
Goodman, G. S., 43–44, 56, 60
Goodstein, C., 31
Gordon, J. R., 208
Gordon, M., 33, 37–38, 41, 46, 48, 50–52, 55, 175, 177, 179, 180, 222, 319
Gore-Felton, C., 11, 62–63
Gorman, J. M., 162
Gorski, R. A., 214
Gothard, J. S., 403
Graduated exposure, 442
Granger, D. A., 403
Grassian, S., 79–81, 221–222, 224
Gray, A., 32, 37, 39–41, 56, 97–98, 143–144, 213
Gray, E., 45, 57, 143
Greenberg, D. M., 28–29
Greene, M. P., 33–34, 39–40, 42, 46, 49, 97, 147
Greene, R. R., 208
Gregory, Bishop W., 10
Gremy, I. M., 25
Grice, D. E., 39
Gries, L. T., 51, 164, 179, 357
Grilo, C. M., 73–74, 82, 93, 148
Grinnel, R. M., Jr., 447
Grinnell, R. M., 33, 40
Grooming behaviors, 442
Grossoehme, D. H., 59
Groth, A. N., 38, 139–140, 233
Grotstein, J. S., 203, 319
Gruber, E., 33, 89
Gruen, R. S., 94
Grunberg, N. E., 193–194
Guidano, V. F., 112
Guilt, 83, 95, 140, 168–169, 180, 183, 185, 188, 193–196, 204–205, 207–208, 232, 234, 238–239, 242, 289, 294, 299, 319, 384, 426, 430
Gully, K. J., 15, 33, 42, 44–46, 53, 55, 68–69, 147–148, 164, 334, 335

Gunnar, M., 70
Gutierres, S. E., 39
Gutman, L. T., 91
Guyon, R., 5

Haaf, R. A., 26, 56, 58, 144
Haas, G. L., 74, 93, 210
Habituated fear response, 140, 149, 174–175, 190, 194, 381, 443
Hack, T. F., 403
Hagglof, B., 233
Haley, G., 25, 73, 37, 39, 42, 47, 74–75, 92, 97, 146, 212
Haley, N., 11, 38, 42, 46, 64, 69, 82, 147
Hall, D. K., 24–26, 97–98, 139, 143, 212–213
Hall, J., 69–72, 148, 160, 164
Hall-Marley, S., 403
Hamane, M., 11, 38, 42, 46, 64, 69, 82, 147
Hamby, S. L., 25, 34, 42, 51
Hamilton, K., 45
Hammett, T. A., 91
Hammond, D. C., 79–80, 102, 121, 124–126, 188, 219, 223, 395
Hamner, M. B., 158
Han, S. S., 403
Handel, W., 112
Hannon, P. J., 82
Hansen, D. J., 48, 50, 54
Hansen, K., 11, 15, 33, 38, 42, 44–46, 53, 55, 68–69, 82, 88–89, 147–148, 164, 238, 334–335
Hanson, I. C., 91
Hanson, R. K., 29, 97–98, 143, 212
Harakal, T., 94
Harber, K. D., 402
Harkavy-Friedman, J., 12
Harkins, K., 160
Harper, D., 71, 214–215
Harrington, D., 14–15, 25, 39, 48, 55, 64–65, 67, 72, 78, 82, 84, 86, 88–89, 92–94, 102, 177, 179, 228, 334
Harris, K., 371
Harris, W., 84
Harrison, J. S., 25, 33–35, 37, 39–42, 44, 46, 64, 67, 75, 81, 87–89, 91–92, 142, 146, 167, 176, 212, 238
Harrison, P. A., 14, 39, 47, 82, 146, 196, 199
Harry, 35, 142
Hart, J., 70
Harter, S., 111
Hartman, C. R., 51, 94, 157, 170–171, 181, 185, 381

Hartman, C., 34–35, 43, 53–54, 69, 73–74, 77–82, 84, 86–89, 92, 92–98, 105, 139, 142, 145, 148, 175, 178, 205, 224, 218, 354
Hartman, G. L., 40, 42, 63, 67, 72–73, 84, 88, 92–94, 168
Hartmann, H., 364
Hartwell, T., 11, 38, 82, 88–89, 238, 335
Harvey, M. R., 150, 223, 355, 363–364, 381
Hashima, P. Y., 177
Haskett, M. E., 55, 175
Hastie, R., 112
Hawkins, R. M. F., 27, 65
Hayden, R., 84
Haywood, T. W., 27
Hazen, A. L., 65, 77
Hazlett, G., 79
Headaches, 69
Heath, A. C., 25, 74–75, 82, 87
Hebden-Curtis, J., 48
Hebert, M., 37–38, 43–46, 55, 68, 102
Hecht, D. A., 48
Hegedus, A. M., 39, 82
Heim, C., 70
Heinrich, 403
Heller, S. S., 104
Hellhammer, D., 160
Hellin, A. H., 322, 346, 363, 387
Helmers, K., 71
Helplessness, 21, 95, 148, 163, 199, 202, 207, 218, 225, 236, 239, 242, 383
Hemorrhoids, 69
Henderson, R., 94
Hendriks, D., 30
Henry, D., 14, 33–34, 40, 46, 65, 72–73, 76–78, 85–86, 90, 134, 143, 147, 168, 212, 334
Henry, J., 11, 38, 53, 56, 143
Henschel, D., 38, 41–42, 44, 90, 164
Heras, P., 39
Herman, J. L., 6, 11, 132, 134, 165–166, 168, 172, 174, 184, 187, 189, 192–194, 196–197, 220, 223, 225, 317, 319, 326, 329–330, 336–338, 340, 343–344, 346–347, 349, 351, 354–355, 363–365, 372, 381, 388, 395–396, 402
Herman-Giddens, M. E., 91
Hernandez, J., 25, 82, 193
Herrenkohl, E. C., 104, 228
Herrenkohl, R. R., 104, 228
Herring, D. J., 25–26, 42, 72–74

Hervada, A. R., 27, 34, 37, 39–40, 42, 44–45, 47, 68, 144
Herzog, D. B., 82
Hetherton, J., 54–55, 57–58, 61, 177
Hibbard, R. A., 12–13, 24, 40, 42, 62–63, 67, 72–74, 81–82, 84, 86, 88–89, 92–96, 148, 168, 218, 228
Higgins, K. V., 24–25, 27, 33, 37, 42, 46, 49, 57, 67, 91, 164
Hilliker, D. R., 44, 178
Hilsenroth, M. J., 403
Hippocampus, 70–71, 108, 120–121, 150, 155–156, 160–162, 170, 179, 200–202, 214–216, 219, 390
  overload, 313, 443
Hislop, J., 14
Histories, 453–460
HIV/AIDS, 91–92
  fear of, 270
Hobbs, C. J., 102
Hobbs, G. F., 68, 102
Hobson, W. F., 139–140
Hodges, J., 213
Hoffman, N. G., 39, 82
Hoffman, T. J., 33, 38, 42, 46–47, 52, 146, 164, 179, 236, 319
Hogg, R. S., 89, 234
Hohnecker, L., 80
Hoier, T. S., 403
Holder, W. M., 58
Hollis, F., 321
Hollon, S. D., 113–114, 132, 205
Holmes, G. R., 11–12, 63, 39, 48, 62, 175, 234
Holmes, W. C., 12, 24, 34, 38–39, 41, 46, 81, 102, 105, 147, 334
Holmstrom, L. L., 20
Holt, J. C., 14, 34, 39–41, 64–65, 73–74, 76, 146, 335
Holt, K. D., 103–104
Holtzen, D., 79–81, 221–222, 224
Homelessness, 94
Homophobia, 61, 83–84, 90, 165, 180, 319
Homosexuality, 165, 176, 233
  confusion over, 239, 307, 309–311
  perpetrator, 38, 53, 61, 82, 84, 88, 100
  stigma of, 12, 53, 271–272
Hood, J. E., 102
Hopper, J. W., 168
Horne, L., 66, 148, 212
Hornstein, N. D., 78

Horowitz, J. M., 42, 46, 48–50, 52–53, 66, 72, 75, 78, 83, 86, 92–93, 106, 212
Horowitz, M. J., 114, 170, 181–182, 224, 227
Horwood, L. J., 66, 102
Hotaling, G., 8, 11, 25, 33–34, 38–41, 44, 48, 50–51, 102, 146, 167, 175, 178–179
Houchens, P., 32, 37, 39–41, 56, 97–98, 143–144, 213
Hoyt, D. R., 14, 25–26, 38–40, 47, 73–74, 85, 94–95, 164, 228
HPA Axis, 70, 152, 155–157, 164, 168, 189
HPA Axis dysregulation, 159–160, 443
Hudson, S. M., 27, 141
Hughes, D. M., 11, 14, 25, 33–34, 37, 40–43, 45–47, 68, 80, 87, 146, 147, 178, 357
Hughes, M., 76–77
Humanistic psychology, 6
Hunter, J. A., 27, 30
Hunter, M., 8, 14, 37, 39–40, 46–47, 63, 73, 81, 84, 86–87, 93, 95, 145–146, 212, 234, 236, 334, 343
Hussey, D. L., 67, 72–73, 83, 88
Huston, R. L., 14, 33–34, 38–39, 46–47, 55, 68, 147
Hutcheson, T., 55, 175
Hutchings, P. S., 33, 38, 41–42, 46–47, 64
Hyde, J. S., 132
Hyperarousal, 66, 76, 78, 81, 159, 162–164, 167, 173–180, 188, 189–190, 194–195, 202, 224, 227–228, 243, 268, 275, 281, 294, 306–307, 367–368, 373, 394, 401–403, 425, 443–444, 452
  defined, 167
  lessening, 444
  reducing, 368–370
  state-dependent psychobiology of, 189–190
Hypersexuality, 89–90
Hypervigilance, 95, 122, 151, 159, 161, 171, 200, 260, 288, 438

Identification, 116, 210–211, 350–351
  projective, 53–54, 115
Implicit memory, 129–131, 201–202, 281, 373
  indelible, 443

Impositions, 424–427, 430
  anticipated outcomes, 426
  definition, 425
  description, 426
Inderbitzenn-Pisaruk, H. 403
Ingersoll, G. M., 24, 42, 73, 81–82, 84, 86, 89, 93–96, 74, 148, 218, 228
Ingram, D. L., 90
Inhelder, B., 111, 113–114, 182
Innis, R. B., 80
Integration, 226–227
Internalization, 116, 297, 299, 430, 443
International Psychoanalytic Conference (Wiesbaden), 4
International Society for Prevention and Treatment of Child Abuse and Neglect, 6
Internet
  "Boylove Manifesto," 9
  role of, 36–37
Interventions, 411–452
  action connection, 414–418
  anxiety, 426–429
  change chart, 411–414
  establishing point of view, 421–424
  evaluation, 446–452
  facts and meaning, 418–421
  impositions, 424–427
  processing the story, 429–432, 439–444
  reframing, 432–434
  self-mastery project, 444–446
  story guidelines, 439–444
  understanding emotions, 434–439
  validation, 429–432
  voicing the experience, 429–432
  whose voice? 421–424
Intimidation, 44, 248, 250, 274, 442
  to enforce concealment, 47, 49–50
Intrapsychic system, 115–116
Introjection, 115–116, 430–432
Intrusion, 442–443
Intrusive thinking, 224–225, 277–278, 287, 294
  reducing, 368–370
  regulating reactions, 377–378
Invalidation, 137, 180–199, 243, 274–275, 280, 338–339, 344–345, 441
  body numbing, 192–193
  case examples, 274–283

clinical notes, 275–283
compulsive behavior, 193–196
defenses, 185–196
definition, 274
denial, 186
depersonalization, 191–192
derealization, 191–192
dissociation, 186–190
isolation, 186
negative consequences, 197–199
positive consequences, 196–197
reducing, 368–370
repression, 190
story guidelines, 441
strategies, 184
suppression, 186
Isolation, 186, 239–240
Isquith, P., K., 57–58, 144, 233
Israel, E., 98
Ito, Y., 71, 214–215, 335
Itskovich, Y., 29

Jackson, H. J., 27, 33, 39, 41–42, 61, 63, 87
Jacobs, J. E., 177
Jacobson, A., 68, 357
Jacobvitz, D., 103–104
Jaffe, A. C., 90
Jamieson, E., 42, 82, 146
Janet, P., 3
Janikowski, T. P., 38
Janoff-Bulman, R., 25, 74, 81, 83, 87, 102, 114, 132, 149, 182–183, 235, 242, 321, 329, 339, 364
Janus, M. D., 24–25, 95, 25–26, 43, 67, 69, 73–74, 78, 83–86, 88, 94–97, 144–145, 178, 205, 212, 218, 228, 230, 236
Jaranson, J. M., , 25, 33, 34, 38–39, 44–47, 52, 74–76, 84–88, 93–94, 96, 102, 146, 168, 176, 188, 210, 228
Jemelka, R. P., 69
Jenike, M. A., 214–215, 329
Jenkins, F. J., 69–71, 160, 164
Jenkins, P., 7–8
Jennings, K. T., 38
Jenny, C., 38, 40, 140
Jensen, E. L., 29
Johnson, C. F., 41
Johnson, J. G., 101
Johnson, J. L., 11, 33, 38, 45, 74, 82, 148, 176, 374
Johnson, J. T., 61
Johnson, N., 10

Johnson, P. E., 35, 89–90, 1420, 240
Johnson, R. L., 15, 37, 39–41, 44, 49, 51, 64, 89–90, 206, 212, 239–240
Johnson, T. C., 31, 33, 98, 338
Joint paralysis, 443
Jolly, J. B., 78
Jones, D. P. H., 51, 56
Jones, J. G., 75–77, 84, 134
Jones, J. J., 72–76, 92, 95
Joseph, J. A., 41
Joseph, R., 121, 155, 179, 202, 216
Journal of Homosexuality, 8
Joy, D., 25, 33–35, 37, 39–42, 44, 64, 67, 75, 81, 87–89, 91–92, 142, 146, 167, 176, 212, 238
Joyce, P. R., 76, 78, 134
Jumper, S. A., 65

Kagan, B., 401
Kahn, T. J., 30
Kalichman, S. C., 61–62
Kalinowski, M., 36
Kandel, E. R., 120, 126–129, 190, 201, 226
Kantrowitz-Gordon, I., 38, 82, 89, 91, 238
Kaplan, G. M., 69
Kaplan, H. I., 219
Kaplan, I., 6
Karger, H., 4
Karlen, A., 131
Karp, C. L., 342
Karpinski, E., 5
Kasl, C. D., 84
Katon, W. J., 69
Kaufman, K. L., 44, 178
Kay, J., 392
Kazelskis, R., 60–61, 110, 318, 321, 364
Keairnes, M., 69
Keary, K., 51, 179, 357
Keck, P. E. Jr., 11, 15, 38, 42, 66, 74–76, 145, 374
Kehrberg, L. L. D., 198
Kelley, S. J., 25, 32, 44
Kellogg, N. D., 33, 37–39, 41–42, 46–47, 52, 64–65, 68, 146–147, 164, 179, 236, 319, 334
Kelly, R., 51
Kelly, R. J., 33, 36
Kempe, C. H., 5–6
Kendall, P. C., 113–114, 132, 205

Kendall-Tackett, K. A., 40, 42, 46, 50, 55, 61, 63, 68, 88, 102, 99, 105, 134
Kennedy, S., 9, 74, 82
Kenning, M., 177
Kenny, M. C., 59, 104, 233
Kernberg, O. F., 111, 364
Keshavan, M. S., 69–73, 76, 78, 92, 160, 164, 214
Kessel, S. M., 88, 91–92
Kessler, R. C., 76–77
Ketcham, K., 8
Kiecolt-Glaser, J. K., 402
Kilcoyne, J., 26, 28, 33, 35, 37, 43, 45, 47, 141–142, 147, 177–178, 206
Kilmer, R. P., 14, 25–26, 38–40, 47, 73–74, 85, 95, 164, 228
Kilpatrick, D. G., 39, 65, 76, 134
Kim, J. H., 121, 215
Kimball, M. 131
Kinard, E. M., 85, 334
Kinscherff, R., 84–85
Kinsey Institute, 5
Kinsey, A. C., 5
Kipke, M. D., 94
Kirby, J. S., 78–79
Kirschbaum, L., 160
Kiser, L. J., 44, 52, 67, 72–73, 76–78, 81, 86, 88, 92, 94, 96–97, 99, 178, 180, 186, 212
Kisiel, C. L., 33–34, 41, 46, 78–79, 143, 146, 167
Kite, M. E., 61
Klajner-Diamond, H., 24, 33, 34, 40, 42, 48, 68–69, 72, 88, 90, 92, 94, 96, 175
Klassen, P., 29
Klein, E., 29
Klein, I., 339
Kling, M. A., 71
Knight, R. A., 27, 29–31, 139–140
Knopp, F. H., 98
Knutson, J. F., 94, 102–103
Kobayashi, J., 30
Koenigsberg, H. W., 162
Kogan, N., 12, 30
Kohlberg, L., 131
Kohut, H., 111, 113, 115, 333, 347, 349, 364
Kolko, D. J., 42, 58, 72, 81, 86, 88, 146, 179, 212, 335
Kollack-Walker, S., 117, 149, 154
Koocher, G. P., 59
Koopman, C., 11, 62–63, 94
Koplin, B., 197
Korbin, J. E., 11, 60
Kornheiser, T., 9

Koss, M. P., 39, 48, 64
Kosten, T. R., 151, 159–160, 165
Kravitz, H. M., 27
Krivacska, J. J., 144, 177
Kroupina, M. G., 126, 222, 329
Krug, R., 25, 88, 210, 236
Krugman, R. D., 25, 31, 213
Krystal, H., 116, 148, 157, 166–
    167, 175, 184, 187, 192, 197,
    199, 365
Krystal, J. H., 15, 71, 119, 123,
    151, 159–160, 163, 165, 169–
    170, 172, 174
Kuban, M., 29
Kupka, R., 11, 15, 38, 42, 66, 74–
    76, 145, 374
Kusama, H., 75, 212

Lab, D. D., 11–13, 62–63, 234
Lackey, L. B., 98
LaFrance, S. R., 94
Laird, M., 84, 228
Lamb, S., 48, 48, 49–52, 178–180,
    207, 233, 334, 357
Lambert, J. D. C., 162
Lambie, I., 28, 140, 213
Lane, B., 91
Lane, S., 140
Langeland, W., 78
Langelier, P., 33
Langley, M., 15, 33, 42, 44–46,
    53, 55, 68–69, 147–148, 164,
    334, 335
Lanktree, C., 50, 403
Lanyado, M., 213
Larose, M. R., 112
Larrieu, J. A., 104
Larson, B., 50
Larzelere, R. E., 403
Lauer, R., 112
Laufer, D., 38, 82, 89, 91, 238
Lawson, C., 145
Lawson, L., 48–50, 72–76, 92, 95,
    179
LeBaron, D., 24, 33, 34, 40, 42,
    48, 68–69, 72, 88, 90, 92, 94,
    96, 175
Lebowitz, L., 355, 363, 381
LeDoux, J. E., 71, 120–123, 128,
    149, 151–154, 158–159, 166,
    168–170, 174, 201–202, 214,
    219–220, 227, 319
Lee, A. F., 27, 29
Lee, A., 28, 140, 213
Lee, J. D. P., 27
Lencz, T., 121, 215
Lesage, A. D., 74
Leserman, J., 69
Lesnick, L., 39, 82

Lethargy, 59
LeTourneau, D., 343
Leverich, G. S., 11, 15, 38, 42,
    66, 74–76, 145, 374
Levesque, R. J. R., 33–34, 37, 41–
    44, 46, 48–50, 63, 68, 143, 176
Levine, M., 12, 57–58, 144, 233
Levitan, R. D., 74
Levy, M. S., 225–226
Lew, M., 8, 13–14, 144–145, 175,
    177, 181, 185, 210–211, 230,
    233, 236, 317, 319, 339
Lewis, D. O., 31, 83, 221, 335
Lewis, I. A., 8, 11, 25, 33–34, 38–
    41, 44, 48, 50–51, 102, 146,
    167, 175, 178–179
Lewis, J. E., 31–32, 64
Lewis, M., 14, 24, 26, 33–34, 41–
    42, 44, 46, 48, 143, 146, 164,
    221
Li, Z., 69
Lichtenberg, J., 59, 333
Licinio, J., 15, 71
Liggan, D. Y., 392
Limbic system, 70–71, 119–122,
    124, 136, 150, 156–159, 163,
    170, 200–202, 214
    response to threat, 152–155
Lin, E., 42, 82, 146
Lindblad, F., 49
Lindegren, M. L., 91
Lindsay, D., 90
Lindstrom-Ufuti, H., 11, 60
Lindy, J., 325, 333, 347–350
Linton, S. J., 69
Liotti, G., 112
Lips, H. M., 60–62, 206, 233–234
Lipshires, L., 105, 145, 177
Lipsitt, L. P., 88, 91–92
Lisak, D., 12, 15, 25, 34, 37, 39,
    41–42, 46–47, 64, 66–67, 73–
    74, 81, 84–88, 90, 93–95, 99,
    133, 145, 147, 154, 157, 176–
    177, 181, 212, 218, 225, 228–
    230, 235–238, 240, 329,
    334–335, 341
Lister, E., 347
Literature
    on male sexual abuse, 23–106
    treatment outcome studies,
    403–404
Little, L., 25, 34, 39, 42
Livingston, R., 72–76, 92, 95
Locke, C., Jr., 62
Locke, G. R., III, 69
Lodico, M. A., 33, 89
Loeb, A., 31–32, 64
Lofland, J., 15
Lofland, L., 15

Loftus, E. F., 8, 129
Long, P. J., 73
Longstreth, G. F., 69
Looman, J., 45
Los Angeles Times, 49
Lothrop, T., 4
Lott, D. A., 124
Lourie, K. J., 76, 88, 91–92, 134
Lovallo, W. R., 116
Lowman, J., 89, 238
Lucenko, B., 11, 14, 25, 33–34,
    37, 39–43, 45–47, 68, 87,
    146–148, 178, 357
Luecke, W. J., 25–26, 46, 53, 84,
    88, 92, 97–98, 145, 148, 210,
    228, 233, 403
Lujan, C., 38
Lumpkin, M., 131
Lundberg, U., 158
Lusignan, R., 140–141
Lussier, P., 141
Luster, L., 34, 37, 41–42, 46–47,
    84–85, 87–88, 147, 212, 225,
    228–230, 236, 335
Luster, T., 89
Lyna, P. R., 90
Lynch, D. L., 51, 164, 179
Lynskey, M. T., 66, 102–104
Lyons, J. S., 33–34, 41, 46, 78–
    79, 143, 146, 167

MacDonald, G., 62
MacDonald, V., 33
MacEachron, A. E., 340–341, 343,
    367, 371, 384
Macedo, C., 84
Macfie, J., 78
MacMillan, H. L., 42, 82, 146
MacMillan, R., 10, 85, 230
Madden, P. A. F., 25, 74–75, 82,
    87
Maes, M., 30
Magnus, E., 71, 214–215
Mahoney, D., 9, 11
Mahoney, M. J., 202, 321
Major, B., 110
Malcom, R., 39
Male sexual abuse (See also
    Child sexual abuse)
    literature on, 23–99
    predictors, 24–26
    protective factors, 103–104
    risk factors, 101–103
Malin, H. M., 59
Malone, K. M., 74, 93, 210
Man/boy love
    attempts to normalize, 11
    first forum on, 6
    NAMBLA, 9

Mandel, F. S., 134, 189
Manjanatha, S., 78
Mann, J. J., 74, 93, 210
Mannarino, A. P., 403–404
Marital discord, 25
Marlatt, G. A., 208
Marmar, C. R., 401
Marriage, K., 25, 73, 37, 39, 42, 47, 74–75, 92, 97, 146, 212
Marshall, W. L., 26–27, 45, 141
Marshall, W. N., 62
Martens, S. L., 56–57
Martin, C. E., 5
Martin, N. G., 25, 74–75, 82, 87, 403
Martindale, S. L., 11, 33, 38, 45, 74, 82, 89, 148, 176, 234, 374
Martino, S., 73–74, 82, 93, 148
Marx, B. P., 73
Masalehdan, A., 69, 71–72
Mason, J. W., 151, 159–160, 165
Mason, W. A., 89
Massachusetts Society for the Prevention of Cruelty to Children, 4
Masson, J. M., 3–4
Masten, A. S., 103
Masturbation, 140, 168, 212–213, 231
    compulsive, 89
    inability to, 294
Mathew, S. J., 162
Mathews, F., 24–26, 34, 97–98, 139, 143, 212–213
Mathews, R., 26, 30, 34, 40
Matthews, J. A., 79, 158, 160, 164, 170, 172, 190, 220
Matthews, J. K., 33
Matthews, R., 33
Matthieu, M., 94
Mattia, J. I., 76–77
May, P., 38
May, R., 321
Mayer, A., 32, 141
Mayer, K., 38, 82, 89, 91, 238
Mayran, L. W., 38
Mazure, C., 80
Mazzucco, A., 27
McBride, K. K., 15, 33, 42, 44–46, 53, 55, 68–69, 147–148, 164, 334, 335
McCann, I. L., 148, 349
McCann, J., 24, 33–34, 46, 68–69, 82–86, 88, 94, 147, 176, 210, 334, 354
McCanne, T. R., 65
McCarthy, G., 80

McCarty, L., 33, 98
McCauley, M. R., 11, 60
McCausland, M., 34, 43, 53–54, 69, 73–74, 78, 81–82, 84, 86, 88, 92, 94–95, 97–98, 105, 139, 142, 145, 148, 175, 178, 205, 218, 354
McClellan, J., 16, 25, 93, 25, 42, 72–73, 76, 78, 81, 94, 98
McColgan, E., 44, 52, 67, 72–73, 76–78, 81, 86, 88, 92, 94, 96–97, 99, 178, 180, 186, 212
McCord, J., 36, 51
McCormack, A., 24–26, 35, 43, 54, 67, 69, 73–74, 77–78, 83–89, 92–97, 144–145, 178, 205, 212, 218, 228, 230, 236
McCoy, M., 28–29
McCurry, C., 16, 25, 93, 25, 42, 72–73, 76, 78, 81, 94, 98
McDonald, S., 30
McDonald, W. L., 40, 42, 45, 164
McElroy, S. I., 11, 15, 38, 42, 66, 74–76, 145, 374
McEwen, B., 69, 71, 157, 164, 319
McFarlane, A. C., 134, 189, 380, 390, 343
McGaugh, J. L., 158, 166, 169, 200–201, 215
McGee, R. A., 27
McGeoch, P. G., 29
McGlashan, T. H., 73–74, 82, 93, 148
McGraw, J. M., 51
McGuire, J., 84
McHugh, M., 55, 59
McKelvey, R. S., 72, 74
McKenzie, N., 37, 39, 44–48, 73, 77–78, 84, 89, 148, 175
McKibben, A., 29, 140–141
McKinney, R. E., Jr., 91
McKirnan, D., 25, 37, 39, 67, 75, 81, 87–89, 91–92, 176, 212, 238
McLaughlin, T., 25, 74–75, 82, 87
McLeer, S. V., 14, 33–34, 40, 46, 65, 72–73, 76–78, 85–86, 88, 90, 134, 143, 147, 168, 212, 334
McMillan, D., 213
McPherson, W. B., 75–77, 84, 134
Megadoren, K. M., 74
Meiselman, K., 6–7, 325, 336, 338, 340, 343, 352, 355, 365, 380, 382, 401
Melchert, T. P., 38, 42, 79–80, 178, 222, 334, 374
Melton, L. J., 69

Memory, 16, 111, 119, 124, 131, 214–215, 319, 323, 325, 329, 365, 367, 373, 377, 381–382, 389–390, 392–395, 401–404, 414, 418, 440–441
    amnesia, 79–81, 188–189, 218–227, 222–223
    continuous, 222–223
    development of, 124–126
    disremembering, 219–221
    explicit, 129–131, 201–202, 373, 443
    "false," 7–9
    forms of, 129–131
    fractionation to integration, 226–227
    hippocampus and, 120–121
    implicit, 129–131, 201–202, 281, 373, 443
    intrusion, 224–225
    limbic system and, 120
    numbing, 224–225
    process, 126–129
    recall, 223–224
    recovered, 79–81
    repression, 115, 190, 267, 323
    retrieval, 128–129, 188–190
    semantic, 125–126
    suppression, 115, 186, 223
    traumatic, 168–173, 200–202, 218–220, 279, 365
Menard, S., 68, 33, 37, 39, 41–42, 46–47, 64–65, 146–147, 164, 334
Mendel, M. P., 12, 24, 34, 37–39, 42–43, 45–47, 50, 64–65, 67–68, 76, 81, 83, 95–96, 74, 145, 147, 165, 168, 177–178, 205, 212, 218, 233, 235, 240, 334
Menn, F., 160
Mental illness, 33
Mental retardation, 33
Meredith, W. H., 33–34, 39, 46–47, 84, 147, 165, 211, 235
Merry, S., 85
Metzner, J. L., 26, 31, 213
Meyer, C., 364
Meyer-Bahlburg, H. F. L., 94
Meyerson, L. A., 73
Mian, M., 24, 33, 34, 40, 42, 48, 68–69, 72, 88, 90, 92, 94, 96, 175
Migraines, 69
Miller, A., 70
Miller, G. D., 39, 67, 71, 82
Miller, J. M., 12
Miller, W. R., 14, 38–39, 104
Miller-Perrin, C. L., 28, 102, 140–141, 143, 364

Mills, A., 12, 175, 233
Mills, T., 67
Miner, M. H., 27, 29–31
Minnesota Multiphasic Personality Inventory, 67
Miranda, R., Jr., 73
Mississippi Supreme Court, 3
Mitchell, K., 36
Mittelman, M., 26, 28, 140, 142
Miyoshi, T. J., 26, 31, 213
Moisan, P. A., 46, 102, 147
Moisan, P. M., 46, 102, 147
Molnar, B. E., 74
Monastersky, C., 26, 30, 32–33, 57, 141, 144
Mondale, W., 6
Money, J., 131
Montaner, J. S. G., 89, 234
Mood disorders, 25, 29, 164
  reducing, 368–370
Moore, B. E., 187, 191
Moore, D., 6, 51
Moran, T., 25, 33–34, 40, 42, 67, 72–73, 86, 88, 92–93, 98, 145
Morgan, C. A., 79
Moritz, G., 25–26, 42, 70–74, 148, 160, 164
Morrell, B., 334
Morris, C. C., 63, 234
Morris, L. A., 340–341, 343, 367, 371, 384
Morris, S., 65, 79–80, 222
Morton, T., 403
Morrow, J., 83, 335
Moser, J. T., 42, 72, 81, 86, 88, 146, 179, 212, 335
Moss, P. M., 25, 33–35, 37, 39–42, 44, 46, 64, 67, 75, 81, 87–89, 91–92, 142, 167, 176, 212, 238
Moulton, F. R., 7
Mraovich, L. R., 39–40
Mulder, R. T., 76, 78, 134
Multiple episodes, 41–42, 68, 84, 164, 442
Multisystemic, multitemporal determinism, 317, 320–321
Munsch, J., 49, 55–56, 175, 177
Munsie-Benson, M., 54, 60
Murnen, S. K., 82
Murphy, S., 29
Murphy, W. D., 26, 28, 97, 140, 142, 144, 212
Myers, J. E. B., 54, 206
Mykelbust, C., 197, 197

Nachman, G., 69
Nagel, D. E., 48–49, 175
Nagy, M. C., 82, 93

Nagy, S., 82, 93
Narayan, M., 214
Nasby, W., 190
Nasjleti, M., 6, 12
National Association of Social Workers, 331
National Center for Victims of Crime, 177
National Center on Child Abuse and Neglect, 40, 58, 175–176
National Child Abuse and Neglect Reporting System, 10
National Child Protection Act of 1993, 8
National Commission on Obscenity and Pornography, 5–6
National Committee to Prevent Child Abuse, 3
National Incidence Study, 39
National Organization of Male Sexual Victimization (NOMSV), 3, 9
National Research Council, 92
National Resource Center on Child Sexual Abuse, 105
National Task Force on Juvenile Sexual Offending, 31
Nausea, 69
Navalta, P., 71
Neels, H., 30
Neisen, J. H., 38, 374
Nelson, C. B., 76–77
Nelson, E. C., 25, 74–75, 82, 87
Nemeroff, C. B., 15, 70–71
Neumark-Sztainer, D., 82
Neurological issues, 318–319
  acetycholine, 162
  after abuse, 69–72
  amygdala, 121–122
  basal ganglia, 122
  brain basics, 117–123
  brainstem, 119, 151–152
  catecholamines, 158–159
  cerebrum, 122–123
  cortex, 122–123, 155–157
  diencephalon, 119–120, 152, 200–202
  dopaminergic neuronal system, 160–161
  dysregulation, 163–164
  effects of sexual abuse, 213–216
  endogenous opioids, 163
  GABA pathways, 161–162
  glial cells, 117–118
  glutamatergic system, 161–162
  hipoocampus, 120–121, 215, 219, 313, 443

HPA axis, 159–160
  limbic system, 120, 152–155
  memory, 124–131
  neurons, 117–118
  neurophysiological dysfunction, 15
  of pedophiles, 30
  response to threat, 150–157
  serotonergic system, 161
  traumatic memories, 168–173, 200–202, 218–220, 279, 365
New York Gay Activist Alliance, 6
New York State Senate and Assembly, 9
New, M., 213
Newberger, C. M., 25
Newberger, E. H., 25
Newport, J., 70
Newton, J. E. O., 75–77, 84, 134
Nichols, J. E., 33–34, 39–40, 42, 46, 49, 97, 147
Niedda, T., 14, 33–34, 40, 46, 65, 72–73, 7678, 85–86, 90, 134, 143, 147, 168, 212, 334
Niemeyer, J. G., 91
Niggemann, E., 90
Night terrors, 293, 300, 377, 414, 443
Nightmares, 293, 300, 438, 443
Nijenjuis, E. R. S., 79
Nolen, W. A., 11, 15, 38, 42, 66, 74–76, 145, 374
Noll, J. G., 48–49, 69, 71–72, 175
Nondisclosure, 51–52, 243
North American Man/Boy Love Association (NAMBLA), 3, 6, 9
Novelly, R. A., 121, 215
Numbing, 224–225, 287, 309, 323, 426, 438
  body, 192–193, 441
  psychic, 262
  reducing, 368–370
Nurius, P. S., 112–113, 129, 312, 364
Nutall, R., 33, 39, 41–42, 61, 63, 87
Nutt, D. J., 161–162

O'Brien, M. J., 31, 97, 212
O'Callaghan, M. G., 60
O'Connor, S., 94
O'Donohue, W., 60
O'Hare, E., 60
O'Shaughnessy, M. V., 89, 234
O'Toole, B. I., 47, 51, 55, 164, 179
Oates, K., 47, 51, 164, 179

Ochberg, F. M., 349
Offen, L., 11–12, 63, 39, 48, 62, 175, 234
Ogawa, J. R., 78
Ohlerking, F., 27, 29
Öhman, A., 153–154
Okamura, A., 39
Olio, K. A., 381, 401
Oliveri, M. K., 36, 51
Olson, P. E., 34, 37, 67, 82, 84–85, 88–89, 93, 96, 212, 228, 230, 237, 242, 335
"Operation Candyman," 10
Oquendo, M., 74, 93, 210
Orientation to treatment, 367–370
Orme, J. G., 322
Ormrod, R., 32, 56
Ornstein, P. A., 129
Orr, D. P., 24, 42, 73, 74, 81–82, 84, 86, 89, 93–96, 148, 218, 228
Orr, S. P., 214–215, 329
Orvaschel, H., 85
Osachuk, 403
Oshins, L., 41
Overcoming fear and anxiety intervention, 428
Overcompliance, 443
Owens, M. J., 15, 70–71
Owens, R. G., 61–62, 132

Paidika: The Journal of Paedophilia, 8
Paine, M. L., 48, 50, 54
Paivio, S. C. 403
Palmer, R. F., 94
Panic attacks, 159, 173, 229, 376, 414, 443
Paolo, A. M., 39
Papanicolaou, A. C., 80, 214–215
Paradis, C., 73–75
Paradis, Y., 29
Paradise, J. E., 99
Parallel processes perspective, 317, 321–322
Paraphilias, 29
"Parents United," 6
Parikh, S. V., 74
Parker, J. F., 11, 60
Parker, R. L., 38, 42, 79–80, 178, 334, 374
Parkinson, P. N., 47
Parra, J. M., 14, 33–34, 37–39, 41–42, 46–47, 55, 64–65, 68, 146–147, 164, 334
Parrila, R. K., 102–103
Patterson, C. J., 207
Pattison, P., 27

Paul, J. P., 11–12, 38, 41, 44–46, 89, 147, 238, 334, 374
Payer, K. L., 38, 40, 140
Pearce, J. W., 336, 342, 346, 403
Pearce, J., 24–26, 97–98, 139, 143, 212–213
Pearlman, L. A., 148, 203, 225, 329, 333, 337, 347, 349–350, 352, 354, 381
Pearlstein, T., 78
Pearlstone, Z., 128
Pedophiles, 29–30
Pedophilia, 27, 108, 139, 156, 442
Peed, S. F., 30
Pelcovitz, D., 134, 189
Pellerin, B., 29
Pelvic paralysis, 443
Pennebaker, J. W., 402
Peplau, L. A., 61
Perceptions
    of professionals, 61–63
    of individuals abused as children, 64–65
    preabuse, 440
    social, 138, 165, 177, 181, 184, 186, 192–193, 197, 204, 206, 209, 213, 216, 220–221, 373, 375–376, 411, 416, 425, 431, 433, 435, 440
Perez, C., 84–85, 228–229
Perfectionism, 228–229
Peridissociation, 78–79
Perpetrators, 26–29
    adolescent, 30–31
    age of, 40
    beliefs imposed by, 386
    child, 31–32
    choosing victims, 141–142
    concealment, 47
    criminal prosecution of, 55–59
    drug/alcohol abuse, 45
    female, 32–33
    fixated, 140–141, 442
    gender, 37–38
    misattribution, 442
    neurology, 30
    pedophiles, 29–30
    penetration of, 442
    perpetrator/boy relationship, 33–34
    rationales of, 45, 142–143
    regressed, 139–140
    selection criteria, 34–35
    selection strategies, 35
    sexual orientation, 38
    siblings, 31
    strangers, 34
    tandem, 33

Perry, B. D., 70, 113, 118–122, 127–128, 131, 148–152, 155, 159–160, 164–165, 167, 169–170, 174, 183, 189, 200, 202, 216, 319, 329
Perry, J. C., 196
Personality disorders, 76
Personality Inventory for Children, 67
Perspectives
    boy's, 317, 329–330, 368–370
    conceptual, 317, 323–324
    developmental, 317, 324–325
    dynamics and effects, 317, 327–328
    ecosystems, 317–320
    establishing, 383, 421–424
    facts and meaning, 317, 328–329
    multisystemic, multitemporal, 317, 320–321
    parallel processes, 317, 321–322
    relational, 317, 325–327
    self-determinative, 317, 330
    strengths, 317, 331
    theoretical, 317, 322–323
Pescosolido, F. J., 81–83, 86–88, 92–93, 95–96, 102, 139, 179, 193, 210–212, 218, 235
Peters, D. K., 75
Peters, J. M., 144
Peters, S. D., 7
Peterson, B. E., 110
Peterson, L., 69, 82, 142
Peterson, M., 7
Petretic-Jackson, P. A., 403
Pezzot-Pearce, T. D., 336, 342, 346, 403
Phillips, R. G., 71
Philosophical assumptions, 317–332
    boy's perspective, 317, 329–330
    conceptual perspective, 317, 323–324
    developmental perspective, 317, 324–325
    dynamics and effects perspective, 317, 327–328
    ecosystems perspective, 317–320
    facts and meaning perspective, 317, 328–329
    multisystemic, multitemporal determinism, 317, 320–321
    parallel processes perspective, 317, 321–322
    relational perspective, 317, 325–327

Philosophical assumptions (*continued*)
self-determinative perspective, 317, 330
strengths perspective, 317, 331
theoretical perspective, 317, 322–323
Physical abuse, 42–43, 99, 146, 442
progression of, 146–147
Physical effects of abuse, 68–72
gagging, 443
gastrointestinal, 69
headaches, 69
joint paralysis, 443
lethargy, 59
neurological, 69–72
pelvic paralysis, 443
sleep disturbances, 94, 164, 371, 443
sleepwalking, 414
somatization, 95–96, 115, 198, 443
Piaget, J., 111, 113–114, 182
Pierce, L. H., 25, 31, 39–41, 44, 46, 53, 55, 90, 146, 148, 177
Pierce, R. L., 25, 31, 39–41, 44, 46, 53, 55, 90, 146, 148, 177
Piers-Harris Self-Concept Scale, 67
Pillemer, D. B., 124–126, 129–130, 169, 202
Pincas, J. H., 221
Pintello, D., 11, 53
Pipe, M. E., 43–44
Pithers, W. D., 32, 37, 39–41, 56, 97–98, 143–144, 213
Pitman, R. K., 214–215, 329
Place, V., 403
Pleck, J. H., 110, 132
Plotsky, P., 70
Plummer, C. A., 144
Plunkett, A. M., 47
Polcari, A., 70–71
Pollack, L., 11–12, 38, 41, 44–46, 89, 147, 238, 334, 374
Pollack, W., 132, 232, 234
Pollard, R. A., 118, 122, 127, 131, 148–151, 164, 170, 189, 216, 329
Pollard, T., 158–159
Polusny, M. A., 80, 222
Pomeroy, W. B., 5
Pope, K. S., 38, 79–80, 221–222
Pornography, 28, 30, 36, 141, 143, 148
exposing children to, 35, 43, 99, 442
Port, L. K., 56

Porter, F. S., 46, 139, 146
Porter, J., 8
Post, R. M., 11, 15, 38, 42, 66, 74–76, 145, 374
Post-sexual abuse trauma, 371
Posttraumatic stress disorder, 25, 65, 70–71, 75–77, 79, 85, 88, 134, 158, 212, 320, 414
Powell, T. A., 14, 34, 39–41, 64–65, 73–74, 76, 146, 335
Power issues, 294, 302, 384
powerlessness, 23, 236–237, 387
Powers, J. L., 26. 55
Powers, P., 34, 43, 53–54, 69, 73–74, 78, 81–82, 84, 86, 88, 92, 94–95, 97–98, 105, 139, 142, 145, 148, 175, 178, 205, 218, 354
Pozansky, O., 29
Prado, L., 56
Premature sexualization, 442
Prentsky, R. A., 27, 29–31, 139–140
Preparatory empathy, 333–361
client's role, 338–339
countertransference, 346–354
defined, 333–334
egalitarian relationship, 339–341
expectancies, 357–360
policies, 360–361
safety and trust, 341–346
SAM knowledge base, 334–336
therapeutic relationship, 336–360
therapeutic window, 354–357
therapist's role, 337–338
transference, 346–348
Pretence, 259
Price, J. L. 403
Priest, R., 39
Prihoda, T. J., 14, 33–34, 38–39, 46–47, 55, 68
"Primetime Live," 8
Pringle, M., 403
Projective identification, 53–54, 115
Prostitution, 94
Protective factors, 103–104
Protter, B., 32–33, 141
Proulx, J., 29, 140–141
Pruitt, D. B., 44, 52, 67, 72–73, 76–78, 81, 86, 88, 92, 94, 96–97, 99, 178, 180, 186, 212
Psychiatric effects of abuse, 75–81
dissociative disorders, 78–79
personality disorders, 76

posttraumatic stress disorder, 76–77
recovered memories, 79–81
trauma symptoms, 77–78
Psychic numbing, 262
Psychic trauma, 16
Psychobiology, 79, 115, 119, 134, 149–164, 193
catecholamines, 158–159
dissociation, 78–79, 115, 164, 186–190, 219–221, 243, 262, 268–270, 275, 313, 319, 322, 371, 373, 441, 443
hyperarousal, 164, 167, 173–180, 189–190, 243, 268, 275, 281, 294, 306–307, 368–370, 373, 443–444
of stress, 149–150
sensitization, 226–227, 288, 306–307, 443
Psychoeducation, 371–382, 407
Pugh, R., 44, 52, 67, 72–73, 76–78, 81, 86, 88, 92, 94, 96–97, 99, 178, 180, 186, 212
Putnam, F. W., 48–49, 71, 78, 111–113, 146, 151, 175, 187, 196–198, 215, 221, 364
Pynoos, R. S., 65, 228, 364, 401

Quadagno, D., 131
Quayle, E., 36
Quimet, M., 29
Quirarte, G. L., 166, 200–201

Rachman, S., 227, 381, 390
Rage, 16, 304, 426, 430
traumatic, 443
Raj, A., 88–89
Ralphe, D., 34, 78, 88
Ramsey-Klawsnik, H., 37
Randall, R. P., 80
Randall, W., 102–103
Range, L. M., 75
Rank, O., 115
Rape trauma syndrome, 20–21, 23
Raskovsky, A., 5
Raskovsky, M., 5
Rasmussen, J. K., , 25, 33, 34, 38–39, 44–47, 52, 74–76, 84–88, 93–94, 96, 102, 146, 168, 176, 188, 210, 228
Rasmussen, L. A., 29
Rationalization, 243
Ratner, P. A., 11, 33, 38, 45, 74, 82, 148, 176, 374
Rauch, S., 214–215, 329
Ray, J. A., 24–26, 32, 42, 53, 57, 98, 139, 178, 354

Ray, S. L., 40, 51, 64, 69, 83, 87, 164, 179, 235, 354
Raymond, N. C., 27, 29
Reay, D., 68
Recall, 223–224
Reconciliation, 137, 200–207, 243
  case examples, 283–293
  clinical notes, 283–293
  definition, 283
  dichotomous thinking, 202–207
  story guidelines, 441
  traumatic memory, 200–202
Recontextualizing. *See* Reframing
Recovered memories, 79–81
Rectal discomfort, 443
Reeker, J., 403
Reenactments, 57, 225–226, 231
Reframing, 7, 372–373, 432–433
  anticipated outcomes, 433
  definition, 433
  description, 433
Regression
  after abuse, 93, 115
  perpetrator, 442
Reinger, A., 55, 59
Reinhart, M. A., 34, 37, 39, 46, 48–49, 68, 144, 146, 175, 179
Reinherz, H. Z., 65
Reiser, E., 64, 87, 230
Relational effects of abuse, 86–88, 230–242
  closed system, 442–443
  control, 236–237
  dichotomous relations, 240–241
  gender identity, 239
  isolation, 239–240
  overresponsibility, 240
  power, 236–237
  risky behaviors, 237–239
  self-concept, 232–235
  sexless relationships, 241–242
  sexualization, 235–236
Relational perspective, 317, 325–327
Remer, R., 11, 63, 178
René Guyon Society, 5
Renshaw, P. F., 70
Repression, 115, 190, 267, 323
Resick, P. A., 403
Resnick, M. D., 15, 74, 82, 89, 93–94, 96, 210, 403
Responsibility, 16, 264, 273, 285
  age and perception, 60–61
  nondisclosure, 51–52
  self-blame, 16, 94–95, 206–207, 240, 379, 443
Retraction, 22
Rew, L., 38, 48, 72, 84, 93–96, 175, 210, 218

Richardson, B., 68, 357
Richardson, E. G., Jr., 79
Richardson, M. F., 33–34, 39, 46–47, 84, 147, 165, 211, 235
Richey, M. F., 214
Richey-Suttles, S., 11, 63, 178
Riegel, D., 3
Rieker, P. P., 7, 67, 165, 181–182, 199, 208, 206, 355, 365, 382, 389
Rimsza, M. E., 90
Rind, B., 3, 9
Risin, L. I., 39, 48, 64
Risk factors, 101–103
  children with disabilities, 102–103
Risky behaviors, 237–239, 344–345
Ritualistic abuse, 33, 35–36, 53–36
Roane, T. H., 11–12, 25, 34, 40, 43–44, 46, 74, 77, 82, 90, 98–99, 102, 142
Robin, R. W., 25, 33, 34, 38–39, 44–47, 52, 74–76, 84–88, 93–94, 96, 102, 146, 168, 176, 188, 210, 228
Robinson, E., 55, 59
Rockwell, L. A., 90
Rodgers, C., 131
Rodriguez, R. A., 31–32, 64
Roesler, T. A., 37–40, 44–48, 50, 73, 77–78, 84, 89, 140, 148, 175
Rogeness, G., 84
Rogosch, M. L., 103–104
Rohan, K. J., 33–34, 39–40, 42, 46, 49, 97, 147
Rohsenow, D. J., 38, 82
Role differential, 442
Roman Catholic priest offenders, 7–8
  case example, 252–254, 263–264, 272–273
Romano, E., 26, 37, 102
Romanski, L., 123
Ronnei, M., 98
Roozendaal, B., 166, 200–201
Rosado, J., 31–32, 64
Rosario, M., 94
Rosenblum, L. A., 162
Ross, C. A., 38
Ross, R. R., 48
Rossetti, S. J., 38, 146, 148
Rotatori, A. F., 102
Roth, S., 124, 134, 189
Rothbaum, B. O., 390
Rotheram-Borus, M. J., 94
Rothschild, B., 127, 162–163

Rouleau, J. L., 26, 28, 140, 142
Rousey, J. T., 91
Rowan, A. B., 85
Rowan, E. L., 33
Rowan, J. B., 33
Rowe, E., 84
Roy, A., 70
Roy-Byrne, P. P., 69
Royce, D. D., 60
Rubinstein, M., 31
Ruchkin, V. V., 233
Rudin, M. M., 32, 38, 141
Rudy, L., 56
Ruggiero, K., 14, 33–34, 40, 46, 65, 72–73, 76–78, 85–86, 90, 134, 143, 147, 168, 212, 334
Running away, 94, 443
Runtz, M., 39–40, 67, 73–74, 76–78, 86, 94–95, 105, 184, 210, 212, 371
Runyon, M., 104
Rush, A. J., 11, 15, 38, 42, 66, 74–76, 145, 374
Rush, F., 7
Russell, D. E. H., 7, 11, 32, 37, 132
Russell, J. A., 163
Russo, J., 69
Russo, N. F., 39
Rutter, M., 103–104
Ryan, G., 26–27, 30–31, 98, 140, 142, 213
Ryan, J. J., 39
Ryan, K. D., 14, 25–26, 38–40, 47, 73–74, 85, 95, 164, 228
Ryan, N. D., 69–73, 76, 78, 92, 160, 164, 214

Saakvitne, K. W., 148, 203, 225, 329, 333, 337, 347, 349–350, 352, 354, 381
Sabotta, E. E., 96
Sachs, H., 84
Sachs, R. G., 221
Sack, W. H., 25, 33–34, 40, 42, 67, 72–73, 86, 88, 92–93, 98, 145
Sacks, M. B., 81
Sadeh, A., 84
Sadock, B., 6
Sadock, B. J., 219
Safer, M. A., 81
Safety, 341–346
Sainton, K., 38
Saleeby, D., 331
Salmon, P., 26, 96
Salter, A. C., 48, 175, 338, 340, 343
Saltzman, L. E., 33–35, 37, 39–42, 44, 46, 64, 142, 146, 167
Salzinger, S., 101

Sanchez, R. P., 60
Sandall, H., 38, 374
Sanders, B., 78
Sanders-Philips, K., 46, 102, 147
Sandfort, T., 8
Sands, D., 38, 48, 72, 84, 93, 95–96, 175, 210, 218
Sanislow, C., 73–74, 82, 93, 148
Sansone, R. A., 82
Sansonnet-Hayden, H., 25, 73, 37, 39, 42, 47, 74–75, 92, 97, 146, 212
Saplonsky, R. M., 69
Saporta, J., 149, 161, 170, 172, 201
Saradjian, J., 27–28, 33–34, 36, 38, 43
Sarlin, C. N., 187, 191
Sarwer, D. B., 39, 44, 46
Sas, L., 33, 34, 42, 44–45, 76–77, 148
Sass, K. J., 121, 215
Satanism, 36
Saunders, B. E., 65, 76, 134, 141, 144, 403
Sauzier, M., 46, 48–49, 52–53, 72, 75, 78, 83, 86, 92–93, 106, 212
Savage, C. R., 214–215, 329
Saxe, G., 133, 226
Saywitz, K. J., 404
Scanlon, J. M., 403
Schaaf, K. K., 65
Schacter, D. L., 129–130
Schechter, M. T., 89, 234
Scheflin, A. W., 79–80, 102, 121, 124–126, 188, 219, 223, 395
Scheidt, D. M., 39, 67, 74, 82
Scheiner, J., 57–58, 144, 233
Schemata, 110–115, 122, 125, 170, 181–184, 202, 205, 208–209, 366, 378, 381–382, 387, 392–394, 401, 404
  abuse-generated, 385–388
  and gender, 131–135
Schiff, M., 27, 45, 50, 67, 73–74, 88, 92–94, 96, 106, 145–146, 205
Schiffer, F., 80, 214–215
Schilder, A. J., 11, 33, 38, 45, 74, 82, 89, 148, 176, 234, 374
Schilling, R. F., 414
Schlosser, S. S., 198
Schnurr, P., 79
Schoepp, D. D., 162
Scholle, R., 14, 33–34, 40, 46, 65, 72–73, 7678, 85–86, 90, 134, 143, 147, 168, 212, 334
Schore, A. N., 70, 111, 117, 124–125, 127, 130, 149, 164, 170, 214, 329, 391–392

Schuerman, J. R., 24, 34, 43, 46, 65, 72, 83, 86, 88, 92, 98, 106, 178, 207, 212, 234
Schulte, L. E., 403
Schwade, J. A., 126, 222, 329
Schwartz, M., 53, 58, 178, 180–181, 233
Schwarzin, H., 39
Schwarzmueller, A., 220, 329
Scott, C. G., 80
Sebold, J., 52, 72, 83, 88, 92–93, 96, 180, 222, 235, 319
Secrecy. See Concealment
Sedlak, A. J., 39, 54
Sedney, M., 131
Sego, S. A., 60
Selection criteria of perpetrators, 34–35
Seleyo, F., 58
Self-blame, 16, 94–95, 206–207, 379, 443
Self-concept, 231, 443
  after abuse, 83–84, 99
  sexual, 232–235
Self-determinative perspective, 317, 330
Self-esteem, 290–291
Self-injurious behaviors, 81, 193–196, 304
  anogenital injuries, 443
  mutilation, 15–16
  reducing, 368–370
Self-mastery project, 398–403, 444–446
  anticipated outcomes, 446
  definition, 444
  description, 444–446
Self-monitoring, 400–401
Self-system
  cognitive-perceptual subsystem, 113–114
  independent of abuse, 111–114
  sense of self, 111–113
Sensitization, 226–227, 288, 306–307, 443
Sensory overload, 281
Sensory symbols, 381–383
Serotonergic system, 161
Serran, G. A., 27, 141
Sewell, P. M., 33, 39–40, 46, 54–55, 69
Sex and Love Addicts Anonymous, 307
Sex
  different from gender, 131–135
Sexless relationships, 241–242
Sexual abuse (See also Child sexual abuse; Male sexual abuse)

case examples, 256–265
defined, 256
story guidelines, 440–443
Sexual Abuse of Males (SAM) model
  acknowledging abuse, 366–367
  action connection, 414–418
  analogy of, 405–409
  anxiety, 426–429
  application, 245–314
  arousal continuum, 150
  assessment, 371
  assumptions of, 109–111
  biophysical subsystem, 116–117
  brain basics, 117–123, 150–157
  case examples, 138–139, 453–460
  caveats, 138
  change chart, 411–414
  claiming gains, 395–397
  cognitive-perceptual system, 113–114
  common dynamics, 442
  compensation, 207–217, 293–302
  concealment, 165–180, 266–274
  costs and benefits, 402–403
  cycle continuation, 217–227, 303–314
  decision to proceed, 370–371
  defenses, 185–199
  development of, 106–108
  differentiating authentic vs. social views, 385–388
  domaminergic neuronal system, 160–161
  dynamics, 139–148, 372–379
  effects of abuse, 64–99, 139–148
  emotional connection, 383–385
  endogenous opioids, 163
  establishing point of view, 383, 421–424
  evaluation, 446–452
  facts and meaning, 418–421
  foundation, 364
  gender differences, 99–101
  grieving loss, 395–397
  hyperarousal, 173–180
  impositions, 424–427
  infusing contextual meaning, 379–385
  interventions for, 411–452
  intrapsychic subsystem, 115–116
  introduction to, 16

invalidation, 180–199, 274–283
justification for, 19
knowledge base, 334–336
limbic system, 152–155
memory, 124–131
neurotransmitter dysregulation, 157–164, 163–164
orientation, 367–370
origins of, 106–107
outcome studies, 403–404
philosophy of practice, 317–332
preparatory empathy, 333–361
processing the story, 392–395, 429–432, 439–444
protective factors, 103–104
rationale, 371–372
reconciliation, 200–207, 283–293
reframing, 432–434
relational effects, 228–242
risk factors, 101–103
self-mastery project, 398–401, 444–446
self-system, 111–114
serotonergic system, 161
sex, gender, and schemas, 131–135
sexual abuse, 146–148, 256–265
sexuality effects, 230–242
story guidelines, 439–444
stress response, 149–150, 157–164
subjection, 139–146, 245–256
therapeutic goal, 365–366
traumatic memories, 166–180, 200–207
treatment objectives, 363–404
understanding emotions, 434–439
utility and applications, 107–108
validation, 388–395, 429–432
"whose voice?", 421–424
workplace effects, 228–230
Sexual compulsion, 89–90
Sexual orientation
conflict, 15
confusion, 239, 443
of perpetrator, 38
Sexual Self-Esteem Scale, 67
Sexuality
control, 236–237
dichotomous relations, 240–241
effects of abuse, 88–90, 230–242
gender identity, 239
isolation, 239–240

overresponsibility, 240
power, 236–237
risky behaviors, 237–239
self-concept, 232–235
sexless relations, 241–242
Sexualization
premature, 442
relational effects of abuse, 235–236
traumatic, 22
Sexually transmitted disease, 89–92, 270, 443
Seymour, F., 28, 140, 213
Sgroi, S. M., 12–13, 46, 139, 146, 330, 364
Shame, 16, 83, 95, 252, 265, 270, 273–274, 293–294, 300, 304, 309, 319, 353–354, 368, 379, 384, 387, 426, 430, 443
lessening, 444
nondisclosure, 51–52
Sharpé, S., 30
Shaw, J. A., 31–32, 64
Shea, T., 78
Shoveller, J. A., 11, 33, 38, 45, 74, 82, 148, 176, 374
Showers, J., 41
Shrier, D. K., 15, 37, 39–41, 44, 49, 51, 64, 89–90, 206, 212, 239–240
Shrimpton, S., 47
Shubin, C. I., 69
Siblings
co-abused, 41
offenders, 31
protecting, 250, 298–299
Siebert, J., 68
Siegel, D. J., 112, 117, 124–130, 148–149, 166, 168–170, 179, 200–202, 214, 218, 220–221, 227, 325, 329, 381–382, 390, 392, 401–402
Siegel, J. M., 39, 67, 72–73, 76, 89, 93, 96, 106, 212
Siekert, G. P., 30
Siever, L. J.,162
Sigmon, S. T., 33–34, 39–40, 42, 46, 49, 97, 147
Silver, D., 333
Silver, H. K., 5
Silverman, A. B., 65
Silverman, F. N., 5
Silverman, J. G., 88–89
Simmons, R., 10
Simon, A. F., 40, 42, 46, 50, 60
Simpson, E., 78
Simpson, T. L., 14, 38–39, 104
Singer, M., 67, 72–73, 83, 88
Sipe, R., 29

Sirles, E. A., 75, 212
Sivers, H., 166
Sjöberg, R. L., 49
Skuse, D., 213
Slap, G. B., 12, 24, 41, 102, 105, 334
Slater, S., 97–98, 212
Sleep disturbances, 94, 164, 443
(See also Nightmares; Night terrors)
assessing, 371
Sleepwalking, 414
Sloane, P., 5
Slusser, M. M., 69
Smaile, E., 15, 65–66
Small, S. A., 89
Smallbone, S. W., 27
Smiljanich, K., 38, 41–42, 44, 90, 164
Smith, B. E., 56
Smith, C., 8, 11, 25, 33–34, 38–41, 44, 48, 50–51, 85, 98, 102, 146, 167, 175, 178–179, 228
Smith, D. M. 403
Smith, D. W., 141, 144
Smith, E. L. P., 162
Smith, H. D., 63, 234
Smith, H., 98
Smith, J. A., 75, 212
Smith, L., 73–75
Smith, P. H., 26, 56, 58, 144
Smith, T. A., 97, 212
Smith, T., 35, 142
Smith, W., 30
Smoking, 81–82
Smolak, L., 82
Snow, B., 32, 36, 48–49, 51–52, 175, 180, 222, 319
Sobsey, D., 102–103
Social intervention, 54–59
Social introversion, 443
Social mythology, 132, 146, 167, 176–178, 181–183, 185, 205–207, 209, 229, 232–235, 239, 247, 255, 257, 267, 275, 280, 290, 297, 319, 323–324, 331, 338, 341, 351–352, 356–357, 374–375, 378–379, 382, 385, 388–389, 393–394, 402, 441–442
beliefs imposed by, 385–386
internalization, 443
recognizing, 372–373
supporting, 283, 285
Social perceptions, 60–61
Social responses to abuse, 54
Sollers, J. J., III, 116
Somatization, 95–96, 115, 198, 443

Songer, D. A., 82
Sonnega, A., 76–77
Sorenson, S. B., 39, 67, 72–73, 76, 89, 93, 96, 106, 212
Sorenson, T., 32, 36
Sorenson, T., 48–49, 51–52, 175, 180, 222, 319
Southwick, S. M., 15, 71, 79, 118–119, 121, 123, 129–130, 150, 155, 158–159, 161, 163–164, 170, 175, 200, 214–216, 219, 329
Southwick, S., 151, 159–160, 165, 169–170, 172, 174
Spaccarelli, S., 184
Spegg, C., 82
Speltz, K., 33–34
Spencer, D. D., 121, 215
Spencer, M. J., 24, 27, 33, 38, 40–42, 46, 68, 75, 83, 91, 93–95, 143
Spencer, T. D., 11, 60, 178, 206, 233, 334
Spiegel, D., 11, 62–63, 72, 171–172, 187, 347
Spiegel, J., 12, 15, 37, 39, 44, 46–47, 50, 52, 83, 90, 94–95, 102, 107, 137, 144–145, 157, 161, 165, 168, 175–177, 180, 185, 192–193, 195, 206–207, 210–212, 218, 222, 233, 235, 239, 319, 335, 352, 358, 364–365, 401–402, 404
Spilsbury, J., 11, 60
Spirituality, 96, 103, 146, 148, 167–168, 182, 368
loss of, 443
Squire, L. R., 120, 126–129, 170, 190, 201, 226
St. Claire, K. K., 91
Staffelbach, D., 85
Staib, L., 80
Stall, R., 11–12, 38, 41, 44–46, 89, 147, 238, 334, 374
Stanwood, G. D., 161
Statham, D. J., 25, 74–75, 82, 87
Statistics, 24
perpetrator gender, 37–38
Status differential, 442
Stauffer, L. B., 403
Steele, B. F., 5
Steele, K., 329, 363, 381
Stein, J. A., 39, 67, 72–73, 76, 89, 93, 96, 106, 212
Stein, M. B., 65, 77
Steinberg, A. M., 228, 364
Steiner, H., 79
Steketee, G., 30
Stephens, B. G., 68

Stephens, M., 33, 40
Stern, A. E., 51, 164, 179, 392
Stevenson, J., 38, 213
Stiffman, A. R., 92
Stigmatization, 23
nondisclosure, 51–52
of homosexuality, 12
upon disclosure, 54
Stoesz, D., 4
Storck, M., 16, 25, 93, 25, 42, 72–73, 76, 78, 81, 94, 98
Story guidelines, 439–444
anticipated outcomes, 443–444
compensation, 442
concealment, 441
cycle continuation, 442
definition, 439
description, 440
disclosure, 443
invalidation, 441
long-term effects, 443
reconciliation, 441
sexual abuse, 440–443
Strathdee, S. A., 89, 234
Straus, M. A., 51, 85, 228
Streiner, D. L., 42, 82, 146
Strengths perspective, 317, 331
Stress
arousal continuum, 150
brain's response, 150–157
chronic, 268, 304, 323
effects on the brain, 213–216
neurotransmission, 157–164
psychobiology of, 149–150
sensations of, 265
Stress-induced analgesia, 163, 171, 218, 238
Stress response cycle, 150–166, 173–174, 189, 227
dysregulated, 443
Strom, G., 67, 72–73, 83, 88
Stroud, D. D., 52–53, 56–57, 233
Stroufe, L. A., 78, 103–104
Strupp, H. H., 321, 333
Struve, J., 12, 143, 144, 176–177, 236
Stuss, D. T., 125–126, 129, 218
Styron, T., 25, 74, 87, 242
Subjection, 137, 139–146, 243
case examples, 245–256
clinical notes, 245–256
defined, 245
impositions, 424–426
story guidelines, 440
Substance abuse, 279, 308, 442–443
as a defense, 81–82, 300, 311–312, 377, 441

by parents, 25
by perpetrators, 27, 29, 33, 45
exposing children to, 35, 250, 260
reducing, 368–370
Suicidality, 74–75
Sullivan, H. S., 111, 115, 349, 364, 403
Sullivan, P. M., 94, 102–103
Sullivan, R., 59, 233
Summit, O., 7
Summit, R., 20–22, 139
Suppes, T., 11, 15, 38, 42, 66, 74–76, 145, 374
Suppression, 115, 186, 223
Surrey, J., 70, 75, 213–214
Survivors Network of those Abused by Priests (SNAP), 3
Sutherland, S. M., 151, 159–161, 163
Suzuki, J. 150, 214, 319, 381
Swanston, H. Y., 47
Swett, C., Jr., 70, 75, 213–214
Swica, Y., 221
Swingle, J. M., 11, 14, 25, 33–34, 37, 39–43, 45–47, 68, 87, 146, 147–148, 178, 357
Syphilis, 90

Tabacoff, R., 27, 30, 142
Talley, N. J., 69
Tan, J. C. H., 11, 60, 178, 206, 233, 334
Tandem perpetrators, 33
Tardif, M., 29
Taska, L., 14, 24, 26, 33–34, 41–42, 44, 46, 48, 143, 146, 164, 207
Taub, E. P., 56
Tavana, J., 55, 175
Tavris, C., 131
Taylor, M., 36
Taylor-Seehafer, M., 94
Teicher, M. H., 70–71, 80, 94, 213–215, 335
Tennessee Self-Concept Scales, 67
Termination, 401–402
Terr, L. C., 81, 124, 128, 134, 168, 171–172, 174, 185, 218, 220–221, 223, 319
Teti, L., 143
Texas Supreme Court, 3
Theoretical models, 20–23
child sexual abuse accommodation syndrome, 21–22
rape trauma syndrome, 20–21
traumagenic dynamics model, 22–23

Theoretical perspective, 317, 322–323
Therapeutic alliance, 16, 325–327, 333–361, 372
client's role, 338–339
countertransference, 346–354
egalitarian, 339–341
expectancies, 357–360
policies, 360–361
safety and trust, 341–346
SAM knowledge base, 334–336
therapist's role, 337–338
transference, 346–348
Therapeutic window, 354–357, 379–382
Therapists
conceptualizations of, 325–327
countertransference, 346–354
egalitarian relationship, 339–341
expectancies, 357–360
perceptions of, 61–63
policies, 360–361
preparatory empathy, 333–336
role of, 333–361, 391–392
safety and trust, 341–346
therapeutic window, 354–357
transference, 346–348
Thoennes, N., 24, 26, 40, 57–58, 144, 206
Thomlinson, B., 33, 40
Thompson, C. W., 10
Thompson, R. J., 25, 33–34, 40, 42, 67, 72–73, 86, 88, 92–93, 98, 145
Thoreson, C., 11, 62–63
Thorstad, D., 6
Threat, 44, 442
brain's response to, 150–157
neurotransmitters and, 157–166
Tidwell, R., 25, 98
Tilelli, J. A., 90
Timnick, L., 49
Titus, T. G., 39, 73, 86, 88, 92–93
Tjaden, P. G., 24, 26, 40, 57–58, 144, 206
Tolving, E., 125–126, 129, 218
Toomey, T. C., 69
Tornusciolo, G., 27, 30, 142
Toth, S. I., 78, 104
Transference, 16, 346–348
traumatic, 347–348
Trappler, B., 73–75
Trauma Symptom Checklist, 67
Trauma Symptom Inventory, 371
Trauma Syndrome Checklist for Children, 49

Trauma
post-sexual abuse, 371
PTSD, 25, 76–77, 134, 320, 414
symptoms, 77–78
Traumagenic dynamics model, 7, 20, 22–23
Traumatic memories, 145, 159, 162, 166, 168–173, 188–189, 191, 200–202, 214, 218–220, 222, 225, 241, 279, 365, 390
invariable, 169–170
manifest, 172–173
sensations, 168–169
state dependent, 170–171
timeless, 171–172
Traumatic rage, 443
Traumatic sexualization, 22
Travin, S., 32–33, 141
Treatment
acknowledging abuse, 365–367
action connection, 414–418
ambivalence, 371–379
anxiety, 426–429
assessment, 371
boy's perspective, 317, 329–330
change chart, 411–414
claiming gains, 365, 395–397
client's role, 338–339
conceptual perspective, 317, 323–324
costs and benefits, 402–403
countertransference, 346–354
decision to proceed, 370–371
demystifying, 372
developmental perspective, 317, 324–325
differentiating authentic vs. social views, 385–388
dynamics and effects perspective, 317, 327–328
ecosystems perspective, 317–320
egalitarian relationship, 339–341
emotional connection, 383–385
establishing point of view, 365, 383, 421–424
evaluation, 446–452
examining dynamics and effects, 372–379
expectancies, 357–360
facts and meaning perspective, 317, 328–329, 418–421
foundation, 364
grieving loss, 365, 395–397
impositions, 424–427

infusing contextual meaning, 365, 379–385
interventions, 411–452
multisystemic, multitemporal determinism, 317, 320–321
objectives, 322, 363–404
orientation, 367–370
outcome studies, 403–404
parallel processes perspective, 317, 321–322
policies, 360–361
preparatory empathy, 333–361
processing the story, 392–395, 429–432, 439–444
rationale, 371–372
reframing, 432–434
relational perspective, 317, 325–327
safety and trust, 341–346
SAM knowledge base, 334–336
self-determinative perspective, 317, 330
self-mastery project, 365, 398–401, 444–446
story guidelines, 439–444
strengths perspective, 317, 331
termination, 401–402
theoretical perspective, 317, 322–323
therapeutic relationship, 336–360
therapeutic window, 354–357
therapist's role, 337–338
transference, 346–348
understanding emotions, 434–439
validation, 365, 388–395, 429–432
whose voice? 421–424
Trickett, P. K., 48–49, 71, 146, 175, 187, 196, 198, 364
Triggers, 399
Tromovitch, P., 3, 9
Trujillo, M., 39
Trust, 341–346
Trute, B., 62
Tubiolo, V. C., 24–25, 27, 33, 37, 42, 46, 49, 57, 67, 91, 164
Tulving, E., 127–129, 214
Turek, D., 90
Tutty, L. M., 14, 53, 64, 78, 83, 85–87, 89–90, 139, 168, 178–179, 181, 185, 206, 210, 212, 230, 232, 235–238, 240, 335, 349, 354
Tyler, K. A., 14, 38, 94
Tzeng, O., 39

U.S. Conference of Catholic Bishops, 10
U.S. Congress and House of Representatives, 9
U.S. Dept. of Health and Human Services, 50, 54, 58
U.S. Dept. of Justice, 27–28, 33, 36–37, 38, 40, 45, 46, 56, 58, 143, 178
Understanding emotions intervention, 434–439
  anticipated outcomes, 439
  definition, 434
  description, 434–436
  experiencing and naming emotions, 434–436
  expressing emotions, 436–439
Unger, J. B., 94
University of Pennsylvania School of Social Work, 10
Urbanski, L., 39
Urinary tract infections, 69
Urquiza, A. J., 15, 24–25, 37, 44, 65, 67, 72–75, 84, 86, 88–89, 92–93, 95, 106, 145–146, 210, 228

Vaillant, G. E., 116, 186, 190, 322
Validation, 429–432
van der Hart, O., 3, 79, 329, 363, 380–381, 390
van der Kolk, B. A., 3, 15, 70–71, 78–81, 117, 120–122, 134, 148–150, 155, 157–158, 161, 163–164, 166, 168–172, 174–175, 184, 189, 191, 193–194, 195–196, 201, 214–215, 218–220, 223, 225, 238, 319, 329, 343–344, 364, 380–381, 390
Van Fleet, J., 39
Van Gijseghem, H., 29
Van Hunsel, F., 30
van Naerssen, A., 8
Van West, D., 30
Velentgas, P., 38, 82, 89, 91, 238
Vermetten, E., 80
Verschoore, A., 64, 67, 82, 84, 86, 89, 92–95, 228
Vigilante, D., 118, 127, 131, 164, 170, 189, 216, 329
Violato, C., 26, 37–38, 47
Violence, 44–45, 262–263, 271, 283, 294 (See also Domestic violence; Physical abuse)
  as identification, 116
Viswanathan, R., 73–75
Voicing the experience, 429–432
  anticipated outcomes, 432
  definition, 430
  description, 420–432
Voris, J., 24, 33–34, 46, 68–69, 82–86, 88, 94, 147, 176, 210, 334, 354
Vulliamy, A. P., 59, 233
Vuz, J., 30

Wade, C., 131
Wagner, W. G., 60–61, 110, 318, 321, 364
Walker, E. A., 69
Walker, J. R., 65, 77
Wall, T., 39–40, 67, 73–74, 76–78, 94–95, 105, 184, 212
Wallen, J., 39, 85
Waller, G., 11, 63, 39, 48, 62, 175, 187, 234
Wallerstein, R., 116
Walsh, C. A., 42, 82, 146
Wang, S., 79, 159, 215
Ward, J. W., 91
Ward, T., 27, 141
Wasyliw, O. E., 27
Watanabe, H., 14, 25–26, 38–40, 47, 73–74, 85, 95, 164, 228
Waterman, C. K., 60, 62, 179, 206
Waterman, J., 32–33, 36, 51
Waternauz, C. M., 25
Watkins, B., 24, 334
Watson, M. S., 29
Watson, M. W., 55, 61, 63
Watson, R., 97, 212
Watts, A. G., 155
Wayland, K., 55, 175
Weaver, T. L., 403
Webb, J. A., 72, 74
Webster, S. W., 55
Weedy, C., 91
Weekes, C., 227, 428
Weeks, R., 98
Wehrspann, W., 24, 33, 34, 40, 42, 48, 68–69, 72, 88, 90, 92, 94, 96, 175
Weihe, V. R., 54, 233, 354
Weinberg, S. K., 5
Weiner, N. A., 10
Weinfield, N. S., 78
Weinrott, M., 31
Weinstein, B., 12
Weinstein, D., 85
Weir, I., 36
Weisaeth, L., 214–215, 343
Weiss, B., 39, 403
Weisz, J. R., 403
Wekerle, C., 33, 34, 42, 44–45, 76–77, 148
Weldy, S. R., 42, 72, 81, 86, 88, 146, 179, 212, 335
Wellman, M. M., 61
Wells, R., 24, 33–34, 46, 69, 82–86, 88, 94, 147, 176, 210, 334, 354
Westenberg, H., 30
Westerberg, V. S., 39
Westerveld, M., 121, 215
Wewerke, S., 126, 222, 329
Wexler, S., 25–26, 42, 72–74
Wheatcroft, M., 36
Wheeler, M. A., 125–126, 129, 218
Wherry, J. N., 78
Whitbeck, L. B., 14, 38, 94
Whitcomb, D., 56–57, 143
White, S. H., 124–126, 129–130, 169, 202, 90–91
Whitfield, C. L., 343
Whose voice?
  antcipated outcomes, 424
  definition, 423
  description, 423–424
  intervention, 421–424
Widom, C., 84–85, 98, 228–229
Widom, D. C., 25–26, 65, 76, 79–80, 97, 134, 210, 222
Wiedeking, C., 131
Williams, B., 213
Williams, L. M., 14, 32–33, 36–38, 47, 64, 87–88, 90, 99, 102, 105, 132, 134, 147, 165, 181, 208, 210, 232, 234, 236–237, 239
Wilson, J. F., 39–40
Wilson, J. P., 325, 333, 347–350
Wilson, R. J., 30
Wilson, S. K., 27
Wind, T. W., 48, 50
Winder, C., 24, 33, 34, 40, 42, 48, 68–69, 72, 88, 90, 92, 94, 96, 175
Windle, M., 39, 67, 74, 82
Windle, R. C., 39, 67, 74, 82
Winnicott, D. W., 333, 336–337, 364
Winter, D. G., 110
Wirtz, S., 68
Wolak, J., 36
Wolde-Tsadik, G., 69
Wolfe, D. A., 27, 33, 34, 42, 44–45, 76–77, 148
Wolfe, F. A., 26, 33, 44
Wolfe, J., 133, 226
Wolfe, L. C., 60
Wolfe, S., 35, 142
Wolfsdorf, B. A., 76–77
Wolpe, J., 322
Wong, M. Y. Y., 42, 82, 146
Wong-Kernberg, L., 39

Wood, J. J., 33
Wood, J. M., 25–27, 33, 38, 49, 51–52, 67, 73–74, 76, 78, 85, 92, 143, 180, 222, 230, 334
Woods, M., 321
Woods, S. C., 16, 26, 33–34, 37, 41–43, 46–47, 49–50, 52, 64, 83, 86–87, 89, 94–95, 147, 165, 180, 212, 222, 235, 319
Woodward, D. J., 214
Workplace effects of abuse, 85, 228–230, 443
World Assumptions Scale, 67
World War II, 4
Worling, J. R., 26, 31, 98, 142
Wraith, R., 228, 364
Wright, G., 160
Wroten, J., 90
Wurtele, S. K., 28, 69, 102, 140–141, 143, 364

Wust, S., 160
Wyatt, G. E., 7
Wynne, J. M., 68, 102

Xagoraris, A., 123

Yalom, I., 321
Yates, J. L., 190
Yeager, C. A., 31, 83, 221, 335
Yehuda, R., 70, 149–150, 154, 159–160, 164, 189, 202, 215
Young, R. E., 25–27, 38–39, 52, 67, 73–74, 76, 78, 85–86, 88, 92–93, 180, 222, 230, 334

Zaidi, L., 50, 403
Zalewski, C., 32, 38, 141
Zautra, A. A. J., 102

Zeena, T. H., 39, 82
Zellman, G., 12, 58, 59, 61–62, 233
Zierler, S., 38, 82, 89, 91, 238
Zigmond, M. J., 161
Zimmerman, L., 89
Zimmerman, M., 76–77
Zinmeister, A. R., 69
Zlotnick, C., 76–78, 91, 134
Zoellner, L. A., 81
Zola, S. M., 155, 201
Zollinger, T. W., 12–13, 62–63
Zucker, K. J., 102
Zuravin, S. J., 11, 14, 25, 39, 48, 53, 55, 72, 78, 82, 88, 93–94, 102, 177, 179, 334
Zurbriggen, E. L., 80
Zverina, J., 39
Zymurgy, Inc., 9